ANTHRACYCLINE ANTIBIOTICS IN CANCER THERAPY

DEVELOPMENTS IN ONCOLOGY 10

ANTHRACYCLINE ANTIBIOTICS IN CANCER THERAPY

Proceedings of the International Symposium
on Anthracycline Antibiotics in Cancer Therapy, New York,
New York, 16 – 18 September 1981

edited by

FRANCO M. MUGGIA
CHARLES W. YOUNG
STEPHEN K. CARTER

1982

MARTINUS NIJHOFF PUBLISHERS

THE HAGUE/BOSTON/LONDON

Distributors:

for the United States and Canada
Kluwer Boston, Inc.
190 Old Derby Street
Hingham, MA 02043
USA

for all other countries
Kluwer Academic Publishers Group
Distribution Center
P.O. Box 322
3300 AH Dordrecht
The Netherlands

ISBN 90-247-2711-1 (this volume)
ISBN 90-247-2338-8 (series)

PRINTED IN THE NETHERLANDS

DEDICATION

AURELIO DI MARCO--A BIOGRAPHICAL SKETCH

This volume is dedicated to Professor Aurelio Di Marco
for his pioneering efforts in the development of anthracycline
antibiotics for cancer therapy. Salient features of his
productive scientific career are described.

Aurelio Di Marco was graduated as medical doctor from the
University of Milan in 1940. In 1945 he was appointed
assistant director and, subsequently, director of the
Department of Microbiology and Experimental Chemotherapy of
the Farmitalia Research Laboratories in Milan. As director,
he organized laboratories for the isolation and identification
of antibacterial antibiotics possibly useful in the treatment
of bacterial infections. He directed his attention to the
classification of mechanisms of action of these agents as well
as those of synthetic products.

Following Waksman's discovery of the antitumor effect of
actinomycins, he turned to the screening of fermentation
broths of streptomycetes on tissue-cultured neoplastic cells
and experimental tumors.

Under his directorship, researchers at the Farmitalia
Research Laboratories isolated and studied Daunomycin, an
antibiotic with strong effect on experimental leukemia.
Structural modifications of this antibiotic were developed
by means of mutations obtained by mutagenic selection of the
primary Daunomycin-producer strain, Streptomyces peucetius.
Cultures of this strain were submitted to mutagenic treatment
and the antitumor effect of the fermentation products was
studied. The biosynthesis product of one of these cultures,
var. caesius, strain 106 FI, was found to show a greater
antitumor activity on the Ehrlich ascites tumor. This

strain was further studied to ascertain its effects on different experimental tumors. A crude analog of this strain with a rather high titer was found that had a strong antitumor action on systems like sarcoma 180, solid myeloma, and Walker carcinosarcoma. Subsequently, the product was chemically characterized by Arcamone and coworkers as the hydroxy- analog of Daunomycin and was named Adriamycin.

The superior activity of Adriamycin on experimental solid tumors, including spontaneous and transplanted murine mammary tumors, was confirmed.

A number of studies on the new antibiotic demonstrated several differences when it was compared to Daunomycin. Pharmacokinetics demonstrated a prolonged average life and different metabolism. There was a stronger activity toward solid tumors, possibly related to less immunosuppression. Recently, these studies were extended to a wide series of structural analogs, with special concern to DNA interaction, their transport, and their effects on the heart.

In addition to this research career, Professor Di Marco pursued an active academic career. He qualified as professor of microbiology in 1952 at the University of Florence and of chemotherapy in 1956 at the University of Milan.

In 1961 Professor Di Marco was appointed assistant director of the Experimental Chemotherapy Services of the National Cancer Institute of Milan and, in 1972, became director of the Division of Experimental Oncology B at this institute. He was also responsible for teaching microbiology at the University of Milan from 1974 to 1977.

His contributions to the medical literature include over 200 papers concerned mainly with studies on new chemotherapeutic agents and their mechanisms of action.

It is fitting that this volume be dedicated to Professor Di Marco as a testimonial of the vast areas of science which have been opened up through his efforts.

CONTRIBUTORS

E. M. ACTON, SRI International, Menlo Park, California 94025

P. A. ANDREWS, Baltimore Cancer Research Center, Baltimore, Maryland 21201

F. ARCAMONE, Farmitalia Carlo Erba, Milan, Italy

E. ARLANDINI, Farmitalia Carlo Erba, Milan, Italy

G. ATASSI, Institut Jules Bordet, Brussels, Belgium

N. R. BACHUR, Baltimore Cancer Research Program, Baltimore, Maryland 21201

L. BALLERINI, Farmitalia Carlo Erba, Milan, Italy

R. BAURAIN, International Institute of Cellular and Molecular Pathology, Brussels, Belgium

O. BAWA, Farmitalia Carlo Erba, Milan, Italy

O. BELLINI, Farmitalia Carlo Erba, Milan, Italy

R. S. BENJAMIN, M. D. Anderson Hospital and Tumor Institute, Houston, Texas 77030

G. BERETTA, Farmitalia Carlo Erba, Milan, Italy

C. BERTAZZOLI, Farmitalia Carlo Erba, Milan, Italy

M. E. BILLINGHAM, Stanford University Medical Center, Stanford, California 94305

R. H. BLUM, New York University Medical Center, New York, New York 10016

G. BLUMENSCHEIN, M. D. Anderson Hospital and Tumor Institute, Houston, Texas 77030

G. BONADONNA, Istituto Nazionale Tumori, Milan, Italy

V. BONFANTE, Istituto Nazionale Tumori, Milan, Italy

J. BOTTINO, New York University Medical Center, New York New York 10016

C. BRAMBILLA, Istituto Nazionale Tumori, Milan, Italy

M. R. BRISTOW, Stanford University Medical Center, Stanford, California 94305

D. BRON, Instutut Jules Bordet, Brussels, Belgium

R. BUZZONI, Istituto Nazionale Tumori, Milan, Italy

S. K. CARTER, Northern California Oncology Group, Palo Alto, California 94304

A. CASAZZA, Farmitalia Carlo Erba, Milan, Italy

E. CASPER, Memorial Sloan-Kettering Cancer Center, New York, New York 10021

G. CASSINELLI, Farmitalia Carlo Erba, Milan, Italy

F. CAVALLI, Ospedale San Giovanni, Bellinzona, Switzerland

S. T. CROOKE, Smith Kline & French Laboratories, Philadelphia, Pennsylvania 19101

G. DAGNINI, Padua G. R. Hospital, Padua, Italy

M. DALMARK, Finsen Institute, Copenhagen, Denmark

P. DEESEN, Memorial Sloan-Kettering Cancer Center, New York, New York 10021

D. DEPREZ-DE CAMPENEERE, International Institute of Cellular and Molecular Pathology, Brussels, Belgium

A. DI MARCO, **Farmitalia Carlo Erba, Milan, Italy**

P. DODION, Instutut Jules Bordet, Brussels, Belgium

J. H. DOROSHOW, City of Hope National Medical Center, Duarte, California 91010

P. DUMONT, Institut Jules Bordet, Brussels, Belgium

V. H. DUVERNAY, Baylor College of Medicine, Houston, Texas 77030

M. J. EGORIN, Baltimore Cancer Research Center, Baltimore, Maryland 21201

M. S. EWER, M. D. Anderson Hospital and Tumor Institute, Houston, Texas 77030

V. J. FERRANS, National Heart, Lung, and Blood Institute, Bethesda, Maryland 20205

E. FERRAZZI, Padua G. R. Hospital, Padua, Italy

M. V. FIORENTINO, Padua G. R. Hospital, Padua, Italy

A. FORNASIERO, Padua G. R. Hospital, Padua, Italy

E. A. FORSSEN, University of Southern California, Los Angeles, California 90033

B. M. FOX, Baltimore Cancer Research Center, Baltimore Maryland 21201

E. FREI III, Sidney Farber Cancer Institute, Boston, Massachusetts 02115

G. GAHRTON, Karolinska Institute, Stockholm 60, Sweden

M. B. GARNICK, Sidney Farber Cancer Institute, Boston, Massachusetts 02115

A. GOLDIN, Georgetown University Hospital, Washington, D.C. 20007

M. D. GREEN, New York University Medical Center, New York, New York 10016

J. D. GRIFFIN, Sidney Farber Cancer Institute, Boston, Massachusetts 02115

H. L. GURTOO, Roswell Park Memorial Institute, Buffalo, New York 14203

M. ISRAEL, Sidney Farber Cancer Institute, Boston, Massachu Massachusetts 02115

B. F. ISSELL, Bristol Laboratories, Syracuse, New York 13201

R. JAENKE, Colorado State University, Fort Collins, Colorado 8052!

R. A. JENSEN, SRI International, Menlo Park, California 94025

B. JONES, Memorial Sloan-Kettering Cancer Center, New York, New York 10021

P. M. KANTER, Roswell Park Memorial Institute, Buffalo, New York 14203

S. KAPLAN, Ospedale San Giovanni, Bellinzona, Switzerland

H. KAPPUS, University of Düsseldorf, Düsseldorf, Germany

Y. KENIS, Institut Jules Bordet, Brussels, Belgium

M. KOHLER, Northern California Oncology Group, Palo Alto, California 94304

K. W. KOHN, National Cancer Institute, Bethesda, Maryland 20205

S. S. LEGHA, M. D. Anderson Hospital and Tumor Institute, Houston, Texas 77070

G. Y. LOCKER, St. Joseph Hospital, Chicago, Illinois 60657

B. H. LONG, Baylor College of Medicine, Houston, Texas 77030

B. LUM, Palo Alto Veterans Administration Center, Palo Alto, California 94304

B. MACKAY, M. D. Anderson Hospital and Tumor Institute, Houston, Texas 77030

G. MARAGLINO, Padua G. R. Hospital, Padua, Italy

R. MARAL, Institut de Cancérologie et d'Immunogénétique, 94800 Villejuif, France

A. J. MARINELLO, Roswell Park Memorial Institute, Buffalo, New York 14203

HANS MARQUARDT, University of Hamburg Medical School, Hamburg, Germany

HILDEGARD MARQUARDT, University of Hamburg Medical School, Hamburg, Germany

A. MARTINI, Farmitalia Carlo Erba, Milan, Italy

M. MASQUELIER, International Institute of Cellular and Molecular Pathology, Brussels, Belgium

G. MATHÉ, Institut de Cancérologie et d'Immunogénétique, 94800 Villejuif, France

M. MATTELAER, Institut Jules Bordet, Brussels, Belgium

M. MENOZZI, Farmitalia Carlo Erba, Milan, Italy

A. MOLITERNI, Istituto Nazionale Tumori, Milan, Italy

F. M. MUGGIA, New York University Medical Center, New York, New York 10016

H. MULIAWAN, University of Dusseldorf, Dusseldorf, Germany

C. E. MYERS, National Cancer Institute, Bethesda, Maryland 20205

N. NAKAZAWA, Baltimore Cancer Research Center, Baltimore, Maryland 21201

C. NICAISE, Institut Jules Bordet, Brussels, Belgium

O. NICOLETTO, Padua G. R. Hospital, Padua, Italy

M. OGAWA, Japanese Foundation for Cancer Research, Toshima-ku, Tokyo, Japan

R. F. OZOLS, National Cancer Institute, Bethesda, Maryland 20205

P. PAGNIN, Padua G. R. Hospital, Padua, Italy

C. PAUL, Karolinska Institute, Stockholm 60, Sweden

M. PAVONE-MACALUSO, Università di Palermo, Palermo, Italy

S. PENCO, Farmitalia Carlo Erba, Milan, Italy

J. H. PETERS, SRI International, Menlo Park, California 94025

C. PETERSON, Karolinska Institute, Stockholm 60, Sweden

F. S. PHILIPS, Memorial Sloan-Kettering Cancer Center, New York, New York 10021

M. PICCART, Institut Jules Bordet, Brussels, Belgium

D. D. PIETRONIGRO, New York University Medical Center, New York, New York 10016

C. PRAGA, Farmitalia Carlo Erba, Milan, Italy

A. W. PRESTAYKO, Smith Kline & French Laboratories, Philadelphia, Pennsylvania 19101

A. RAHMAN, Georgetown University Hospital, Washington, D.C. 20007

N. W. REVIS, Oak Ridge Research Institute, Oak Ridge, Tennessee 37830

M. ROBERT-NICOUD, Universität Göttingen, D-3400 Göttingen, Germany

K. E. ROGERS, University of Southern California, Los Angeles, California 90033

A. ROSSI, Istituto Nazionale Tumori, Milan, Italy

M. ROZENCWEIG, Institut Jules Bordet, Brussels, Belgium

M. RUDLING, Karolinska Institute, Stockholm 60, Sweden

M. J. SACK, Sidney Farber Cancer Institute, Boston, Massachusetts 02115

U. SAMMARTINI, Farmitalia Carlo Erba, Milan, Italy

P. SCHEIN, Georgetown University Hospital, Washington, D.C. 20007

M. E. SCHEULEN, University of Essen Medical School, Essen, Germany

H. S. SCHWARTZ, Roswell Park Memorial Institute, Buffalo, New York 14203

F. SPREAFICO, Instituto de Ricerche Farmacologiche "Mario Negri," Milan, Italy

J. L. SPEYER, New York University Medical Center, New York, New York 10016

F. E. STOCKDALE, Stanford University Medical Center, Stanford, California 94305

P. STRIJKMANS, Institut Jules Bordet, Brussels, Belgium

D. TABANELLI, Farmitalia Carlo Erba, Milan, Italy

C. TIHON, Bristol Laboratories, Syracuse, New York 13201

P. TOGNI, Ospedale San Giovanni, Bellinzona, Switzerland

Z. A. TÖKÈS, University of Southern California, Los Angeles, California 90033

F. M. TORTI, Stanford University Medical Center, Stanford, California 94305

M. G. TOSANA, Farmitalia Carlo Erba, Milan, Italy

A. TROUET, International Institute of Cellular and Molecular Pathology, Brussels, Belgium

P. VALAGUSSA, Istituto Nazionale Tumori, Milan, Italy

M. VALDIVIESO, M. D. Anderson Hospital and Tumor Institute, Houston, Texas 77030

L. VALENTINI, Farmitalia Carlo Erba, Milan, Italy

D. VAN ECHO, Baltimore Cancer Research Center, Baltimore, Maryland 21201

E. VANNINI, Farmitalia Carlo Erba, Milan, Italy

M. VARINI, Ospedale San Giovanni, Bellinzona, Switzerland

O. VINANTE, Padua G. R. Hospital, Padua, Italy

S. VITOLS, Karolinska Institute, Stockholm 60, Sweden

D. D. VON HOFF, University of Texas Health Science Center, San Antonio, Texas 78284

S. WALLACE, M. D. Anderson Hospital and Tumor Institute, Houston, Texas 77030

R. WARRELL, Memorial Sloan-Kettering Cancer Center, New York, New York 10021

J. WERNZ, New York University Medical Center, New York, New York 10016

J. WESTENDORF, University of Hamburg Medical School, Hamburg, Germany

M. WHITACRE, Baltimore Cancer Research Center, Baltimore, Maryland 21201

R. WITTES, Memorial Sloan-Kettering Cancer Center, New York, New York 10021

C. W. YOUNG, Memorial Sloan-Kettering Cancer Center, New York, New York 10021

R. C. YOUNG, National Cancer Institute, Bethesda, Maryland 20205

P. ZANON, Farmitalia Carlo Erba, Milan, Italy

L. A. ZWELLING, National Cancer Institute, Bethesda, Maryland 20205

PREFACE

F. M. MUGGIA

When faced with the inadequacies of current cancer treatment, we prefer to look at what the future may hold. Quite often, we take for granted the past, preferring research into totally new areas. However, the persistent development of fertile soil may yield surprising rewards for those who choose to build on the knowledge of the past--hence, this symposium on anthracycline antibiotics.

Although the anthracycline antibiotics represent much of the present and future of cancer treatment, their actual use ɪ stretches back barely two decades to the pioneering efforts of Aurelio Di Marco, who characterized the antitumor properties of daunomycin and adriamycin.* The clinical application of these two compounds heralded a decade of excitement among oncologists dealing with pediatric tumors, breast cancer, leukemias, and lymphomas, and opened new hope for patients afflicted with sarcomas and a variety of other tumors that had been deemed resistant to chemotherapy. These successes were tempered with the realization that the antitumor effect of anthracyclines could be achieved at times only at the very high price of risking cardiac decompensation and, almost invariably, with the occurrence of alopecia and other acute toxicities.

This record of past achievements and problems has slowly given way to a present increasingly illuminated by our ability to modify the distressing toxicities of these agents. Detailed clinical studies supplemented by ingenious laboratory models have gradually elucidated mechanisms and risk factors implicated in the cardiomyopathy. Advances in cardiac monitoring

---

*Throughout this volume, the authors have used the terms Adriamycin and doxorubicin and the terms daunomycin and daunorubicin interchangeably.

have helped to define, identify, and prevent cardiac damage prior to symptomatic manifestations. Necrosis resulting from extravasation is being similarly studied. Finally, acute intolerance may be minimized by dose schedule alterations, which are now possible through improved techniques of drug delivery into high-flow venous systems.

Less erratic and serious toxicities from current anthracyclines will have predictably beneficial effects on important clinical applications. For example, studies of adjuvant therapy in breast cancer, soft tissue sarcomas, and bone sarcomas will be able to utilize doxorubicin optimally once toxicity risks have been more precisely defined. Another consequence will be the ability to treat patients who at present are automatically precluded from receiving anthracyclines because of preexisting heart disease. When treatment is applied for diseases which are prevalent in the elderly, such as prostatic cancer, exclusions currently probably outnumber patients placed on treatment.

Soon to enter more widespread trial are several anthracycline derivatives that differ from doxorubicin in a variety of interesting aspects. Drugs active by the oral route, others with possibly more selectivity to solid tumors, and still others exhibiting unique biochemical properties, attenuated toxicities, or lack of cross-resistance are in active preclinical and clinical development. Clinical studies are confirming some of the laboratory observations, and, therefore, will provide excellent feedback toward further drug development.

The more distant future holds prospects that are no less exciting. Fundamental biological processes are being unraveled by the study of anthracyclines, as prototypal anticancer drugs continue to be developed in many laboratories. From the simplistic view of their action through intercalation into DNA chains, we have continually added to knowledge of their complexity, as exhibited by membrane disturbances, free radical activation, generation of activated oxygen species, and the iron-anthracycline complexes. The prospects of separating antitumor from toxic manifestations have stimulated a number of experiments in the laboratory and in the clinic. Still undefined but perhaps of greatest importance to the future of cancer therapeutics is the basis for the antitumor selectivity of the anthracyclines and its relationship to hypoxia and other general metabolic alterations of malignancy. Thus, the trails of investigations with the anthracycline antibiotics continue to expand toward therapeutic horizons barely apparent only a decade ago.

CONTENTS

SECTION 1

BIOLOGICAL EFFECTS

INTRODUCTION

F. S. PHILIPS

This volume is based upon papers presented at an International Symposium on Anthracycline Antibiotics in Cancer Therapy that was held in New York City, 16-18 September 1981. Cosponsors of the Symposium were New York University Post-Graduate Medical School and New York University Cancer Center.

I was invited by the organizing committee of the Symposium to deliver the keynote address. My immediate reaction to the invitation was that of an individual who views a "keynote address" as a speech given at a political convention in a manner calculated to present the issues of primary interest to those assembled and aimed toward arousing great enthusiasm and much emotion. If that, in fact, was the organizing committee's charge to me, then it was likely sorely disappointed; for I am not by nature an inspirator. Had I been a different individual, I might have begun as follows: "Fellow members of this international party that stands for all that is wonderful about the anthracyclines, this party of Aurelio Di Marco, this party of Federico Arcamone, this party of all those splendid individuals who have been inspired by them and who believe so firmly in the basic tenets of our common faith in these quite splendid antibiotics, this party of /et cetera, et cetera/!" Take heart, I did not so begin even though I confess that I am by conviction deeply committed to the objectives of this important Symposium.

I preferred, rather, to begin with a quotation from Claude Bernard, that giant of the nineteenth century who in my opinion fathered many of our modern biomedical disciplines, not the least of which is pharmacology. That quotation has served me well as a guiding inspiration for my research career in cancer chemotherapy. He wrote in 1865 as follows (1):

"But when we reach the limits of vivisection we have other means
of going deeper and dealing with the elementary parts of organ-
isms where the elementary properties of vital phenomena have
their seat. We may introduce poisons into the circulation,
which carry their specific action to one or another histological
unit. . . . Poisons are veritable reagents of life, extremely
delicate instruments which dissect vital units. I believe
myself the first to consider the study of poisons from this point
of view, for I am of the opinion that studious attention to
agents which alter histological units should form the common
foundation of general physiology, pathology, and therapeutics."

For many, Bernard's word "poisons" may be offensive if meant
to include drugs having useful therapeutic activity. Perhaps
the more squeamish might prefer Adrien Albert's reference to
drugs as selectively toxic agents that cause injury to one kind
of living matter without harming another kind (2). For me,
"selective poisons" will do; for drugs act by virtue of their
capacity to inhibit, interrupt, disable, or destroy a physiological or biochemical function in a discriminating manner that
results in therapeutic benefit. The more exquisite the selectivity, the more beneficial is the result.

My introduction to the meaning of Bernard's aphorism began
nearly 40 years ago when in 1942 I was invited by Alfred Gilman
and Louis Goodman to assist them in their secret wartime
research that was aimed toward understanding the mechanism
of action of war gases and developing appropriate antidotes
or other therapeutic measures to reduce casualties. Little
did I know at the time, but that event marked the beginning
of my research in cancer chemotherapy; for both of these outstanding pharmacologists had already conceived of the possibility that the nitrogen mustards might possess therapeutic
activity against neoplasms of lymphoid origin. At that time,
as is now a matter of record, the nitrogen mustards were <u>bona
fide</u> war gases among the armaments of most military powers
and likely to serve a deadly purpose at any moment. Fortunately
the deadly military potential was never realized. But in the
early part of 1943, cautious clinical trials began at Yale with

the outcome that is now well known, namely, that nitrogen
mustards have therapeutic activity against lymphomatous
diseases (3).

In 1946 at the conclusion of World War II, I was invited
to join with Gilman in the preparation of a manuscript for publication in Science that might serve to introduce the general
biomedical community to the unpublished wartime research that
had resulted in the discovery of active antitumor agents (3).
Clearly, these were the first cancer chemotherapeutic drugs,
apart from sex hormones, that had the potential for widespread
therapeutic utility against human cancer. Certain comments
from that publication are worth considering. The basis for
the discovery came from the observation that "the marked effects
of the mustards on lymphoid tissue, coupled with the finding
that actively proliferating cells are selectively vulnerable
to the cytotoxic action of the mustards, suggested the therapeutic use of these compounds in the treatment of neoplasms of
lymphoid tissue." It was the high selectivity of the nitrogen
mustards against proliferating cells in vivo that intrigued
me and seemed so in keeping with Bernard's view that poisons
(or drugs) are "extremely delicate instruments which dissect
vital units."

Gilman and I had other comments that are still timely: "The
action of the available nitrogen mustards on lymphoid tissue
has not yet reached that degree of specificity which precludes
undesirable actions on the hematopoietic system. . . . However,
if care is taken with dosage, an adequate clinical response may
be obtained without affecting to a serious degree the formed
elements of the blood." Finally, we concluded hopefully that
"the previous successes which have characterized the evolution
of chemotherapeutic agents by chemical alteration of a parent
compound may be duplicated in the case of the β-chloroethyl
amines. The result would be a compound having a sufficiently
specific toxic action for certain types of proliferative cells
to possess therapeutic value."

Thirty-five years have elapsed since the appearance of our
essay. In this period all of us have seen an astounding

burgeoning of useful antineoplastic drugs that have expanded
our capacity to treat a wide variety of human cancers in a
manner that is heartwarming to those relatively few investigators who dreamed in those early days of a truly successful
cancer chemotherapy. That success has been achieved is no
longer questioned; that new successes continue to appear stimulates all of us involved worldwide in cancer treatment that we
are engaged in a useful, productive endeavor. Yet we must
admit that we have not achieved the original goal of finding
drugs that are specific poisons for neoplastic proliferating
cells. All antitumor agents discovered since 1946 are cytotoxic to normal host cells. Most are, like the nitrogen
mustards, selectively damaging to proliferating cells without
true specificity for neoplastic proliferations. Many have
other undesirable sites of cytotoxic action which appear unrelated to the proliferative capacity of the susceptible host
cell, for example, the cardiac muscle cell, so uniquely susceptible to damage by anthracycline antibiotics, or the renal
tubular epithelium that is destroyed by cisplatin.

The goal of developing drugs which are highly specific in
attacking neoplastic proliferations remains a forlorn hope.
The conception of such a possibility implies that there are
in tumor cells vital targets for drug action which have no counterpart among the biochemical and physiological functions of
nonneoplastic host cells. Greenstein in 1954 stated the problem
must succinctly when he concluded in his treatise on the biochemistry of cancer (4) that "the tumor is a new tissue with a
metabolic pattern which, though peculiar to itself in an overall sense, comprises enzymes which function qualitatively like
similar enzymes in normal tissues." In expressing the implication of this conclusion for developing tumor-specific thera
peutic agents, he went on to state, "It is not improbable that,
like the antibacterial drugs, the successful chemotherapeutic
agents will be those most destructive to cells undergoing active
metabolism and division. Cells in this category are found in
non-neoplastic as well as in neoplastic tissues." Furthermore,
"no agent has been found as yet to be completely effective in

the treatment of cancer, whether in mouse or man. There are
only agents which have more favorable ratios than others for
the maximum tolerated dose, and the use of different agents,
either consecutively or in combination, appears to be the
most frequently effective procedure." Greenstein's
sagacious remarks are as cogent today as they were in 1954.

In view of what I have said above, must one conclude that
it is unlikely that we can ever explain satisfactorily the
therapeutic efficacy of anticancer drugs, or to put it another
way, their selectivity of action in vivo? Lest there be any
misunderstanding, I wish to make it clear that I am not refer-
ring to explanations of mechanisms of cytotoxic action in
susceptible cells. Such mechanisms deal with the biochemical
lesions induced by drugs as the consequence of their reaction
with relevant cellular target(s). To quote R. A. Peters (5),
"a biochemical lesion can be defined as the biochemical change
or defect which directly precedes pathological change or
dysfunction." The annals of cancer chemotherapeutic research
are replete with elegant studies aimed at delineating biochemical lesions. A long-accepted and outstanding paradigm
is the research that has dealt with the inhibition of dihydro-
folate reductase by methotrexate. Other examples were amply
provided during the first day of the Symposium, wherein the
focus was the interaction between cytotoxic anthracyclines and
macromolecular targets, particularly, though not exclusively,
DNA. Elucidation of mechanism of action, though a necessary
step in the right direction, is not sufficient to provide
understanding of the basis for therapeutic selectivity.
This is true for chemotherapeutic agents which are targeted
against vital functions that are present in both host and
parasitic cells; it is particularly so for antitumor drugs,
since these are not directed exclusively against tumor-specific
functions.

Determination of the basis for the therapeutic efficacy
of antitumor agents is a complex pharmacological problem that
has not in my opinion received sufficient attention by cancer
researchers. Werkheiser and Moran (6) and Schwartz and

Mihich (7) have addressed the problem in scholarly essays
in which they have ably summarized the many possible factors
which, acting singly or in concert, might conceivably result
in therapeutically selective outcomes. Yet there are relatively
few examples of investigations that have been focussed on direct
study of the problem in vivo. Sirotnak et al. (8) and Chou
et al. (9) have compared sensitive leukemic cells and the most
susceptible host tissue in mice treated with therapeutically
efficacious doses of methotrexate and ara-C. Their studies
demonstrated that there are in vivo significantly greater
levels of accumulation or persistance of methotrexate or of
the active nucleotide ara-CTP in mouse leukemic cells than in
host tissues. Presumably, favorable differences in cell-
concentrating mechanisms are responsible for the therapeutic
activity of the agents in mouse leukemia. Whether such favorable differences account for the therapeutic utility of the
same drugs against human cancer is a question that has not yet
been addressed.

I am not at present overly optimistic that studies with
other cancer chemotherapeutic agents will result in so straight-
forward and surprisingly simple an explanation for beneficial
selectivity as preferential drug accumulation by tumor cells.
As a case in point, there is to my knowledge no notable evidence
showing that anthracyclines accumulate and persist in susceptible
tumors to a greater extent than in host tissues.

Even though direct study of the selective mechanisms responsible for therapeutic efficacy is not an easy task because of
the complexity of the possible factors involved, I am convinced
that it is worth pursuing. Satisfactory explanations can be
intellectually rewarding; but, more importantly, the search
for such explanations can be expected to offer useful suggestions for improvements in therapy.

For some time I have had the impression that, as practiced
by our segment of biomedical research, study of the mechanism
of cytotoxic action of antitumor agents has been for the most
part like a one-sided coin. The simile is obviously nonsensical
the concept of a one-sided coin is fantastical unless the minter

deliberately or accidently chooses to leave the reverse side
blank. To most cancer chemotherapists, the blank side, host
toxicity, has been and still is distasteful. Since host toxicity
has been the primary object of my research career, I have frequently responded to the feelings of my worthy colleagues in
cancer chemotherapy with a sense of loneliness. Clearly, all
known antitumor drugs have two-sided activity; they do selectively
damage tumor cells, but they also damage selectively host tissues.
Intensive effort directed toward understanding selectivity of
action in host cells could be rewarding; for it might open up
other avenues of access toward improving therapeutic efficacy.
From my vantage point, I do perceive that the kind of effort
may now be beginning in earnest. Thus, a significant portion
of the Symposium was focused on the cardiotoxicity of anthracycline antibiotics. The search for the biochemical lesion
responsible for cardiotoxic effects is thriving and engendering
wide interest. Bioassay for cardiotoxicity now appears to be
as essential in the development of newer anthracyclines as are
tests for antitumor activity. I am hopeful that such effort
will soon result in anthracycline derivatives that cause little
or no cardiac damage while retaining high selectivity against
tumors. It is worth noting that greater focus on host toxicity
is becoming the fashion in developing new antitumor platinum-
containing coordination complexes (10). Here as much emphasis
is being given to tests for emetic activity and nephrotoxicity
as to bioassay for antitumor activity.

I shall end my remarks with a few speculations about future
approaches toward the greater understanding of selective antitumor activity. Several lines of current endeavor in cell
biology are suggestive. These are concerned with regulatory
factors involved in growth control of animal cells. For
example, Pardee and his associates, citing their work and
that of others, have compelling evidence for the existence of
a labile regulatory protein which is synthesized early in the
G_1 phase of the mitotic cycle and which determines whether or
not cells will procede through the mitotic cycle. Partial
inhibition of the synthesis of the regulator will delay progress

through G_1. Severe restriction of synthesis will arrest
cells in early G_1 and, if prolonged, may force some into the
quiescent G_0 state. Pardee and his colleagues suggest further
that the decontrolled growth of tumor cells results from changes
in the regulatory system such that the controlling protein is
more stable or its synthesis less dependent on control by
inducing factors (11). Supposing their hypotheses to be
true, would it not seem reasonable to ask whether cancer
chemotherapeutic agents might in some direct or indirect manner
adversely affect the synthesis of the growth regulatory protein
to a greater extent in nonmalignant than in tumor cells? The
consequence of such a differential inhibition, which need
only be quantitative in origin, would be the retention of a
significantly greater portion of normal, host cells than of
tumor cells in early G_1 or quiescent G_0 where they would be
protected from selective damage from drugs that act destructively
in later phases of the mitotic cycle. The result would be a
greater and, hence, more therapeutically efficacious killing
of tumor cell populations.

Other speculation about selectivity of antitumor action has
occurred to me in thoughts about the significance of the
angiogenesis factor. This regulatory substance, demonstrably
elaborated by certain experimental tumors, serves to stimulate
the proliferation of host capillary endothelium (12) Function-
ally, it is the impetus for provision by the host of an
adequate vascularity, a contigency essential for the progressive
growth of tumor cell population. That the capillary endothelium
of tumors must proliferate if tumor growth is to be sustained
is obvious. But the extent of the proliferative activity
involved is quite surprising. For example, Tannock has shown
that the thymidine-labelling index of capillary endothelium
in growing mouse mammary tumors is of the order of 10% (13).
Certainly such high proliferative activity implies that tumor
capillary endothelium is at great risk of destruction by cancer
chemotherapeutic agents. The damage would be highly selective;
for the proliferation of endothelium in normal host organs,
though finite, is quite low. It would seem that the effect

of antitumor agents on tumor capillary endothelium would be
a proper object of investigation; for such study might shed
further light on the nature of selective tumor drugs.

I have mentioned the above speculations not solely because
I believe in their merit. Rather, I mean to suggest that continued progress in research concerned with the cell and molecular
biology of tumors will almost certainly uncover valuable new
information about the nature of the regulatory aberrations
responsible for malignant growth. Open-eyed attention on the
part of cancer chemotherapists to such new information should
ensure that it will be applied sagaciously in the development
of truly selective and, therefore, highly efficacious antitumor
drugs. I am confident that we shall see the day when we have
those "poisons" of Claude Bernard that have "specific action"
on the "histological unit" that is cancer.

REFERENCES

1. Bernard C. 1957. An introduction to the study of experimental
   medicine. New York, Dover Publications, Inc.
2. Albert A. 1973. Selective toxicity. The physico-chemical basis
   of therapy. 5th ed. London, Chapman and Hall.
3. Gilman A, Philips FS. 1946. The biological actions and therapeutic
   applications of the B-chloroethyl amines and sulfides. Science
   103: 409-415.
4. Greenstein JP. 1954. Biochemistry of cancer. 2nd ed. New
   York, Academic Press.
5. Peters RA. 1967. The biochemical lesion in thiamine deficiency.
   In Biochemical lesions and their clinical significance. Boston,
   Little Brown.
6. Werkheiser WC, Moran RG. 1973. The dynamic multifactional basis
   for selectivity of antitumor agents: General principles. In
   Mihich E, ed. Drug resistance and selectivity. Biochemical and
   cellular basis. New York, Academic Press, pp. 1-40.
7. Schwartz HS, Mihich E. 1973. Species and tissue differences in
   drug selectivity. In Mihich E, ed. Drug resistance and selectivity.
   Biochemical and cellular basis. New York, Academic Press,
   pp. 413-452.
8. Sirotnak FM, Chello PL, Degraw JI, Piper JR, Montgomery JA. 1981.
   Membrane transport and the molecular basis for selective antitumor
   action of folate analogs. In Sartorelli AC, Lazo JS, Bertino JR,
   eds. Molecular actions and targets for cancer chemotherapeutic
   agents. New York, Academic Press, pp. 349-384.
9. Chou TC, Hutchison DJ, Schmid FA, Philips FS. 1975. Metabolism
   and selective effects of 1-B-D-arabinofuranosylcytosine in L1210
   and host tissues in vivo. Cancer Res. 35: 225-236.

10. Prestayko AW, Crooke ST, Carter SK, eds. 1980.
    Cisplatin: Current status and new developments.
    New York, Academic Press.
11. Rossow PW, Riddle VGH, Pardee AB. 1979. Synthesis of
    labile serum-dependent protein in early G_1 controls
    animal cell growth. Proc. Natl. Acad. Sci. USA 76:
    4446-4450.
12. Langer R, Folkman J. 1981. Angiogenesis inhibitors.
    In Sartorelli AC, Lazo JS, Bertino JF, eds. Molecular
    actions and targets for cancer chemotherapeutic agents.
    New York, Academic Press, pp. 511-525.
13. Tannock IF. 1970. Population kinetics of carcinoma cells,
    capillary endothelial cells, and fibroblasts in a
    transplanted mouse mammary tumor. Cancer Res. 30:
    2470-2476.

ANTITUMOR ACTIVITY OF ANTHRACYCLINES: EXPERIMENTAL STUDIES

A. M. CASAZZA

1.   INTRODUCTION

Among the numerous classes of antitumor agents identified so far, anthracyclines have played a major role because of the high antileukemic effectiveness of daunorubicin (DNR) and doxorubicin (DX) and because of the rather large spectrum of antitumor activity of DX, which is active both against leukemias and solid tumors. Interest in this class of compounds has grown considerably from 1963, date of the first report on DNR (1), and many research groups are actively engaged in the investigation of new anthracycline molecules, with the aim of finding compounds that show a higher antitumor effectiveness of a more favorable therapeutic index in comparison with DNR and DX. Most of the new molecules are being investigated for their antitumor activity against experimental tumor systems, mainly of mice, as this evaluation is one of the fundamental steps in the study of new anthracycline analogs (2). In this review, I will summarize the experience gained by studies on the antitumor activity of DNR, DX, and several new derivatives selected on the basis of interesting biological or pharmacological properties (3).

2.   ANTITUMOR ACTIVITY OF DNR AND DX

2.1. Ascitic tumors

Ascitic tumors are generally used as primary screening models. Table 1 shows the results obtained by several authors on ascitic tumors of mice and rats after treatment with optimal doses (doses which cause the maximal anti-tumor activity without toxic effects) of DNR and DX administered according to different schedules. Both compounds are highly active; in general, DX is more active than is DNR. As regards the optimal doses, the one of DNR is in general lower than that of DX. This is due to the high toxicity of DNR injected i.p.

Table 1. Comparison of DX with DNR against ascitic tumors

Tumor	Schedule	DNR O.D.[a]	DNR T/C(%)[b]	DX O.D.[a]	DX T/C(%)[b]	Refs.
Ll210 leukemia	dl	2.5	150	10	151	4
		4	168	5	241	5
		2.9	144	6.6	159	6
P288 leukemia	qd, 1 to 5	1	140	2	240	7
P388 leukemia	q6hr x 3, dl	2	195	4	545	4
B16 melanoma	dl	5	159	13.3	204	8
	qd, 1 to 9	0.5	94	1	188	
	q4d,1,5,9	2	47	2	88	
Ehrlich carcinoma	qd, 1 to 5	2.5	180	2.5	280	9
Sarcoma 180	dl	0.25	222	0.5	227	10

a, Optimal dose (mg/kg, i.p.).
b, Median survival time of treated mice/controls x 100.

2.2. Solid tumors

Ascitic tumors in experimental animals are very useful as screening models, but differ from human cancer as 1) the tumor is localized and disseminates only in the late stages of the disease; 2) the treatment is mainly carried out i.p., giving irritation of the peritoneum (and this is particularly true for anthracyclines) and gives somewhat optimistic results, as the drug can reach the target cells very quickly. It was felt, therefore, that experiments in which the drugs were injected i.v. could be of greater relevance. Also it was important to investigate the response of solid tumors of different origins and of different histological types. Table 2 summarizes some of the many experimental data obtained with DNR and DX against solid tumors. In these experiments, the superiority of DX versus DNR is particularly evident. In particular, it is interesting to note the high antitumor activity of DX injected i.v. against spontaneous and transplanted mammary carcinoma of C3H mice; DX produces inhibition of tumor development and regression of already established tumors up to 90%. The activity depends on the schedule of the i.v. treatment, the most effective treatment being every other day x 12 with a low dose (as reported in Table 2), or treatment on a weekly schedule for 3-4 weeks with a higher dose (6 mg/kg) (11).

Table 2. Comparison of DX with DNR against mouse solid tumors

Tumor	Schedule	DNR			DX			Refs.
		O.D.[a]	T/C %[b]	% inhib.[c]	O.D.	T/C %	% inhib.	
Sarcoma 180	qd,1 to 8	3.25		50	2.5		69	10
Transplanted mammary ca.	q2d,1 to 11 17 to 27	2.6	160		2.5	210		11
Spontaneous mammary ca.	q2d,1 to 11 17 to 27	3.25		34	2.25		76	
MSV-induced sarcoma	qd, 3 to 10	3.25		37	2.25		46	12
MS-2 sarcoma	6,10,14,18	4	107	38	3.5	132	68	13
	qw x 5	5.3	124	40	6.6	130	65	
	q3d x 5	6	129	61	4	131	69	
Colon 38								
advanced	q3-4d x 4	10.0		60	7,5		94	14
early	q4d x 3				5.0		91	

(a), (b) see Table 1. (c) Inhibition of tumor growth, % over untreated controls.

Another important experimental model investigated by us was the sarcoma induced by Moloney Sarcoma Virus (MSV). In this experimental system, not only DX is more active than DNR, but also it does not inhibit the regression which takes place spontaneously in the controls because of immunological mechanisms (12). These data induced us to think that DX, even if more toxic than DNR when administered i.v., could have a different effect on immune response, thus hampering less than DNR the immunological host mechanisms which can operate and can be very important for the final success of antitumor therapy. This hypothesis was also advanced by Schwartz and Grindey (7) and was confirmed in experimental studies carried out by us and by other Authors (15,16,17).

Recently, DX was found to be highly active against several human tumors heterotransplanted into Balb/c nude mice, such as breast cancer, one oat-cell carcinoma of lung, melanoma, prostate cancer and sarcoma (18). DNR did not show such a high antitumor activity in these experimental systems (Giuliani F.; personal communication). The high antitumor effectiveness of DX in nude mice suggests that the differences in the immunomodulating activity in respect to DNR is not the only reason for the outstanding antitumor effectiveness of DX. DNR was found to differ from DX for the pharmacokinetic properties in the whole animal (19) and at the cellular level (20,21). Probably in relation to the lower partition coefficient between water and lipids, DX is taken up by the cells in vitro more slowly and less than DNR; however, according to some Authors, it localizes mainly into the cell nucleus, while DNR remains in great amounts confined into the cytoplasm (21). In mice, the most important finding is that DX remains for longer time than DNR in the tissues, and particularly in the spleen (19). This result can explain the higher toxicity of DX versus DNR injected i.v., but the high antitumor activity of DX against solid tumors can be only partially explained by drug levels in the tumor tissue.

As regards solid tumors, one important aspect is the possibility of influencing by chemotherapeutic treatment not only the primary tumor, but also (and mainly) the micrometastatic foci which can already be present at the time of tumor diagnosis. We have therefore made an effort to set up experimental systems that can allow the detection of: 1) activity on the primary solid tumor; 2) activity on metastases; 3) activity on metastases in combination with surgery.

Table 3. Antimetastatic activity of DX, alone or in combination, against lung metastases by MS-2 sarcoma in mice.

Schedule of treatment[a]	Drug[b]	% of mice cured[c]
1,4,7	DX	25*
	ICRF-159	0
	DX + ICRF-159	90**
15,18,21	DX	9
	ICRF-159	9
	DX + ICRF-159	60*
1,4,7,15,18,21	DX	46
	ICRF-159	10
	DX + ICRF-159	45

(a) Surgery on day 13. (b) DX i.v., 4 mg/kg; ICRF-159 i.p., 50 mg/kg. (c) Evaluated by bioassay on lung of mice killed 20-26 days after tumor implant into footpad. * $p < 0.05$; ** $p < 0.01$, Mussett test.

The model chosen was the MS-2 sarcoma (originally derived from a MSV-induced sarcoma), which spontaneously metastasizes to the lung (13). DX is active against lung metastases, particularly when administered in combination with other chemotherapeutic drugs like the antimetastatic agent ICRF-159, before the time of surgical tumor amputation (Table 3) (22).

2.3. Leukemias
Another important field of the tumor pathology in humans is represented by hematological malignancies. We considered

the ascitic leukemias, as previously noticed, as too artificial models, and we have investigated the antileukemic activity of anthracyclines on transplanted Gross leukemia, which
is: a) originally virus-induced; b) transplanted i.v., giving
a disseminated disease. Our results have shown that both DNR
and DX have a high antileukemic activity, which depends on
the schedule of treatment (2).

3. ANTITUMOR ACTIVITY OF SELECTED ANTHRACYCLINE ANALOGS
    The preclinical tests conducted to date for experimental
evaluation of anthracycline analogs have been previously reviewed (2). As regards antitumor activity, the general approach to these studies was to set up experimental models
which could allow the identification of new anthracycline
analogs having in respect to the parent compounds, either
greater antitumor activity against tumors already sensitive
to anthracyclines, or activity against tumors with natural or
acquired resistance. I will here describe the antitumor effectiveness against experimental tumors of some anthracycline
analogs which have been selected because of outstanding antitumor properties or because of a higher therapeutic index in
respect to DX.

3.1. 4'-Epidoxorubicin
    4'-Epidoxorubicin (4'-epiDX) was first described in 1975
by Arcamone et al. (23), and subsequently experimentally
investigated for antitumor activity (14,23,24,25,26,27); mechanism of action (28,29); pharmacokinetic properties (24,30,31,
32); toxic effects (24,33,34); and effect on immune systems(35).
    In general, the experimental studies suggested that 4'-epiDX
is as potent as DX, exerting its antitumor activity at the same
doses as DX, but slightly less toxic and less cardiotoxic,
being therefore endowed with a higher therapeutic index than
DX. For example, in mice bearing P388 leukemia, DX shows an
LD10 $\simeq$ 7 mg/kg and an ED$_{200}$ (dose that caused a 200% increase
of life span) $\simeq$ 6.4, while 4'-epiDX shows an LD10 12 mg/kg
and an ED$_{200}$ = 6.6 mg/kg. The latter appears therefore endowed,
in this system, with a therapeutic ratio (ratio LD10/ED$_{200}$)
equal to 1.81, distinctly higher than the one showed by DX,
which is equal to 1.09 (24). 4'-EpiDX shows a therapeutic
index slightly higher than that of DX also when the cardiotoxic doses are compared to antitumor doses; the Minimal Cumulative Cardiotoxic Dose of DX in mice is 11 mg/kg, and the
one of 4'-epiDX is 14 mg/kg, while the Optimal Cumulative
Antitumor Dose is 15 mg/kg for both compounds; the therapeutic
index is therefore in the system here considered, 0.73 for DX
and 0.93 for 4'-epiDX (33). Several experiments carried out

against mammary carcinoma of C3H mice and MSV-induced sarcoma, and against the spontaneous lung metastases given by Lewis Lung carcinoma and MS-2 sarcoma, showed that 4'-epiDX has the same potency and, at the optimal dose, the same antitumor activity as DX (24). In some experiments, because of the lower general toxicity of 4'-epiDX vs DX, it was possible to administer higher doses of the new derivative than of DX, and to obtain a more favourable therapeutic activity. This was observed, for example, on Lewis Lung carcinoma and MS-2 sarcoma lung metastases: the administration of 4'-epiDX after the surgical removal of the primary tumor, cured 50% and 100% of the mice, respectively (24,25). In these experimental systems, the high antitumor effect given by 4'-epiDX can be due to the increased dose administered and to the fact that, as described elsewhere in this volume (3) $/^{-14}C/$ 4'-epiDX exhibits significantly higher initial concentration of radioactivity than $/^{-14}C/$ DX in rats lungs. It will be interesting to know if 4'-epiDX is superior to DX in the therapy of human lung metastases.

Table 4. Antitumor activity of DX and some new anthracycline derivatives against early murine colon 38 adenocarcinoma [a].

Compound[b]	Dose (mg/kg)	T/C %[c]	% inhib.[d]	Toxicity[e]
DX	6	119,186	74,61	0/6
	9	175,186	95,95	13/16
4'-epiDX	9	229,142	94,76	1/6
	13.5	162,248	98,98	11/16
4'-deoxyDX	4	>278,273	91,89	0/6
	6	>278,171	97,96	10/16
4'-O-methylDX	4	157,244	91,89	0/6
	6	>278,288	94,99	6/16

(a) Data of two experiments. (b) Treatment i.v. q7d x 4, starting on Day 1 after tumor inoculation. (c) See Table 1. (d) See Table 2. (e) Evaluated in non-tumored mice, observed for 90 days.

No dose-related tissue uptake studies have been carried out up to now, but it is rational to think that by increasing the dose, it is possible to increase the antitumor effect. We have observed such an effect in experiments carried out on the colon 38 adenocarcinoma transplanted s.c. in mice: 4'-epiDX, at the dose of 9 mg/kg administered once a week for four weeks, is tolerated and produces an inhibition of tumor growth higher

than that given by DX at the maximal tolerated dose of 6 mg/kg
(Table 4) (14).

This result is of interest because of the sensitivity to
4'-epiDX of some human colon tumors observed in patients (36,
37), but is in contrast with the lack of antitumor activity
of 4'-epiDX on some human colon tumors heterotransplanted in
nude mice (27). It is possible that the sensitivity to 4'-epiDX
treatment is a property of only some colon tumors, and a larger
investigation on a broad spectrum of tumors is needed in order
to answer to this question. On the other hand, it was shown
in two different experimental studies that, after administration of the same dose of the two compounds, similar drug levels
are found in tumor tissue (24,32) at initial times, but 4'-epiDX
seems to be less firmly bound than DX to this tissue or its
subcellular functions, as at later times after treatment
slightly higher concentrations of DX than of 4'-epiDX are present in the tumor. Therefore the increase of the dose of 4'-epiDX
over that of DX can give advantages which are not clearly demonstrable in all the experiments.

As regards the immunodepressive activity in mice, 4'-epiDX
is, like DX, active in depressing IgM and IgG antibody response,
and not active on allograft survival; it slightly reduces the
delayed hypersensitivity reaction to sheep red blood cells, a
reaction which is not influenced by DX (35). The pattern of
immunodepressing effect given by 4'-epiDX is therefore similar
to that of DX.

In conclusion the antitumor activity of 4'-epiDX seems so
far very similar to that of DX, the two compounds having about
equal spectrum of antitumor effectiveness and equal activity
at the same doses on experimental tumors; whether the slight
differences observed are predictive of differences in the clinical effectiveness remains to be shown. The lower general toxicity of 4'-epiDX vs DX was observed both in experimental
studies (24,33) and in patients (37,38,39), and correlates
well with the lower spleen concentration and faster elimination
of 4'-epiDX vs DX (31,38) and possibly also with its higher
rate of metabolism (32). This correlation between experimental and clinical findings is of high interest.

3.2. 4-Demethoxydaunorubicin

4-Demethoxydaunorubicin (4-dmDNR) was first described in
1976 by Arcamone and coworkers (40) and subsequently investigated for antitumor activity (40,41,42); cytotoxicity and mechanism of action (43); pharmacokinetic properties (44, 45);
oncogenicity and cell transformation (46) and toxicological
properties (33). 4-DmDNR showed higher affinity of binding to
DNA than DNR (2) and higher cell uptake in vitro (43). The

cytotoxic effect in vitro and the induction of DNA breaks
caused by 4-dmDNR are higher than those given by DNR and DX
(43,47); inhibition of DNA synthesis, as measured by tritiated
thymidine incorporation, was equal to that caused by DNR in
one study (43) and higher in other studies (45,47). In parallel with the cytotoxicity data, a higher potency of 4-dmDNR
in comparison with DNR and DX was observed in animals (2,33).
Another important feature of 4-dmDNR is its absorption by the
gastrointestinal tract (44) and its ability to exert antitumor
activity also when administered (41,42).

The antitumor activity of 4-dmDNR was investigated mainly
against experimental leukemias (42). It is interesting to observe that the ratio between the antitumor activity (at optimal
non toxic doses) of 4-dmDNR and the antitumor activity of DNR
or DX, differs depending on the type of experimental leukemia
investigated, and on the route of tumor implantation and of
drug treatment. The most relevant data in this regard are reported in Table 5.

Table 5. Antileukemic activity of 4-dmDNR in comparison with
DNR and DX. Comparison at optimal non toxic doses
($\leqslant LD_{10}$)[a].

Tumor		Treatment			T/C[b]	Ratio[c]
Leukemia	Route	Route	Days	Drug	%	
P388	ip	ip	1	DNR	197	
				4-dmDNR	147	<
L1210	ip	ip	1	DX	157	
				DNR	156	
				4-dmDNR	146	=
	iv	iv	1	DX	162	
				4-dmDNR	>750	>
			3,7,11	DX	114	
				DNR	114	
				4-dmDNR	150	>
Gross (2x10^6)	iv	iv	1	DX	217	
				DNR	167	
				4-dmDNR	225	>
Gross (10^2)	iv	iv	1	DX	50^d	
				DNR	83^d	
				4-dmDNR	100^d	>

(a) Data from Ref. 42. (b) See Table 1. (c) Relative antitumor
activity of 4-dmDNR and DX or DNR. (d) % of surviving mice.

4-DmDNR is less active than DNR against the ascitic P388
leukemia, and as active as DNR and DX against ascitic L1210
leukemia. However, when L1210 leukemia cells are injected

i.v., 4-dmDNR administered i.v. on Day 1 is definitely more active than DNR and DX, and it is also active against the late tumor, while DNR and DX are not. Higher antitumor effectiveness than that of DNR and DX against i.v.-injected L1210 leukemia was also observed with 4-demethoxydoxorubicin (2), and seems therefore a general property of 4-demethoxyanthracyclines.

It has been reported that 4-dmDNR is two times more active than DNR and 3-4 times more active than DX on DNA and RNA synthesis of L1210 leukemia cells in vitro (45). It is possible that the high inhibition of macromolecular synthesis correlates with the high antitumor activity against i.v.-injected L1210 leukemia, and that in the ip-ip experiments the high antitumor effectiveness of 4-dmDNR cannot be shown because of the important toxic effect of i.p. injected anthracyclines (48). Cell uptake and intracellular distribution of 4-demethoxyanthra-cyclines must also be considered. In experimental conditions in which DNR and DX cytofluorescence is localized in cell nuclei, 4-dmDNR cytofluorescence is localized in the cytoplasm (45); however, in another study, carried out by fluorescence micro-scopy using a laser for excitation, it was reported that both 4-dmDNR and DNR cytofluorescence is localized in the nuclei of HeLa cells (49). This aspect should therefore be more deeply investigated.

L1210 leukemia is rather resistant to DNR and DX therapy; the high effectiveness of 4-dmDNR on this type of tumor stim-ulated researches on P388/DX (P388 leukemia resistant to DX). 4-DmDNR is not active in vivo on this tumor line bearing ac-quired resistance to anthracyclines (26); however, in in vitro experiments, 4-dmDNR has an interesting cytotoxic activity on P388/DX leukemia cells, as the ratio between ID_{50} on P388/DX and ID_{50} on P388, is 75 for DX, 85 for DNR, and 35 for 4-dmDNR (50). It is possible that because of the increased cell uptake and possibly retention (47) 4-dmDNR is more active than DNR on resistant or partially resistant leukemia cells.

Another interesting observation is the very high effective-ness of 4-dmDNR in mice injected with a low number of Gross leukemia cells. Not only 100% of the animals are cured by the maximal tolerated dose (2.5 mg/kg), but this effect is present in a range of tolerated doses, from 1.7 to 2.5 mg/kg. No dose of DNR or DX could cure all the animals. •

When the mice are injected with a high number of Gross leukemia cells (2×10^6 cells/mouse), the increase of survival time given by 4-dmDNR administered iv on Day 1 is about equal to that given by DX and slightly superior to that given by DNR (Table 5). In our experimental Gross leukemia the median tumor cell doubling time is 0.33 days, as calculated on the base of a titration with 10-fold dilutions of cancer cells, according to Skipper et al. (51).

As the median survival time (in days) of controls inoculated with 2×10^6 tumor cells is 6 days, and treatment was
performed on Day 1 the total tumor cell decrease during treatment is 7 logs with DX, 4 logs with DNR, and 8 logs with 4-
dmDNR. The slight differences observed in the increase of life
span caused by the three anthracyclines here compared (Table
5) reflect a difference in terms of cell kill. The high tumor
cell kill by 4-dmDNR suggests that stepwise selection of specifically drug resistant tumor cells is not occurring after
4-dmDNR single treatment (51).

All together, these data stimulate further investigations
on 4-dmDNR against other experimental leukemias resistant to
DX and DNR, and suggest the possibility that 4-dmDNR might
have some effect on DNR and DX resistant human leukemias.

As regards solid tumors, the data so far obtained showed
that 4-dmDNR was, in general, as active as DNR. Therefore the
activity is lower than that of DX against those tumors which
are particularly sensitive to DX activity, like mammary carcinoma and MSV-induced sarcoma. However, on MS-2 sarcoma and
180 sarcoma, 4-dmDNR shows an antitumor activity of the same
order of magnitude as that of DX. 4-DmDNR has a good activity
against 180 sarcoma also when it is administered by oral route.
These data are of interest, and stimulate further experimental
studies.

3.3. 4'-Deoxydoxorubicin

4'-Deoxydoxorubicin (4'-deoxyDX) is a new DX analog lacking
the hydroxyl group in position 4' of the aminosugar (52).
This compound has been investigated for antitumor activity
(27,33,52,53,54,55,56,57), cytotoxicity and mechanism of action
(29), pharmacokinetic properties (31,58,59) and toxicity, with
particular attention for cardiac toxicity (33,53).

The most interesting properties of 4'-deoxyDX are: 1) lack
of clear cardiotoxic dose-dependent effects in all the experimental animals so far investigated: CD 1 mice (33), C3H mice
(53), rabbits (33); 2) selectivity of the antitumor effect,
which, at the optimal doses, is equal to that of DX against
several experimental tumors, such as Gross leukemia and MS-2
sarcoma, lower than that of DX against B16 melanoma, and
higher than that of DX against colon 26 and 38 adenocarcino-
mas (56). In nude mice heterotransplanted with human colon
tumors, it was observed that the antitumor effectiveness of
4'-deoxyDX is definitely superior to that of DX (27,54). The
data against solid tumors are of extreme interest, and deserve
a detailed description. DX and 4'-deoxyDX were given i.v.
every week for a total of four weeks, starting when the tumor

was palpable. Only the results obtained at the Optimal Doses
are here reported.

Table 6. Effects of DX and 4'-deoxyDX against melanomas

| Compound | % inhibition[a] | | | |
| | Human[b] | | | Mouse |
	T 242	T 354	T 355	B16
DX[c]	87	56	51	95
4'-deoxyDX[d]	76	42	33	83

(a) See Table 2. (b) Data obtained in nude
mice (57). (c) O.D. 10 mg/kg iv, q7dx4. (d)
O.D. 6 mg/kg iv, q7dx4.

Table 6 reports the data obtained by Giuliani et al. against
human melanomas transplanted in nude mice (57), and against
the mouse melanoma B16, injected s.c. In all these systems,
it is peculiar to observe the high effectiveness of DX, which
is known as not active in melanoma patients, and the fact
that 4'-deoxyDX is less active than DX.

Table 7. Effects of DX and 4'-deoxyDX against mammary
carcinomas

| Compound | % inhibition[a] | | | |
| | Human[b] | | | Mouse |
	T 112	T 378	T 386	C3H
DX[c]	88	96	90	-72[d]
4'-deoxyDX[e]	93	65	67	-52

(a) See Table 2. (b) Data obtained in nude
mice (57). (c) O.D. (mg/kg)=10 in nude mice,
7.5 in C3H mice. (d) % regression of tumor
volume. (e) O.D. (mg/kg)=6 in nude mice, 6.25
in C3H mice.

Table 7 reports the data obtained against human mammary carcinomas transplanted into nude mice (57), and against the spontaneous mammary carcinoma of C3H female mice at its 3rd trans-
plant. These tumors are highly sensitive to the DX activity,
in good correlation with the clinical data. 4'-DeoxyDX also
shows a very good antitumor activity, but some tumors seem
less sensitive to 4'-deoxyDX than to DX.

Table 8. Effects of DX and 4'-deoxyDX against colon carcinomas

| Compound | % inhibition[a] | | | | | |
| | Human[b] | | | | Mouse | |
	T 183	T 219	T 374	T 380	26	38
DX[c]	19	63[d]	44	33	52	67
4'-deoxyDX[e]	65	>99	72	59	67	90

(a) See Table 2. (b) Data obtained in nude mice (27).
(c) O.D. (mg/kg)=10 in nude mice, 6 in conventional mice.
(d) At 6.6 mg/kg. (e) O.D. (mg/kg)=6 in nude mice, 4 in
conventional mice.

Table 8 reports the data obtained against human colon adenocarcinoma transplanted into nude mice (27), and against two
colon tumors of conventional mice: the undifferentiated carcinoma 26 and the adenocarcinoma 38. The effects against colon
38 carcinoma are also shown in Table 4. The effectiveness of
DX is definitely lower than that exerted against the highly
sensitive mammary carcinoma, and only in two tumors the inhibition is higher than 50%. On the contrary, in all the colon
tumors tested 4'-deoxyDX causes inhibition higher than 50%,
and the two tumors whose growth is sensitive to DX (the human
tumor T 219 and the mouse tumor 38), are inhibited by 4'-
deoxyDX by 90% or more. Another DX derivative modified in
position 4' of the aminosugar, that is 4'-O-methylDX, was
particularly effective against colon tumors (Table 4).

In conclusion, these data show that 4'-deoxyDX is a peculiar new anthracycline derivative, showing a different spectrum of antitumor activity in comparison with DX. In an attempt to explain these differences, we have investigated the
pharmacokinetic properties of 4'-deoxyDX and DX in mice bearing solid tumors. The preliminary data so far obtained do not
seem to allow an explanation of the selective antitumor effect
of 4'-deoxyDX against colon tumors: after administration
of DX or 4'-deoxyDX equal levels of drug equivalents are
found in a human colon tumor transplanted in nude mice, as
well as in colon 38 carcinoma transplanted in conventional
mice (58).

4'-DeoxyDX, as well as the other new derivatives described
here, has been compared to DX also in human tumor stem cell
assay (60). In these experiments, 4'-deoxyDX shows a cytotoxic
effect in vitro higher than that of DX against all the tumors
tested, which included breast, ovarian, and lung tumors. The
effect of 4'-deoxyDX against three ovarian tumors seems particularly interesting, as these tumors are scarcely sensitive
to DX. These data suggest that the selective antitumor activity

of 4'-deoxyDX against colon tumors and possibly against ovarian tumors can be due to a particular effect of the drug at
the tumor cell level, rather than to different pharmacokinetic
properties in comparison with DX in the whole animal. Further
in vitro and in vivo studies are desirable, as well as the
advancement of this anthracycline analog into phase I clinical
trials.

4. CONCLUSIONS

The data here reported show that modifications in the chemical structure of DNR and DX can alter the biological activity
of these compounds, leading to new anthracycline analogs
having interestingly favourable therapeutic properties. The
main characteristics of the new analogs discussed here are
presented in Table 9.

Table 9. Comparison with DX

Compound	Potency	Antitumor activity (at MTD)					Cardio-toxicity	T.I.
		Leuk ip iv	Mam-mary	Colon	Mela-noma	MS-2		
4-dmDNR	↑	= ↑	↓	=			↑	↑
4'-epiDX	=	= =	=	=	=	=	↓	↑
4'-deoxyDX	↑	= =	=	↑	↓	=	↓	↑

Besides the variations in potency (the relationships among ability of binding to DNA, cytotoxic effects in vitro and potency
in vivo have been already discussed (3)),the first important
observation is that antitumor effectiveness of anthracyclines
can be different, depending on the molecule and on the type
of tumors investigated. In fact, 4'-epiDX shows the same spectrum of antitumor effectiveness as DX; 4-dmDNR is particularly
active against disseminated leukemias; and 4'-deoxyDX is selectively less active than DX against melanoma B16 and more
active than DX against colon tumors. The reasons for these
differences are not yet understood. It does not seem that
variations in drug uptake by tumor cells can completely explain these properties, even if high uptake and particularly
high retention by the tumor cells can be of importance for
the activity against resistant tumors. The balance of effects
of the drug against tumor cells, normal cells and host immune
systems is probably conditioning the final therapeutic result;
and we still do not have a clear comprehension of how this
balance works for DNR and DX, which have been investigated
for a long time. We can only say, at this point, that the
experimental studies have been in some way predictive of the
antitumor activity in humans: DNR is definitely less active

than DX against solid tumors in mice and in parallel it is less active in humans. However, the high antitumor activity of DX against B16 melanoma, and also against some human melanomas transplanted in nude mice (18) is not paralleled by the clinical results. It is therefore of interest to know whether the selective antitumor activity observed in experimental studies with the anthracyclines here described will be observed and confirmed in humans.

The second important observation in that cardiotoxicity can be dissociated from potency and from antitumor activity. Particularly interesting in this regards is 4'-deoxyDX, which is more potent than DX, more active against some solid tumors, and definitely less cardiotoxic.

In our studies (31), we have found a good correlation between pharmacokinetic properties and general and cardiac toxicity of anthracyclines. A relation was found between peak level and AUC (Area Under the Curve) at 48h in the spleen, and general toxicity evaluated as LD_{50} i.v. As pointed out previously, such a relation seems to be present also in humans, at least for 4'-epiDX, which in patients is better tolerated than DX and is eliminated more rapidly than DX (38).

In our studies (31) the extent of cardiotoxicity evaluated in mice treated chronically correlated well with the AUC in the heart at 48 h (31). It is not yet clear whether cardiac toxicity and antitumor activity of anthracyclines are effects sustained by the same mechanism of action, as pointed out in a recent review by Di Marco (61).

The different pharmacokinetic properties of the anthracyclines here considered can very well be accompanied by different ability to interfere with subcellular components in addition to DNA, such as cellular chromatin, mitochondria, cell membrane, etc. The availability of compounds, such as the three new anthracyclines here described, showing profound differences compared to DX, is very interesting in this respect, and stimulates further investigation in experimental systems as well as in patients.

REFERENCES

1. Di Marco A, Gaetani M, Dorigotti L, Soldati M, Bellini O. 1963. Tumori, 49, 203.
2. Casazza AM. 1979. Cancer Treat. Rep. 63, 835.
3. Arcamone F, Casazza AM, Cassinelli G, Di Marco A, Penco S. Symposium on Anthracycline Antibiotics in Cancer Therapy, New York, September 16-18, 1981.
4. Sandberg JS, Howsden FL, Di Marco A, Goldin A. 1970. Cancer Chemother. Rep., 54, 1.

5. Kitaura K, Watanabe Y. 1972. Jap. J. Antib., $\underline{25}$, 65.
6. Di Marco A, Casazza AM, Giuliani F, Pratesi G, Arcamone F, Bernardi L, Franchi G, Giardino P, Patelli B, Penco S. 1978. Cancer Treat. Rep., $\underline{62}$, 375.
7. Schwartz HS, Grindey GB. 1973. Cancer Res., $\underline{33}$, 1837.
8. Goldin A. 1978. Rec. Res. Cancer Res., $\underline{63}$, 99.
9. Di Marco A, Gaetani M, Scarpinato BM. 1969. Cancer Chemother. Rep., $\underline{53}$, 33.
10. Di Marco A, Casazza AM, Dasdia T, Giuliani F, Lenaz L, Necco A, Soranzo C. 1973. Cancer Chemother. Rep., $\underline{57}$, 269.
11. Di Marco A, Lenaz L, Casazza AM, Scarpinato BM. 1972. Cancer Chemother. Rep., $\underline{56}$, 153.
12. Casazza AM, Di Marco A, Di Cuonzo G. 1971. Cancer Res., $\underline{31}$, 1971.
13. Giuliani F, Di Marco A, Casazza AM, Savi G. 1979. Europ. J. Cancer, $\underline{15}$, 715.
14. Savi G, Casazza AM. 1981. 12th Int. Congress Chemother., Florence, July 19-24, 1981, Abstracts, 258.
15. Casazza AM, Isetta AM, Giuliani F, Di Marco A. 1975. Adriamycin Review. European Press Medikon, Ghent, Belgium, 123.
16. Vecchi A, Mantovani A, Tagliabue A, Spreafico F. 1976. Cancer Res., $\underline{36}$, 1222.
17. Ehrke MJ, Cohen SA, Mihich E. 1978. Cancer Res., $\underline{38}$, 521.
18. Giuliani FC, Zirvi KA, Kaplan NO. 1981. Cancer Res., $\underline{41}$, 325.
19. Di Fronzo G, Gambetta RA, Lenaz L. 1971. Eur. J. Clin. Biol. Res., $\underline{16}$, 572.
20. Meriwether WD, Bachur NR. 1972. Cancer Res., $\underline{32}$, 1137.
21. Noel G, Trouet A, Zenebergh A, Tulkens P. 1975. Adriamycin Review. European Press Medikon, Ghent, Belgium, 99.
22. Giuliani F, Casazza AM, Di Marco A, Savi G. 1981. Cancer Treat. Rep., $\underline{65}$, 267.
23. Arcamone F, Penco S, Vigevani A, Redaelli S, Franchi G, Di Marco A, Casazza AM, Dasdia T, Formelli F, Necco A, Soranzo C. 1975. J Med. Chem., $\underline{18}$, 703.
24. Casazza AM, Di Marco A, Bertazzoli C, Formelli F, Giuliani F, Pratesi G. 1978. Current Chemotherapy. Am. Soc. Microbiology, Washington, 1257.
25. Giuliani F, Bellini O, Casazza AM, Formelli F, Savi G, Di Marco A. 1978. Europ. J. Cancer, $\underline{14}$, 555.
26. Johnson RK, Chitnis MP, Embrey WM, Gregory EB. 1978. Cancer Treat. Rep., $\underline{62}$, 1535.
27. Giuliani FC, Kaplan NO. 1980. Cancer Res., $\underline{40}$, 4682.
28. Di Marco A, Casazza AM, Gambetta R, Supino R, Zunino F. 1976. Cancer Res., $\underline{36}$, 1962.

29. Di Marco A, Casazza AM, Dasdia T, Necco A, Pratesi G, Rivolta P, Velcich A, Zaccara A, Zunino F. 1977. Chem. Biol. Interactions, 19, 291.

30. Arcamone F, Di Marco A, Casazza AM. 1978. Adv. Cancer Chemother. Japan Sci. Soc. Press, Tokyo and University Park Press, Baltimore, 297.

31. Formelli F, Casazza AM. 1981. 12th Int. Congress Chemother., Florence, July 19-24, 1981, Abstracts, 114.

32. Broggini M, Colombo T, Martini A, Donelli MG. 1980. Cancer Treat. Rep., 64, 897.

33. Casazza AM, Di Marco A, Bonadonna G, Bonfante V, Bertazzoli C, Bellini O, Pratesi G, Sala L, Ballerini L. 1980. Anthracyclines: current status and new developments. New York, Academic Press, 403.

34. Villani F, Favalli L, Piccinini F. 1980. Tumori, 66, 689.

35. Isetta AM, Trizio D. 1981. 12th Int. Congress Chemother., Florence, July 19-24, 1981, Abstracts, 115.

36. Robustelli della Cuna G, Pavesi L, Cuzzoni Q, Ganzina F, Tramarin R. 1981. 12th Int. Congress Chemother, Florence, July 19-24, 1981, Abstracts, 75.

37. Bonfante V, Villani F., Bonadonna G. Cancer Chemother. Pharmacol. (submitted).

38. Natale M, Brambilla M, Lucchini S, Martini A, Moro E, Pacciarini MA, Tamassia V, Vago G, Trabattoni A. 1981. 12th Int. Congress Chemother., Florence, July 19-24, 1981, Abstracts, 114.

39. Hourteloup and the Clinical Screening Cooperative Group of EORTC. 1981. 12th Int. Congress Chemother., Florence, July 19-24, 1981, Abstracts, 115.

40. Arcamone F, Bernardi L, Giardino P, Patelli B, Di Marco A, Casazza AM, Pratesi G, Reggiani P. 1976. Cancer Treat. Rep., 60, 829.

41. Di Marco A, Casazza AM, Pratesi G. 1977. Cancer Treat. Rep., 61, 893.

42. Casazza AM, Pratesi G, Giuliani F, Di Marco A. 1980. Tumori, 66, 549.

43. Supino R, Necco A, Dasdia T, Casazza AM, Di Marco A. 1977. Cancer Res., 37, 4523.

44. Formelli F, Casazza AM, Di Marco A, Mariani A, Pollini C. 1979. Cancer Chemother. Pharmacol., 3, 261.

45. Egorin MJ, Clawson RE, Cohen JL, Ross LA, Bachur NR. 1980. Cancer Res., 40, 4669.

46. Marquardt H, Philips FS, Marquardt H, Sternberg SS. 1979. Proc. Am. Ass. Cancer Res., 20, 45.

47. Kanter PM, Schwartz HS. 1979. Cancer Res., 39, 3661.

48. Lenaz L, Di Marco A. 1976. Cancer Chemother. Rep., 60, 99.

49. Bottiroli G, Prosperi E, Dasdia T. 1981. Basic Appl. Histochem., 25 (Suppl.), 43.
50. Geroni C, Casazza AM. Unpublished data.
51. Skipper HE, Schabel FM, Lloyd HL. 1979. Adv. Cancer Chemother., 1, 205.
52. Arcamone F, Penco S, Redaelli S. 1976. J. Med. Chem., 19, 1424.
53. Casazza AM, Bellini O, Savi G, Di Marco A. 1981. Proc.. Am. Ass. Cancer Res.; 22, 267.
54. Giuliani FC, Zirvi KA, Kaplan NO, Goldin A. 1981. Int. J. Cancer, 27, 5.
55. Savi G., Casazza AM, Giuliani F. 1981. Tumori (Suppl.), 67, 183.
56. Casazza AM, Savi G, Pratesi G. 1981. 12th Int. Congress Chemother., Florence, July 19-24, 1981, Abstracts, 73.
57. Giuliani FC, Coirin AK, Rice MR, Kaplan NO. Cancer Treat. Rep. (in press).
58. Formelli F, Fumagalli A, Giuliani F, Casazza AM, Kaplan NO. 1981. Proc. Am. Ass. Cancer Res., 22, 267.
59. Formelli F, Pollini C, Casazza AM, Di Marco A, Mariani A. 1981. Cancer Chemother. Pharmacol., 5, 139.
60. Salmon SE, Liu RM, Casazza AM. Cancer Chemother. Pharmacol. (in press).
61. Di Marco A. 1980. Chemiot. Oncol. 4, 5.

ANTHRACYCLINE ANTITUMOR ANTIBIOTICS: THEIR CARCINOGENICITY AND
THEIR MUTAGENICITY

J. WESTENDORF, HILDEGARD MARQUARDT, AND HANS MARQUARDT*

1. INTRODUCTION

The long-term toxicity of antitumor agents, i.e., their oncogenicity and their mutagenicity, is a subject of growing concern because
of the increased survival of cancer patients which modern chemotherapy
has made possible. It has been one of the intriguing results of
cancer research that many active antineoplastic agents have been
found to be carcinogenic. It is now well established that many
antitumor substances are oncogenic in cells in culture (1) and in
laboratory animals (2, 3); and, from observations in patients being
given such compounds for nonmalignant diseases and after transplantation surgery as well as from the occurrence of second neoplasms
after chemotherapy of a primary neoplasm, it can be suspected that
many are also carcinogenic in man (4). This report attempts to
consolidate the available data on the genotoxic effects of one
important class of antitumor agents, i.e., the anthracycline
antibiotics.

2. ADRIAMYCIN AND DAUNOMYCIN

2.1. Oncogenicity

Both adriamycin and daunomycin have been shown to induce mammary
carcinomas amd mammary fibroadenomas in female and male Sprague-Dawley
rats after single i.v. doses (5-9). The mammary-tumorigenic activity
of both agents compares well with that of irradiation (10) and of
the potent polycyclic aromatic hydrocarbon 7,12-dimethylbenz(a)anthracene

*Direct correspondence to this author.

(11). In one report renal tumors, too, were observed following a single i.v. administration of daunomycin (6). In addition, in vitro studies demonstrated the high potential of
adriamycin and daunomycin to induce malignant transformation
of fibroblastic cells in culture (8, 12). It is noteworthy
that actinomycin D, which exhibits strong binding interac -
tions with DNA of an intercalative nature similar to those
of the anthracyclines, shows only limited tumorigenicity and
minimal transformation capacity (8).

Since it is known that antioxidant radical-scavengers
can prevent adriamycin-induced cardiotoxicity (13), we attempted to also inhibit anthracycline-induced oncogenicity
by such treatment (14). However, a dose-regimen of cysteamine
which resulted in suppression of the oncogenic effects of the
polycyclic aromatic hydrocarbon, 7,12-dimethylbenz(a)anthra-
cene (15), did neither affect adriamycin-induced mammary
tumorigenesis nor malignant transformation caused by the
antibiotic (Tables 1 and 2).

Table 1.   Effect of cysteamine-HCl on adriamycin-induced
            mammary tumorigenesis in female Sprague-Dawley
            rats

Cysteamine-HCl[a]	Adriamycin, i.v. (mg/kg)	Rats with mammary tumors
-	0	5/18
-	5	21/30
+	0	5/16
+	5	22/29

[a] Experimental conditions and treatment with cysteamine-HCl
   as in reference no. 15.

Table 2. Effect of cysteamine-HCl on adriamycin-induced ma-
          lignant transformation of mouse M2 fibroblasts

Cysteamine-HCl[a]	Adriamycin (μg/ml)	Plating Efficiency (%)	No.of transformed foci per no. of dishes treated
-	0	29	0/12
-	0.001	25	8/12
-	0.005	19	13/11
-	0.01	8	20/12
+	0	28	0/12
+	0.001	26	7/11
+	0.005	19	13/12
+	0.01	9	17/18

[a] Experimental conditions and treatment with cysteamine-HCl
    as in reference no. 15.

2.2. DNA Interaction

The physico-chemical characteristics of the anthra -
cycline-DNA complex, the biological consequences of the
anthracycline-DNA interaction as well as free radical damage
caused by anthracyclines will be discussed in other chapters
of this volume. We will limit our discussion here to those
aspects of the anthracycline-DNA interaction relevant to
carcinogenesis, i.e., particularly to the question of a
covalent anthracycline-DNA interaction and to some results
of DNA repair studies.

It is now generally accepted that the ultimate forms of
chemical carcinogens - often following metabolic activation -
are strong electrophilic reactants which interact covalently
with nucleophilic cellular macromolecules, i.e., DNA, RNA and
proteins (16). In the case of carcinogenic anthracyclines,
however, there is as yet no evidence for such a covalent
interaction with DNA. The anthracyclines may thus be carcinogenic through tight non-covalent binding (16). In agreement
with this suggestion, our preliminary data suggest that
adriamycin is merely detoxified by microsomal metabolism and
that its intercalation into DNA without covalent interactions
may initiate oncogenesis (17). Adriamycin binds to DNA, presumably by intercalation (18),it can be removed from DNA by

extraction of the complex with water-saturated phenol (19). Our results show that, in a test-tube assay, addition of rat liver microsomes will reduce this non-covalent interaction between the agent and DNA (Tables 3 and 4).

Table 3. Effect of postmitochondrial cell fraction on the adriamycin-DNA interaction

Adriamycin	nmoles ^{3}H-adriamycin[a]/mg DNA after incubation[b] (min)			
	5	15	30	60
50	29	35		49
100	51	64		81
200	00	108	123	155
200+heat-inact. S9[c]		112	121	151
200+active S9		117	94	26

[a] ^{3}H-adriamycin (sp.act., 13.8 µCi/µmole), gift of Dr. F. Arcamone, Farmitalia - Carlo Erba, Italy.

[b] 4 mg calf thymus DNA/6 ml incubation mixture.

[c] S9, postmitochondrial cell fraction from rat liver (5 mg protein/ml incubation mixture) prepared according to reference no. 20.

Table 4. Effect of purified microsomes on the adriamycin-DNA interaction

Adriamycin (µg/ml)	nmoles ^{3}H-adriamycin[a]/mg DNA after incubation[b] (min)		
	5	60	300
100+heat-inact. microsomes	44,46,65	59,59,77	50,54,81
100+microsomes without cofactors	42,52	49,66	58
100+active microsomes			
0.6 mg protein/ml	53,55	31,33	19,21
1.2 mg protein/ml	48,52,66	21,23,33	1,4,17
2.4 mg protein/ml	49	25	16

[a] ^{3}H-adriamycin (sp.act., 13.8 µCi/µmole), gift of Dr. F. Arcamone, Farmitalia - Carlo Erba, Italy.

[b] 4 mg calf thymus DNA/6 ml incubation mixture.

[c] Purified microsomes prepared according to reference no. 21.

In in vitro short-term tests, adriamycin induces frame-shift mutants in Salmonella typhimurium TA98 (see below) and malignant transformation in mouse M2 fibroblasts (see above). Addition of rat liver postmitochondrial cell fraction to the bacterial assay (Table 5) and induction of microsomal enzyme activity by 2,5-diphenyloxazole in M2 cells (Table 6) decreases these biological effects. Conversely, inhibition of microsomal enzyme activity in M2 cells by α-naphthoflavone or SKF-525A increases the yield of drug-induced transfor - mations (Table 6). These results await further confirmation, particularly in view of the observation that photoirradiation of the daunomycin-DNA complex generates a firm linkage between daunomycin and DNA (19). It should also be noted that irreversible binding of adriamycin to protein following microsomal activation has been reported (22).

Table 5. Effect of postmitochondrial cell fraction on adriamycin-induced mutagenesis. Ames Assay with Salmonella typhimurium (TA98)

Adriamycin (μg/plate)	$His^+/10^6$ Survivors	
	without S9	with S9
0	1.6	0.5
0.2	1.6	1.4
2	5.7	1.3
10	24.2	5.3
20	65.4	14.9
30	122.5	26.7
40	272.3	119.0

Procedures according to reference no. 20. (S9 from aroclor-induced rat liver, 400 μg protein/plate.) Each result is a composite of those from two separate experiments.

Table 6. Effect of inducers and inhibitors of microsomal enzyme activity on adriamycin-induced cytotoxicity and malignant transformation in mouse M2 fibroblasts

Pretreatment	Plat.Eff. (%) after Adriamycin (μg/ml)				Transf. Foci/No. Dishes after Adriamycin (μg/ml)			
	0	0.001	0.005	0.01	0	0.001	0.005	0.01
None	23	18	14	8	0/12	6/12	12/12	8/12
PPO (2.5 μg/ml)	22	23	21	19	0/12	0/12	3/12	1/12
ANF (1.5 μg/ml)	23	12	9	1	0/12	21/12	17/12	-
SKF-525A (10 μg/ml)	19	18	4	0	0/12	11/12	26/12	-

Inducer: PPO (2,5-diphenyloxazole) was present in cultures only during 24 hr preceding adriamycin treatment. Inhibitors, SKF-525A and ANF (α-naphthoflavone) were present during that time and during the 24 hr period of adriamycin treatment.

As a consequence of their interactions with DNA and chromosomes, chemical carcinogens usually cause DNA damage, such as single- and double strand breaks and chromosomal aberrations, and DNA repair. For the anthracyclines these effects will be reviewed in other chapters of this volume. In general, adriamycin and daunomycin, too, have been reported to induce DNA damage (23, 24, 25) and cyto-genetic toxicity including sister chromatid exchanges (23, 26). In contrast, it seems that the activity of adriamycin to induce DNA repair processes is limited (27, 28). Our own preliminary results (unpublished) also show that adriamycin and daunomycin are weakly active in inducing unscheduled DNA synthesis in primary Sprague-Dawley rat liver cells in vitro (29) but are strong inhibitors of DNA repair induced by N-methyl-N'-nitro-N-nitrosoguanidine.

2.3. Mutagenicity

Adriamycin and daunomycin are clearly mutagenic in bacterial and mammalian cell assays. Adriamycin and dauno-mycin were shown to be active mutagens (without microsomal activation) in Salmonella typhimurium (30, 31, 32). In Saccharomyces cerevisiae, however, daunomycin though re-combinogenic was not mutagenic (33). In agreement with the findings with Salmonella typh., both, adriamycin and dauno-mycin are potent mutagens in a mammalian cell mutagenesis assay employing V79 Chinese hamster cells (8). In this assay, both antibiotics were as active as the standard mutagen, N-methyl-N'-nitro-N-nitrosoguanidine.

3. DERIVATIVES OF ADRIAMYCIN AND DAUNOMYCIN

3.1. 4-Demethoxydaunomycin

4-Demethoxydaunomycin is a new analog of daunomycin with higher antitumor activity than the parent compound (34). Our results demonstrate that 4-demethoxydaunomycin is a potent carcinogen: After single i.v. administration, the agent was at least as active at inducing mammary tumors in female Sprague-Dawley rats as adriamycin or daunomycin (35,Table 7).

Table 7.   Induction of mammary tumors in female Sprague-
Dawley rats by 4-demethoxydaunomycin

Treatment[a]	Rats with tumors[b]		
	Mammary fibroadenomas	Mammary adenocarcinomas	Other tumors
Control	1	0	0
Adriamycin 5 mg/kg	14	3	3
4-Demethoxy-daunomycin 1.8 mg/kg	5	10	0

[a] Compounds, gift of Dr. F. Arcamone, Farmitalia - Carlo Erba, Italy.
Single i.v. injections of equally toxic doses.
[b] Observation period, one year. 20 rats per group.

The agent was shown to intercalate into DNA with an
affinity equivalent to that of daunomycin (36). As our
studies show, the agent is also a mutagen in a bacterial
mutagenesis assay with the strain TA98 of Salmonella typhimurium (Table 8).

Table 8.   Mutagenic activity of 4-demethoxydaunomycin with
strain TA98 of Salmonella typhimurium

Compound	Concentration (μg/plate)	Relative Survivors(%) -S9	+S9	His$^+$Revertants/10^6Surv. -S9	+S9
Control		100	100	1.6	0.5
Adriamycin	0.2	100	100	1.6	1.5
	2.0	100	100	5.7	1.3
	20.0	78	91	65.4	14.9
4-Demethoxy-daunomycin	0.2	100	100	2.5	1.9
	2.0	100	100	7.6	7.5
	20.0	75	82	27.0	27.0

Procedures according to reference no. 20. Compounds, gift of
Dr. F. Arcamone, Farmitalia - Carlo Erba, Italy.

   With this compound the _in vitro_ short-term tests employing mammalian cells are clearly not correlated to the _in vivo_
carcinogenicity and the mutagenicity in bacteria described
above: Our findings show that 4-demethoxydaunomycin is devoid of mutagenic activity in V79 Chinese hamster cells
(Table 9) and devoid of transforming activity in M2 mouse
fibroblasts (Table 10). It is noteworthy that the agent,
though non-mutagenic in V79 cells, did induce sister chromatid exchanges· in these cells (35).

Table 9.   Induction of mutagenesis in V79 Chinese hamster
           cells by 4-demethoxydaunomycin

Compound	Concentration (µg/ml)	Plating Efficiency (%)	8-Azaguanine-resistant colonies/10^5 Survivors
Control		93	4.8
N-methyl-N'-nitro-N-nitro-soguanidine	0.5	26	305.2
Adriamycin	0.01	56	53.7
	0.05	28	195.7
Daunomycin	0.01	61	90.7
	0.05	23	282.6
4-Demethoxy-daunomycin	0.001	77	4.8
	0.005	44	13.3
	0.01	13	4.1
	0.02	9	5.3

Procedures according to reference no. 8. Expression time,
48 hrs. (which was found to be optimal). Compounds, gift of
Dr. F. Arcamone, Farmitalia - Carlo Erba, Italy.

Table 10.   Induction of malignant transformation in M2 mouse
fibroblasts by 4-demethoxydaunomycin

Compound	Concentration (μg/ml)	Plating Efficiency (%)	Transformed Foci per	
			#treat.dishes	10^3 Surviv.
Control		46	0/9	0
N-methyl-N'-nitro-N-nitro-soguanidine	0.5	29	9/8	3.9
Adriamycin	0.001	35	5/12	1.2
	0.005	26	13/12	4.2
Daunomycin	0.001	37	6/8	2.0
	0.005	25	8/8	4.0
4-Demethoxy-daunomycin	0.0001	39	0/6	0
	0.0005	35	0/11	0
	0.001	30	0/12	0
	0.005	7	2/12	0.24

Procedures according to reference no. 8. Compounds, gift of
Dr. F. Arcamone, Farmitalia - Carlo Erba, Italy.

3.2. Other Analogs

The available data on the oncogenicity/mutagenicity of
various other analogs of adriamycin and daunomycin are
scarce, indeed. Our own results with compounds supplied by
Dr. F. Arcamone, Farmitalia - Carlo Erba, Italy are summarized in Table 11.

It appears from these data that antitumor activity and at
least mutagenicity with adriamycin, daunomycin and their
derivatives are closely related biological parameters.

Table 11. Mutagenicity of anthracycline derivatives

Compound[a]	Antitumor activity[b]	Mutagenicity in Salm.typh.(TA98)	V79 Chinese hamster cells
Daunomycin	+	+	+
Adriamycin	+	+	+
1'-epi-adria-mycin	-	-	-
4-demethoxy-7(R)9(R) (1'S) daunomycin	-	-	-
4'-epi-adria-mycin	+	+	+
4-demethoxy-adriamycin	+	+	+
3',4'-di-epi-4'-O-methyl-daunomycin	-(+)	-[c]	-
3',4'-di-epi-4'-O-methyl-adriamycin	+	+[c]	+

[a] Compounds, gift of Dr. F. Arcamone, Farmitalia - Carlo Erba, Italy.

[b] Dr. F. Arcamone and Dr. A.M. Casazza, Farmitalia - Carlo Erba, Italy.

[c] Previously seen (unpublished) by Dr. I. de Carneri, Farmitalia - Carlo Erba, Italy.

4.   OTHER ANTHRACYCLINE ANTITUMOR ANTIBIOTICS

4.1. 5-Iminodaunomycin

5-Iminodaunomycin is a quinone-modified anthracycline analog with retained antitumor activity but with reduced cardiotoxicity (37). Though found non-mutagenic in strain TA98 of Salmonella typh. (37), our data show that this agent is a potent mutagen in V79 Chinese hamster cells (Table 12).

Table 12.   Mutagenicity of 5-iminodaunomycin in V79 Chinese
            hamster cells

Compound	Concentration (µg/ml)	Relative Survival (%)	8-Azaguanine-resistant colonies per 10^5 surv.
Control		100	8.5
N-methyl-N'-nitro-N-nitro-soguanidine	0.2	57	82.8
	0.4	48	126.7
5-Iminodauno-mycin	0.001	100	7.5
	0.005	100	8.4
	0.01	100	15.3
	0.05	100	40.7
	0.1	57	90.3
	0.5	0	-

Compound, gift of Dr. H.B. Wood jr., NCI (US PHS). Procedures
according to reference no. 8.

4.2. 7-con-O-Methylnogarol

7-con-O-Methylnogarol is an anthracycline with good
antitumor activity but with reduced affinity for DNA binding
(38). Our results, however, show that the agent is,neverthe-
less, a potent mutagen in V79 Chinese hamster cells
(Table 13).

Table 13.   Mutagenicity of 7-con-O-methylnogarol in V79
            Chinese hamster cells

Compound	Concentration (µg/ml)	Relative Survival (%)	8-Azaguanine resistant colonies per 10^5 surv.
Control		100	1.1
N-methyl-N'-nitro-N-nitro-soguanidine	0.4	46	206.7
7-con-O-Methylnogarol	0.01	76	20.2
	0.03	54	32.2
	0.05	49	62.7
	0.08	35	101.1
	0.1	30	158.5

Compound, gift of Dr. J.P. McGovren, Upjohn Company, Kalamazoo, Mi., USA. Procedures according to reference no. 8.

4.3. Carminomycin

Carminomycin is an anthracycline analog which differs from daunomycin by the absence of a methoxy-group at C_4. The antibiotic is at least as active as an antitumor agent as daunomycin (39). In our studies with Salmonella typh. the agent (gift of Dr. L. Lenaz, International Div. of Bristol Myers Co., New York, N.Y., USA)proved to be mutagenic in strains TA98 and TA100 of Salmonella typh. with and without addition of rat liver S9.

4.4. Marcellomycin

Marcellomycin is a new anthracycline antitumor antibiotic. We found this agent to be non-mutagenic in strains TA98 and TA100 of Salmonella typh. with and without addition of rat liver S9 (Table 14).

Table 14. Mutagenic activity of marcellomycin in Salmonella typhimurium

Bacteria	Compound	Concentration (µg/plate)	Relat.Surv.(%) -S9	+S9	His+-Revert./Plate -S9	+S9
TA98	Control		100	100	17	23
	Marcellomycin	1	100	100	16	28
		20	55	100	20	15
		40	42	75	14	19
		80	29	68	13	20
		100	2	66	2	27
	Aminofluorene	250	92	78	325	813
TA100	Control		100	100	124	118
	Marcellomycin	20	32	60	84	90
		40	13	51	75	89
		80	2	42	26	74
	N-methyl-N'-nitro-N-nitro-soguanidine	2	67	–	>1,000	–

Procedures according to reference no. 20. Marcellomycin, gift of Dr. L. Lenaz, International Div., Bristol Myers Co., New York, N.Y., USA.

4.5. Aclacinomycin A

Aclacinomycin A is composed of the aklavinone aglycone
linked via glycosidic bondage to a triglycoside. The agent
possesses potent antitumor activity and, compared to adriamycin, minimal cardiotoxicity (40, 41, 42). Similar to
actinomycin D, aclacinomycin A inhibits RNA synthesis at
about 10-fold lower concentrations than those required to
inhibit DNA synthesis (42). In contrast, adriamycin and
daunomycin inhibit DNA and RNA synthesis at approximately
equal concentrations (42). It is striking to note that these
biochemical effects are reflected in the oncogenicity of the
agents. While adriamycin and daunomycin are potent oncogens
and mutagens (see above), the tumorigenicity of actinomycin D
in vivo is limited and its capacity to induce malignant
transformation and mutations in mammalian cells in vitro is
minimal (8). Likewise, aclacinomycin A proved to be devoid
of mutagenic activity in Salmonella typh. (41, 43, own unpublished results) and in V79 Chinese hamster cells in vitro
(Table 15).

Table 15. Mutagenicity of aclacinomycin A in V79 Chinese
hamster cells

Compound	Concentration (µg/ml)	Relative Survival (%)	8-Azaguanine-resistant colonies per 10^5 survivors
Control		100	3.0
N-methyl-N'-nitro-N-nitro-soguanidine	0.2	57	214.7
Aclacino-mycin A	0.05	100	1.6
	0.1	78	7.4
	0.5	21	5.9
	1.0	0	0

Compound, gift of Dr. T.Oki, Sanraku-Ocean Co., Ltd.,
Fujisawa, Japan. Procedures according to reference no. 8.

5. CONCLUSIONS

The existing data demonstrate the high oncogenic potential of most of the anthracycline antitumor antibiotics. Such results suggest that patients treated with these substances should be closely monitored in anticipation of the possible appearance of newly induced tumors and that the drugs should be restricted to the therapy of diseases with poor prognosis.

The mechanisms of action by which anthracyclines elicit their oncogenic effects are unknown. Though it is not established that DNA is the critical target in chemical carcinogenesis (44), the findings with anthracyclines, too, point toward DNA as the initial cellular target of chemical carcinogens. It is now generally believed that, in their ultimate state, carcinogens or their metabolically activated derivatives are chemically reactive electrophilic substances that react covalently with nucleophilic macromolecules, i.e., DNA (16). In contrast, from the available data it can be concluded that the anthracyclines are carcinogenic through a tight non-covalent interaction with DNA.

Naturally, generalizations on structure-activity relationships are biologically most interesting. However, in spite of the several hundred anthracycline analogs produced so far, such generalizations have been slow to develop. With regard to oncogenicity/mutagenicity the most interesting such relationship involves the number of sugars present in the glycosidic side chain. Class I anthracyclines with a single sugar, such as adriamycin and daunomycin, inhibit RNA synthesis at nearly the same concentrations required to inhibit DNA synthesis. Antitumor antibiotics of this type are highly oncogenic and mutagenic. On the other hand, class II anthracyclines with multiple sugars, such as marcellomycin and aclacinomycin, behave like actinomycin D and inhibit RNA synthesis at lower concentrations than is required to inhibit DNA synthesis. These RNA-selective anthracyclines, as

well as actinomycin D, apparently, are devoid of mutagenic
activity. It will be most interesting to study their oncogenic potential in vivo and in vitro. Another group of interest are the N-alkylated anthracyclines. It has been noted
that N-alkylation converts class I anthracyclines into RNA
selective agents with properties similar to class II agents
(45). One such agent, dibenzyl-daunomycin, is a potent antitumor agent which reportedly does not bind to DNA and is non-
mutagenic (45). However, these very preliminary findings
urgently await confirmation.

Finally, the data with actinomycin D, adriamycin and
daunomycin also demonstrate a satisfactory correlation between in vivo tumorigenicity and in vitro assays for malignant transformation and mutagenesis. This correlation supports the use of the in vitro tests as rapid screening assays for carcinogenic potential which are advantageous, for
instance, in developing derivatives with antitumor activity
but with reduced oncogenic potential. However, as documented
by the results with 4-demethoxydaunomycin, in certain instances poor correlations must be anticipated between in
vivo tumorigenicity and activity in in vitro short-term tests
as well as among different short-term tests. This conclusion
necessitates the use of a battery of short-term tests to
detect the potential for carcinogenicity of chemicals.

REFERENCES

1. Marquardt H and Marquardt H. 1977. Induction of malignant
   transformation and mutagenesis in cell cultures by cancer
   chemotherapeutic agents. Cancer, 40 : 1930-1934.

2. Sieber SM and Adamson RH. 1975. The clastogenic, mutagenic, teratogenic and carcinogenic effects of various
   antineoplastic agents. In "Pharmacological Basis of
   Cancer Chemotherapy", Williams and Wilkins Publ., Baltimore, pp. 401-468.

3. Sieber SM and Adamson RH. 1975. Toxicity of antineoplastic agents in man: Chromosomal aberrations, anti-
   fertility effects, congenital malformations and carcinogenic potential. Adv. Cancer Res., 22 : 57-155.

4. Weisburger JH, Griswold jr. DP, Prejean JD, Casey AE,
   Wood jr HB,and Weisburger EK. 1975. The carcinogenic
   properties of some of the principal drugs used in clinical cancer chemotherapy. Recent Results Cancer Res., 52 :
   1-17.

5. Bertazzoli C, Chieli T,and Solcia E. 1971. Different
   incidence of breast carcinomas or fibroadenomas in daunomycin or adriamycin treated rats. Experienta, 27 : 1209-
   1210.

6. Sternberg SS, Philips FS, and Cronin AP. 1972. Renal
   tumors and other lesions following a single intravenous
   injection of daunomycin. Cancer Res., 32 : 1029-1036.

7. Philips FS, Gilladoga A, Marquardt H, Sternberg SS, and
   Vidal PM. 1975. Some observations on the toxicity of
   adriamycin. Cancer Chemotherap. Rep. Part 3, 6 : 177-181.

8. Marquardt H, Philips FS, and Sternberg SS. 1976. Tumorigenicity in vivo and induction of malignant transformation and mutagenesis in cell cultures by adriamycin and
   daunomycin. Cancer Res., 36 : 2065-2069.

9. Bucciarelli E. 1981. Mammary tumor induction in male and
   female Sprague-Dawley rats by adriamycin and daunomycin.
   J. Natl. Cancer Inst., 66 : 81-84.

10. Shellabarger CJ, Bond VP, and Cronkite EP. 1960. Studies
    on radiation-induced mammary gland neoplasia in the rat.
    Rad. Res., 13 : 242-249.

11. Philips FS and Sternberg SS. 1975. Tests for tumor induc-
    tion by antitumor agents. Recent Results Cancer Res., 52:
    29-35.

12. Price PJ, Su WA, Skeen PC, Chirigos MA, and Huebner RJ.
    1975. Transforming potential of the anticancer drug
    adriamycin. Science, 187 : 1200-1201.

13. Bertazzoli C, Sala L, Solicia E, and Ghione M. 1975.
    Experimental adriamycin cardiotoxicity prevented by
    ubiquinone in vivo in rabbits. IRCS Med. Science,3 : 468.

14. Notman J, Marquardt H, and Zedeck MS. 1980. Cardiac
    effects and tumor induction in rats receiving a single
    injection of adriamycin with and without treatment with
    cysteamine. Proc.Amer.Assoc.Cancer Res., 21 : 309.

15. Marquardt H, Sapozink MD, and Zedeck MS. 1974. Inhibition
    by cysteamine-HCl of oncogenesis induced by 7,12-dimethyl-
    benz(a)anthracene without affecting toxicity. Cancer Res.,
    34 : 3387-3390.

16. Miller EC. 1978. Some current perspectives on chemical
    carcinogenesis in humans and experimental animals:
    Presidential address. Cancer Res., 38 : 1479-1496.

17. Marquardt H, Baker S, Grab D, and Marquardt H. 1977.
    Oncogenic and mutagenic activity of adriamycin decreased
    by microsomal metabolism. Proc.Amer.Assoc.Cancer Res.,
    18 : 13.

18. DiMarco A and Arcamone F. 1975. DNA-complexing anti-
    biotics: Daunomycin, adriamycin and their derivatives.
    Arzneimittelforsch., 25 : 368-375.

19. DiMarco A, Zunino F, Orezzi P,and Gambetta R. 1972.
    Interaction of daunomycin with nucleic acids: Effect of
    photoirradiation of the complex. Experientia, 28 : 327-
    328.

20. Ames BN, McCann J, and Yamasaki E. 1975. Methods for
    detecting carcinogens and mutagens with the Salmonella/
    mammalian microsome mutagenicity test. Mutat. Res., 31 :
    347-364.

21. Scornik OA, Hoagland MB, Pfefferkorn LC, and Bishop EA.
    1967. Inhibition of protein synthesis in rat liver
    microsome fractions. J.Biol.Chem., 242 : 131-139.

22. Ghezzi P, Donelli MG, Pantarotto C, Facchinetti T, and
    Garattini S. 1981. Evidence for covalent binding of
    adriamycin to rat liver microsomal proteins. Biochem.
    Pharmacol., 30 : 175-177.

23. Vig BK. 1977. Genetic toxicology of mitomycin C, actino-
    mycins, daunomycin and adriamycin. Mutat.Res., 49 : 189-
    238.

24. Schwartz HS. 1975. DNA breaks in P-288 tumor cells in
    mice after treatment with daunorubicin and adriamycin.
    Res. Commun.Chem.Pathol.Pharmacol., 10 : 51-64.

25. Lee YC and Byfield JE. 1976. Induction of DNA degrada-
    tion in vivo by adriamycin. J.Natl.Cancer Inst., 57 :
    221-224.

26. Kusyk CJ and Hsu TC. 1976. Adriamycin-induced chromo-
    some damage: Elevated frequencies of isochromatid aber-
    rations in G2 and S phases. Experientia, 32 : 1513-1514.

27. Fialkoff H, Goodman MF, and Seraydarian MW. 1979. Differential effect of adriamycin on DNA replicative and repair synthesis in cultured neonatal rat cardiac cells. Cancer Res., _39_ : 1321-1327.

28. Anderson WA, Moreau PL, and Devoret R. 1980. Induction of prophage λ by daunorubicin and derivatives. Correlation with antineoplastic activity. Mutat. Res., _77_ : 197-208.

29. Montesano R, Bartsch H, and Tomatis L (eds.). 1980. Long-term and short-term screening assays for carcinogens: A critical appraisal. IARC Monographs, Supplement 2, IARC, Lyon; pp. 210-211.

30. Pani B, Monti-Bragadin C, and Samer L. 1975. Effect of excision repair system on antibacterial and mutagenic activity of daunomycin and other intercalating agents in Salmonella typhimurium. Experientia, _31_ : 787-788.

31. Marquardt H. 1978. Chemical oncogenesis: Mammalian cell culture studies. Staub-Reinhaltung der Luft, _38_ : 258-265.

32. Seino Y, Nagao M, Yahagi T, Hoshi A, Kawachi T, and Sugimura T. 1978. Mutagenicity of several classes of antitumor agents to Salmonella typhimurium TA98, TA100, and TA92. Cancer Res., _38_ : 2148-2156.

33. Hannan MA and Nasim A. 1978. Mutagenicity and recombinogenicity of daunomycin in Saccharomyces cerevisiae. Cancer Letters, _5_ : 319-324.

34. DiMarco A, Casazza AM, and Pratesi G. 1977. Antitumor activity of 4-demethoxydaunorubicin administered orally. Cancer Treatment Reports, _61_ : 893-894.

35. Marquardt H, Philips FS, Marquardt H, and Sternberg SS. 1979. Oncogenicity of 4-demethoxydaunomycin: Lack of correlation among in vitro short-term tests and between in vitro and in vivo findings. Proc.Amer.Assoc.Cancer Res., _20_ : 45.

36. Plumbridge TW and Brown JR. 1978. Studies on the mode of interaction of 4'-epi-adriamycin and 4-demethoxydaunomycin with DNA. Biochem.Pharmacol., _27_ : 1881-1882.

37. Tong GL, Henry DW, and Acton EM. 1979. 5-Iminodaunorubicin. Reduced cardiotoxic properties in an antitumor anthracycline. J.med.Chem., _22_ : 34-40.

38. Li LH, Kuentzel SL, Murch LL, Pschigoda LM, and Krueger WC. 1979. Comparative biological and biochemical effects of nogalamycin and its analogs on L1210 leukemia. Cancer Res., _39_ : 4816-4822.

39. Gause GF, Brazhnikova MG, and Shorin VA. 1974. A new antitumor antibiotic, carminomycin. Cancer Chemotherapy Reports (Part 1), 58 : 255-256.

40. Hori S, Shirai M, Hirano S, Oki T, Inui T, Tsukagoshi S, Ishizuka M, Takeuchi T, and Umezawa H. 1977. Antitumor activity of new anthracycline antibiotics, aclacinomycinA and its analogs, and their toxicity. Gann, 68 : 685-690.

41. Oki T, Takeuchi T, Oka S, and Umezawa H. 1980. Current status of Japanese studies with the new anthracycline antibiotic aclacinomycinA. Recent Res. Cancer Res., 74 : 207-216.

42. Oki T, Takeuchi T, Oka S, and Umezawa H. 1981. New anthracycline antibiotic aclacinomycinA: Experimental studies and correlations with clinical trials. Recent Res. Cancer Res., 76 : 21-40.

43. Umezawa K, Sawamura M, Matsushima T, and Sugimura T. 1978. Mutagenicity of aclacinomycinA and daunomycin derivatives. Cancer Res., 38 : 1782-1784.

44. Marquardt H. 1979. DNA - The critical target in chemical carcinogenesis ? In:"Chemical Carcinogens and DNA", Grover PL (ed.), CRC Press, Inc., Boca Raton, Florida; pp 159-179.

45. Tong GL, Wu HY, Smith TH, and Henry DW. 1979. Adriamycin analogs. 3. Synthesis of N-alkylated anthracyclines with enhanced efficacy and reduced cardiotoxicity. J.med.Chem., 22 : 912-918.

THE IMMUNOLOGICAL ACTIVITY OF ANTHRACYCLINES

F. SPREAFICO

1. INTRODUCTION

The aim of this article is to review a series of results
obtained by this group in the past years on the immunological
effects of anthracyclines, centering on the two clinically most
widely used compounds of the group, i.e. Doxorubicin (DX) and its
earlier analog Daunorubicin (DM). An interest in the immunopharmacology of cancer chemotherapeutic agents finds its justification at different levels. In the first place, it is well accepted
that drug-induced immunodepression is an important causative
component of the infectious complications associated with cancer
chemotherapy. Immunological derangements may also play a role
in the higher risk of second malignancies observed in patients
submitted to protracted treatment with cytotoxic compounds (1).
Since host reactivities play a complex, multifaceted role in
the control of neoplastic progression, immunomodulation by cancer
chemotherapeutic agents can also represent a determinant of the
therapeutic effectiveness of these compounds. In this connection,
the term modulation emphasizes the concept that the effects of
anticancer cytotoxic chemicals on the immune apparatus should not
be viewed solely in terms of depression but rather in the light
of a more complex interaction (2). Investigations of such
aspects can thus be of interest not only for obtaining a better
knowledge of the pharmacotoxicological properties of these drugs
and in guiding towards the development of better analogs, but
also in the elucidation of the mode of action of cancer chemotherapeutic agents and thus ultimately, in providing a sounder
basis for their most efficacious employ. In this regard, the
anthracyclines DX and DM can be regarded as useful model compounds

2. HOST REACTIVITY AND ANTHRACYCLINES EFFECTIVENESS

Our original motive in attempting a characterization of the
immunopharmacological profiles of DX and DM was to obtain insight
into the possible mechanism(s) sustaining the higher antineoplastic efficacy of the former agent observed by various groups
in a range of animal models. At that time known differences
in metabolism and pharmacokinetics between the two analogs,
believed to possess analogous molecular modes of action, could
not in our opinion satisfactorily account for this in vivo
differential, the quandary being compounded by the comparable
in vitro cytotoxic capacity of the two chemicals when conditions
simulating their relatively long tissue persistence were employed.
On the other hand, initial results of this group (3-5) had
revealed in rodents differences between DX and DM in their
immunodepressive activity not explainable by differences in
their acute toxicity. For instance, whereas the acute LD_{50} and
the inhibition of bone marrow stem cells were comparable for
both agents in mice, DM was more depressive than DX of T-dependent cell-mediated reactivities, i.e. those believed to be preferentially at play in the resistance to tumor grafts, and of
secondary humoral antibody responses, known to be more T-lympho-
cyte dependent than primary responses. Differences between DX
and DM were also observed in their capacity to interfere with
the response to T-independent stimuli. On such a basis, the
hypothesis was then advanced that quantitative and/or qualitative
differences between these drugs in their interaction with host
reactivity could have been of importance in imparting their
different therapeutic effectiveness. In other words, it was
hypothesized that the higher in vivo activity of DX resulted
from a better capacity of the DX-treated than of the DM-host
to react immunologically against the tumor thus obtaining a
"synergism" between host-dependent neoplasm inhibition and
direct cancer cell killing by the chemical.

Evidence in support of this line of reasoning was obtained
comparing the antineoplastic efficacy of DX and DM, employed
at single optimal doses, in mice transplanted with lymphomas
of different immunogenicity (6). As shown by the representative

data of Fig. 1, the antitumoral effectiveness of DM was not significantly influenced by tumor immunogenicity whereas DX efficacy was obviously dependent on this factor as for instance revealed by the markedly different results seen between the non-immunogenic L1210 Cr subline and the highly immunogenic Ha subline of the same lymphoma. The in vitro sensitivity of these sublines to both drugs was comparable. The antineoplastic effectiveness of DX and DM was also compared in mice whose immune capacity had previously been reduced by procedures such as thymectomy, antilymphocyte serum or treatment with DTIC, which in rodents is a very powerful inhibitor of thymus-dependent re-activities while not significantly affecting natural cell-mediated cytotoxicity (7,8). In analogy with previous initial findings (9), it was found (Table 1) that the therapeutic activity of DM was comparable in normal and immunodepressed hosts. In contrast, the efficacy of DX against immunogenic tumors, but not versus non-immunogenic ones, was significantly reduced in immunodepressed animals. The DTIC-resistance of the L1210 Ha subline gave us the opportunity of additionally exploring the effect on DX activity of immunodepression applied after chemotherapy. Since,

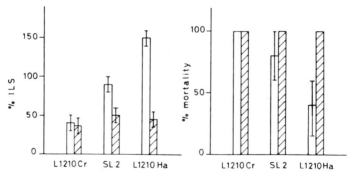

A   **B**

FIGURE 1. Antineoplastic effectiveness of Doxorubicin (A) and Daunorubicin (B) on murine lymphomas of different immunogenicity. Tumor cells (10^5 cells i.p.) were transplanted on day 0 and drugs (10 mg/kg i.v.) injected on day 1. Results are mean of 5 expts. and mortality was evaluated at 120 days. Immunogenicity was assessed in terms of the highest no. of tumor cells specifically rejected by mice inoculated i.p. 10 d. previously with 10^7 x-irradiated lymphoma cells. Values were $<10^2$ cells for L1210 Cr, 10^3 for SL2 lymphoma and 10^5 cells for L1210 Ha leukemia.

Table 1. Antileukemic activity of Doxorubicin (DX) and Daunorubicin (DM) in normal, and DTIC-immunodepressed mice

Exp. group	Day of treatment	L1210 Cr MST	L1210 Cr %LTS	SL2 MST	SL2 %LTS	L1210 Ha MST	L1210 Ha %LTS
Control	-	8.1	0	15.1	0	10.9	0
DTIC	-5	8.7	0	14.6	0	9.8	0
DX	+1	11.5	0	27.5	40#	28.5	60#
DTIC + DX	-5 +1	11.8	0	22.5	0	19.0	0
DM	+1	11.0	0	18.9	0	16.5	0
DTIC + DM	-5 +1	11.4	0	18.6	0	15.5	0

p 0.01

CD2F1 mice were transplanted i.p. on day 0 with 10^5 tumor cells; DX and DM (10 mg/kg) were given i.v.; DTIC (imidazole-4-carboxamide, 5-(3,3-dimethyl-1--triazeno) was given i.p. at 180 mg/kg.

MST = median survival time in days; LTS = long-term (> 120 d) survivors.

in the system employed, DTIC administration as late as 9 days after DX had significantly reduced this drug's effectiveness (Table 2), it can be suggested that in animals eventually cured by DX, a number of tumor cells were not permanently inhibited by the drug but were held in check by host mechanisms. Whether this state of operative "dormancy" is sustained by predominantly cytostatic defense mechanisms, as could be mediated by cytostatically rather than cytolytically active macrophages, or by a true equilibrium between tumor cell multiplication and host-mediated cell lysis is undetermined, although the elucidation of the basic mechanism(s) of such a condition could be of interest at both fundamental and applied levels. The correlation between tumor immunogenicity and DX activity in vivo together with the decrease in effectiveness of this drug in immunologically non-responsive hosts in which the therapeutic advantage of DX over DM can totally disappear, appears, therefore, to support the contention that host reactivity against the tumor is contributory to the antineoplastic effectiveness of these compounds, as per our original hypothesis. In this context, it seems worth mentioning that this conclusion does not apply exclusively to anthracyclines. As reviewed elsewhere (2), also for a number of other widely employed agents (e.g., cyclophospha-mide, Melphalan, BCNU, methotrexate, cis-diamminodichloroplatinum) experimental evidence has been obtained that the full expression of antineoplastic activity is, at least in part, dependent upon the participation of host reactivity.

As expected, interaction with immunity is not the only determinant of differences in efficacy among anthracyclines, as, for instance, exemplified by N-trifluoroacetyladriamycin-14-valerate (AD32), a derivative shown by this and other groups to be therapeutically superior to DX in mice (10). Although the antitumoral activity of AD32 was reduced in immunodepressed hosts, indicating that antineoplastic mechanisms were not totally abrogated by effective drug treatments, this compound was signifi-cantly more active than was DX on poorly or non-immunogenic tumors (11). Considering also that AD32 is significantly more immunodepressive than is DX, these findings suggest that the superiority in murine tumor models of the former compound derives

Table 2. Effect of treatment with Silica and of DTIC-immuno-
depression applied after chemotherapy on Doxorubicin (DX)
effectiveness in the L1210 Ha leukemia in $CD2F_1$ mice.

DX day 1	DTIC on day	Silica on days	MST (days)	%LTS
–	–	–	11	0
+	–	–	22	80
+	–5	–	19	0[+]
+	+5	–	20	0[+]
+	+10	–	26	20[+]
+	+20	–	17	80
–	+5	–	11	0
+	–	0.2	16	0[+]
+	–	–2.0	18	0[+]
–	–	–2.0	10	0[+]
+	–	–	33	80

[+] p < 0.01 compared to DX alone
In the DTIC and Silica expts, i.p. tumor inoculum was 10^5 and
10^4 cells, respectively, on day 0, DX dose being 10 and 12.5
mg/kg i.v. respectively. DTIC was given at 180 mg/kg i.p.
and Silica at 3 mg/mouse i.v.

from a greater direct cell killing capacity and/or more favourable
pharmacokinetic-metabolic properties. As indicated by the
results of Table 3, the newer derivative 4'-deoxydoxorubicin
(4'-deoxy DX) appears to behave as DX in its comparative activity
on immunogenic and non-immunogenic lymphomas. In contrast however
with DM, 4-demethoxydaunorubicin (4-demetDM) was found to be
significantly more effective on the immunogenic L1210 Ha subline
than on the Cr subline, a finding which may suggest a lower interference of antitumor resistance mechanisms by this derivative
than with the parent drug DM. A detailed comparative analysis of
the immunological activities of these newer derivatives is
however still in progress.

3. EFFECT OF ANTHRACYCLINES ON DIFFERENT IMMUNOCYTES
As an extension of the studies described above and in the
general objective of clarifying the relative role of the various
host antitumor mechanisms in determining the effectiveness of DX
and DM, it was necessary to analyze the sensitivity of the
different populations and subsets of immune cells to these

Table 3. Effect of 4'-deoxydoxorubicin and 4-demethoxydaunorubicin on L1210 leukemia sublines of different immunogenicity.

Drug	Dose (mg/kg i.v.)	L1210 Cr		L1210 Ha	
		%T/C	%LTS	%T/C	%LTS
DX	12	141	0	258	50
4'-deoxyDX	6	143	0	311	25
	4	140	0	213	0
	2	105	0	155	0
DM	14	131	0	144	0
4-demetDM	2.8	153	0	483	40
	2.0	141	0	416	30
	1.2	129	0	314	20

10^5 leukemia cells transplanted i.p. on day 0; drugs on day 1

compounds. As mentioned, DX was found to be significantly less inhibitory than DM of T lymphocyte-dependent reactivities, a finding not apparently related to a different intrinsic sensitivity of these elements to the two drugs as these were comparable in their effect in vitro on resting or mitogen-stimulated murine T and B cells (12). In contrast, these agents differed markedly in their effect on macrophages, DM being clearly more toxic for these cells both in vitro (Table 4) and in vivo (Table 5). Not only treatment with DM was in fact associated with significantly greater reductions in the number of these cells in lymphoid organs (4) but in addition this drug more profoundly impaired the functional activity of surviving macrophages as assessed for instance by their phagocytic ability (13) or by their capacity to express non-specific cytotoxicity towards neoplastic cells after treatment with macrophage stimulants or spontaneously (12,14). Whereas the participation of activated macrophages in host resistance towards neoplastic growth and dissemination is well known, more recent is the finding (15) that in mice and men also normal elements of the monocyte-macrophage lineage can spontaneously damage transformed (but not untransformed) target cells, a mechanism also of probable importance in natural resistance against cancer and infections. Whereas DM was clearly inhibitory, table 6 shows that equitoxic doses of in vivo DX did not significantly impair these macrophage activities

Table 4. Spleen macrophage ($\times 10^6$) numbers after Doxorubicin (DX) and Daunorubicin (DM) injection (15 mg/kg i.v.) in mice.

Day after treatment	Control	DX	DM
1	11.1 + 1.2	12.2 + 0.7	6.7 + 1.0[+]
4	13.0 + 0.9	10.9 + 1.3	5.5 + 1.7[+]
8	12.3 + 1.2	9.6 + 1.6	5.4 + 1.5[+]

[+] $p < 0.05$

Table 5. Effect of Doxorubicin and Daunorubicin on the survival of murine macrophages

Drug	µg/ml	^{86}Rb uptake (cpm) 3h	24h
DX	0	15,310 + 850	12,710 + 410
	0.1		
	0.2	14,520 + 280	10,310 + 890
	0.5	13,460 + 640	9,860 + 760
DM	0.1		
	0.2	8,480 + 210[+]	2,010 + 80[+]
	0.5	1,200 + 110[+]	250 + 20[+]

[+] $p < 0.05$
Exposure to drugs in vitro was for 3 and 24 h

Table 6. Effect of anthracyclines and other cancer chemotherapeutic agents on macrophage-mediated and NK cell-dependent cytotoxic activity in mice.

Drug	Dose (mg/kg)	% decrease in specific cytotoxicity macroph. spont.	BCG-activated	NK
DX	10	0	3	4
DM	10	35[+]	44[+]	22[+]
Aza	250	52[+]	56[+]	48[+]
Cy	150	2	5	58[+]
DTIC	150	60[+]	67[+]	6

[+] $p < 0.01$
Targets for spleen macrophages cytolytic activity were mKSATU5 cells (A:T ratio 20:1 incubation 48 h) whereas YAC1 lymphoma cells used for spleen NK activity (A:T 20:1, incubation 4 h). Tests were performed 2 d after drug injection; BCG given 7 d before drugs. Aza = Azathioprine; Cy = Cyclophosphamide.

on a unit cell number basis. The effect of DX on the in vivo
induction of macrophage-mediated cytostasis by stimulants such
as C.parvum is however dependent on the relative timing between
the two agents (16). If both compounds are administered at
close intervals (e.g. 1,2 days) the induction of cytotoxicity
measured 6 to 14 days later was reduced, whereas DX given 3-7
days prior to C.parvum did not interfere with cytostatic activity
levels. Indeed, in several experiments, higher cytotoxicity
levels were seen in animals given both agents viz. those treated
with C.parvum alone, possibly as a result of rebound proliferation of macrophage precursors. An increased tumor cell inhibitor
capacity of peritoneal macrophages after DX treatment has also
been described by others (17) paralleling the higher relative
proportion of these cells in lymphoid organs (12,18,19). The
relative resistance to DX of macrophage cells is also supported
by the non reduction of antibody-dependent cellular cytotoxicity
(ADCC) against neoplastic and non-tumorous cells (19,20), a
function which is largely mediated by phagocytic-adherent element
Although direct data are limited, it may be noted that the data
in rodents seem to have a counterpart in humans. In vitro exposure to DX has recently been observed to increase the generation
in culture of cytotoxic monocytes (21) and in our hands chemotherapy with combinations including DX did not reduce in ovarian
cancer patients antibody-dependent and independent cytotoxicity
against tumor cells (22). In addition to its possible importance
in the antineoplastic efficacy of DX versus DM as discussed
later, the modulation of macrophage activity by DX is presumably
of relevance in the effects of DX on other immunological changes
described after its administration. At least in selected experimental conditions, DX has in fact been found to produce augmente
generations of cytotoxic T lymphocytes and of PHA or LPS-induced
lymphocyte colonies (5,18,23,24). Monocytes-macrophages are
known to play a role in these immune reactivities, although the
effect of DX on suppressor cells could also be of importance.

Although the kinetics of cell depletion in the spleen after
DX and DM is related to the different rates of accumulation and
total drug levels, and the extent of cell loss seen with DX in

the mouse peritoneal cavity, spleen and lymphnodes is inversely
correlated (2) with drug concentrations at these sites (and interestingly, with their macrophage content), still hypothetical
are however the mechanism(s) through which DM can kill mature,
non-replicating macrophages _in vitro_ and responsible for the differential _in vivo_ sensitivity of these cells to DM and DX. Since
higher drug levels were measured in lysosomes after DM than DX
(25), a greater accumulation of the former agent into lysosome-
rich mature macrophages could be a determining factor, possibly
in association with the known capacity of these drugs to interact
with membranes (26). The inhibition of protein synthesis seen
with anthracyclines could be important in the interference seen
with DM in macrophage cytotoxicity as protein synthesis is
necessary for the expression of this activity by human and
murine elements.

Differences in sensitivity to DX and DM are not limited only
to macrophages but extend to other populations of immunocytes.
No significant inhibition of Natural Killer (NK) cell activity
in the spleen, lymphnodes and peritoneal cavity was in fact
seen after DX treatment in mice (27,28) whereas clear reductions
were seen with DM (Table 3). It should be noted that although
no reductions were found with DX on a unit cell number basis,
lower numbers of mononuclear cells were however recovered from
these animals, the depletion being comparatively greatest in
the spleen and lowest in the peritoneal cavity as a consequence
of unequal drug distribution-persistence at these sites (29).
A reduction in total NK activity was accordingly observable also
with DX although of significantly lower extent than seen with
equitoxic doses of DM. Therefore, although in selected conditions
increases in macrophage-mediated and NK-dependent (e.g. _in vivo_
radioresistant antitumor responses (30)) activities can be
observed, one deals in reality with conditions of relative
rather than absolute sparing of such elements after DX injections.
In addition to giving further evidence of the heterogeneity among
antitumoral compounds even of the same class in their effect on
immunocytes, the data of Table 4 provide an example of the
possible usefulness of this type of investigation in under-

standing the mode of action of drugs. The divergent results
seen between DX and AD32 in their effects on NK and macrophage-
mediated cytotoxicity are against the possibility that the
latter agent acts essentially by releasing DX, a possibility
disproven also by more recent direct metabolic data (31). The
contrasting sensitivity of NK cells and macrophages to at least
some drugs (e.g. DTIC and Cyclophosphamide) incidentally gives
support to the concept that these elements, both credited with
an important role in natural resistance mechanisms, belong to
different lineages. Evidence has in fact been advanced for
a T-cell origin of at least some NK cells (32). The basis for
the differential susceptibility of NK activity to DX and DM is
again undetermined.

A further type of immune cells for which a divergent sensitivity to DX and DM has been revealed is represented by regulatory
immunocytes. It is now widely accepted that an activation of
immunologically specific and/or nonspecific suppressors identifie
by most groups with T lymphocytes and macrophages, respectively,
could be a crucial element in the pathogenesis of neoplastic
progression (33) by antagonizing the generation and expression
of antitumor effector mechanisms. Investigating firstly the
sensitivity of specific T-suppressor cells involved in the
regulation of the humoral response to the T-dependent antigen
sheep erythrocytes (Ts-abs), it was found (34) that DM inhibited
the expression of suppressor activity only when used at toxic
doses (Fig. 2). In contrast, DX was clearly inhibitory as
judged by the inability of cells obtained from drug-treated
mice to suppress the humoral response to sheep erythrocytes
(SRBC) of syngeneic hosts, an inhibition which, in the conditions
used, lasted for 2 weeks after a single antileukemically optimal
dose. Since cells from animals treated with DX after, concomi-
tantly with, as well as prior to the suppressor-inducing stimulus
were incapable of transferring suppression in syngeneic recipients,
it appeared that this agent can interfere not only with the
generation-expression of "activated" suppressors but could
also interfere with the precursor elements of this regulatory
mechanism. Somewhat different results were on the other hand

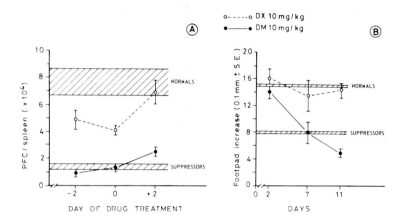

FIGURE 2. Effect of Doxorubicin (DX) and Daunorubicin (DM) on Ts-abs (A) and Ts-dth (B) dependent activity in mice. Ts were induced injecting 10^{10} SRBC on day 0. For Ts-abs, $3 \cdot 10^7$ spleno-cytes were injected on day 5 into syngeneic recipients challenged simultaneously with 10^8 SRBC, response in recipients being evaluated 4 d later. For Ts-dth, splenocytes were transferred on day 14 to recipients simultaneously sensitized with $2 \cdot 10^7$ SRBC s.c.; a 10^8 SRBC s.c. challenge was applied 5 d later and response evaluated after further 24 h.

obtained when DM and DX effects were evaluated on specific T-suppressors involved in the regulation of cell-mediated, delayed type hypersensitivity reactions (Ts-dth) to the same antigen (8). In fact, DX was again markedly inhibitory of these cells as well as of their precursors, but inhibition of "induced" Ts-dth transferable activity(but not of their precursors) was seen also with DM. Preliminary findings seem to indicate that 4'-deoxyDX behaves qualitatively like DX on these activities. It may be of interest that a different sensitivity of Ts-dth and Ts-abs has been documented also with other antitumorals (8), suggestive of the existence of definite differences in the cellular composition of these regulatory networks, and that these agents are qualitatively and quantitatively quite hetero-geneous in their effect on suppressor activity. It may be additionally mentioned that, as might have been expected from previous results, DX and DM gave contrasting results when macro-phage-mediated non-specific suppressor activity was investigated measuring inhibition of lymphocyte mitogenic response. As for

other drugs (2), the mechanisms responsible for the differential
sensitivity of T-dependent suppressor cell activities to DX and
DM are essentially unknown, also in view of the still large
ignorance of the kinetic characteristics of these cells and their
precursors at rest and after stimulation. In view however of
the ineffectiveness of DM in the same conditions in which DX
was clearly active (e.g. on precursors and induced Ts-abs), it
is difficult to accept that only the proliferative characteristics of
the target population play a role in the observed differences.
Possibly other factors at present only conjectural (different
rates of drug persistence and consequent ability to repair cell
damage, toxic mechanisms other than cell death) are also involved in determining the different immunopharmacological profiles of DX and DM. In view of recent findings (35) favouring
the possibility that within T-regulatory circuits more than one
cell sustain the induction and actual mediation of suppressive
signals, it is also undetermined whether these drugs affect
only one or more than one of the cells comprising the network.

4. IMMUNOCYTE POPULATIONS AND DOXORUBICIN ACTIVITY

Results described above have provided evidence in support
of the conclusion that a qualitatively-quantitatively different
interaction with host reactivity can be of importance in the
therapeutic efficacy of at least some anthracyclines, and that
these agents even when chemically closely related as DX and
DM, can possess markedly different immunopharmacological
characteristics. It was accordingly of interest to extend the
studies and investigate the relative role played by different
immunocytes and dependent effector mechanisms in the antineoplastic activity of DX. In this regard it is appropriate
to emphasize that such types of analyses are hampered by the
complex web of functional interactions existing among the cells
of the immune system, current difficulties in analyzing separately each component of the integrated networks of the immune
complex and the still large uncertainty as to the relative
in vivo importance of the various host anti-tumor reactivities.
Conclusions advanced from such investigations are therefore to

be viewed essentially as operational and suggestive.

A possible role for the different sensitivity to DX and DM
of NK cells could be suggested by the finding that DX displayed
a greater therapeutic capacity towards a NK-sensitive lymphoma
in mouse strains physiologically possessing a "high" NK activity
than in strains with low or undetectable natural cell-mediated
cytotoxicity (36). However, because of the known regulatory
influences exerted by macrophages on NK cells, this evidence
should still be considered as inconclusive. Accordingly, whether
the relative resistance of these cells to DX is therapeutically
relevant is still unclear. Although the sensitivity to DX and
the relative resistance to DM of at least some T-dependent
suppressor mechanisms could in principle be an important determinant of the in vivo superiority of the former agent seen in many
neoplastic models, no direct evidence on this point is at present
available. Similarly indirect is the evidence in support for
a possible role of a differential interaction of the two analogs
at the level of T-dependent effector mechanisms, suggested for
instance by the decreased DX effectiveness in thymectomized mice,
and, more indirectly, by the lower inhibition by DX than by DM of
tumor allograft resistance (3,5). Host reactivity to allo-
antigens is generally considered to be related to T-dependent
reactivity to tumor-associated antigens. Less informative in
this respect is the reduced DX effectiveness found in DTIC-pre-
treated hosts since DTIC, which is strongly depressive in mice
of T-dependent reactivities while sparing NK cytotoxicity and
radioresistant antitumor resistance, also impairs macrophagic
cytotoxicity.

With the proviso that the close functional interplay between
macrophages and other immunocytes (e.g. T cells) caution against
drawing definitive conclusions, more direct evidence has on the
other hand been obtained in favour of the importance of macrophages in the differential in antineoplastic effectiveness
between DX and DM. This conclusion is supported by the finding
(Table 2) that the therapeutic activity of DX in mice transplanted with the immunogenic L1210 Ha leukemia was markedly
reduced in hosts pretreated with silica particles (6). By

virtue of their capacity to accumulate into macrophages, these
non-degradable particles possess a selective toxicity for these
cells which are ultimately destroyed. Decreases in DX activity
also in the moderately immunogenic SL2 lymphoma were similarly
observed employing another macrophage toxin, carrageenan, which,
like silica, did not appreciably influence DX pharmacokinetics.
In contrast, neither of these compounds significantly affected
DX activity in the non-immunogenic L1210 Cr system, or influenced
DM effectiveness on either immunogenic or non-immunogenic tumors.
These observations appear thus consistent with the possibility
that a relative sparing by DX of mononuclear phagocytes, possibly
activated as a consequence of an immune response to immunogenic
tumors, contributed to the antineoplastic activity of this anthra
cycline. Macrophages recovered from DX-treated, "cured" L1210 Ha
transplanted mice showed enhanced non-specific cytotoxic capacity
(6). In indirect support of this interpretation are also the
findings obtained when DX or DM were combined in vivo with
macrophage stimulators such as C.parvum or BCG (16,20,37). In
various leukemia-lymphomas and solid tumor models a significantly
better antineoplastic efficacy was found when DX was combined
with these immunopotentiators whereas no therapeutic advantage
was obtained when DM was employed in the chemotherapy arm of
the combination. Given the greater in vivo and in vitro toxicity
of DM for macrophages, the therapeutic synergism of DX with
C.parvum or BCG can be attributed to the relative sparing by
the latter anthracycline of phagocytes. This contention is
reinforced by the fact that, as discussed elsewhere (16,20),
the schedules of chemotherapy and C.parvum immunotherapy which
were synergistic in vivo were also those which did not interfere
(indeed, could enhance) with the expression of the cytotoxic
activity of macrophages. Conversely, in vivo non synergistic
schedules were associated with impaired macrophage-dependent
cytotoxicity. In addition, the therapeutic synergism of the
DX-C.parvum combination was abolished (Table 7) by treatment
of the animals with silica.

Table 7. Effect of treatment with Silica on the effectiveness
of Doxorubicin-C.parvum combination in the SL2 lymphoma

DX	C.parvum	Silica	MST[a]	% LTS
-	-	-	14	O
+	-	-	23	O
+	-	+	17	O
+	+	-	33	50
+	+	+	18	O

DX (10 mg/kg i.v.) on day 1; C.parvum (0.7 mg i.v.) day -7;
Silica (3 mg i.v.) on day 0 and 2.
a, Median survival time in days.

5. CONCLUSIONS

   Results discussed in this review appear to warrant a series
of conclusions of basic and applied relevance. In the first
place, the contention seems justified that the qualitative and
quantitative characteristics of the interaction with host
defences of anthracyclines can indeed be an important determinant
of their therapeutic effectiveness. The study of this biological effect can thus be useful to us, not only for permitting
a better comprehension of the mode of action and pharmacotoxicological properties of such compounds but also for assisting
in the development of novel more active and safer analogs. A
further more general conclusion regards the distinct individua-
lity which can exist between even closely structurally related
cytotoxic chemicals in their immunopharmacological profiles.
In view of the fact that such agents are no longer to be
considered in the strict optics of immunodepression since they
can exert more complex immunomodulatory effects, a better
understanding of the still largely unclear mechanistic aspects
of this heterogeneity appears of interest. It appears not
unreasonable in fact to expect that through such type of investigations a more in depth knowledge can be obtained on
various aspects of the cell biology of antitumorals and thus reveal
information of importance towards the most effective employment of
such compounds, for instance in guiding the choice of drugs to
be associated in combination chemotherapy or in the frame of
more complex multimodality therapeutic strategies.

66

REFERENCES

1. Harris CC. 1979. A delayed complication of cancer therapy: Cancer.
   J Natl Cancer Inst 63: 275-277.
2. Spreafico F, Mantovani A. 1981. Immunomodulation by cancer chemotherapeutic agents and antineoplastic activity. In: Pathobiology Annual,
   1980, (HL Ioachin ed.) New York, Raven Press, in press.
3. Vecchi A, Mantovani A, Tagliabue A, Spreafico F. 1976 . A characterization
   of the immunosuppressive activity of adriamycin and daunomycin on
   humoral antibody production and tumor allograft rejection. Cancer Res
   36: 1222-1227.
4. Mantovani A, Tagliabue A, Vecchi A, Spreafico F. 1976 . Effects of
   adriamycin and daunomycin on spleen cell populations in normal and
   tumor allografted mice. Eur J Cancer 12: 381-387.
5. Mantovani A, Vecchi A, Tagliabue A, Spreafico F. 1976 . The effects
   of adriamycin and daunomycin on antitumoral immune effector mechanisms
   in an allogeneic system. Eur J Cancer 12: 371-379.
6. Mantovani A, Polentarutti N, Luini W, Peri G, Spreafico F. 1979 . The
   role of host defense mechanisms in the antitumor activity of adriamycin
   and daunomycin in mice. J Natl Cancer Inst 63: 61-66.
7. Vecchi A, Fioretti MC, Mantovani A, Barzi A, Spreafico F. 1976 . The
   immunodepressive and hemototoxic activity of imidazole-4-carboxamide,5-
   (3,3-dimethyl-1-triazeno) in mice. Transplantation 22: 619-624.
8. Spreafico F, Vecchi A, Conti G, Sironi M. 1981. On the heterogeneity
   of immunotherapeutic agents. In: Advances Immunopharmacology (J Hadden,
   L Chedid, P Mullen, F Spreafico eds.) New York, Pergamon Press pp. 51-63.
9. Schwartz HS, Grindey GB. 1973. Adriamycin and daunorubicin: A comparison
   of antitumor activities and tissue uptake in mice following immunosuppression. Cancer Res 33: 1837-1844.
10. Vecchi A, Cairo M, Mantovani A, Sironi M, Spreafico F. 1978. Comparative
    antineoplastic activity of adriamycin and N-trifluoroacetyladriamycin-
    14-valerate. Cancer Treat Rep 62: 111-117.
11. Vecchi A, Spreafico F, Sironi M, Cairo M, Garattini S. 1980. The
    immunodepressive and hematotoxic activities of N-trifluoro-acetyl-adriamyc:
    14-valerate. Eur J Cancer 16: 1289-1296.
12. Mantovani A. 1977. In vitro and in vivo cytotoxicity of adriamycin and
    daunomycin for murine macrophages. Cancer Res 37: 815-820.
13. Facchinetti T, Raz A, Goldman R. 1978. A differential interaction of
    daunomycin, adriamycin, and N-trifluoroacetyladriamycin-14-valerate
    with mouse peritoneal macrophages. Cancer Res 38: 3944-3949.
14. Mantovani A, Luini W, Candiani GP, Spreafico F. 1980 . Effect of
    chemotherapeutic agents on natural and BCG-stimulated macrophage
    cytotoxicity in mice. Int J Immunopharmacol 2: 333-339.
15. Mantovani A, Jerrells TR, Dean JH, Herberman RB. 1979 . Cytolytic and
    cytostatic activity on tumor cells of circulating human monocytes. Int
    J Cancer 23: 18-27.
16. Spreafico F. 1980. Heterogeneity of the interaction of anticancer agents
    with the immune system and its possible relevance in chemoimmunotherapy.
    Oncology 37: suppl. 1, 9-18.
17. Stoychkov JN, Schultz RM, Chirigos MA, Pavlidis NA, Goldin A. 1979.
    Effects of adriamycin and cyclophosphamide treatment on induction of
    macrophage cytotoxic function in mice. Cancer Res 39: 3014-3017.
18. Orsini FR, Pavelic Z, Mihich E. 1977. Increased primary cell mediated
    immunity in culture subsequent to adriamycin or daunorubicin treatment
    of spleen donor mice. Cancer Res 37: 1719-1726.

19. Cohen SA, Ehrke MJ, Mihich E. 1980. Selectivity of immunomodulation by adriamycin. Adv Enzyme Regul 18: 335-346.
20. Mantovani A, Vecchi A, Tagliabue A, Spreafico F. 1979 . The effect of chemotherapeutic agents on host defence mechanisms: Ist relevance for chemoimmunotherapy combinations. In: Tumor-Associated and their Specific Immune Response (F Spreafico, R Arnon eds.) New York, Academic Press pp. 271-286.
21. Kleinerman ES, Muchmore AV. 1981. Effect of various cancer chemotherapeutic agents on naturally occurring human spontaneous monocyte-mediated cytotoxicity (SMMC). Proc Am Ass Cancer Res 22: 277.
22. Mantovani A, Peri G, Polentarutti N, Allavena P, Bordignon C, Sessa C, Mangioni C. 1980 . Natural cytotoxicity on tumor cells of human monocytes and macrophages. In: Natural-Cell Mediated Immunity against Tumors (RB Herberman ed.) New York, Academic Press pp. 1271-1293.
23. Orsini FR, Henderson ES. 1980. Doxorubicin and daunorubicin modulation of macrophages,T and B lymphocytes (anthracycline lymphocyte modulation). Immunopharmacology 2: 375-384.
24. Tomazic V, Ehrke MJ, Mihich E. 1980. Modulation of the cytotoxic response against allogeneic tumor cells in culture by adriamycin. Cancer Res 40: 2748-2755.
25. Noel G, Trouet A, Zenebergh A, Tulkens P. 1975. Comparative cell pharmacokinetics of daunorubicin and adriamycin. In: Adriamycin Review, EORTC International Symposium, Brussels, May 1974,Ghent, European Press pp. 99-105.
26. Goldman R, Facchinetti T, Bach D, Raz A, Shinitzky M. 1978. A differential interaction of daunomycin, adriamycin and their derivatives with human erythrocytes and phospholipid bilayers. Biochim Biophys Acta 512: 254-269.
27. Mantovani A, Luini W, Peri G, Vecchi A, Spreafico F. 1978. Effect of chemotherapeutic agents on natural cell-mediated cytotoxicity in mice. J Natl Cancer Inst 61: 1255-1261.
28. Santoni A, Riccardi C, Sorci V, Herberman RB. 1980. Effects of adriamycin on the activity of mouse natural killer cells. J Immunol 124: 2329-2335.
29. Mantovani A, Tagliabue A. 1981. Modulation of mononuclear phagocytes by cancer chemotherapeutic agents. In: The Reticuloendothelial System: A Comprehensive Treatise, vol VIII: Cancer (H Friedman, RB Herberman eds.) New York, Plenum Press in press.
30. Riccardi C, Bartocci A, Puccetti P, Spreafico F, Bonmassar E, Goldin A. 1979 . Combined effects of antineoplastic agents and anti-lymphoma allograft reactions. Eur J Cancer 16: 23-33.
31. Abbruzzi R, Rizzardini M, Benigni A, Barbieri B, Donelli MG, Salmona M. 1980. Possible relevance of N- trifluoroacetyladriamycin (AD 41) in the antitumoral activity of N-trifluoroacetyladriamycin-14-valerate (AD 32) in tumor bearing mice. I. Pharmacokinetic evidence. Cancer Treat Rep 64: 873-878.
32. Herberman RB (ed.). 1980. Natural Cell-Mediated Immunity Against Tumors. New York, Academic Press.
33. Naor D. 1979. Suppressor cells: Permitters and Promoters of malignancy? Adv Cancer Res 29: 45-125.
34. Anaclerio A, Conti G, Goggi G, Honorati MC, Ruggeri A, Moras ML, Spreafico F. 1980. Effect of cytotoxic agents on suppressor cells in mice. Eur J Cancer 16: 53-58.
35. Benacerraf B. 1980. Genetic control of the specificity of T lymphocytes and their regulatory products. In: Progress in Immunology IV (M Fongereau, J Dausset eds.) New York, Academic Press pp. 420-430.

36. Spreafico F. 1980. The heterogeneity of the interaction between cancer chemotherapeutic agents and host resistance mechanisms. Recent Results Cancer Res 75: 200–206.
37. Tagliabue A, Polentarutti N, Vecchi A, Mantovani A, Spreafico F. 1977. Combination chemo-immunotherapy with adriamycin in experimental tumor systems. Eur J Cancer 13: 657–665.

SECTION 2

MECHANISM OF ACTION

INTRODUCTION

N. R. BACHUR

We are very furtunate to have the contributions of established leaders
in the study of anthracycline mechanism of action who are continuing their
enlightening studies. In addition, we have new and exciting voices to add
to our knowledge of anthracycline actions.

Beginning this section on mechanism of action is Dr. Federico Arcamone
who describes the physicochemical characteristics of the anthracycline
complexing with DNA. Dr. Arcamone's work, which is well known, began with
the earliest studies of the anthracycline structural characterization and
analog development. He describes the binding characteristics and the molecular
conformation of the anthracyclines in relation to intercalation and action.
Through outstanding advances in the synthetic arena, Dr. Arcamone compares a
large number of analogs with differing affinities for DNA.

Dr. Kurt Kohn is an authority in the effects of drugs on cellular DNA.
His development of the alkaline elution technique for investigation of DNA
breakage is well known. Dr. Kohn's studies on the types of strand breaks and
modifications in DNA structure that are caused by anthracycline action are
discussed in detail and compared to different DNA binding drugs. In recent
advances, Dr. Kohn and his coworkers related protein binding and more specifically topoisomerase binding to the single-strand breaks as being important
to our understanding of the mechanism of actions of anthracyclines.

Moving a step toward the understanding of the chemistry and biochemical
modifications that are possible with anthracycline antibiotics in the cell,
I discuss the nature of the anthraquinone nucleus, its physicochemical
characteristics, and the potentials available to the cell in metabolic
modification and free radical formation.

At the level of the giant chromosome, Dr. Michel Robert-Nicoud demonstrates
differential binding characteristics that occur with anthracycline antibiotics
to the polytene chromosomes. Dr. Robert-Nicoud's investigations show remark-

able differences among anthracycline antibiotics to these large nuclear structures.

Moving a step in the direction of other anthracycline-caused marcomolecular events such as inhibition of nucleolar RNA synthesis, Dr. Archie Prestayko describes studies from the research program at the Bristol Laboratories. By defining the class I and class II types of anthracyclines, we see additional differentiation of the specificity of action of anthracycline antibiotics.

Dr. Herbert Schwartz examines the metabolic transformations of anthracyclines produced by membranous microsomal preparations. He has studied the effects of metabolic inhibitors and specificity in the metabolic pathways of daunorubicin, Adriamycin, and carminomycin.

In studying the cellular transport of the anthracyclines and the interactions of the anthracyclines at the cellular membrane for a number of years, Dr. Peterson is concerned as to whether cellular uptake affects the specific action of anthracyclines; for example, is it because of differential uptake and retention that Adriamycin is more effective than daunorubicin in solid tumors? Dr. Peterson has investigated the active efflux mechanism and anthracycline cellular accumulation and transport and explains the observations concerning cellular accumulation and localization according to DNA and protein binding of the anthracyclines.

In his studies on myocardial physiological chemistry, Dr. Revis points to aberrant calcium flux as the toxic phenomenon related to cardiotoxicity. Certainly ionic effects may be important as effects of anthracycline mechanism of action.

Dr. Scheulen has investigated the question of acute lipid peroxidation as measured by ethane expiration in anthracycline-treated animals. Those data and their relationship to specificity of action and to free radical production are interesting foils to the lipid peroxidation theory of action.

Dr. Dalmark has fundamental data on the uptake of anthracyclines into cells and the physicochemical relationships with cellular membranes that govern this uptake.

From these interesting contributors, we see quite clearly that the actions of anthracyclines are expressed in many ways. These unique antibiotic molecules have high specificities, yet multiple effects, in the cell. Small changes in the molecule can negate the molecule's actions and cytotoxicities. Small changes can modify the types of cytotoxicity and the types of effects that are seen. It is important that we see the broad spectrum of effects that anthracyclines create in cells; and this, I believe, is the key to the understanding of these effective antibiotic molecules--toxins that have multiple functions and multiple actions. We have inherited these toxins from nature and have found them to be useful in man as a means of alleviating malignant growth. We do not understand which of the actions, if any, are responsible for the selective cytotoxicity against malignant cells. It is our cause to examine these data and to find those actions that are responsible for the antitumor action of the anthracyclines. It is hoped that we will be able to build new molecules or to use old ones more knowledgeably to reduce the toxic side effects and to increase the efficacy of anthracycline antibiotics in the treatment of human disease.

DOXORUBICIN AND RELATED COMPOUNDS.   I.   PHYSICOCHEMICAL CHARACTERIZATION
OF THE DNA COMPLEX

F. ARCAMONE, E. ARLANDINI, M. MENOZZI, L. VALENTINI, AND E. VANNINI

1.   INTRODUCTION

The study of molecular interactions between drugs and biological macromolecules in solution has received considerable attention in recent years.
Researchers in this field of biophysical chemistry, although well aware of
the different situation present in in vivo systems (those that show a complexity of molecular structures in a dynamic state and in a polyphasic system
as that represented by living cells), believe that information obtained at
the molecular level is a prerequisite for the complete understanding of the
mechanism of action of drugs.   From the standpoint of the medicinal chemist,
any molecular property related to biological activity is of great interest;
a knowledge of structural requirements that exhibit a given property allows
an understanding of the chemical modifications needed to optimize desired
pharmacological behavior within a given class of related compounds.   This is
particularly important in the case of the antitumor anthracyclines.   Even
though hundreds of new compounds have been made available for biological
evaluation and a variety of pharmacological properties of the parent compounds
have been investigated in different laboratories, programs aimed at the
development of new analogs are still based solely on empirical considerations
that have been derived from results obtained in standard biological screening
systems.

Evidence that indicates that DNA is a major site of action of the antitumor anthracyclines is the result of several studies, both in cell cultures
and animal systems (1-4).   Studies of cell cultures have demonstrated 1) a
nuclear localization of the drugs, 2) alteration of DNA template functions,
3) chromosomal damage, mutation, and cell transformation, and 4) DNA fragmentation as direct consequences of the exposure of cells to the anthracyclines.   Animal and clinical studies have demonstrated that treatment with
anthracyclines causes 1) impairment of the synthesis of nucleic acid in
tumors and other tissues, including the heart, 2) nucleolar alterations in

heart and liver cells of the rat, 3) carcinogenicity in rodents, 4) fragmentation of tumor cell DNA, and 5) chromosomal abnormalities.

These observations have focused the attention of biochemists and biophysical chemists on the ability of antitumor anthracyclines to bind to DNA
in solution, a property originally reported by Di Marco and his coworkers (5).
Current views accept the conclusion that the stronger binding process of
doxorubicin and related drugs to DNA, as revealed at low-drug-to-DNA molar
ratios, corresponds to the formation of an intercalation complex (6).
The intercalation complex has been studied by a variety of techniques (7).
These are based on alterations of properties of the drug as a consequence of
complexation and include ultraviolet and visible spectroscopy, fluorescence
spectroscopy, circular dichroism, high resolution NMR spectroscopy, polarography, equilibrium dialysis, and solvent distribution; or are based on properties of the macromolecule and include thermal denaturation, ultracentrifugation, viscometry, and inhibition of enzyme reactions. Other methods used
to study the intercalation complex are calorimetry and X-ray diffractometry.
As for the two major points of interest for the structure-activity relationships studies, namely quantitative evaluation of the affinity of the drugs
for the DNA biopolymer and the structural details of the complex itself,
conclusive data cannot be derived from the literature, although a considerable
amount of information is accumulating in this regard. In a total of 10
published studies (8-17), it was shown that the apparent stability constant
of the doxorubicin calf thymus DNA (double stranded) complex, K_{app}, was in
the range 0.37 to 11.6 $1 \cdot mol^{-1} \cdot 10^{6}$, and the apparent number of binding sites
per nucleotide, n_{app}, was in the range of 0.09 to 0.25. A similar range
of K_{app} values has been reported for daunorubicin in different studies
based on spectrophotometric and spectrofluorometric titrations, equilibrium
dialysis, solvent distribution, and polarography, the deviations reflecting
differences in experimental conditions, ionic strength, DNA preparations,
and Scatchard linear plot treatment of the results (1-6, 9, 12, 14, 16, 18-
22).

Although different X-ray diffraction studies of daunorubicin and its derivatives afford a coherent representation of the overall molecular conformation in the solid state for the free drugs (1-6, 23-25), only two studies
concerning the doxorubicin-DNA complex are available (26,27). These studies
allow the conclusion that the cyclohexene ring A is in the half-chair conformation, in agreement with NMR findings on different derivatives in

solution (7), the sugar moiety being nearly perpendicular in respect to the planar chromophoric system. Such deductions are also in agreement with the standard semiempirical approach, which allowed Neidle and Taylor (28) to draw the energy surface for daunorubicin as a function of torsion angles C8-C7-O7-C1' and C7-O7-C1'-O5'. A consequence of these observations is the conclusion that, since daunorubicin has been found to adopt the same conformation in different crystallographic environments and in solution, the same conformation probably is the biologically active one at the receptor site. The study by Pigram et al. (27) consisted of the fiber X-ray analysis of the daunorubicin-calf thymus double helical DNA intercalation complex, and the results suggested the sugar moiety in the wide groove, the amino group interacting with a phosphate anion two base pairs away from the intercalation site. The Quigley et al. study (26) consisted, instead, of an X-ray crystal diffraction analysis at the atomic resolution of the intercalation complex between daunorubicin and the hexadeoxynucleotide d(CpGpTpApCpG). According to the results, the planar aglycone was oriented at right angles to the long dimension of the base pairs, whereas the sugar moiety was in the narrow groove, no electrostatic interaction being displayed by the amino group. However, OH-9 and O13 were involved in hydrogen bonds, the size of the binding site being three base pairs.

The small upfield shifts of ring D protons in the high resolution PMR spectra of the mixture of poly (dA-dT) or dG-dC-dG-dC and daunorubicin at DNA-P to drug molar ratios ≥ 5 allowed the conclusion that anthracycline ring D does not overlap with the nearest-neighbor bases (29,30). In a recent study (31), confirmation of the location of ring B in the shielding region of base pairs was obtained from the large upfield shift of H-11 of 11-deoxydoxorubicin upon intercalation in poly (dA-dT). Furthermore, the shift of thymidine CH_3-5 upon complexation suggested that, unlike the acridines, the orientation of the anthracycline chromophore is perpendicular to the direction of the Watson-Crick hydrogen bonds. Phillips and Roberts (32) arrived at similar conclusions.

In our laboratory we have become interested recently in the use of physicochemical techniques as additional sources of information regarding new analogs. We report here about an investigation that was aimed at defining the formation constants of the doxorubicin-DNA complex, and about an evaluation of data from our laboratory concerning a number of representative analogs of the antitumor anthracyclines that sought to establish the molecular requirements for complex formation.

2. THE DIMERIZATION OF DAUNORUBICIN AND DOXORUBICIN

During the course of investigations currently being carried out in our laboratory on interactions between doxorubicin and pharmacologically important biopolymers, we found that we had to take drug dimerization into account. The self-association of daunorubicin and doxorubicin has been the subject of different publications (22, 33-37) in which a variety of results apparently related to the different conditions and methodologies used have been reported. We have determined the dimerization constants of the said compounds, employing the spectrophotometric method and using interferential filters in order to cut off the fluorescence radiation which seemed to be a source of error not considered in previous spectrophotometric studies.

Figure 1 shows the differences among specific absorption spectra of doxorubicin at various concentrations in pH 7 phosphate buffer and the curves of molar absorptivity versus concentration in the same buffer according to two different experimental procedures. Unknown parameters, i.e., the molar absorptivity of monomeric and dimeric species and the dimerization constants, were estimated by nonlinear curve fitting procedures. The results are presented in Table 1.

a: $1.72 \cdot 10^{-6} \underline{M}$
b: $1.72 \cdot 10^{-5} \underline{M}$
c: $1.72 \cdot 10^{-4} \underline{M}$

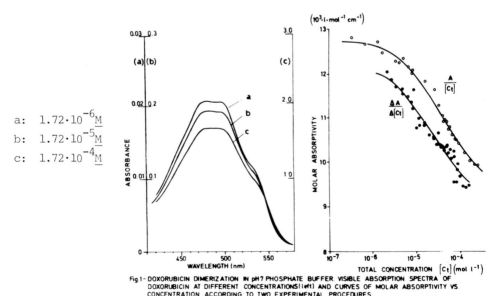

Fig.1- DOXORUBICIN DIMERIZATION IN pH 7 PHOSPHATE BUFFER. VISIBLE ABSORPTION SPECTRA OF DOXORUBICIN AT DIFFERENT CONCENTRATIONS (left) AND CURVES OF MOLAR ABSORPTIVITY VS. CONCENTRATION ACCORDING TO TWO EXPERIMENTAL PROCEDURES.

Table 1. Dimerization constants K_d of daunorubicin and doxorubicin in
different buffers

Buffer	Ionic strength	$K_d \times 10^4$ l·mol^{-1}	
		daunorubicin	doxorubicin
Phosphate	0.05	1.25 ± 0.48	1.53 ± 0.32
Tris · HCl	0.05	1.13 ± 0.30	2.10 ± 0.34
Tris · HCl + NaCl	0.19	1.70 ± 0.47	2.39 ± 0.39

3. EQUILIBRIUM DIALYSIS EXPERIMENTS AT DIFFERENT DNA CONCENTRATIONS

The scope of this part of our study was the determination of the curve
of formation of the doxorubicin-DNA complex, i.e., the variation of the
number of drug molecules bound per nucleotide, r, versus the logarithm of
the concentration of monomeric free drug, Log cf, over the wide possible
range of r and cf values. All of the said values are related to the
stronger binding process, namely, the formation of the intercalation complex.
Toward this end, equilibrium dialysis experiments were carried out with a
·Kontron Diapack apparatus, using Sigma calf-thymus DNA type I at concentrations varying from 10^{-6} to 10^{-3} M (as DNA-P) and ^{14}C-doxorubicin as the ligand
Both the macromolecule and the ligand were mixed in the inner compartment,
and dialysis was performed for 26 hours at 25° C. Buffer was pH 7 Tris · HCl
0.05 M plus NaCl 0.15 M ionic strength, μ= 0.19). Radioactivity of samples
of solution from the two compartments was measured in a Packard Tricarb
model B 2450 scintillation spectrometer. RiaLuma (Lumac, Basel) was used as
the scintillation medium, and the channel ratio method was used for quenching
correction. Although radiochemical purity of the $\sqrt{14-^{14}C}$ -doxorubicin
sample was ≥98% and no specific impurity could be revealed by radiochromato-
graphic analysis, measurements involving external total drug concentration
at equilibrium (c_e values) lower than 2% of the total internal concentration
of the drug were discarded to avoid interference from trace contaminants.

The results of equilibrium dialysis experiments are presented in Figure 2,
showing the plot of r versus Log cf, the latter being deduced from the total
concentration in the external compartment corrected.. Dimerization was taken
into account to give the actual concentration of free monomeric drug. The
full line represents the best fitting curve obtained on the basis of a model
corresponding to two classes of independent binding sites. The model was
chosen as a first nonlinear approach to the treatment of the experimental
data.

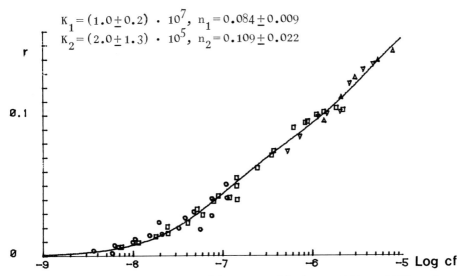

FIGURE 2. Binding curve of doxorubicin to calf-thymus DNA at different concentrations (as DNA-P): 0.93 and $1.18 \cdot 10^{-6}$M (O); 1.05, 1.02 and 1.03. 10^{-5}M (□); $0.91 \cdot 10^{-4}$M (∇); $0.88 \cdot 10^{-3}$M (Δ).

The pure visible spectrum of bound drug could be determined by measurement of the differential spectra of solutions of appropriate composition. Solutions having the same composition as the internal dialysis compartment were read against solutions having the same composition as the corresponding external compartment. The spectrum of bound drug at two different r values, the one (Figure 3A) corresponding to a point within the first half of the binding curve, the second (Figure 3B) to a point within the second half of the same, were superimposable, indicating that, at least as far as the electronic system of the chromophore is concerned, the type of drug-macromolecule interaction is probably the same (i.e., intercalation) in the whole range of r studied. A comparison of the spectrum of bound drug with that of the free monomeric and dimeric species shows the marked bathochromic shift caused by intercalation and the considerable difference between the DNA bound and the monomeric and the dimeric chromophores. Two different pathlength curvettes (5 cm and 1 cm) were used to obtain spectra shown in Figure 3C in order to allow subtraction of the contribution due to the other species to the absorption of the measured sample. As for the binding parameters derived by the nonlinear curve fitting procedure, it may be noted that the

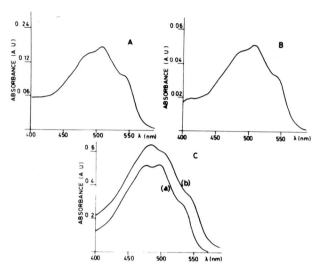

Fig 3 - ABSORPTION SPECTRA OF DNA BOUND DOXORUBICIN (A)r = 0 046, c_e = 2 76 · 10^{-7} M,
(B)r = 0.136, c_e = 5 75 · 10^{-6} M   AND (C) OF DOXORUBICIN MONOMER, 0 82 · 10^{-5} M (curve a)
AND DIMER, 3 54 · 10^{-5} M (curve b) AS OBTAINED BY DIFFERENTIAL SPECTROPHOTOMETRY

size of the binding site ($n_1 + n_2$ = 0.193) corresponding to 2.6 base pairs
is in reasonable agreement with the size deduced from X-ray crystallographic
data reported above. Available information does not allow preferences
between a model consisting of more than one independent class of binding
sites and a model consisting of a single class of binding sites with
negative cooperativity (or a model containing both features). However, we
plan to extend this investigation to other pharmacologically important
anthracyclines in order to perform more accurate comparisons with the
clinically useful compounds. On the other hand, when comparing the binding
properties of a large number of new analogs (widely different in chemical
structure and presumably in the structural and conformational details of the
corresponding DNA complex), we shall probably find other experimental schemes
not involving radiolabeled compounds to be adequate.

4. CHARACTERIZATION OF THE DNA BINDING ABILITY OF THE ANALOGS BY PHYSICO-
CHEMICAL METHODS

The use of physicochemical methods for the evaluation of DNA binding
properties of chemically modified anthracyclines has been reported in
different papers (8,12,13).

Thirty daunorubicin and doxorubicin analogs have been classified recently
(38) by apparent binding constant as measured by the equilibrium dialysis

method with 10^{-3} M (as DNA-P) being used, total ligand concentrations in
the range $7 \cdot 10^{-5}$ M to $7 \cdot 10^{-7}$ M, and the Scatchard linearization procedure
for determination of binding parameters (12,13). The classifications were
based on the affinity of the analog for calf-thymus DNA relative to that
of doxorubicin. The K_{app} values were taken as a measure of the said affinity,
and those compounds that showed K_{app} values greater than 80% the K_{app} value
of doxorubicin in identical experimental conditions were classified as
possessing a "high relative affinity." Similarly, those compounds that
showed K_{app} values in the 50% to 80% range or lower than 50% were classified
as belonging to the "intermediate" or "low relative affinity" groups,
respectively. Still unpublished results obtained according to the same
experimental procedure allowed the further classification of 10(R)-methoxy-
daunorubicin, 4'-O-acosaminyldaunorubicin in the "high," 4'-O-daunosaminyl-
daunorubicin, 7-O-(3-amino-2,3,6-trideoxy-L ribo-hexofuranosyl) daunomycinone,
11-deoxydoxorubicin in the "intermediate," and 11-deoxydaunorubicin in the
"low relative affinity" group.

Viscometry as a useful technique for the study of DNA binding properties
of the antitumor anthracyclines has received considerable attention, notwith-
standing an awareness of the complexity and an incomplete knowledge of the
relationships between viscosity and the structural or conformational features
of biopolymer molecules in solution. From the results of different investigations, researchers have been able to establish a relationship between
the formation of an intercalation complex and the enhancement of viscosity
of DNA solutions as evaluated, using the low shear rate viscometers now
commercially available (8,39,40). Tables 2 to 5 show the effects of
anthracycline derivatives on the specific measured viscosity of native
calf-thymus DNA prepared according to the method of Zamenhoff (41). Drug
concentrations were $5.2 \cdot 10^{-5}$ M and DNA was $5.2 \cdot 10^{-4}$ M as DNA-P. Data are
expressed as ratios of specific viscosities of treated (η'sp) and untreated
(ηsp) DNA, measurements being performed at 25° C with a Zimm-Crothers low
shear viscometer (shear stress $3.5 \cdot 10^{-3}$ dyne/cm^2).

With the exception of the L-ribo isomer of doxorubicin and of doxorubicinol, all compounds classified in the "high relative affinity" group,
in the experimental conditions used, increased by a factor greater than 1.9
the specific viscosity of DNA. In the "intermediate relative affinity"
group, the enhancement of DNA viscosity has been expressed by a factor in
the range of 1.51 to 2.01, with the exception of 9,10-anhydrodaunorubicin,

Table 2. Effect of anthracycline derivatives belonging
to the "high relative affinity" group on spe-
cific viscosity of $0.52 \cdot 10^{-3}\underline{M}$ (as DNA-P) native
calf-thymus DNA

Compound $(5.2 \cdot 10^{-5}\underline{M})$	η'_{sp}/η_{sp}
10(R)-methoxydaunorubicin	2.47
4-Demethoxydaunorubicin	2.33
Daunorubicin	2.16
Doxorubicin	2.03
4'-Deoxydoxorubicin	2.03
4'-Epidoxorubicin	1.90
3',4'-Diepidoxorubicin	1.83
13-Dihydrodoxorubicin (doxorubicinol)	1.75

Table 3. Effect of anthracycline derivatives belonging
to the "intermediate relative affinity" group
on specific viscosity of $0.52 \cdot 10^{-3}\underline{M}$ (as DNA-P)
native calf-thymus DNA

Compound $(5.2 \cdot 10^{-5}\underline{M})$	η'_{sp}/η_{sp}
9-Deoxydoxorubicin	2.01
9-Deoxydaunorubicin	2.01
4'-O-Methyldaunorubicin	2.01
Doxorubicin, 14-O-glycolate	1.89
4'-O-Methyldoxorubicin	1.88
3',4'-Diepidaunorubicin	1.88
7-O-(3-Amino-2,3,6-trideoxy-α-$\underline{L}$-ribo-hexofuranosyl)-daunomycinone	1.82
4'-Daunosaminyldaunorubicin	1.81
14-Morpholinodaunorubicin	1.73
3',4'-Diepi-6'-hydroxydaunorubicin	1.70
11-Deoxydoxorubicin	1.54
9-Deacetyldaunorubicin	1.51
9,10-Anhydrodaunorubicin	1.20

Table 4. Effect of anthracycline derivatives belonging
to the "low relative affinity" group on viscosity of calf-thymus DNA

Compound	η'_{sp}/η_{sp}
4'-Epi-4'-O-methyldaunorubicin	1.80
11-Deoxydaunorubicin	1.62
3'-Epi-daunorubicin	1.60
3',4'-Diepi-6'-hydroxydoxorubicin	1.55
1'-Epidoxorubicin	1.43
9-Deacetyl-9-epidaunorubicin	1.42
N-Acetyldoxorubicin	1.18

Table 5. Effect of anthracycline derivatives of unknown affinity for DNA on viscosity of calf-
thymus DNA

Compound	η'_{sp}/η_{sp}
10(R)-Methoxydoxorubicin	3.42
3'-Epi-6'-hydroxydaunorubicin	2.37
10(S)-Methoxydaunorubicin	1.47
N-Acetyldaunorubicin	1.16

which displayed a very small effect. The effect on DNA viscosity shown by
compounds classified in the "low relative affinity" group was lower than that
shown by the majority of derivatives of the "intermediate relative affinity"
group with the exception of a 4'-O-methyl derivative whose $\eta'sp/\eta sp$ value
was comparable with the average value of those of the preceding group. From
these observations we may deduce that a classification based on the K_{app}
values is generally confirmed by the rheological measurements (Figure 4),
the latter allowing a differentiation of the analogs within each group.
Whether this differentiation was caused by inappropriate classification
of some analogs or by diversified structures of the different DNA complex
remains to be established.

84

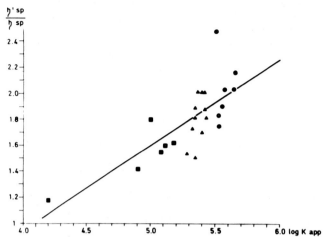

Fig 4 - PLOT OF η'_{sp}/η_{sp} VALUES (SEE TABLES 3 TO 5) VS LOG K_{app} OF DIFFERENT ANTHRACYCLINES DETERMINATED AT IONIC STRENGTH I = 0.196 (Arlandini et al., 1977 and 1980; Penco et al.,1977 and unpublished data from Authors laboratory). COMPOUNDS ARE DIVIDED IN THE "HIGH"(●),"INTERMEDIATE"(▲) AND "LOW"(■) "RELATIVE AFFINITY" GROUPS. CORRELATION FACTOR FOR LINEAR REGRESSION: 0.75.

REFERENCES

1. Di Marco A, Arcamone F, Zunino F. 1974. Vol. 3, pp 101-128 in: "Antibiotics" (Corcoran JW and Hahn FE, Eds), Springer Verlag, Berlin, Heidelberg, New York.
2. Di Marco A. 1975. Cancer Chemother. Rep. 6, 91.
3. Di Marco A, Arcamone F. 1975. pp 11-24 in "Adriamycin review" (M. Staquet et al. Eds.), European Press Medikon, Ghent, Belgium.
4. Arcamone F. 1981. Vol. 17 Med. Chemistry Series, Academic Press, N.Y.
5. Calendi E, Di Marco A, Reggiani M, Scarpinato MB, Valentini L. 1965. Biochem. Biophys. Acta, 103, 25.
6. Neidle S. 1978. Vol. II part D, pp 240-278 in "Topics in Antibiotic Chemistry" (P. Sammers, Ed.), Ellis Horwood Ltd., Chichester.
7. Arcamone F. 1978. see ref. 6 pp 100-239.
8. Zunino F, Gambetta R, Di Marco A, Zaccara A. 1972. Biochim. Biophys. Acta, 277, 489.
9. Di Marco A, Casazza AM, Gambetta R, Supino R, Zunino F. 1976. Cancer Res., 36, 1962.
10. Di Marco A, Casazza AM, Dasdia T, Necco A, Pratesi G, Rivolta P, Velcich A, Zaccara A, Zunino F. 1977. Chem. Biol. Interactions 19, 291.
11. Tsou KC, Yip KF. 1976. Cancer Res., 36, 3367.
12. Arlandini E, Vigevani A, Arcamone F. 1977. Il Farmaco, Ed. Sci. 32, 315.
13. Arlandini E, Vigevani A, Arcamone F. 1980. Il Farmaco, Ed. Sci. 35, 65.
14. Byrn SR, Dolch GD. 1978. J. Pharm. Sci. 67, 688.
15. Plumbridge TW, Brown JR. 1979. Biochim. Biophys. Acta 563, 181.
16. Schneider YJ, Baurain R, Zenebergh A, Trouet A. 1979. Cancer Chemother. Pharmacol. 2, 7.
17. Duvernay VH, Pachter JA, Crooke ST. 1979. Biochemistry, 18, 4024.
18. Barthelemy-Clavey V, Maurizot JC, Sicard PJ. 1973. Biochemie, 55, 859.
19. Zunino F, Gambetta R, Di Marco A, Luoni G, Zaccara A. 1976. Biochim. Biophys. Res. Comm., 69, 744.

20. Parr GD, McNulty H. 1978. J. Pharm. Pharmacol. 31, 65P.
21. Molinier-Jumel C, Malfoy B, Reynaud JA, Aubel-Sadron G. 1978. Bioch. Biophys. Res. Comm. 84, 441.
22. Schütz H, Gollmick FA, Stutter E. 1979. Studia Biophysica 75, 147.
23. Angiuli R, Foresti E, Riva di Sanseverino L, Isaacs NW, Kennard O, Motherwell WDS, Wampler DL, Arcamone F. 1971. Nature New Biol. 234, 78.
24. Neidle S, Taylor G. 1977. Biochim. Biophys. Acta 479, 450.
25. Courseille C, Busetta B, Geoffre S, Hospital M. 1979. Acta Cristallographica 35 B, 364.
26. Quigley GJ, Wang AGJ, Ughetto G. 1980. Proc. Natl. Acad. Sci. USA 77, 7204.
27. Pigram WJ, Fuller W, Hamilton LD. 1972. Nature New Biol. 235, 17.
28. Neidle S, Taylor L. 1979. Febs Letters 107, 348.
29. Patel DJ, Canuel LL. 1978. Eur. J. Biochem. 90, 247.
30. Patel DJ. 1979. Biopolymers 18, 553.
31. Patel DJ, Kozlowski SA, Rice JA. Proc. Natl. Acad. Sci. USA, in press.
32. Phillips DR, Roberts GCK. 1980. Biochemistry 19, 4795.
33. Barthelemy-Clavey V, Maurizot JC, Dimicoli JL, Sicard P. 1974. Febs Letters 46, 5.
34. Crescenzi V, Quadrifoglio F. 1975. In: Polyelectrolytes and their Applications (Rembaum A, Sélègny E, Eds.) pp 217-220.
35. Eksborg S. 1978. J. Chromatogr. 10, 638.
36. Martin SR. 1980. Biopolymers 19, 713.
37. Goormachtigh E, Chatelain P, Caspers J, Ruysschaert JM. 1980. Biochim. Biophys. Acta 597, 1.
38. Arcamone F. 1981. Paper presented at the Symposium on Anthracyclines, Paris, June 24-25, 1981.
39. Saucier JM, Festy B, Le Pecq JB. 1971. Biochimie 53, 973.
40. Gabbay EJ. 1976. Quantum Biology Symp. No. 3, 217.
41. Zamenhoff S. 1958. In: "Biochemical Preparations" (Westling C, Ed.), Vol. 6, p. 8, Wiley, New York.

CONSEQUENCES OF DNA INTERCALATION: PROTEIN-ASSOCIATED DNA
STRAND BREAKS

K.W. KOHN AND L.A. ZWELLING

1. INTRODUCTION

The intercalation complex of anthracyclines and DNA,
previously inferred on the basis of hydrodynamic and optical
measurements (1, 2), has recently been given a detailed
structural representation by X-ray diffraction analysis (3).
A general effect of intercalation is a reduction of winding of
the DNA helix. The unwinding angle for daunorubicin (DNR)[*]
was estimated from solution studies on superhelical DNA to be
near 11°. The X-ray diffraction structure of Quigley et al.
(3) yielded a value of 8°, which is in reasonable agreement
with the solution studies, but much less than the value of 26°
for simple intercalators such as ethidium. A surprising
feature of the X-ray structure was that the unwinding by DNR
does not occur between the base pairs immediately on either
side of the intercalator, but rather is associated with the
base pairs one removed from the intercalator. The unwinding
effect of intercalation in DNA in intact cells would be
expected to distort chromatin structure and could bring into
play the action of topoisomerase enzymes which could relieve
the distortion.

This article concerns the formation in intercalator-treated
cells of DNA "lesions" that may be a representation of
topoisomerase action. The therapeutically most significant
question is whether these "lesions" help or detract (or neither)

---

[*] Abbreviations: SSB, single-strand break; DSB, double-strand
break; DPC, DNA-protein crosslink; ADR, adriamycin; DNR,
daunorubicin; 5imDNR, 5-imino-daunorubicin; m-AMSA, 4'-(9-
acridinylamino)-methanesulfon-m-anisidide.

from the ability of cells to survive intercalator action. A
second question is whether the formation of these "lesions" in
cells can serve as a useful indicator of drug action.

2. SINGLE-STRAND BREAKS (SSB) AND DNA-PROTEIN CROSSLINKS (DPC)

Measurements of DNA single-strand size by alkaline sedimentation had indicated that treatment of mammalian cells with ADR
leads to the formation of SSB's (4, 5). However, when analogous
studies were carried out using the alkaline elution method (6,
7), no SSB's were at first detected (8). This was surprising,
because the alkaline elution procedure was at least 5 times
as sensitive as alkaline sedimentation in detecting SSB's
caused by X-ray. In the alkaline elution procedure, DNA single-
strands elute from filters at an average rate that increases
as strand length decreases. The polyvinylchloride filters that
were used in these assays, however, also have the property of
adsorbing protein molecules; if the drug treatment caused DPC's,
as well as SSB's, the elution of DNA single-strand segments
could be prevented (9). Alkaline elution assays were therefore also performed using proteinase K to remove DPC's. Using
proteinase K, the presence of SSB's in ADR-treated cells was
readily demonstrated (8).

Typical results are illustrated in figure 1. In the assays
without proteinase K (left panel), ADR caused no significant
increase in DNA elution compared to untreated cells, whereas
the SSB's produced by 300 R of X-ray caused a large increase
in elution rate. The effect of X-ray on DNA elution in ADR-
treated cells, however, was reduced; the assays with proteinase
K (right panel) indicate that this was due to the formation of
DPC's. Proteinase K produced little change in the DNA elution
of control cells or of X-irradiated cells. In the ADR-treated
cells, however, there was a large increase in DNA elution.
Furthermore, the combined treatment with ADR followed by 300 R
now gave an additive effect on elution rate. (ADR alone
produced an effect comparable to 300 R, and the combined
treatment produced an effect comparable to 600 R.)

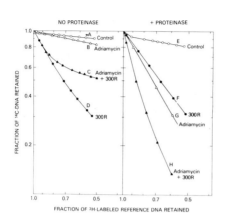 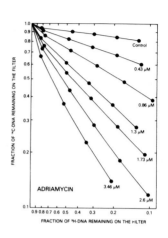

FIGURE 1   FIGURE 2

FIGURE 1. Effects of ADR on DNA in mouse leukemia Ll210 cells. Cells, prelabeled with ^{14}C-thymidine, were exposed to 2.8 μM ADR for 1 hr. Following removal of drug, the cells were (when indicated) exposed to 300 R of X-ray at ice temperature. The cells were then deposited on 2 μm pore-size polyvinylchloride filters, washed with phosphate-buffered saline, lysed with 0.2% Sarkosyl, 2 M NaCl, 0.04 M EDTA (pH 10), and eluted with tetra-propylammonium hydroxide-0.02M EDTA (pH 12.1) at 0.04 ml/min (6, 7). As an internal standard, ^{3}H-thymidine-labeled cells, irradiated with 150 R, were mixed with the ^{14}C-labeled cells prior to deposition on the filter. The retention of ^{3}H-DNA, plotted logarithmically on the horizontal axis, serves as a corrected elution time scale. (The elution kinetics for X-irradiated cells are approximately first-order with respect to time, and the apparent elution rate constant is proportional to X-ray dose.) (From Ross et al. (8).)

Figure 2. Increased DNA alkaline elution produced by treatment of Ll210 cells with the indicated concentrations of ADR for 1 hr. Assays utilized proteinase K and were performed as described in figure 1, except that polycarbonate filters were used in order to further reduce protein adsorption effects, and the ^{3}H-labeled internal standard cells received 300 R of X-ray. (From Zwelling et al. (11).)

When assayed under conditions which eliminate the effects of DPC's, ADR produces a clear dose-dependent increase elution rate (10, 11) (figure 2). The SSB frequencies produced by various ADR concentrations were estimated by calibrating the elution rates relative to the effect of X-ray. Assuming an efficiency for X-ray-induced SSB's of 0.9×10^{-9} per nucleotide per rad (12), treatment with 1 μM ADR for 1 hr produced approximately 0.7 SSB per 10^7 nucleotides (1,400 SSB's per cell).

In summary, the assays with proteinase K show that ADR produces SSB's; the assays without proteinase K indicate that the ADR-induced SSB's are completely hidden by DPC's. An equal frequency of SSB's induced by X-ray, however, is only partially hidden by the DPC's. This suggests that the ADR-induced SSB's are distributed differently than X-ray-induced SSB's. Since the latter may be assumed to be randomly distributed, the distribution of the former is probably non-random

3. EQUIVALENCE AND LOCALIZATION

What is the relationship, if any, between the SSB's and DPC's produced by ADR? That there is a relationship was suggested by the finding that the ADR-induced SSB's are completely obscured by the DPC's, whereas an equivalent frequency of X-ray-induced SSB's are only partially obscured. This suggested that the ADR-induced SSB's and DPC's are localized relative to each other.

In order to pursue this question further, it was necessary to measure the frequency of DPC's, as well as SSB's. This was done by means of a modification of the alkaline elution technique, in which a relatively high dose of X-ray (3,000 R) is used to break the DNA randomly into relatively short single-strand segments (9). The segments are short enough to elute rapidly from the filter. However, those segments that are linked to protein are retained on the filter due to protein adsorption. The frequency of DPC's can then be calculated, using a simple probability model, from the fraction of the DNA retained on the filter.

The results showed that the frequencies of ADR-induced SSB's and DPC's in L1210 cells were approximately equivalent (well within a factor of 2 of each other) (10, 11). We have recently obtained similar results--i.e., SSB's requiring proteinase K to bring them out, and approximate equivalence of SSB's and DPC's--using another anthracycline, 5imDNR (13). We have encountered this equivalence between SSB's and DPC's in a sufficient variety of intercalating agents, differing widely in cytotoxicity (vide infra), to be confident that the equivalence is not an accident, but rather is a manifestation of a specific mechanism.

4. RELATIONSHIP BETWEEN SSB'S AND DPC'S.

Figure 3 shows 4 models for possible relationships between equal frequencies of SSB's and DPC's.

In A, the SSB's and DPC's are distributed randomly and independently of each other. In this model, some of the DNA single-strand segments would by chance be free of DPC's and therefore should elute even without the use of proteinase K. This is contrary to experiment; therefore, this model is excluded.

In B, one, and only one, protein molecule is linked some-where along each single-strand segment. Although this model fits the experimental data, it is difficult to envision a mechanism that would regulate a one-protein-to-one-segment relation, except by a circumstance such as model C.

Model C is a special case of model B, with a protein molecule linked to one terminus (3' or 5') of each SSB. This is an attractive model, because mechanisms of formation can readily be proposed (10).

The final alternative, D, assumes that a protein molecule bridges across each SSB. This model fits the alkaline elution data. However, contrary to models B and C, the cross-bridges would prevent the detection of SSB's by alkaline sedimentation assays in which proteinase is not used. Reduced sedimentation of DNA from ADR-treated cells has been observed (4, 5), but at relatively high drug doses which may have caused secondary breakdown of DNA in dying cells. Using the much less toxic intercalating agent, m-AMSA, which exhibits the same phenomenon

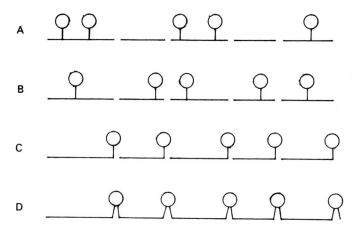

Figure 3. Possible relationship between equivalent frequencies of SSB's and DPC's.

of protein-associated strand breaks as does ADR, we have found that SSB's that were completely hidden in alkaline elution assays without proteinase were clearly visible and accounted for in alkaline sedimentation assays (11). Hence, model D is excluded, at least for some intercalating agents.

Our studies point to model C as the characteristic DNA "lesion" of intercalator-treated cells.

5. SPECIFICITY FOR INTERCALATION

Protein-associated SSB's--i.e., SSB's detected by alkaline elution only when proteinase is used, and associated with an equal frequency of DPC's--have been demonstrated in cells treated with the following intercalating agents: ADR (10, 11), ellipticine (10), m-AMSA (11), 5imDNR (13) and dihydroxy-anthracenedione (14). These compounds cover a wide range of chemical structures and cytotoxic potencies. In addition, for the following intercalating agents, proteinase-dependent SSB's were demonstrated, but DPC frequencies were not determined: actinomycin, DNR, ethidium, lucanthone (10). The non-inter-calative DNA binders, anthramycin and chromomycin, did not produce proteinase-dependent SSB's (10).

Hence protein-associated SSB's may be specific for interca-lating agents.

It has been reported, however, that ADR derivatives, such as AD32, which bear a trifluoroacetyl substitution on the sugar amino group, produce protein-associated SSB's, but fail to bind to purified DNA (15, 16). Upon incubation of AD32 with cells, no conversion to ADR was detected, although some unidentified products appeared (16). It is conceivable that the N-tri-fluoroacetyl-ADR compounds can bind to DNA in chromatin, even though there appears to be no binding to purified DNA. This possibility is conceivable in view of the X-ray structure finding (3) that, contrary to previous supposition, the sugar amino group of DNR need not be intimately associated with a particular DNA phosphate group. Thus the positive charge on the amino group, required for binding to pure DNA, may act in a more general way than by intimate ion binding, and the positive charge on the amino group may not be essential in the presence of positively charged histones.

6. DOUBLE-STRAND BREAKS (DSB)

Some of the protein-associated strand breaks produced by intercalators appear to be of the DSB variety (17). That is, SSB's sometimes exist in both strands of the DNA helix sufficiently close to each other that a double-strand cleavage occurs under non-denaturing conditions. Such DSB's can be assayed by elution from filters at pH 9.6, which is well below the pH required to separate the strands of the DNA helix (18). The assays are calibrated relative to the effect of X-ray, which also produces DSB's. However, since the efficiency of DSB production by X-ray is uncertain, we cannot at present assign precise values of DSB lesion frequencies. Nevertheless, the ratio of DSB/SSB produced by a given drug can be determined relative to the ratio produced by X-ray. On this relative scale of DSB/SSB, the effect of X-ray is assigned the value 1.0 (Table 1).

Table 1.

Agent	Relative DSB/SSB/ ratio[a]
X-ray	(1.0)
m-AMSA	1.9
actinomycin D	4.4
ADR	5.4
5imDNR	8.3
ellipticine	13.2

---

[a]Assayed by DNA elution at pH 9.6 (DSB) and pH 12.1 (SSB), each assay being calibrated relative to the effect of X-ray.

We have determined the relative values of DSB/SSB for 5 intercalating agents, including 2 anthracyclines (11, 13) (Table 1). The DSB/SSB ratios varied greatly for different intercalating agents, and were in all cases larger than for X-ray. (The ratio for ellipticine is high enough for it to be possible that all of the breaks are of the DSB type.)

The widely different DSB/SSB ratios for different inter-calators suggest that DSB's and SSB's are produced by different mechanisms.

7. KINETICS OF FORMATION AND REVERSAL

In the presence of ADR at 37°, protein-associated SSB's increased linearly for 1 hr (figure 4). At 4° or 25°, however, the formation of these SSB's was almost completely inhibited. After washing the cells to remove drug, the SSB's persisted for many hours; after 24 hr at 37°, approximately 50% of the original SSB's remained (11).

The interpretation of these results rests on the kinetics of ADR uptake and egress, as well as on the kinetics of formation and reversal of the SSB's. The nearly linear formation kinetics of SSB's at 37° (figure 4) could be due to rate-limiting uptake of ADR into mouse leukemia cells (19), and the poor reversal of the SSB's could be due to the slow and incomplete egress of the drug from the cells (19). The nearly complete inhibition of SSB formation at 25°, however, may not be due to an uptake effect, because ADR uptake in Ehrlich ascites cells was reported to have little temperature

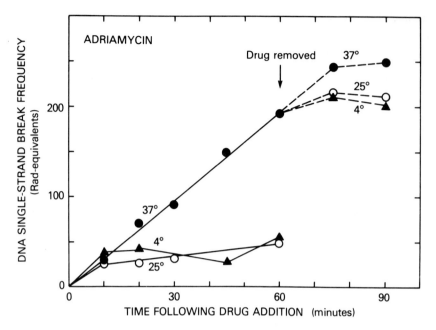

Figure 4. Kinetics of protein-associated SSB formation in
L1210 cells exposed to 3.5 μM ADR at 37° (●), 25° (o), or
4° (▲). After (60 min, arrow), the cells were washed and
resuspended in fresh media at the indicated temperatures.
(From Zwelling et al. (11).)

dependence (20).

In contrast to ADR, the protein-associated SSB's produced
by m-AMSA rise rapidly to a steady state within 10 min, and,
upon washing the cells, the SSB's disappear rapidly (within 10-
30 min) (11). Both the formation and the reversal of the m-AMSA
induced SSB's are completely inhibited at 4°. The anthracycline
5imDNR behaves in these respects like m-AMSA, although the
rates of SSB formation and reversal are somewhat slower than
in the case of m-AMSA (13). The results suggest that all 3
compounds may produce the same classes of protein-associated
DNA breaks by similar mechanisms, but that the over-all kinetics
of break formation and reversal varies with the transport
characteristics of each drug.

8. RELATION TO CYTOTOXICITY

When ADR and m-AMSA were compared at doses producing the
same frequencies of protein-associated SSB's or DSB's ADR

was found to be much more cytotoxic (1-hr drug treatment, colony-forming assay) (11). This is not surprising, in view of the persistence of ADR in the cells, as opposed to the rapid egress of m-AMSA. A more appropriate comparison, however, was obtained using 5imDNR instead of ADR, because the SSB's produced by 5imDNR reversed within 1 hr after washing the cells (13). Nevertheless, when colony survival was gauged either relative to SSB's or to DSB's, 5imDNR was still substantially more cytotoxic to L1210 cells than was m-AMSA.

These results suggest that anthracyclines, such as 5imDNR, kill cells by some mechanism unrelated to protein-associated DNA strand breaks. However, these DNA "lesions" may have cytotoxic significance in the case of other intercalators, including perhaps other anthracyclines. It is also possible that these DNA "lesions" represent a physiologic protective mechanism that allows cells to withstand DNA torsion resulting from intercalation. This possibility can be investigated by comparative studies of cell types having different sensitivities to intercalating agents.

9. SUMMARY, CONCLUSIONS, HYPOTHESES

Our evidence indicates that anthracyclines, as well as other DNA intercalating agents, produce, in mammalian cells, characteristic DNA "lesions," consisting of strand breaks associated in some specific manner with DNA-protein crosslinks. The simplest structural hypothesis consistent with the evidence is that a protein becomes covalently linked to the 3' or 5' terminus of each single-strand break. An attractive possibility is that the linked protein is, in fact, an enzyme which produces a strand break and, at the same time, becomes linked to one terminus of the break. Such a mechanism is known for topo-isomerase enzymes, which become covalently linked to the 3' terminus (21). Some topoisomerases produce single-strand breaks, whereas others produce double-strand breaks. Our finding that intercalators induce the formation of both types of breaks suggest that both types of topoisomerases can be involved. Intercalating agents would be expected to produce DNA torsional stress, due to their tendancy to unwind the DNA helix, and topoisomerases would tend to relieve this torsional stress. We hypothesize that protein-associated DNA breaks may be indicators of topoisomerase action in response to DNA intercalation, and may relieve the detrimental effects of DNA torsion produced by these drugs.

REFERENCES

1. DiMarco A, Arcamone F, Zunino F. 1974. In: Antibiotics, eds. Corcoran JW Hahn FE (Springer, Berlin). Vol. 3, pp. 101-128.
2. Neidle S. 1979. Prog. Med. Chem. 16: 151-220.
3. Quigley GJ, Wang AHJ, Ughetto G, Van der Marel G, van Boom JH, Rich A. 1980. Proc. Natl. Acad. Sci. USA 77: 7204-7208.
4. Schwartz HS. 1976. J. Medicine 7: 33-46.
5. Lee YC, Byfield JE. 1976. J. Natl. Cancer Inst. 57: 221-224.
6. Kohn KW 1979. In: Meth. Cancer Res, eds. DeVita VT & Busch H (Academic Press, New York). Vol. 16, pp. 291-345.
7. Kohn, KW, Ewig RA, Erickson LC, Zwelling LA. 1981. In: DNA Repair, A Laboratory Manual of Research Procedures, eds. Friedberg EC & Hanawalt PC (Marcel Dekker, New York). Vol. 1, part B, pp. 379-401.
8. Ross WE, Glaubiger DL, Kohn KW. 1978. Biochim. Biophys. Acta 519: 23-30.
9. Kohn KW, Ewig RA. 1979. Biochim. Biophys. Acta 562: 32-40.
10. Ross WE, Glaubiger DL, Kohn KW. 1979. Biochim. Biophys. Acta 562: 41-40.
11. Zwelling LA, Michaels S, Erickson LC, Ungerleider RS, Nichols M, Kohn KW. 1981. Biochemistry, in press.
12. Kohn KW, Erickson LC, Ewig RA, Friedman CA. 1976. Biochemistry 15: 4629-4737.
13. Zwelling LA, Kerrigan D, Michaels S. Submitted for publication.
14. Cohen LF, Glaubiger DL, Kann HE, Kohn KW. 1980. Proc. Amer. Assoc. Cancer Res. 21: 277.
15. Brox L, Gowans B, Belch A. 1980. Can. J. Biochem. 58: 720-725.
16. Levin M, Silber R, Israel M, Goldfeder A, Kherpal K, Potmesil M. 1981. Cancer Res. 41: 1006-1010.
17. Ross WE, Bradley MO, 1981. Biochim. Biophys. Acta 654: 129-135.
18. Bradley MO, Kohn KW. 1979. Nucleic Acids Res. 7: 793-804.
19. Inaba M, Johnson RK. 1978. Biochem. Pharmacol. 27: 2123-2130.
20. Skovsgaard T. 1978. Biochem. Pharmacol. 27: 1221-1227.
21. Gellert M. 1981. Ann. Rev. Biochem. 50: 879-910.

FREE RADICAL DAMAGE

N. R. BACHUR

Scientists have observed that a disproportionate number of natural products and synthetic products which contain quinone groups are cytotoxic both to tumors and to bacteria. From this vantage, proposals have been made that quinones are involved in a biochemically mediated reductive mechanism that plays a part in their cytotoxic action.

It is unlikely to be coincidental that so many of the cytotoxic natural products are quinones, and this makes a great deal of sense when the quinone ring and its chemical properties are considered from the biochemist's point of view. A quinone ring is capable of simple reversible oxidation and reduction through single electron transfer steps. Although quinones were believed to be reduced in the cell in a concerted two electron transfer to hydroquinone, it was established recently that the quinones were generally reduced _in vivo_ through single electron transfer steps so that a one electron reduced intermediate, the semiquinone, a free radical, exists. The semiquinone may be reduced to the hydroquinone in the reducing environment of the cell.

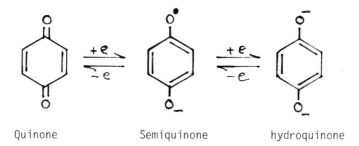

Quinone   Semiquinone   hydroquinone

Whereas the concept of a free radical mechanism involved in the mechanism of action of anthracycline antibiotics is relatively new, this concept has been applied to other antibiotic classes. Several years ago, scientists who studied the antibacterial drugs streptonigrin and mitomycin C proposed that these agents were reduced in bacteria to a free radical form which was capable of generating secondary free radicals. The secondary free radicals were speculated to be responsible for killing the target bacteria. Both mitomycin C and streptonigrin also showed activity as anticancer agents in mouse tumor screening.

Quinones are very photoactive, indicating that they have the propensity for homolytic type reactions, i.e., for free radical formation. Their ability to polymerize under light activation is classic organic chemistry. Recently, the photochemical properties of the anthracycline antibiotics have been studied with some success. This series of studies originated in the laboratory of Professor DiMarco who reported that daunorubicin and DNA formed a stable complex under UV activation and had a modified absorption spectrum (1). The DNA-daunorubicin complex resisted enzymatic digestion of the DNA by DNAse and could be isolated on silica gel chromatography. These studies demonstrated that ultraviolet irradiation activated the anthracycline molecule to produce a stable combination of the daunorubicin and DNA, presumably with the formation of a covalent bond. Subsequently, photoactivation studies of anthracyclines have been carried out by several other investigators (2,3,4). These investigators have shown that adriamycin, daunorubicin, and rubidazone form covalent bonds to DNA and produce photo-adducts which are stable to various forms of solvent extraction, ionic challenge, and acid and alkaline treatment. The drug binding is catalyzed not only by ultraviolet light but also by visible light at approximately 470 nm, which is the peak visible absorption for the anthracyclines. Isolation of the products of the photoactivation DNA reaction has yielded predominately aglycones; deoxyaglycone type structures with loss of the 9-position acetyl group as well as drug polymers which are presumed an inactive species. Another interesting observation has been that hydrogen peroxide is produced with UV irradiation of daunorubicin. This is another indication that oxygen is interacting with the anthracycline structure and undergoing redox reactions presumably through homolytic type reactions which produce free radical intermediates.

Besides the photochemical reactions that have been described with anthracyclines alone or with anthracyclines and macromolecules such as DNA, there is photodynamic action of the anthracyclines to react with DNA of bacterial and animal viruses, with resultant inactivation of these viruses (5).

These chemical and photochemical characteristics of the anthracycline antibiotics indicate that these molecules possess a high degree of reactivity through homolytic type reactions; through free radical reactions that are the realm of photochemistry. In determining the unique chemical properties of the anthracycline ring systems and the biochemical properties of this planar ring system, we will be lead to an understanding of the total mechanisms of action of anthracycline antibiotics.

Of course, the planar ring system also lends itself to other characteristics in the biological system. Anthracyclines are clearly intercalating agents which bind in a very neat fit between stacked bases of double helical DNA. This characteristic has been reported extensively as the primary mode of action of the anthracycline antibiotics through the inhibition of DNA bioprocessing. Certainly, the hydrophobic and charged nature of the planar ring system would also lead to binding to other parts in the cell besides the intercalative region between stacked base pairs.

It was with the concept of the reactivity of the anthracycline system that our laboratory approached the problem of understanding what occurs at a molecular level with the anthracycline antibiotics. Although we can simply state that the anthracycline system is a fine recipient of a single electron and is converted to a free radical intermediate which can then pass on its electron, our experimental data indicate that the free radical reactions of anthracyclines are very complex. It is for this reason of complexity that we are forced to understand that anthracyclines are not simply quinones that enter the cell and short-circuit the electron transfer system. Rather the anthracycline antibiotics are very intricate and delicately sculpted molecules which have the potential for numerous reactions. This will be discussed further in other chapters that describe the structure-activity relationships of many of the anthracycline antibiotic systems.

In our study of the biochemical free radical production in the cell, we were concerned with the modes by which anthracyclines were activated to free radical state. Perhaps in controlling the activation process we may be able to modify drug action.

Various organelles in the cell possess the capability of free radical production with anthracyclines. From our studies, we find that microsomes have the highest specific activity for free radical production followed by nuclei and mitochondria (6,7). There may be a problem with the permeability of the anthracycline through the mitochondrial membrane and the availability of pyridine nucleotides inside the mitochondria for sufficient reduction of anthracyclines. For the production of anthracycline free radicals, the organelles require reduced pyridine nucleotide as electron donor such as NADPH.

Microsomes from all tested tissues of rats and mice as well as nuclei from rat and mice cells show capability of free radical production from the anthracycines, although at different rates and specific activities. Our limited investigation of malignant cells and free radical production indicates that their microsomes have a high rate of free radical production. However, precise quantitative estimates have not yet been done.

From our experimental data the enzymes that reside in nuclei, mitochondria, and microsomes which catalyze the production of anthracycline free radicals are primarily flavoproteins, operating through the reduction pathway (8). Although it is conceivable that anthracycline free radicals can be obtained through an oxidative pathway we have not seen that occur. NADPH cytochrome P450 reductase which is found both in the microsome and nuclear membranes, has the highest activity for catalysis of anthracycline free radical reduction. This enzyme requires NADPH, and is presumably the major enzyme operating _in vivo_. Other flavoproteins which catalyze the formation of the free radical intermediates are xanthine oxidase, which was isolated from bovine milk, nitrate reductase and NADH cytochrome C reductase.

Once the anthracycline free radicals are formed, the question arises what type radical damage could occur to produce the cytotoxicity within the cell. The type which was heralded most by previous scientists has been what I call "secondary" form of free radical, i.e., free radicals such as superoxide or hydroxyl radical generated by the anthracycline free radical (9). These "secondary" free radicals can react with intracellular target and damage or destroy macromolecules. Evidence for this type of reaction has been demonstrated previously within other systems and is shown by the studies of Berlin and Hazeltine in collaboration with our laboratory (10). Using purified NADPH cytochrome P450 reductase system, Berlin and Hazeltine activated anthracycline in the presence of known sequence, labeled plasmid DNA. A large amount of cleavage occurred under these conditions very early in the reaction and was associated with the presence of oxygen. The complete enzymatic system was required to demonstrate DNA breakage; reduced pyridine nucleotide, the anthracycline, and the active enzyme as well as oxygen. When the oxygen in the reaction mixture was consumed, the DNA breakage stopped. In addition, when these reactions were run under anaerobic conditions, no DNA cleavage or minimal DNA cleavage was observed. From these experiments oxygen necessary in this system for the DNA breakage. Not only is double-stranded D broken, but single-stranded DNA is an excellent substrate for the cleavage reaction which minimizes the need for drug intercalation. This study yields clear evidence that the anthracyclines are activating oxygen presumably to superoxide and/or to hydroxyl radical level. The hydroxyl radical is presumably a more effective reactant than superoxide and would be the more likely candidate for DNA breakage. There may be something special about the anthracycline types of quinones that activate oxygen very specifically to high energy radicals.

Besides the propensity of the anthracyclines to produce active oxygen, the early studies of Schwartz and others who worked with other quinone antibiotics such as the mitomycins pointed to the production of activated quinone molecules. These very elaborate molecules react directly in addition to transferring electron to oxygen, and they yield additional types of reactions such as seen with the photo adducts of anthracyclines to DNA. The anthracycline structure is very specific; and although there are variations among anthracyclines which show interesting differences in mode of action, length of action, in selectivity to cells, and in toxicity and efficacy, a common uniting structural feature among all of the anthracyclines is their quinone system. Reduction of the anthracycline molecules yields a primary free radical that may react with intracellular macromolecules such as DNA. Evidence for the retention of anthracycline molecules in vivo dates back quite a few years when we demonstrated that radioactive daunorubicin would bind to acid insoluble tissue residue which resisted liberation by organic solvent and acid washing (11). This was our first suggestion that anthracyclines may bind irreversibly to tissue components, although at that time we were not aware of the mechanism by which this may occur. Subsequently, other scientists have shown anthracyclines to bind to tissue components. Most recently, investigators at Mario Negri, Milan, have shown radioactive adriamycin binds to microsomal protein on activation presumably through the free radical mechanism (12).

The work coming from the Yale laboratories of Dr. Sartorelli one of the pioneers in the concept of reductive alkylation applies to the anthracyclines. They have shown that adriamycin is much more effective against tissue cultured cells under hypoxic conditions (13). This is of course, a very complicated experiment to interpret; however, when compared to other types of agents, adriamycin works more effectively in the absence of oxygen. In these cells it appears that oxygen may interfere with adriamycin action. It may be acting as a scavenger to deactivate adriamycin radicals.

Anthracycline molecules are unique. They have a high degree of homolytic type reactivity. They are readily activated in biochemical systems, and they produce secondary free radicals that can damage DNA or other macromolecules. In addition, they may react directly as free radicals with macromolecules for which they were tailored by nature as very effective cytotoxic weapons.

It is clear that the anthracyclines are not just quinones. Although many quinones are cytotoxic against bacteria and other cells, the anthracyclines are very specific quinone molecules. They have been tailored over the eons of time in nature, and they have been designed to be very effective killing agents for the streptomyces. I would be surprised if the anthracyclines acted only in one mode. Rather, I suspect that they operate at several levels. For a microorganism it might be advantageous to have a toxin which is mounting an attack requiring its defenses against two or more different modes of action. We know anthracyclines can act by binding to DNA and inhibiting DNA processing. I propose that anthracyclines also produce primary radicals which are specifically tailored to damage cells at a specific locale, and secondary radicals which are cytotoxic through oxygen and perhaps other acceptor molecules at the specific site where protective mechanisms may be sparse or absent.

REFERENCES

1. Di Marco A, Zunino F, Orezzi P, Gambetta RA. 1972. Experimentia 28: 32?
2. Daugherty JP, Hixon SC, Yielding KL. 1979. Biochem. Biophys. Acta 565:?
3. Grey PJ, Phillips DR. 1980. Photochemistry and Photobiology 32: 621.
4. Williams BA, Tritton TR. 1981. Photochemistry and Photobiology 34: 131.
5. Sanfilippo A, Schioppacassi G, Morvillo M, Ghione M. 1968. J. Microbiol. 16: 49.
6. Bachur NR, Gordon SL, Gee M. 1977. Molec. Pharmacol. 13: 901.
7. Bachur NR, Friedman RD, Gee M. 1979. Proc. AACR 20: 128.
8. Pan S, Pedersen L, Bachur NR. 1981. Molec. Pharmacol. 19: 184.
9. Myers CE, McGuire WP, Liss RH, Iffim I, Grotzonger K, Young RC. 1977. Science 197: 165.
10. Berlin V, Haseltine WA. 1981. J. Biol. Chem. 256: 4747.
11. Bachur NR, Moore AL, Bernstein JG, Liu A. 1970. Cancer Chemother. Rep. 54: 89.
12. Ghezzi P, Donelli MG, Pantarotto C, Faccinetti T, Garattini S. 1981. Biochem. Pharmacol. 30: 175.
13. Teicher BA, Lazo JS, Sartorelli A. 1981. Cancer Res. 41: 73.

INTRACELLULAR, INTRANUCLEAR, AND SUBCHROMOSOMAL LOCALIZATION
OF ANTHRACYCLINE ANTIBIOTICS

M. ROBERT-NICOUD AND N. BACHUR

1. INTRODUCTION

Although it is generally accepted that the anthracycline
antibiotics exert their antineoplastic action by interacting
directly with the genetic material through DNA binding, hence
inhibiting such processes as DNA replication, transcription,
and repair mechanisms, studies on their mode of interaction
with nucleic acids have not provided satisfactory explanations
for the differences observed in the therapeutic efficiency
and spectrum of action of the various compounds; even new
analogs and derivatives which display differing nuclear and
DNA binding properties cannot have their characteristics
reconciled with their cytotoxic activity (1-5).

This poor understanding is partly due to the difficulties
encountered in attempting to follow in vivo the exact sequence
of events that occur after administration of the drugs, and to
the fact that results obtained in vitro may not reflect the in
vivo situation. In particular, numerous in vitro studies on the
interaction of anthracyclines with nucleic acids have neglected
the fact that, in the cell nucleus, the DNA is not present in a
naked state, but forms nucleoprotein complexes arranged in chromosomal substructures at various levels of their supramolecular
organization (6). This fact may prove to be critical to the differences seen among the various anthracycline antibiotics. Moreover, the ionic milieu surrounding the chromosomes is known to
affect their structural and functional state (7,8), and it is
expected that ions also drastically influence the interactions of
the drugs with chromosomal components (9). Therefore, in vitro
experiments should be carried out under conditions as close as
possible to the physiological ones.

The polytene chromosomes found in dipteran larvae, due to their size and their structural and functional characteristics, provide a unique opportunity to investigate in situ the intra-nuclear and subchromosomal distribution of anthracycline anti-biotics by means of fluorescence microscopy and autoradiography. These giant chromosomes are composed of thousands of chromatids arranged in a cablelike structure up to 200 μm in length and 10 μm in diameter (Fig. 1). The close juxtaposition of the homologous chromomeres accounts for the formation of the typical banding pattern which is a constant feature of the chromosomes and allows an easy recognition of chromosomal loci (10). A further advantage of the giant chromosomes is that gene activity is detectable under the microscope by morphological criteria; inactive bands are in a condensed state while active bands decondense to form puffs which, as shown by autoradiography, are sites of RNA synthesis (11). Moreover, techniques are available for the isolation of unfixed polytene nuclei and chromosomes which render possible studies on the direct action of drugs on their structural and functional state (12).

We have investigated the distribution of anthracycline anti-biotics with different molecular structures in explanted sali-vary glands of the midge Chironomus thummi as well as their binding properties in isolated polytene nuclei by means of fluorescence microscopy and autoradiography. Furthermore, in order to enable us to interprete more accurately the results of our microscopic observations, we have examined the effects of various chromosomal components on the fluorescence properties of the drugs.

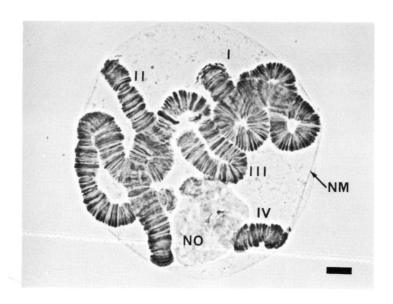

FIGURE 1. Isolated salivary gland nucleus of <u>Chironomus</u>
<u>thummi</u>. Aceto-orcein squash. I-IV: polytene chromosomes,
NO: nucleolus, NM: nuclear membrane. Magn.: bar denotes 10 μm.

2. MATERIAL AND METHODS

2.1. Explanted salivary glands

Salivary glands were explanted from 4th instar larvae of
<u>Chironomus thummi</u> and incubated with anthracyclines ($0.5 \cdot 10^{-4}\underline{M}$)
dissolved in insect saline (87 m$\underline{M}$ NaCl, 3,2 m$\underline{M}$ KCl, 1,3 m$\underline{M}$
CaCl$_2$, 1 m$\underline{M}$ MgCl$_2$ and 10 m$\underline{M}$ Tris-HCl pH 7,3). After periods
of incubation varying from 15 min to 2 hr the glands were
washed in saline solution and examined in the fluorescence
microscope without fixation.

2.2. Isolated polytene nuclei

Unfixed polytene nuclei were isolated from explanted salivary glands by the technique of Robert (12). The isolated
nuclei were incubated with anthracyclines ($0.5 \cdot 10^{-4}\underline{M}$) dissolved
in insect saline. After periods of incubation varying from
15 min to 2 hr, the nuclei were washed in saline solution,
gently squashed and examined in the fluorescence microscope
without fixation.

2.3. Fluorescence microscopy

A Zeiss fluorescence photomicroscope was used for the observation of explanted salivary glands and isolated nuclei. The light source was a high pressure mercury lamp and the filter combination used in most cases was: BG 12, Zeiss 44 & 53.

2.4. Autoradiography

Tritiated daunomycin (New England Nuclear) with a specific activity of 2.3 Ci/mM was used in this study. Explanted salivary glands and isolated nuclei were incubated with ^{3}H-daunomycin dissolved in insect saline for periods varying from 15 min to 2 hr. They were then washed in saline solution, fixed in 45 % acetic acid, stained in aceto-orcein and squashed The preparations were washed in ethanol for 1 hr, postfixed in formalin and processed for autoradiography. A liquid emulsion (Kodak NTB 2) was used and the exposition time was 2 weeks.

2.5 Isolated chromatin, DNA, RNA and chromosomal proteins

Chromatin and DNA were isolated from calf thymus according to the techniques described by Rubin and Moudrianakis (13). RNA was high molecular weight yeast RNA (pA) purchased from Serva, Heidelberg. Histones were obtained from calf thymus chromatin by salt extraction according to Eickbush et al. (14).

2.6. Fluorescence quenching

Fluorescence intensity was measured in an Aminco fluorescence spectrophotometer. The measurements were made at excitation and emission wave lengths optimal for the various compounds tested. Chromosomal components and the drugs were dissolved in solutions of low ionic strength (1 mM Tris-HCl, pH 7.8).

2.7. Drugs

All drugs, except 7-O-methyl nogarol, were obtained from the Developmental Therapeutics Program, National Cancer Institute N.I.H., Bethesda, Maryland. 7-O-methyl nogarol was provided by the Upjohn Company, Kalamazoo, Michigan.

3. RESULTS

3.1. Distribution of anthracyclines in explanted salivary glands

Explanted salivary glands incubated in the presence of anthracycline antibiotics display two basic patterns of fluorescence distribution, nuclear and cytoplasmic.

In the case of daunomycin, N,N-dimethyl daunomycin and adriamycin, the characteristic red-orange fluorescence of the antibiotics is found located primarily in the cell nucleus, the fluorescence intensity in the cytoplasm being lowest for adriamycin (Fig. 2A; Table 1). Inside the nuclei, the fluorescence is associated with the chromosomes and, to a lesser extent, with the nucleolus.

On the other hand, after incubation of explanted salivary glands with aclacinomycin, carminomycin and 7-O-methyl nogarol, the fluorescence is found mainly in the cytoplasm while little or no fluorescence is detectable inside the nucleus (Fig. 2B; Table 1).

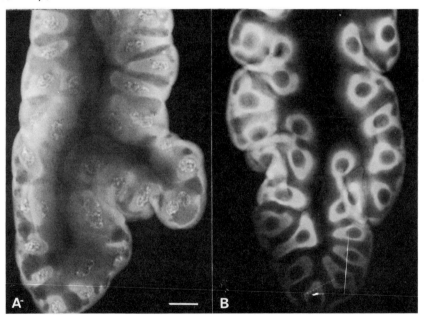

FIGURE 2. Anthracycline fluorescence pattern in explanted salivary glands after incubation with A) adriamycin and B) carminomycin. Drug concentration: $0.5 \cdot 10^{-4}$ M. Magn.: bar denotes 100 μm.

Table 1. Fluorescence distribution patterns of anthracyclines in explanted salivary glands and isolated polytene nuclei of <u>Chironomus thummi</u>.

| | Fluorescence intensity in: | | | |
| | A) Explanted salivary glands | | B) Isolated polytene nuclei | |
	cytoplasm	nuclei	chromosomes	nucleolus
Daunomycin	+ −	+	+	+ −
N,N-dimethyl daunomycin	+ −	+	+	+ −
Adriamycin	−	+ +	+ +	+
Aclacinomycin	+ +	−	−	−
Carminomycin	+ +	−	−	−
7-O-methyl nogarol	+ +	+ −	−	+ −

3.2. <u>Distribution of anthracyclines in isolated polytene nuclei</u>

Isolated salivary gland nuclei behave in a similar manner as nuclei <u>in situ.</u> After incubation in the presence of daunomycin, <u>N,N</u>-dimethyl daunomycin and adriamycin, a strong fluorescence can be observed inside the nuclei, associated with the chromosomes and, to a variable extent, with the nucleolus (Fig. 3; Table 1), the intensity of the nucleolar fluorescence being highest in the case of adriamycin. The fluorescence banding pattern displayed by the chromosomes corresponds to the banding pattern observed with phase contrast optics; however, a particularly intensive fluorescence can be observed in the heterochromatic regions associated with the centromeres of the chromosomes I − III (Fig.3).

On the other hand, after incubation of isolated salivary gland nuclei in the presence of aclacinomycin, carminomycin and 7-O-methyl nogarol, no or only low intensity fluorescence can be seen over chromosomal and nucleolar regions. In the case of 7-O-methyl nogarol, a preferential localization of fluorescence in the nucleolus is detectable.

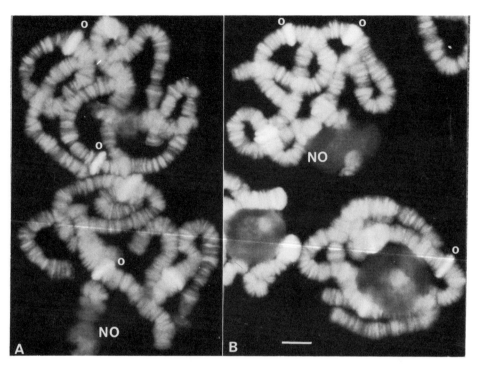

FIGURE 3. Anthracycline fluorescence patterns in isolated
unfixed salivary gland nuclei after incubation with A) daunomycin and B) adriamycin. Drug concentration: $0.5 \cdot 10^{-4}$M.
Magn.: bar denotes 20 μm. NO: nucleolus, o: centromeres.

3.3. Nucleic acid- and protein- mediated effects on the fluorescence of anthracyclines

Spectrofluorometric measurements of the fluorescence intensity of anthracycline antibiotics in the presence of nucleic
acids and chromosomal proteins demonstrate that purified DNA
and, to a lesser extent, isolated chromatin drastically reduce
the fluorescence intensity of the drugs, as shown in Fig. 4
in the case of daunomycin. The degree of quenching mediated
by RNA is lower and, on the other hand, addition of chromosomal proteins results in a slight increase of the fluorescence
intensity (Fig. 4).

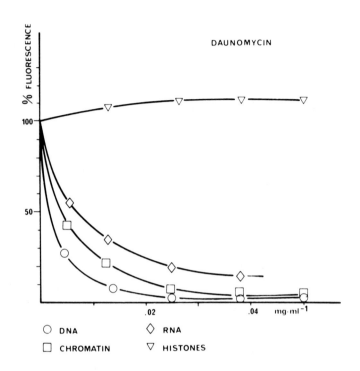

FIGURE 4. Nucleic acid- and protein- mediated effects on the fluorescence of daunomycin. The fluorescence intensity is expressed as a % of the value obtained for a solution of free drug. Drug concentration: 10^{-5} $\underline{M}$.

The degree of quenching mediated by nucleic acids differs depending on the molecular structure of the antibiotic tested. In the presence of DNA, it is maximal for carminomycin and decreases in the order carminomycin > aclacinomycin ≃ daunomycin > N,N-dimethyl daunomycin > 7-O-methyl nogarol > adriamycin (Fig. 5). The sequence is different in the case of RNA; here, the degree of quenching decreases in the order carminomycin > adriamycin ≃ daunomycin > N,N-dimethyl daunomycin > 7-O-methyl nogarol > aclacinomycin (Fig. 6).

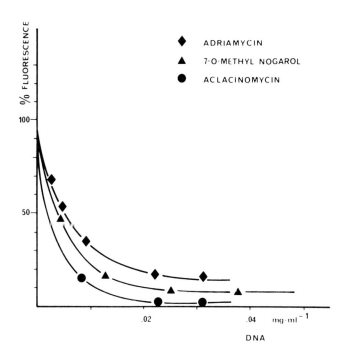

FIGURE 5. DNA-mediated quenching of the anthracyclines fluorescence. The fluorescence intensity is expressed as % of the
value obtained for a solution of free drug. Drug concentration:
10^{-5} M.

It should be pointed out here that these measurements were
made under unphysiological ionic conditions (low ionic strength).
Further experiments, not described here, have shown that the
ionic environment, in particular divalent cations, strongly
influences the degree of quenching mediated by chromosomal
components. Unfortunately, under physiological ionic conditions, the chromatin assumes a condensed state and light
scattering effects render any accurate measurement of the
fluorescence intensity difficult.

112

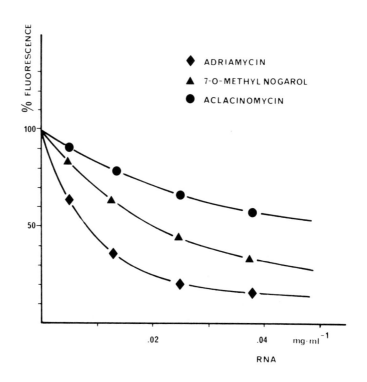

FIGURE 6. RNA-mediated quenching of the anthracyclines fluorescence. The fluorescence intensity is expressed as % of the
value obtained for a solution of free drug. Drug concentration:
10^{-5} M.

3.4. Autoradiographic studies on the distribution of ^{3}H-dauno-mycin in isolated salivary gland nuclei

Isolated salivary gland nuclei incubated in the presence
of tritiated daunomycin and processed for autoradiography display a distribution of silver grains over most chromosomal
regions (Fig. 7). A particularly intensive incorporation of
radioactive drug molecules can be observed in the nucleolus
organizer region located on chromosome IV.

Unfortunately, no comparison with the distribution patterns
of other anthracycline compounds could be made in this study
since only ^{3}H-daunomycin was available to us.

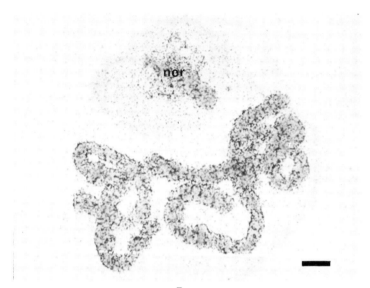

FIGURE 7. Incorporation of ^{3}H-daunomycin into isolated salivary gland nuclei. Autoradiography. nor: nucleolus organizer
region of chromosome IV. Magn.: bar denotes 20 µm.

4. DISCUSSION

Insect larval organs with polytene chromosomes provide a
unique opportunity to study the intracellular, intranuclear
and subchromosomal distribution of antineoplastic agents such
as the anthracycline antibiotics which can easily be detected
by taking advantage of their fluorescence' properties.

Our results indicate that the various compounds tested in
this study fall into two categories: those which, as assessed
by fluorescence microscopy, appear to be located primarily in
the cell nucleus (daunomycin, N,N-dimethyl daunomycin and adriamycin), and those which appear to be preferentially distributed
in the cytoplasm (aclacinomycin, carminomycin and 7-O-methyl
nogarol).

The differences observed in the distribution pattern of
these antibiotics could be due to preferential affinities of
the drugs for various cellular components, to differential
quenching effects and/or to selective transport phenomena.

In order to test these hypotheses, we have determined the degree of fluorescence quenching elicited in vitro by cellular components. The relative quenching efficiency of DNA, RNA and chromatin differs depending on the molecular structure of the drug. Such drug specific effects could provide at least a partial explanation for the differing distribution patterns seen in the fluorescence microscope; e.g., the aclacinomycin fluorescence is quenched to a higher degree by DNA than that of adriamycin while, in the case of RNA, the inverse is observed. These differential quenching effects could account for the apparent preferential localization of aclacinomycin in the cytoplasm and the nuclear localization of adriamycin. However, studies by Egorin et al. (15) have shown that the quenching of other "cytoplasmic" drugs, not tested here, was comparable to that of "nuclear" ones; furthermore, binding studies carried out under various ionic conditions in our laboratory have indicated that some "cytoplasmic" drugs bind to isolated chromatin to the same extent as "nuclear" ones. It should be pointed out here that the presence of the methoxy group at carbon 4 appears to be critical for the nuclear localization of anthracyclines.

Autoradiographic studies on the distribution of radioactive labeled antibiotic molecules could help to solve the problems since, with this technique, the true distribution pattern is not masked by quenching effects. However, the autoradiographic procedure requires a fixation of the preparations which may result in a differential extraction of the drugs from cellular compartments. On the other hand, this technique is especially useful to study the distribution of strongly interacting antibiotic molecules.

The results of our autoradiographic experiments show that, in addition to a general labeling of the chromosomes, radioactive daunomycin is preferentially incorporated in the nucleolus organizer region located on chromosome IV. Effects of anthracyclines on the structural state of the nucleolus have been reported by Daskal (16) and the ribosomal RNA synthesis is known to be particularly sensitive to certain compounds (17).

Our results also demonstrate that the fluorescence pattern observed in isolated unfixed polytene chromosomes closely resembles the banding pattern seen with phase contrast optics, i.e., the mass distribution pattern of the nucleoproteins along the chromosomes. However, a particularly intensive fluorescence is displayed by the heterochromatic bands in the centromeric regions of the chromosomes. These regions are known to contain AT-rich DNA sequences (10). As in the case of the human chromosomes where the anthracyclines produce a fluorescence banding pattern identical to the quinacrine banding pattern (18), our results could be, at least partially, explained by differences in the DNA base composition of certain chromosomal regions. However, a nonrandom distribution of certain types of chromosomal proteins could also be responsible for the banding pattern observed with fluorescence microscopy. In fact, results not described here have revealed differential effects of some chromosomal proteins on the fluorescence properties of certain anthracycline antibiotics.

Our study demonstrates that extreme caution is needed when interpreting the results of cytofluorescence observations. An accurate interpretation requires the exact knowledge of the effects mediated by cellular components and by environmental factors on the fluorescence properties of the antibiotics. However, since the fluorescence techniques offer the unique opportunity to visualize drug molecules in situ and to study their interactions with nucleoproteins in their native state and in their natural environment, they should be used as often as possible when testing the potentialities of new drugs, though always in connection with other techniques. Insect organs with polytene chromosomes are particularly suited for such studies since the interactions and the effects of the antibiotics can easily be investigated at the cellular, nuclear, chromosomal and subchromosomal levels using a single system.

ACKNOWLEDGMENTS

We wish to thank Dr. E.N. Moudrianakis in whose laboratory the experiments were carried out for his support and advice.

116

REFERENCES

1. Bachur N. 1976. In: Sartorelli AC ed., Cancer Chemotherapy, ACS Symp. Ser. 30, Amer. Chem. Soc., Wash. DC., pp. 58-70.
2. Brown JR. 1978. Progr. Med. Chem. $\underline{15}$, 126-164.
3. Crooke ST, Reich SD eds. 1979. Anthracyclines. Current status and new developments. Academic Press, New York.
4. Di Marco A, Arcamone F. 1975. Arzneim.-Forsch. $\underline{25}$, 368-375.
5. Henry DW. 1976. In: Sartorelli AC ed., Cancer Chemotherapy, ACS Symp. Ser. 30, Amer. Chem. Soc., Wash. DC., pp. 15-57.
6. Ts'o POP ed. 1977. The molecular biology of the mammalian genetic apparatus. North-Holland Publ. Co., Amsterdam.
7. Robert M. 1971. Chromosoma (Berl.) $\underline{36}$, 1-33.
8. Lezzi M, Robert M. 1972. In: Beermann W. ed., Results and problems in cell differentiation, Vol. 4, pp. 35-57. Springer Verlag, Berlin Heidelberg, New York.
9. Sigel H. ed. 1980. Metal ions in biological systems, Vol. 11, Metal complexes as anticancer agents. M. Dekker Inc., New York, Basel.
10. Bostock CJ, Sumner AT. 1978. The eukaryotic chromosome. North Holland Publ. Co., Amsterdam, New York, Oxford.
11. Beermann W. ed. 1972. Developmental studies on giant chromosomes. Results and problems in cell differentiation, Vol. 4. Springer Verlag, Berlin, Heidelberg, New York.
12. Robert M. 1975. In: Presscott DM ed., Methods in Cell Biology Vol. 9, 377-390.
13. Rubin RL, Moudrianakis EN. 1975. Biochemistry $\underline{14}$, 1718-1726.
14. Eickbush TH, Watson DK, Moudrianakis EN. 1976. Cell $\underline{9}$, 785-7
15. Egorin MJ, Clawson RE, Cohen JL, Ross LA, Bachur NR. 1980. Cancer Res. $\underline{40}$, 4669-4676.
16. Daskal Y. 1979. In: Busch H, Crooke ST, Daskal Y eds., Effects of drugs on the cell nucleus. Acad. Press, New York.
17. Crooke ST. 1979. In: Busch H, Crooke ST, Daskal Y eds., Effects of drugs on the cell nucleus. Acad. Press, New York.
18. Johnston FP, Jorgenson KT, Lin CC, van de Sande JH. 1978. Chromosoma (Berl.) $\underline{68}$, 115-129.

EFFECTS OF ANTHRACYCLINES ON MACROMOLECULES AND THEIR SYNTHESES

A. W. PRESTAYKO, V. H. DUVERNAY, B. H. LONG, AND S. T. CROOKE

1. INTRODUCTION

The cytotoxicity of anthracyclines has been attributed to their ability to inhibit DNA-dependent nucleic acid synthesis by intercalation into DNA (1-3). Exposure of cells in culture to anthracyclines at low concentrations (0.1-10 μM) produces marked inhibition of both DNA and RNA synthesis without appreciable effects on protein synthesis at comparable doses (4-13). In general, preribosomal RNA synthesis is thought to be more sensitive to inhibition by anthracyclines than is total cell RNA synthesis (5, 11-14). These results have led to the grouping of anthracyclines into two mechanistic classes: Class I, those anthracyclines that yield similar IC_{50} values for inhibition of DNA, total RNA, and nucleolar RNA synthesis; and Class II, those that are selective for the inhibition of nucleolar RNA synthesis (11).

Effects on messenger RNA (mRNA) synthesis have not been extensively studied. Crook et al. (9) reported that daunomycin, while exerting little inhibition of heterogeneous nuclear RNA (hnRNA--precursor of mRNA) synthesis, appeared to alter physical characteristics of the hnRNA. Such a change may manifest itself by the interference of mRNA appearance in the cytoplasm without actual inhibition of RNA synthesis.

Previous studies (1, 12, 13) have suggested different deoxyribonucleotide sequence specificities for binding of anthracycline analogs to DNA. Adriamycin had an absolute requirement for GC-sequence in DNA, while marcellomycin demonstrated preference for binding to AT-rich sequences in DNA. This paper will provide data on nucleotide sequence specificity for binding in addition to studies on inhibition of nucleic acid synthesis by anthracyclines.

Figures 1 and 2 demonstrate the general chemical structure and structural modifications of the Adriamycin (ADM)-daunomycin (DNM) class of anthracyclines (Class I) and of the aclacinomycin (ACM)-cinerubin A (Class II), respectively. Class I anthracyclines are characterized by a

C-13 carbonyl group, the lack of a substituent on C-10, and the presence of only one amino sugar daunosamine attached to the aglycone at C-7. Class II anthracyclines are characterized by the lack of a carbonyl function at C-13, the presence of a carbomethoxy group at C-10, and the presence of an amino sugar rhodosamine. With the exception of pyrromycin, all of the compounds in this class possess di- or trisaccharides at position C-7 of the aglycone.

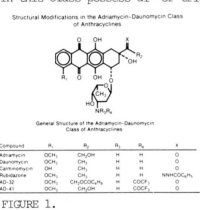

Structural Modifications in the Adriamycin-Daunomycin Class of Anthracyclines

General Structure of the Adriamycin-Daunomycin Class of Anthracyclines

Compound	R₁	R₂	R₃	R₄	X
Adriamycin	OCH₃	CH₂OH	H	H	O
Daunomycin	OCH₃	CH₃	H	H	O
Carminomycin	OH	CH₃	H	H	O
Rubidazone	OCH₃	CH₃	H	H	NNHCOC₆H₅
AD-32	OCH₃	CH₂OCOC₄H₉	H	COCF₃	O
AD-41	OCH₃	CH₂OH	H	COCF₃	O

FIGURE 1.

General structure of the cinerubin A-aclacinomycin class of anthracyclines

Structural Modifications in the cinerubin-aclacinomycin class of anthracyclines

Compound	R₁	R₂	R₃
Pyrromycin	OH	H	H
Musettamycin	OH	DF	H
Marcellomycin	OH	DF-DF	H
Cinerubin A	OH	DF-C	H
Aclacinomycin	H	DF-C	H

FIGURE 2.

2. EFFECTS ON NUCLEOLAR PRERIBOSOMAL RNA SYNTHESIS

Table 1 summarizes results of studies (11, 13) on the inhibition of RNA and DNA synthesis by several anthracyclines in Novikoff hepatoma cells.

Table 1. Inhibition of RNA synthesis by anthracyclines

Anthracycline	IC_{50} Nucleolar RNA (μM)	DNA/whole cell RNA	DNA/nucleoolar RNA
Adriamycin	6.0	1.5	1.7
Carminomycin	13.06	1.00	1.60
Pyrromycin	6.15	2.69	1.70
Marcellomycin	0.009	8.42	1311
Musettamycin	0.014	11.63	457
Aclacinomycin	0.037	7.24	191

The Class II anthracyclines demonstrate a greater selectivity toward inhibition of nucleolar RNA synthesis than do Class I anthracyclines. In addition, structure-activity studies of anthracycline analogs (12) demonstrated that the presence of a carbomethoxy moiety at C-10 of the aglycone was essential for a compound effectively to inhibit nucleolar RNA synthesis. Figure 3 shows that descarbomethoxy marcellomycin is approximately 1000-fold less effective than is marcellomycin in inhibiting nucleolar RNA synthesis. These studies also showed that descarbomethoxy marcellomycin was much less toxic to cultured Novikoff hepatoma cells than was marcellomycin.

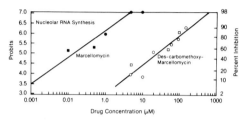

FIGURE 3. Effect of MCM and descarbomethoxy MCM on nucleolar RNA synthesis.

3. EFFECTS OF ANTHRACYCLINES ON PREMESSENGER RNA (HnRNA)

To further elucidate the mechanism of action of the anthracyclines, we chose to investigate the likelihood that some anthracyclines may have a preference for the inhibition of either RNA synthesis--RNA processing to rRNA and mRNA within nuclei or the transport of processed mRNA to the cytoplasm. We approached this question by determining the effects of structurally different anthracycline analogs on the appearance of newly synthesized total RNA and mRNA in the cytoplasm of uninduced Friend erythroleukemia cells. Figures 4 and 5 describe the experimental protocol in which we used whole cells and the cytoplasmic fraction, respectively.

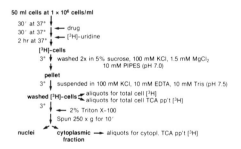

FIGURE 4.

Table 2 shows the IC_{50} values for inhibition of RNA synthesis of anthracyclines, Adriamycin (ADM), daunomycin (DNM), carminomycin (CMM), 4' demethoxy (4d-DNM), pyrromycin (PYM), marcellomycin (MCM), and aclacinomycin (ACM). For the most part, there are greater differences between the effects of different drugs than are exhibited by the same drug on different RNA populations. The Class II anthracyclines MCM and ACM inhibited RNA synthesis by 50% at 60 μM, which is 20- 50-fold lower than that of the Class I anthracyclines DNM and ADM.

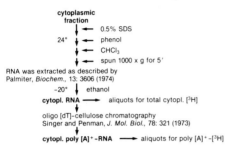

cytoplasmic fraction

24° ← 0.5% SDS
← phenol
← CHCl₃
← spun 1000 x g for 5′

RNA was extracted as described by
Palmiter, *Biochem.*, 13: 3606 (1974)

-20° ↓ ethanol

cytopl. RNA → aliquots for total cytopl. [³H]

oligo [dT]-cellulose chromatography
Singer and Penman, *J. Mol. Biol.*, 78: 321 (1973)

cytopl. poly [A]⁺-RNA → aliquots for poly [A]⁺-[³H]

FIGURE 5.

Table 2. Determination of IC_{50} values of drugs (μM) upon RNA synthesis and appearance of total RNA and poly (A+)-RNA into the cytoplasm

Drug	Total cell RNA synthesis	Appearance into cytoplasm		
		Total RNA	Poly (A+) RNA	ratio $\frac{\text{Poly (A+) RNA}}{\text{Total RNA}}$
ADM	2.88	1.34	3.34	1.7
DNM	1.19	0.37	1.19	3.2
CMM	0.33	0.14	0.38	2.7
4D-DNM	0.45	0.13	0.77	5.9
PYM	0.33	0.12	0.46	3.8
MCM	0.06	0.03	0.18	6.0
ACM	0.06	0.02	0.11	5.5

IC_{50} values for the inhibition of the appearance of total RNA into the cytoplasm were consistently one-half to one-third of the respective IC_{50} values for total cellular RNA synthesis inhibition. This observation could be construed to suggest that all anthracycline studies exert a similar inhibition upon posttranscriptional modifications and/or transport of RNA to the cytoplasm.

These studies confirm the greater sensitivity of nucleolar RNA synthesis to Class II anthracyclines in erythroleukemia cells and suggest that inhibition of posttranscriptional events may occur in cells exposed to PYM, MCM, and ACM, but at higher concentrations than are required for inhibition of RNA synthesis.

4. DNA NUCLEOTIDE BINDING SPECIFICITY OF ANTHRACYCLINES

The effects of anthracyclines on synthesis of macromolecules is most likely related to DNA-anthracycline interactions. Numerous reports have been published on DNA-anthracycline interactions (see this volume for reviews). Recent work (13) has demonstrated that ADM has an absolute GC-sequence requirement for DNA binding, while MCM shows a clear preference for AT-rich sequences of DNA. Figure 6 shows the results of that study.

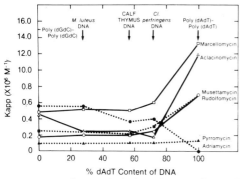

FIGURE 6. DNA nucleotide sequence preference for anthracycline binding.

Recently we initiated a series of experiments to investigate nucleotide sequence specificity of anthracycline binding to DNA. Restriction endonucleases were used to examine the DNA-interactions of anthracyclines. Specifically, the nucleotide sequence-specificities of ADM and MCM were studied and compared to compounds with known sequence specificities. The restriction endonucleases employed in this study were Hae III, which has been shown to have recognition-cleavage site of GG-CC (14-16), and Eco RI*. The latter enzyme has a recognition-cleavage site which has been shown to be AA-TT (17-18), which is slightly different from that of Eco RI*. Eco RI* activity is obtained under specific conditions of low salt and high pH (18).

The restriction endonuclease assays were carried out at 25° C in reactant volumes ranging from 50 to 100 µl and were usually initiated by the addition of enzyme followed by incubation at 25° C. The standard Eco RI* reaction mixture contained 10 mM tris-HCl, pH 8.5, 2 mM $MgCl_2$, and 40% glycerol, ccc-(form I)-PM-2DNA, and Eco RI* at a concentration of 4 units/µg of DNA. The standard Hae III reaction mixture contained 20 mM tris-HCl pH 7.5, 6 mM $MgCl_2$, 0.5 mM dithiothreitol, ccc-(form I)-PM-2-DNA and Hae III at a concentration of 2 units/ g of DNA. After incubation at 25° C, the reaction was terminated by addition of an equal volume of a "stopping solution" containing 40 mM ethylenediamine-tetraacetic acid, disodium salt (EDTA), 70% (v/v) glycerol, 0.05% (w/v) bromphenol blue at pH 7.5. Reaction

122

products were analyzed by electrophoresis on 1% agarose horizontal slab gels as previously described (19). After electrophoresis, the gels were stained with 0.5 µg/ml ethidium bromide in electrophoresis buffer and then were photographed during ultraviolet irradiation. The negative films of the gels were scanned with an RFT Scanning Densitometer, model 2955 (Transidyne General Corporation, Ann Arbor, Michigan).

One unit of activity of Eco RI* was defined as the amount of enzyme needed to digest 1 µg of phage λ DNA in 1 hour at 37° C. One unit of Hae III activity was defined as the amount of enzyme needed to digest 1 µg of X174 RF DNA in 1 hour at 37° C.

To verify that AT and GC sequence specific binding agents can prevent restriction endonuclease cleavage at these sites, we used AT-specific netropsin sulfate and GC-specific olivomycin. Figure 7a compares the effects of netropsin sulfate and olivomycin on the enzyme activity of Hae III. As expected, olivomycin inhibited Hae III endonucleolytic activity at concentrations between 20 µM and 35 µM. However, netropsin sulfate exhibited no significant effect on Hae III activity at concentrations as high as 50 µM. As shown in Figure 7b, the activity of the AT-specific enzyme Eco RI* was inhibited by netropsin sulfate at concentrations between 5 µM and 10 µM, while concentrations of olivomycin as high as 50 µM exhibited no significant inhibitory effect. Control (undigested) PM-2 DNA is shown in the center lane.

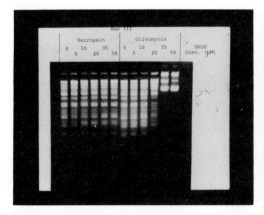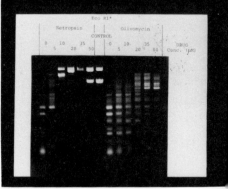

FIGURE 7a, b. Agarose gel electrophoretic patterns of PM-2 DNA digested with Hae III and Eco RI* after incubation of the DNA with varying concentrations of netropsin sulfate and olivomycin.

To establish that Adriamycin and marcellomycin have no direct effect

on endonuclease activity, we incubated the drugs with Eco RI* and Hae III
for 24 hours prior to initiation of incubation with DNA-anthracycline
complexes. The results (not shown) indicate that DNA cleavage patterns
were not affected by the preincubation procedure. Figure 8 shows the
agarose gel electrophoretic patterns of DNA restriction fragments generated
by digestion of DNA-anthracycline complexes with ECO RI*. MCM inhibited
the endonucleolytic activity of ECO RI* at concentrations between 35 mM
and 50 μM, while no significant inhibition of enzyme activity was observed
for ADM at concentrations up to 50 μM. The results were reversed when
Hae III was used in the incubations; i.e., ADM blocked enzyme cleavage,
while MCM had no effect on the pattern of digested DNA products up to
50 M MCM (data not shown).

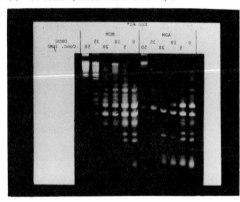

FIGURE 8. Agarose gel electrophoretic patterns of PM-2 DNA
digested with Eco RI* after
incubation of the DNA with varying
concentrations of Adriamycin and
marcellomycin.

These results are in agreement with the sequence preferences of ADM (GC)
and MCM (AT), which have been previously reported (13). Thus, the
efficacy of this assay to facilitate studies on DNA-binding compounds
has been demonstrated, and the sequence specificities of the agents
studied were accurately reproduced by the current assay system. The
sensitivity and application of this assay system can be markedly expanded
by varying the recognition/cleavage sites of the endonucleases employed.

ACKNOWLEDGMENT

The author would like to acknowledge the typing assistance of
Kathryn Butterworth.

REFERENCES

1. Di Marco A, Arcamone F, Zunino F. 1975. Antibiotics III: Mechanism of action of antimicrobial and antitumor agents (JW Corcoran and FE Hahn, eds.). Springer-Verlag, New York, pp. 101-128.
2. Schwartz HS. 1976. J. Med. 7: 33-46.
3. Lown JW, Sim SK, Majumdar KD, Chang RY. 1977. Biochem. Biophys. Res. Commun. 76: 705-710.
4. Rusconi A, Calendi E. 1966. Biochem. Biophys. Acta 119: 413-415.
5. Di Marco A, Silvestrini R, Di Marco S, Dasdia T. 1965. J. Cell Biol. 27: 545-550.
6. Theologides A, Yarbro JW, Kennedy BJ. 1968. Cancer 21: 15-21.
7. Rusconi A, Di Marco A. 1968. Cancer Res. 29: 1507-1511.
8. Meriwether WD, Bachur NR. 1972. Cancer Res. 32: 1137-1142.
9. Crook LE, Rees KR, Cohen A. 1972. Biochem. Pharmacol. 21: 281-286.
10. Henry DW. 1975. Cancer chemotherapy (AC Gartorelli, ed.). 169th meeting of the American Chemical Society, Division of Medicinal Chemistry Symposium, Washington, D.C., pp. 15-57.
11. Crooke LE, Rees KR, Cohen A. 1972. Biochem. Pharmacol. 21: 281-286.
12. DuVernay VH, Essery JM, Doyle TW, Bradner WT, Crooke ST. 1979. Mol. Pharmacol. 15: 341-356.
13. DuVernay VH, Mong S, Crooke ST. 1980. Antibiotics V: Biosynthesis of antibiotics (JW Corcoran and FE Hahn, eds.). Springer-Verlag, New York, pp. 101-128.
14. Danø K, Frederiksen S, Hellung-Larsen P. 1972. Cancer Res. 32: 1307-1314.
15. Blakesley RW, Dodgson JB, Nes IF, Wells RD. 1977. J. Biol. Chem. 252: 730-806.
16. Mann MB, Smith HO. 1977. Nucleic Acid Res. 4: 4211-4221.
17. Polisky B, Greene P, Garfin DE, McCarthy BJ, Goodman HM, Boyer HW. 1975. Proc. Nat. Acad. Sci. USA 72: 3310-3314.
18. Mayer H. 1978. FEBS Lett. 90: 341-344.
19. Strong JE, Crooke ST. 1978. Cancer Res. 38: 3322-3326.

BIOTRANSFORMATIONS OF ANTHRACYCLINES IN THE SMOOTH ENDOPLASMIC RETICULUM
OF RAT LIVER

H. S. SCHWARTZ, P. M. KANTER, A. J. MARINELLO, AND H. L. GURTOO

In 1967, Di Marco and Rusconi[1] reported the first evidence of biotransformations of daunorubicin (Dm) along with some rather remarkable actions of
the agent on DNA and chromosomes of cells in culture. Since the time of these
early observations, a great deal more has been learned about Dm metabolic
biotransformations in subcellular preparations[2-4] and through urinary and
biliary excretion of these products[6-7]. The metabolism of Dm is now
associated with free radical reactions[7-9], and there are rather strong
suggestions that free radical intermediates may also generate DNA damage[10-12],
which may in turn be associated with growth inhibition[13]. Thus, it seems
that we are rapidly approaching a convergence in our understanding of the
interrelationships between biotransformation and mechanism of cytotoxicity
of the anthracyclines.

The study by Di Marco and Rusconi[1] suggested formation of at least two
metabolites from Dm incubated with rat liver supernatant and microsomes.
The first, a water-soluble component, was probably daunorubicinol (Dmol),
and the other appears from its lipophilicity to be one or more aglycones.
Subsequently, Dmol was identified from liver supernatant incubations[2]
and the 7-deO and 7-HO aglycones of Dm from microsomes, using NADPH as a
cofactor under anaerobic conditions[3]. There seem now to be major routes
of transformations for Dm: reduction of the C-13 to the primary alcohol (Dmol)
by the soluble aldoketo reductase, hydrolytic cleavage to form 7-HO aglycones, and reductive cleavage to the 7-deO aglycones. In addition, Dm (and
Adriamycin) also contain a methoxyl group at the C-4 positions, which like
C-7 may be cleaved reductively to form 4-demethoxy derivatives (4d Dm) or
hydrolytically to form the 4-OH compounds. In the case of Dm, the 4-OH
derivative is also known as carminomycin (Cm) and the aglycones may be
referred to as 7-HO-Cma, 7-deO-Cma, etc. Besides these products, a number

126

of conjugated forms have been identified in bile. It should be pointed out
that among these is the 4-O-sulphate which can only result from a free
radical mechanism.

Known and likely aglycones of Dm from these reactions are shown in
Fig. 1 omitting conjugates, semiquinones, other free radicals and intermediary
structures. The aglycones (as well as Dmol) shown in broken boxes have been
identified in the urine of patients treated with Dm, and the heavy arrows
indicate the proposed major route of metabolic biotransformation as suggested
by Takanashi and Bachur[5]. The agents in Fig. 1 that are underlined include
those that have been found in our preparations incubated anaerobically with
NADPH. These preparations include normal rat fresh and aged (6 mos, -70°C)
liver microsomes, microsomes from phenobarbital-treated rats (PBMC) as well
as from purified cytochrome P450, cytochrome P450 reductase, and liver supernatant (alone and in combinations). As shown, 10 of the 12 likely aglycones
are accounted for in in vitro liver preparations. The 2 that have not been
found at this time are the 7-HO aglycones of 4dDma and 4dDmola.

In kinetic studies with washed rat liver microsomes[4], the first aglycone (group I) formed is 7-deO-Dm. Similarly, carminomycin is also converted
first to 7-deO-Cma by the same system. In the Dm sequence, 7-deO-Dm is then
reduced to 7-deO-Dmola (group II), and the pathway follows first-order kineti
for a linear sequence. With the appearance of 7-deO-Dmola, we also find
7-HO-Dma (II) and 7-HO-Dmola (II). This sequence occurs with all of the
rat liver microsomes that have been tested.

Following the I→II sequence, a group III of aglycones is formed. These
are seen most readily in normal MC, and are almost completely absent from
incubations with PBMC and from aged MC preparations. Two of the 3 or more
in this group are 7-deO-4dDma and 7-deO-Cma. When formation of group III
is limited as in aged microsomes or PBMC, there is a build up of precursors
in groups I and II. This is our present view of the sequential appearances
of Dm aglycones formed by microsomes during anaerobic incubations with NADPH
and it appears generally consistent with pathways proposed from excreted
products[5].

There is at this time considerable interest in the group I aglycones
which form rapidly from Dm and Cm during anaerobic incubations. The primary
product in this group is the 7-deO aglycone and its formation involves a
free radical mechanism. For this reason these aglycones are thought to
contribute to the incursions of DNA damage. The implication is that formati

METABOLIC FORMATION OF Dm AGLYCONES IN LIVER

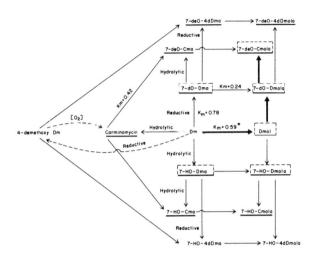

FIGURE 1. The proposed metabolic pathways of daunorubicin (Dm) to daunorubicinol (Dmol) and carminomycin (Cm) and to aglycones(shown by light arrows)
are from anaerobic incubations of Dm and rat liver microsomes with NADPH and
an isocitric dehydrogenase generating system. Underlined compounds have
been identified as products of microsomal metabolism; those in broken boxes
have been identified in urine of treated patients by Takanashi and Bachur (4A)
and the heavy arrows indicate their proposed major pathway. Speculative
pathways for 4-demethoxy Dm are shown as broken arrows. Km values are those
determined in vitro and (*) as in (4) and (5), respectively.

of the 7-deO aglycones are partial contributors to the cytotoxicity of the parent compounds and a number of observations tend to support a determinant role for these products. Table 1 for example shows the kinetic constants for the initial rates of formation of 7-deO-Dma and 7-deO-Cma from Dm and Cm, respectively, measured under comparable conditions with microsomes from normal rat liver.

Table 1. Initial Anaerobic Reaction Kinetics for Daunorubicin (Dm) and Carminomycin (Cm) in Rat Liver Microsomes[*]

		App K_m (mM)	App V_{max} (nmol/min/mg)
a)	Dm (loss)	0.78	37
	7-deO-Dma (formed)	1.04	39
b)	Cm (loss)	0.42	111
	7-deO-Cma (formed)	0.39	102

[*] Reaction conditions as described in (4).

The striking difference is that the apparent affinities and maximum velocities for these conversions are 2 or 3 fold higher for Cm than for Dm. This difference is at least consistent with the relatively greater potency of Cm, as compared to Dm, with respect to DNA damage and growth inhibition in cultured mammalian cells[13]. Yet it is also interesting that these two agents, Cm and Dm, form common metabolites: 7-deO-Cma, 7-HO-Cma, and 7-deO-Cmola (unpublished observation).

Another line of evidence also supports the notion that 7-deO aglycones may contribute to lethality in animals. Fig. 2 shows that SKF525A increases the rate of Dm metabolism by raising the accumulation of 7-deO-Dma by 3-fold or more while having little or no effect on the formation of identified components in group II and inhibiting appearance of those in group III. Should such an accumulation of 7-deO-Dma occur in animals, it would tend to increase drug potency if the aglycone is indeed one of the cytotoxic determinants. This is supported by data with mice given single toxic doses (ip) of Dm 2 hours after pretreatment with SKF525 A at a dose level (30 mg/kg) which is not toxic by itself. The data indicate a probable contribution of 7-deO-Dma to the acute lethality of Dm; doses of the Dm alone at 10, 15 and 22.5 mg/kg produce progressively shorter average survival times; pretreatment

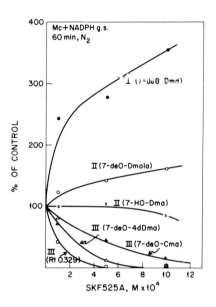

FIGURE 2. The effects of varying concentrations of SKF525A on biotransformations of Dm in anaerobic incubations of rat liver microsomes with NADPH and
an isocitrate dehydrogenase generating system (g.s.). The conditions and
abbreviations are as described in the text and in Figure 1.

with SKF525-A further decreases survival times by about 10, 20 and 30%, respectively. The possibility that this aglycone also contributes to the delayed toxicity of Dm cannot be ruled out at this time because Dm has a prolonged retention in liver and other organs whereas the biologic half-life of SKF525-A is shorter, relative to Dm.

The studies with SKF525 A, described above, may also provide some clues to the mechanisms of biotransformation of the anthracyclines. The inhibition of formation of group III metabolites suggests that these are formed in association with cytochrome P-450 whereas the initial reductive cleavage to form the 7-deO aglycones is carried out by the cytochrome P-450 reductase.

The metabolic transformations of Dm are generally those that might be expected from the products found in urine and bile of patients and animals, and the pattern is qualitatively similar to that found after Adriamycin (Am) administration[14]. An important difference is that rates of formation of 7-deO aglycone and the associated free radicals are more rapid for Dm than for Am, which is also consistent with the greater toxicity of Dm in animals and again implies a determinant role of these products in cytotoxicity. Although the studies here have concentrated on anaerobic biotransformation of Dm in smooth endoplasmic reticular structures, it should be pointed out that other membrane effects are apparent from model studies with neutral and negatively charged unsaturated lipids (15; unpublished observations) and with erythrocytes[16]. These also involve free radicals which, as with cytochrome P450 reductase[14], are generated aerobically by the anthracyclines.

ACKNOWLEDGMENTS

The authors are pleased to express their gratitude to Dr. N. Bachur for spirited discussions, helpful in the preparation of this manuscript.

The studies reported here have been supported in part by grants from the National Cancer Institute (CA-24778) and from the American Cancer Society.

REFERENCES

1. DiMarco A, Rusconi A. 1967. Gann Monograph 2: 23-33.
2. Bachur N. 1971. J. Pharmacol. Exp. Ther. 177: 573-578.
3. Asbell MA, Schwartzbach E, Bullock FJ, Yesair DW. 1972. J. Pharmacol. Exp. Ther. 182: 63-69.
4. Schwartz HS, Parker NB. 1981. Cancer Res. 41: 2343-2348.
5. Takanashi S, Bachur N. 1975. J. Pharmacol. Exp. Ther. 195: 41-49.
6. Chan KK, Watson E. 1978. J. Pharm. Sci. 67: 1748-1752.

7.   Handa K, Sato S. 1975. Gann 66: 43-47.
8.   Goodman J, Hochstein P. 1977. BBRC 77: 797-803.
9.   Bachur N, Gordon S, Gee MV. 1978. Cancer Res. 38: 1745-1750.
10. Schwartz HS. 1976. Biomedicine (Paris) 24: 317-323.
11. Lown JW, Sim S-K, Majumdar KC, Chang R-Y. 1977. BBRC 76: 705-710.
12. Sato S. Iwaizumi M, Handa K, Tamura Y. 1977. Gann 68: 603-608.
13. Kanter PK, Schwartz HS. 1979. Cancer Res. 39: 3661-3672.
14. Bachur N. 1979. Cancer Treat. Rep. 63: 817-820.
15. Schwartz HS, Kanter PK. 1979. Europ. J. Cancer 15: 923-928.
16. Schwartz HS, Schiopacassi G, Kanter P . 1978. Antibiotics. Chemother. 23: 247-254.

TRANSPORT AND STORAGE OF ANTHRACYCLINES IN EXPERIMENTAL SYSTEMS AND HUMAN
LEUKEMIA

C. PETERSON, C. PAUL, G. GAHRTON, S. VITOLS, AND M. RUDLING

1. INTRODUCTION

1.1. Toxicity mechanisms

The mechanisms underlying therapeutic and toxic effects of the anthracyclines are not fully understood. The cytotoxicity of the first generation
anthracyclines, daunorubicin (DNR) and doxorubicin (DOX), which accumulate
extensively in the cell nuclei (1,2), can be explained by intercalation of
drug molecules in the DNA double helix, thereby preventing replication and
transcription (3,4). However, some of the new derivatives including N-
trifluoroacetyl-adriamycin-14-valerate (AD 32) and aclacinomycin A do not
accumulate in the cell nuclei (2) but are still very cytotoxic, indicating
that mechanisms other than direct interaction with nuclear DNA are involved.
Recent studies indicate that anthracyclines cause formation of free radicals
(5) which, by reacting with intracellular macromolecules, could explain toxic
effects of the drugs. Other mechanisms such as interaction with cell membranes may also contribute to the cycotoxicity of the anthracyclines (6).

Important differences have been observed in the spectrum of clinical
activity between DNR and its 14-hydroxy derivative, DOX. Thus, DOX probably
has the broadest activity spectrum of all cancer chemotherapeutics available
today, with effects on a great number of solid tumors (7). On the other hand
DNR is the most active single agent in the treatment of acute nonlymphoblasti
leukemia (ANLL) (7). A lower response rate has been reported for DOX as a
single agent in the treatment of ANLL (8) which, however, may be due to differences in patient selection. A more detailed knowledge of the molecular
mechanisms involved in the cytotoxicity of the anthracyclines as well as the
reason for the difference in the activity spectrum between DNR and DOX should
be useful for the extensive work going on to develop new anthracyclines with
better therapeutic and less toxic effects.

1.2. Drug concentrations in the target cells

A decisive factor for the clinical effects of a cancer chemotherapeutic agent is the concentration of the drug and its active metabolites reached in cells, which are targets for the therapeutic and toxic effects of the drug. Several studies have shown that, in vitro, the intracellular accumulation of DNR clearly exceeds that of DOX (1,4). DNR also exerts a greater inhibitory effect on DNA and RNA biosynthesis (4).

During the last few years we have compared the membrane transport and intracellular storage of DNR and DOX in various types of cultured and isolated cells. In vivo studies have also been performed during treatment of patients with ANLL. This permits a direct comparison between the plasma pharmacokinetics of the drugs and the pharmacokinetics in a compartment which can be regarded as a target for the therapy, namely the circulating leukemic blast cells which easily can be isolated from blood and bone marrow samples. We have also studied the possibilities of increasing the drug concentration in the target cells by administering the drugs associated with DNA or low density lipoprotein (LDL) as carriers.

2. IN VITRO STUDIES

2.1. Intracellular accumulation of free and DNA-linked DNR and DOX

Cultured rat embryo fibroblasts, human and chicken erythrocytes and isolated human leukemic cells have been incubated with free and DNA-linked DNR and DOX to steady-state conditions. Cell counts and drug concentrations were chosen so that cellular uptake did not reduce the drug concentration in the incubation medium by more than 30 %. The drugs were assayed by total fluorescence since under in vitro conditions very little metabolism occurs as determined by high performance liquid chromatography (9). The ratios between the intracellular drug concentration and the concentration in the incubation medium at steady-state have been calculated assuming uniform intracellular distribution (table 1). The volumes of the fibroblasts and the leukemic cells were calculated from the protein content assuming that 1 mg of cell protein corresponds to a cell volume of 5 μl (10). The value used for the volume of human red blood cells was 90 μ^3/cell. Since the chicken red blood cells contained twice as much hemoglobin as the human cells, a volume of 180 μ^3/cell has been used in the calculations. The results show that there is an extensive accumulation of DNR and DOX in nucleated cells but not in human red blood cells. In all cell types, the accumulation of free drug exceeded that of DNA-linked.

Table 1. Calculated ratios between the intracellular concentrations of DNR and DOX at steady-state and the concentrations in the incubation medium

INCUBATION CONDITIONS	DNR	DOX	DNR-DNA	DOX-DNA
Rat fibroblasts in culture 17.5 μM, 5 ml medium/mg cell protein	800	150	210	25
Human red blood cells 40 μM, 3×10^7 cells/ml	17	13	0.6	0.2
Chicken red blood cells 20 μM, 3×10^6 cells/ml	1100	540	150	30
Human leukemic cells 1.75 μM, 10^6 cells/ml	1500	560	610	230

2.2. Mechanisms underlying intracellular drug accumulation

The extensive intracellular accumulation of DNR and DOX does not seem to be caused by an active inward transport mechanism. On the contrary, evidence has been presented for an active efflux mechanism across the plasma membrane. Thus the presence of metabolic inhibitors during incubations of cultured cells increased the intracellular accumulation of DNR and DOX (11,12,13,14). Furthermore, metabolic inhibitors reduced the efflux of DNR and DOX from preloaded cells (12,14,15). Based on experimental results, calculations have been presented indicating that the drug concentration in the cytosol in fact is lower than in the incubation medium (12). Despite this, the extensive intracellular accumulation can be understood since fluorescence microscopy of cells incubated with DNR and DOX have shown that the drugs are highly concentrated in nuclei and cytoplasmic granules (2). Subcellular fractionation studies of cultured fibroblasts have shown that the drug-containing granules are lysosomes (1). However, subcellular fractionation of human leukemic cells has shown that in these cells, DNR and DOX are stored in nuclei only (9). The nuclear trapping of DNR and DOX can easily be explained by the high affinity of the drugs for DNA. In the lysosomes, the drugs being weak bases are probably stored in protonated form as a result of the acid milieu (16). The reason for the difference in subcellular localization of the drugs between rat fibroblasts and human leukemic cells is at present unclear. In all cell types studied, the intracellular accumulation of DNR exceeds that of DOX whereas the affinity of DOX for DNA in vitro exceeds that of DNR (17). The difference in cellular accumulation of DNR and DOX can be explained by a "leak and pump" model for drug transport across the plasma membrane (12,13,15). According to this hypothesis drug influx occurs as passive diffusion of non-ionized drug. Since DNR is more lipophilic than DOX, the diffusion of DNR will be faster. Because of the active efflux mechanism, the concentration of both drugs in the cell sap will be very low, but it will be higher for DNR than for DOX. Equilibration with the storage compartments in the nuclei and in the lysosomes will lead to an extensive intracellular drug accumulation. A schematic picture of the hypothesis is shown in figure 1.

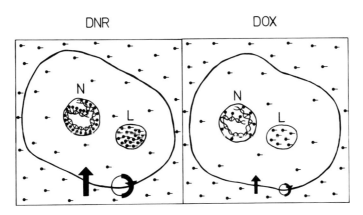

FIGURE 1. Schematic drawing of the "leak and pump" model for the accumulation of anthracyclines in cultured fibroblasts. The drugs enter the cells by diffusion, DNR faster than DOX due to its higher lipophilicity. Intracellular drug is trapped in nuclei (N) or lysosomes (L) or extruded across the plasma membrane by an active efflux mechanism.

Results from experimental systems indicate that development of anthracycline-resistant cell lines is accompanied by an enhanced activity of the active efflux system (14,18). However, it is not known if this mechanism is involved in clinically observed drug resistance.

3. PHARMACOKINETIC STUDIES IN ACUTE LEUKEMIA

To compare the therapeutic and toxic effects of free and DNA-linked DNR in combination with cytosine arabinoside, the Leukemia Group of Central Sweden has performed a randomized clinical study during the last few years (19). Some patients who for certain reasons (e.g. previous chemotherapy) were excluded from the randomized study, have been treated with free or DNA-linked DOX. Parallel with this clinical study, we have compared the pharmacokinetics of DNR and DOX as well as of free and DNA-linked drugs in plasma and in leukemic cells. Blood samples were obtained during 13 treatment courses with i.v. infusions of free

or DNA-linked DNR or DOX (1.5 mg/kg body weight) involving 10 patients with
ANLL and 8,000-200,000 blast cells/mm^3 in the peripheral blood. The DNA-com-
plexes were prepared as described by Paul et al.(19). Leukemic cells were isolated by centrifugation on Ficoll-metrizoate as described previously (20). DNR,
DOX and their reduced metabolites were assayed by high performance liquid chromatography in a straight-phase system as previously described (9).

3.1. DNR in plasma and in leukemic cells

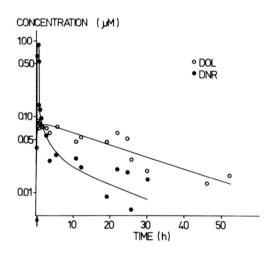

FIGURE 2. Plasma concentrations of DNR and daunorubicinol in patient S-A. H.
after an i.v. infusion of DNR.

Figure 2 shows a typical plasma concentration curve of DNR and its reduced
metabolite, daunorubicinol in a patient with acute myeloblastic leukemia after
intravenous infusion of DNR (1.5 mg/kg body weight during 40 min). The plasma
disappearance of DNR was at least biphasic with an initial rapid decay (t½
about 2 min) followed by a slow elimination phase with a t½ of more than 10
hours. Already a few minutes after the infusion the plasma concentration of
daunorubicinol exceeded that of the parent compound and the concentration declined slowly (t½ about 20 hours).

The corresponding drug concentrations in leukemic cells isolated from the
blood samples are shown in Figure 3. Assuming that one mg of cell protein corresponds to a cell volume of 5 μl, it can be calculated that the concentration
of DNR in the leukemic cells at the end of the infusion was about 175 times

higher than that in plasma. Daunorubicinol did not reach the same concentration in the leukemic cells as that of the parent compound until about 50 hours after the infusion. The calculated ratio between the intracellular and plasma concentrations of daunorubicinol was much lower than for DNR.

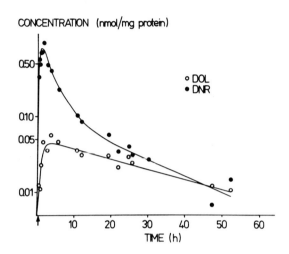

FIGURE 3. Concentrations of DNR and daunorubicinol in the leukemic cells in peripheral blood from patient S-A. H.

3.2. DNA-linked DNR in plasma and in leukemic cells

Figures 4 and 5 show the concentrations of DNR and daunorubicinol in plasma and leukemic cells during treatment of a patient with acute myeloblastic leukemia with DNA-linked DNR (1.5 mg/kg during 4 hours). Although the DNR-DNA solution, because of high viscosity, was infused at a slower rate than the free drug, the plasma concentrations of DNR and daunorubicinol reached higher values than those observed during treatment with the free drug. The plasma decay of DNR was slower ($t\frac{1}{2}$ of the initial phase: 5 to 10 min) than after infusion of free DNR. The concentrations of DNR and daunorubicinol in the leukemic cells were similar during treatment with free and DNA-linked DNR. Table 2 shows that DNA-linking of DNR markedly reduced the clearance and the apparent volume of distribution of the drug. There were pronounced interindividual variations in the pharmacokinetics among the patients.

In combination with cytosine arabinoside, free and DNA-linked DNR were equally effective in inducing remission in patients with acute non-lymphoblastic leukemia (about 70 % complete remissions) (19). Evidence has been presented

138

that DNA-linked DNR is less cardiotoxic than the free drug (19,21). The reduced
toxicity can be explained by our pharmacokinetic data since the higher plasma
concentrations reached during treatment with the DNA-complex indicate a lower
initial tissue uptake probably leading to reduced peak concentrations in cardiac tissue.

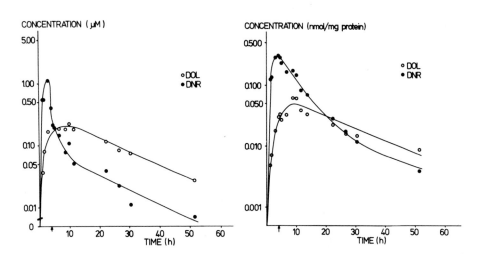

FIGURES 4 AND 5. Concentrations of DNR and daunorubicinol in plasma (left) and
in the leukemic cells in peripheral blood (right) from patient G.A. after an
i.v. infusion of DNA-linked DNR.

Table 2. Plasma pharmacokinetic parameters in patients receiving DNR and DNR-
DNA.

Patient	Treatment	Clearance $(1 \times h^{-1} \times kg^{-1})$	Vd $(1/kg)$
I	DNR	2.00	53.8
II	DNR	0.86	52.8
III	DNR	1.16	48.3
IV	DNR	4.58	30.0
V	DNR	1.98	20.0
	Mean values:	2.12	41.0
VI	DNR-DNA	0.56	10.6
VII	DNR-DNA	1.08	26.2
VIII	DNR-DNA	1.57	16.7
	Mean values:	1.07	17.8

3.3. Free and DNA-linked DOX in plasma and leukemic cells

Two patients, who had been excluded from the randomized clinical trial, were treated with DOX in one course and DOX-DNA in the following course (in both cases 1.5 mg/kg, free drug infused during 40 min and the DNA-complex during 4 hours). The interval between the courses was three weeks, and no remaining DOX could be detected in blood samples obtained immediately before the infusion of DOX-DNA. Figure 6 shows the plasma concentrations of DOX after infusion of free and DNA-linked DOX to one of the patients. In both cases, the plasma decay seemed biphasic. After treatment with the DNA-linked drug, DOX reached a higher peak concentration and could be detected longer. The reduced metabolite, doxorubicinol, could be detected only after infusion of the DNA-complex.

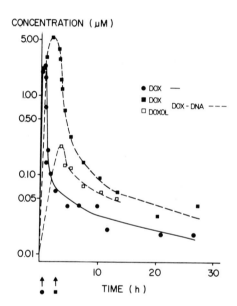

FIGURE 6. Plasma concentrations of DOX and doxorubicinol in patient T.G. after i.v. infusions of free and DNA-linked DOX.

Table 3 summarizes the plasma pharmacokinetic data in patients treated with free and DNA-linked DOX. The reduction in clearance and distribution volume by administering DOX as a DNA-complex was greater than the changes caused by administering DNR as a DNA-complex. The difference in the plasma pharmacokinetics of free and DNA-linked DOX was accompanied by a difference in the concentrations in the leukemic cells. Ten to 15 hours after the infusion and for at least 30 hours the concentration of DOX in the leukemic cells was about three times higher after administration of the drug as a DNA-complex than after infusion of free DOX (figure 7). No doxorubicinol could be found intracellularly.

Table 3. Plasma pharmacokinetic parameters in patients receiving DOX and DOX-DNA.

Patient	Treatment	Clearance $(1 \times h^{-1} \times kg^{-1})$	Vd $(1/kg)$
IX	DOX	1.02	20.4
III	DOX	1.27	54.5
X	DOX	1.29	26.6
	Mean values:	1.19	33.8
X	DOX-DNA	0.18	2.7
III	DOX-DNA	0.25	7.7
	Mean values:	0.22	5.2

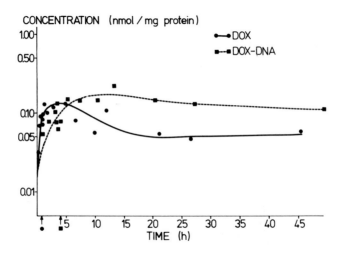

FIGURE 7. Concentration of DOX in the leukemic cells in peripheral blood from patient T.G. after treatment with free and DNA-linked DOX, respectively.

Whether or not the higher intracellular concentration of DOX observed in th leukemic cells after administration of the drug as a DNA-complex leads to a better therapeutic effect is not known at present. However, a randomized clin cal trial has now been initiated to compare the effects of free and DNA-linke DOX.

3.4. Mechanism of cellular uptake of DNA-linked anthracyclines

It was originally proposed that DNA-linked anthracyclines enter the cells endocytosis and that DNA is then digested in the lysosomes (23). After incuba tion of cultured fibroblasts with DNA-linked DNR, the drug could be recovered in nuclei and lysosomes (22). However, the presence of DNR in the lysosomes cannot be taken as evidence that the complex enters the cells by endocytosis since free DNR accumulates also in the lysosomes of cultured fibroblasts (1). After incubation of human leukemic cells with DNA-linked DNR and subsequent subcellular fractionation we could not find any DNR in the lysosomes (9). As after incubation with free DNR, all intracellular drug was found in the nuclei. Furthermore, after injection of ^{125}I-DNA-linked drugs to mice, there was a pronounced discrepancy between the plasma decays of radioactivity and of DNR (24). We therefore believe that the anthracycline-DNA-complexes mainly serve as slow-release preparations of the anthracyclines. This can explain the greater modification of the pharmacokinetics of DOX as compared to DNR since DOX has higher affinity for DNA (17).

3.5. Comparison of the pharmacokinetics of DNR and DOX

One patient who was excluded from the randomized trial was treated with DNR in one course and DOX in the following course about 3 weeks later in both cases 1.5 mg/kg during 45 min).

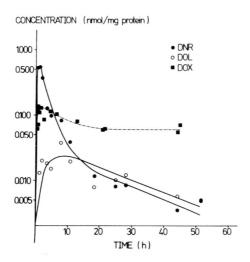

FIGURE 8. Concentrations of DNR, daunorubicinol and DOX in leukemic cells in peripheral blood from patient K.S. isolated during one treatment course with DNR and another with DOX.

Figure 8 shows the drug concentrations in the leukemic cells during and after the infusions. The peak concentration was much higher for DNR presumably due to the higher lipophilicity of this drug leading to a faster equilibration across the plasma membrane. On the other hand, DOX was retained much longer in the leukemic cells, which can be explained by the higher affinity of DOX for DN (17). Recent results on the toxicity of DNR on granulocyte-macrophage committed stem cells from NMRI-mice as assayed by their colony-forming ability in semi-solid agar show that, at identical areas for the intracellular drug concentration versus time curves, DNR is more toxic when present at a high concentration for a short time compared to a lower concentration for a longer period (25). This indicates that the higher peak concentration in the leukemic cells observed during treatment with DNR compared to treatment with DOX may be of importance in the killing of the cells. On the other hand, the longer intracellular retention of DOX may be of value in killing more slowly growing solid tumor cells. Therefore our pharmacokinetic results give a possible explanation for the difference in the spectrum of clinical activity between DNR and DOX.

4. LOW DENSITY LIPOPROTEIN AS A CARRIER OF ANTHRACYCLINES

Recently we have focused our interest on the possibilities of using plasma l density lipoprotein (LDL) as a carrier for cytotoxic drugs. LDL is the major cholesterol-carrying lipoprotein of human plasma (26). The LDL-particles that can be isolated from human plasma by ultracentrifugation in the density range 1.019-1.063 g/ml have a molecular weight of about 2.5×10^6 consisting of a lipic core of esterified cholesterol surrounded by a polar shell of protein, phospholipid and free cholesterol (26). It has been found that various types of normal human cells have a cell surface receptor that binds LDL with high affinity (26). Once bound to the receptor, LDL is internalized by endocytosis and de-livered to lysosomes where the cholesteryl esters are hydrolyzed so that free cholesterol can be made available for use by the cells. Evidence has been presented that leukemic cells from patients with acute myelogenous leukemia (AML) have a higher receptor-mediated uptake and degradation of LDL as compared to mononuclear cells from healthy individuals (27).

4.1. LDL-receptor activity in leukemic cells

In order to further investigate the possibilities of using LDL as a carrier for cytotoxic drugs, we have compared the high-affinity degradation of ^{125}I-LD in various types of freshly isolated normal and malignant blood and bone marrc cells (Figure 9). Mature polymorphonuclear granulocytes have a low receptor-me-diated degradation of ^{125}I-LDL as have non-separated bone marrow cells from healthy subjects. The values are of the same magnitude as for freshly isolated mononuclear cells. Moreover, we have confirmed previous results that leukemic cells from most AML patients have a much greater high-affinity degradation. There was no difference in receptor-mediated degradation of ^{125}I-LDL between leukemic cells isolated from peripheral blood and from bone marrow samples of the same patients. On the other hand, leukemic cells from patients with acute lymphoblastic leukemia have a low receptor-mediated degradation of ^{125}I-LDL, showing that the enhanced receptor activity is not a general property of malignant cells.

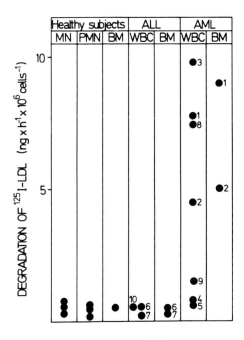

FIGURE 9. High affinity degradation of ^{125}I-LDL by white blood cells from healthy subjects and patients with acute lymphoblastic leukemia (ALL) and acute myelogenous leukemia (AML).

4.2. Toxicity of LDL-incorporated anthracyclines

As a preliminary test of the possibilities of incorporating lipophilic cancer chemotherapeutics into LDL-particles, we have incubated LDL isolated by ultracentrifugation of serum from healthy individuals with DNR or aclacinomycin A and then separated LDL-incorporated from non-incorporated drug by gel filtration on Sephadex G-25 fine. The toxicity of LDL-aclacinomycin A was tested on the clonogenic activity of human leukemic cells in semisolid agar after incubation of the cells with the drug-LDL preparation. As shown in Figure 10,

LDL-incorporated aclacinomycin A inhibited the colony-forming ability of the leukemic cells. This effect could be reversed by the addition of LDL in 10-fold excess during the incubation which indicates that the toxicity was caused by receptor-mediated uptake of LDL-incorporated drug.

The toxicity of LDL-incorporated DNR was tested on the growth of human malignant glioma cells in culture, a cell type which also has been found to exhibit a high LDL-receptor activity (28). As shown in figure 11, LDL-incorporated DNR inhibited the growth of the cells and the effect could be counteracted by the addition of LDL in excess.

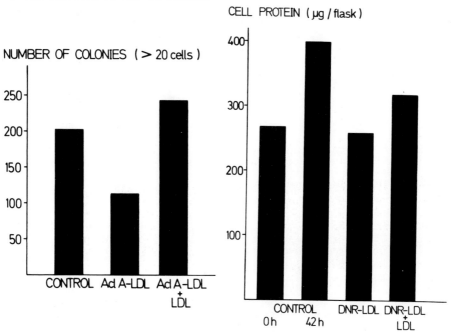

FIGURES 10 AND 11. Toxicity of LDL-incorporated aclacinomycin A (0.6 μM) on the colony-forming ability of leukemic cells (left) and of LDL-incorporated DNR (1 μM) on the growth of human malignant glioma cells in culture (right).

Studies are now in progress investigating the optimal conditions for incorporation of various cytotoxic drugs in LDL.

ACKNOWLEDGMENTS

This study was supported by grants from the Swedish Medical Research Council (No. 14X-05964), the Karolinska Institute and Åke Wibergs Foundation. We are indebted to Miss Iréne Granath, Mrs. Britt Sundman-Engberg, and Mrs. Sif Hultgren for excellent technical assistance.

REFERENCES

1. Noël G, Peterson C, Trouet A, Tulkens P, 1978. Uptake and subcellular localization of daunorubicin and adriamycin in cultured fibroblasts. Eur J Cancer 14, 363-368.
2. Egorin MJ, Clawson RE, Cohen JL, Ross LA, Bachur NR. 1980. Cytofluorescence localization of anthracycline antibiotics. Cancer Res 40, 4669-4676.
3. Pigram WJ, Fuller W, Hamilton LD. 1972. Stereochemistry of intercalation interaction of daunomycin with DNA. Nature New Biol 235, 17-19.
4. Bachur NR, Steele M, Meriwether WD, Hildebrand RC. 1976. Cellular pharmacodynamics of several anthracycline antibiotics. J Med Chem 19, 651-654.
5. Bachur NR, Gordon SL, Gee MV, Kon H. 1979. NADPH cytochrome P-450 reductase activation of quinone anticancer agents to free radicals. Proc Natl Acad Sci USA 76, 954-957.
6. Schioppacassi G, Schwartz HS. 1977. Membrane actions of daunorubicin in mammalian erythrocytes. Res Commun Chem Pathol Pharmacol 18, 519-531.
7. Wiernik PH. 1980. Current status of adriamycin and daunorubicin in cancer treatment. In Anthracyclines: Current status and new developments (Crooke ST, Reich SD, eds), Academic Press Inc, New York, 273-294.
8. Wilson HE, Bodey DP, Moon TE, et al. 1977. Adriamycin therapy in previously treated adult acute leukemia. Cancer Treat Rep 61, 905-907.
9. Peterson C, Paul C, Gahrton G. 1981. Anthracycline-DNA complexes as slow release preparations in the treatment of acute leukemia. In Controlled release of pesticides and pharmaceuticals. (Lewis DH, ed) Plenum Press, New York. 49-65.
10. Tulkens P, Trouet A. 1972. Uptake and intracellular localization of streptomycin in the lysosomes of cultured fibroblasts. Arch Int Physiol Biochem 80, 623-624.
11. Danö K. 1973. Active outward transport of daunomycin in resistant Ehrlich ascites tumor cells. Biochem Biophys Acta 323, 466-483.
12. Skovsgaard T. 1977. Transport and binding of daunorubicin, adriamycin, and rubidazone in Ehrlich ascites tumour cells. Biochem Pharmacol 26, 215-222.
13. Peterson C, Trouet A. 1978. Transport and storage of daunorubicin and doxorubicin in cultured fibroblasts. Cancer Res 38, 4645-46.
14. Inaba M, Kobayashi H, Sakurai Y, Johnson RK. 1979. Active efflux of daunorubicin and adriamycin in sensitive and resistant sublines of P 388 leukemia. Cancer Res 39, 2200-2203.
15. Peterson C, Baurain R, Trouet A. 1980. The mechanism for cellular uptake, storage and release of daunorubicin. Biochem Pharmacol 29, 1687-1692.
16. De Duve C, De Basy T, Poole B, Trouet A, Tulkens P, Van Hoof F. 1974. Lysosomotropic agents. Biochem Pharmacol 23, 2495-2531.
17. Schneider Y-J, Baurain R, Zeneberg A, Trouet A. 1979. DNA-binding parameters of daunorubicin and doxorubicin in the conditions used for studying the interaction of anthracycline-DNA complexes with cells in vitro. Cancer Chemother Pharmacol 2, 7-10.
18. Skovsgaard T. 1978. Mechanism of resistance to daunorubicin in Ehrlich ascites tumor cells. Cancer Res 38, 1785-1791.
19. Paul C, Björkholm M, Engstedt L, et al. Comparison of daunorubicin and daunorubicin-DNA complex in the treatment of acute nonlymphoblastic leukemia. Cancer Chemother Pharmacol, In press.
20. Paul C, Baurain R, Gahrton G, Peterson C. 1980. Determination of daunorubicin and its main metabolites in plasma, urine and leukemic cells in patients with acute myeloblastic leukemia. Cancer Lett 9, 263-269.

146

21. Paul C, Lönnqvist B, Gahrton G, Lockner D, Peterson C. Reducing the cardiotoxicity of anthracyclines by complex-binding to DNA. Report of Three Cases. Cancer, In press.
22. Peterson C, Noël G, Zeneberg A, Trouet A, 1979. Uptake of daunorubicin-DNA complex in cultured fibroblasts. Cancer Chemother Pharmacol 2, 3-6.
23. Trouet A, Deprez-de Campeneere D, de Duve C. 1972. Chemotherapy through lysosomes with DNA-daunorubicin complex. Nature New Biol 239, 110-112.
24. Deprez-De Campeneere D, Baurain R, Huybrechts M, Trouet A. 1979. Comparati study in mice of the toxicity, pharmacology and therapeutic activity of daunorubicin-DNA and doxorubicin-DNA complexes. Cancer Chemother Pharmacol 2, 25-30.
25. Andersson B, Beran M, Tribukait B, Peterson C. Significance of cellular pharmacokinetics for the cytotoxic effects of daunorubicin. Submitted to Cancer Res.
26. Goldstein JL, Brown MS. 1977. The low-density lipoprotein pathway and its relation to atherosclerosis. Ann Rev Biochem 46, 897-930.
27. Ho YK, Smith RG, Brown MS, Goldstein JL. 1978. Low density lipoprotein (LDL) receptor activity in human acute myelogenous leukemia cells. Blood 52, 1099-1114.
28. Rudling M, Peterson C. To be published.

CALCIUM FLUX AND METABOLISM IN THE PIGEON HEART FOLLOWING
DOXORUBICIN TREATMENT: A STUDY OF ACUTE CHANGES

N. W. REVIS

1. INTRODUCTION

Doxorubicin (Adriamycin, an antibiotic of the anthracycline
group, is highly efficacious in the treatment of a variety of
malignant disorders (1,2); however, its efficacy is partly dependent upon high cumulative dosages. At high dosages, a significant
number of patients are reported to develop an irreversible cardiomyopathy (3,4), which has limited the use of this anthracycline
in cancer chemotherapy. The cardiotoxic effects of doxorubicin
include cardiomegaly, EKG abnormalities, myocardial fibrosis, and
heart failure. Morphological changes of myocardial cells observed when this anthracycline is used include mitochondrial
swelling, intramitochondrial dense inclusion bodies (i.e.,
calcium-phosphate crystals), condensation of chromatin, a marked
decrease in glycogen granules, and an increase in the intracellular concentration of calcium (5,6). That calcium accumulates
in the myocardial cell following doxorubicin treatment is interesting because several investigators have observed a decrease in
the influx of calcium into mitochondria (7), red blood cells (8),
and the guinea pig atria (9) in the presence of this anthracycline. These apparent conflicting reports may be explained by
the following observations. It has been reported that doxorubicin chelates divalent cations such as calcium. If this suggestion is correct, one would expect that the available free
calcium would be reduced in a solution that contained both cal-

Research sponsored by the Office of Health and Environmental
Research, U.S. Department of Energy, under contract W-7405-eng-26
with the Union Carbide Corporation. By acceptance of this
article, the publisher or recipient acknowledges the right of the
U.S. government to retain a nonexclusive, royalty-free license
in and to any copyright covering the article.

cium and doxorubicin, which would effectively reduce the cellular influx of calcium. The inhibitory effect of doxorubicin on calcium flux has been observed in in vitro studies over a relatively short period of time (i.e., 60 minutes), whereas the reports that describe the accumulation of calcium in myocardial cells occurred following the long-term (i.e., months) treatment with doxorubicin. Myers et al. (10) have shown that membrane lipid peroxidation occurs in the heart following the long-term treatment with doxorubicin. Since the peroxidation of membrane lipids is associated with alteration in the permeability of these membranes, the observed increase in cellular calcium may result from changes in the permeability of the sarcolemma to calcium. Thus, the initial effects of doxorubicin on calcium influx into myocardial cells may be inhibitory due to the ability of this anthracycline to chelate calcium, whereas the secondary effect may be an increase in the concentration of calcium in the myocardial cells due to a change in the permeability of the cell membrane.

The present studies were performed to determine in vivo the initial and secondary acute effects of doxorubicin on the influx of calcium into myocardial cells. Studies are also described that show the effect of doxorubicin on a calcium-activated neutral protease from cardiac tissue. These latter studies were performed in an attempt to explain the loss of myofibrilular structures in myocardial cells following doxorubicin treatment.

2. MATERIALS AND METHODS

Male white Carneax pigeons 3 months of age were obtained from from Palmetto Pigeon Plant (Summter, S.C.) and were observed for signs of respiratory or intestinal infections for at least 14 days prior to the beginning of this study. After this period, pigeons were placed into a restrainer and the brachiocephalic artery and vein were exposed. A cannula (PE 50) was then introduced into the artery and vein and advanced into the left and right ventricle, respectively. Ventricular pressure was recorded with a Gould Statham (P23) pressure transducer that was attached to a Grass polygraph. The left ventricular pressure signal was fed to a Grass differentiator and dp/dt (i.e., the rate of pressure development in the left ventricle) was recorded.

After ventricular pressure had stabilized (usually within 30 minutes), saline or doxorubicin in saline (i.e., 3.0 or 6.0 mg/kg body weight) was infused over 4 minutes (1 ml/min); and, at various time intervals, ventricular pressure, dp/dt, and blood samples (0.5 ml) were taken. From the blood samples, plasma was isolated and creatine phosphokinase determined (11). At the end of the experimental period, pigeons were killed by injection of air. This was followed by a brief period of perfusion with Ringer's solution (minus calcium). Those pigeons in which morphological studies were to be performed were killed by perfusion of buffered formalin fixative for 10 minutes.

In some studies, $^{45}Ca^{2+}$ in saline (10 μCi) was infused through the cannula at various time intervals following doxorubicin treatment. Forty minutes after $^{45}Ca^{2+}$ had been infused, pigeons were killed by injection of air and then perfused with saline. The heart was removed and trimmed of fat, and a block of the left ventricular free wall was lyophilized and then hydrolyzed in nitric acid at 400° C for 24 hours. An aliquot of the hydrolysate was used to determine total calcium (Perkin-Elmer flame photometer) and $^{45}Ca^{2+}$ (liquid scintillation counter).

In studies in which the calcium-activated neutral protease was to be determined, the following method was employed. The pigeon heart was homogenized in 20 mM tris-acetate buffer (pH 7.0) containing 3 mM EDTA in a Virtis 45 homogenizer. The homogenate was filtered through four layers of cheesecloth and the filtrate was centrifuged at 50,000 g for 100 minutes. All of the procedures described above were carried out at 4° C.

Calcium-activated neutral protease (CANP) was assayed (12) by its ability to release material soluble in 100 mm KCl at pH 7.0 from intact myofibrils (i.e., pigeon myofibrils that had been isolated according to the procedure of Goll et al. /13/ with the omission of Triton X-100). The incubation mixture contained 100 mM KCl, 20 mM tris-acetate pH 7.0, 10 mM

2-mercaptoethanol, 8 mM $CaCl_2$, 4.0 mg purified myofibrils/ml, and 1 mg of enzyme (i.e., 50,000 g supernatant) protein in a total volume of 2.5 ml. Control tubes contained the same solutions except that 8 mm EDTA was substituted for 8 mM $CaCl_2$. After 24 hours at 30° C, each sample was centrifuged at 35,000 g for 30 minutes and the absorbency of the supernatant was measured at 278 nm. The difference in absorbance at 278 nm between sample and ·control tubes was used to calculate the specific CANP activity as ΔOD_{278} nm/mg protein 24 hours.

For morphological studies, heart tissue was prepared for light and electron microscope studies as previously described (14). The results described below were analyzed by student t test, and the differences between values of group means were considered significant only if the analysis of variance indicated a probability of less than 0.05.

3. RESULTS

These studies were performed to determine the effects of doxorubicin on calcium flux in myocardial cells from the pigeon. Ventricular pressure and dp/dt are both controlled in part by contraction of the myocardial cells. Contraction is initiated by the movement of calcium from the excellular space across the sarcolemma and from the sarcoplasmic reticulum. Thus, by measuring ventricular pressure and dp/dt, one can assess the effect of calcium flux in myocardial cells. Figure 1 shows a tracing of ventricular pressure and dp/dt from a control pigeon. These tracings were reproducible over the experimental period of 30 hours.

When doxorubicin was infused, left ventricular pressure remained steady during the first 30 minutes; thereafter, pressure gradually decreased below control values (Figure 2). The decrease was maximal in both groups for 60 minutes after doxorubicin had been infused. This effect appeared to be dose dependent in that the higher dose of doxorubicin (i.e., 6.0 mg/kg) was more effective in reducing ventricular pressure. Six hours after doxorubicin treatment, ventricular pressure gradually returned to control value, and by 30 hours post-

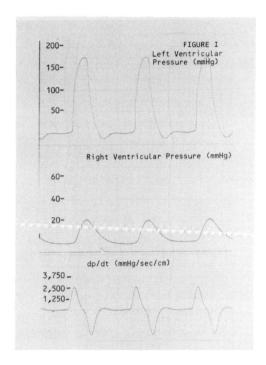

FIGURE 1. An example of ventricular pressure, dp/dt, and right ventricular pressure from a control pigeon 30 hours after saline had been infused.

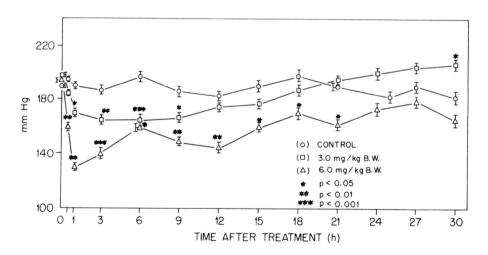

FIGURE 2. The effects of doxorubicin on systolic pressure in the pigeon. For detailed conditions, see "Materials and Methods" section. For each treatment group, 10 pigeons were used. Results are expressed as mean ± SEM.

treatment pressure in both experimental groups had reached the control level. Similar results were observed for dp/dt (Figure 3).

When total calcium in the heart was determined, a significant reduction was observed in the heart 60 minutes after 6.0 mg of doxorubicin had been infused (Figure 4). In pigeons treated with 3.0 mg, total calcium in the heart was decreased, but this reduction was not significant. In contrast to the initial effect (i.e., 60 minutes posttreatment), total calcium in the heart of both experimental groups was significantly increased 30 hours posttreatment. This secondary effect of doxorubicin may be related to the observed change in plasma CPK (Figure 5). The level of this enzyme began to increase in both groups 6-12 hours after doxorubicin treatment. By 24 hours posttreatment, the plasma level of this enzyme had begun to return to control values.

In an attempt to extend the observations on total calcium in the heart following doxorubicin treatment, $^{45}Ca^{2+}$ was infused at 0.20, 11.20, and 29.20 hours after doxorubicin had been infused. At 1, 12, and 30 hours, hearts were removed and $^{45}Ca^{2+}$ determined. We have previously observed that 90% of $^{45}Ca^{2+}$ is clear from the blood within 40 minutes of injection. Results (Table 1) show that the accumulation of $^{45}Ca^{2+}$ in the pigeon heart following doxorubicin treatment is depressed 1 hour after treatment and significantly increased 30 hours after treatment, which would support the results described above on the level of calcium in the heart after treatment with doxorubicin.

Previous morphological studies of the heart show a decrease and disorganization of myofibrilular structures in animals treated with doxorubicin. Figure 6a, b shows that, in the pigeon heart treated with doxorubicin, myofibrilular disorganization occurred after 30 hours of treatment. This morphological change was observed only 18 to 30 hours after treatment. Those factor(s) responsible for the change in the myofibrilular structures were sought by determination of a calcium-activated neutral protease specific to muscle tissue. The activity of this enzyme was significantly increased 12 hours after 6.0 mg of doxorubicin had been injected (Figure 7). At 30 hours posttreatment, both experimental groups showed a significant increase in the activity of this enzyme.

DISCUSSION

The present studies were performed to determine the in vivo effect of doxorubicin on calcium flux in myocardial cells. Sixty minutes after 6.0 mg

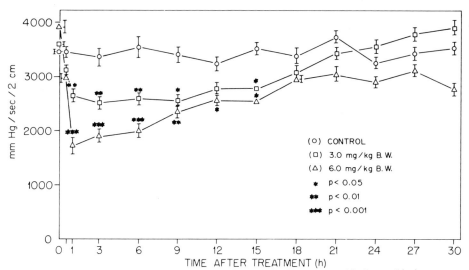

FIGURE 3. The effects of doxorubicin on dp/dt. Detailed conditions are described in "Materials and Methods." For each treatment group, 10 pigeons were used. Results are expressed as mean ± SEM.

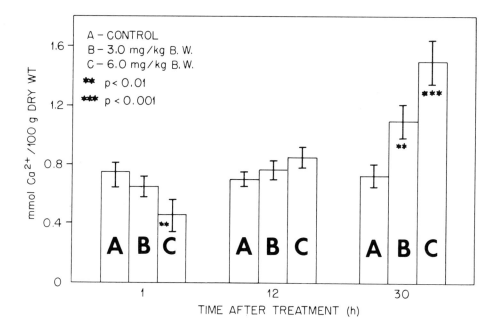

FIGURE 4. The concentration of calcium in the heart of doxorubicin-treated pigeons. Tissue calcium was determined as described in "Materials and Methods." At each time point (i.e., 1, 12, and 30 hours), at least six pigeons were used. Results are expressed as mean ± SEM.

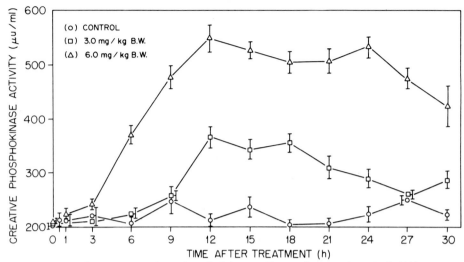

FIGURE 5. Plasma creatine phosphokinase from pigeons treated with doxorubicin. For each treatment group, 10 pigeons were used. Results are expressed as mean ± SEM.

Table 1. The effect of doxorubicin on the accumulation of $^{45}Ca^{2+}$ in the pigeon heart

Treatment	Time (hours) after doxorubicin treatment	cpm/gram wet weight
Control	1	898 ± 70
	12	1132 ± 130
	30	1280 ± 160
Doxorubicin 3.0 mg/kg	1	648 ± 90
	12	1800 ± 200[a]
	30	2460 ± 325[b]
Doxorubicin 6.0 mg/kg	1	543 ± 84[c]
	12	2630 ± 435[b]
	30	4001 ± 680[b]

Note: Doxorubicin was infused into the left ventricle and at 1, 12, and 30 hours after doxorubicin treatment, $^{45}Ca^{2+}$ (10μCi) in saline was injected into the left ventricle and pigeons were killed 45 minutes after $^{45}Ca^{2+}$ treatment. For each experiment point, six pigeons were used. Results are expressed as mean ± SEM.

a, p less than 0.01.
b, p less than 0.001.
c, p less than 0.05.

FIGURE 6a.

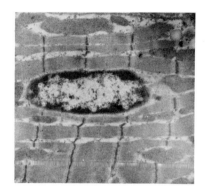

FIGURE 6b.

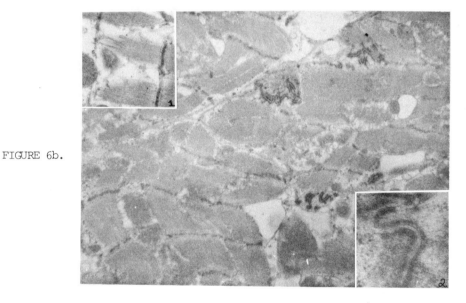

FIGURE 6. a, Ultrastructure of control pigeon heart 30 hours after
saline had been infused, X8500; b, 30 hours after 6.0 mg doxorubicin
had been infused. Note fragmentation of Z-disc, X5500; inset 1, note
fragmentation of Z-disc, X8500; inset 2, note fragmentation of the
intercalated disc, X28,000.

of doxorubicin had been infused, a significant reduction in ventricular pressure, dp/dt, and the concentration of total calcium and $^{45}Ca^{2+}$ in the heart was observed. These results suggest that doxorubicin inhibits the influx of calcium into myocardial cells. This suggestion is supported by several in vitro studies. For example, Herman et al. (15) observed a significant reduction in ventricular contraction in the isolated dog heart perfused with doxorubicin. This anthracycline has also been shown to inhibit the uptake of calcium by mitochondria (7) and red blood cells (8). Since doxorubicin is ineffective in altering the flux of calcium from the sarcoplasmic reticulum (16), it may inhibit calcium flux at the level of the sarcolemma.

In contrast to the results observed at 60 minutes, total calcium and $^{45}Ca^{2+}$ 30 hours after doxorubicin had been infused significantly increased in both experimental groups. The results observed at 30 hours appeared to contradict the suggestion that doxorubicin inhibits calcium flux. However, as tissue calcium increased, the permeability of the myocardial cell also increased (as determined by plasma CPK). These results suggest that doxorubicin has at least two effects on myocardial cells; i.e., 1) inhibition in the influx of calcium, and 2) an alteration in the permeability of the sarcolemma. Presumably these effects occur simultaneously in the myocardium and depend upon the extracellular and intracellular concentration of doxorubicin, respectively.

Lipid peroxidation of the sarcolemma may be responsible for the observed increase in the permeability of myocardial cells (10). Several investigators have suggested that doxorubicin induces lipid peroxidation through the free radical mechanism (17). The peroxidation of membrane lipid can result in change in the permeability of membranes (18). Thus, one may presume that the delay in the accumulation of tissue calcium is directly related to the intracellular concentration of doxorubicin.

In many types of myopathies, the initial alterations observed ultrastructurally are swollen mitochondria and degradation of the Z-disc, intercalated disc, and I bands (19). These ultrastructural changes are currently thought to be related to an impairment of the sarcolemma's ability to control the flux of calcium (20). The increase in the sarcoplasmic concentration of calcium is reported to stimulate a Ca^{2+}-activated cardiac protease which degrades α-actinin, a protein associated with the Z-disc and intercalated disc (21). The results from this study support this

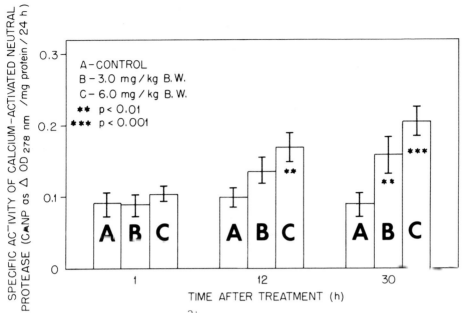

FIGURE 7. The activity of Ca^{2+}-activated neutral protease from pigeon heart following doxorubicin treatment. Assay conditions are described in "Materials and Methods." At each time point (i.e., 1, 12, and 30 hours), five pigeons were used. Results are expressed as mean $\pm$ SEM.

hypothesis, in that we observed biochemically a significant increase in the activity of this protease and ultrastructurally the apparent fragmentation of the Z-disc and intercalated disc.

These results suggest that doxorubicin initially inhibits the flux of calcium across the sarcolemma. As the intracellular concentration of doxorubicin increases, the permeability of the sarcolemma becomes impaired, which results in an increase in the flux of calcium.

REFERENCES

1. Blum RH, Carter SK. 1974. Adriamycin: a new anticancer drug with significant clinical activity. Ann. Intern. Med. 80: 249-259.
2. Di Marco A, Gaetani M, Scarpinato B. 1969. Adriamycin (NSC-123, 127): a new antibiotic with antitumor activity. Cancer Chemother. Rep. 53: 33-37.
3. Lefrank EA, Pitha J, Rosenheim S. 1975. Adriamycin cardiomyopathy. Cancer Chemother. Rep. 6(2): 203-208.
4. Minow RA, Banjamin RS, Gottliev JA. 1975. Adriamycin cardiomyopathy: an overflow with determination of risk factors. Cancer Chemother. Rep. 6(2): 195-201.
5. Young DM. 1975. Pathologic effects of adriamycin in experimental

systems. Cancer Chemother. Rep. 6: 159-175.

6. Jaenke, RS. 1974. An anthracycline antibiotic-induced cardiomyopathy in rabbits. Lab. Invest. 30: 292-304.

7. Revis NW, Marusic N. 1979. Effects of doxorubicin and its aglycone metabolite on calcium sequestration by rabbit heart, liver and kidney mitochondria. Life Sci. 2: 1055-1064.

8. Bossa R, Ceganti M, Dubini F, Galatulas I, Tofanetti O. 1974. Interferences between doxorubicin and calcium. Int. Res. Commun. Syst. 2: 1508-1511.

9. Bossa R, Galatulas I, Mantosani E. 1977. Cardio-toxicity of daunomycin and adriamycin. Neoplasma 24: 405-409.

10. Myers CE, McGuire WP, Young LC. 1976. Adriamycin amelioration of toxicity by α-tocopherol. Cancer Chemother. Rep. 60: 951-963.

11. Rosalki SB. 1967. An improved procedure for serum creatine phosphokinase determination. J. Lab. Clin. Med. 69: 696-705.

12. Dayton WR, Reville WJ, Groll DE, Stromer MH. 1967. A Ca^{2+}-activated protease possibility involved in myofibrillar protein turnover. Partial characterization of the purified enzyme. Biochemistry 15: 2159-2167.

13. Goll, DE, Young RB, Stromer MH. 1974. Proceedings of the 27th Annual Reciprocal Meat Conference, Chicago, National Livestock and Meat Board, p. 250.

14. Revis NW, Marusic N. 1979. Sequestration of $^{45}Ca^{2+}$ by mitochondria from rabbit heart, liver and kidney after doxorubicin or doxorubicin/digoxin treatment. Exp. Mol. Pathol. 3: 440-451.

15. Herman EH, Ramakant M, Mhatre LP, Vaman S. 1972. Prevention of the cardiotoxic effects of adriamycin and daunomycin in the isolated dog heart. Proc. Soc. Exp. Biol. Med. 140: 234-239.

16. Moore L, Landon E, Cooney DA. 1977. Inhibition of the cardiac mitochondrial calcium. Biochem. Med. 18: 131-138.

17. Pyor WA. 1966. Free radicals. New York, McGraw-Hill Book Co.

18. Leibowitz ME, Johnson MC. 1971. Relation of lipid peroxidation to the loss of cations trapped in liposomes. J. Lipid Res. 12: 662-670.

19. Yates JC, Dhalla NH. 1975. Structural and functional changes associated with failure and recovery of hearts after perfusion with calcium-free medium. J. Mol. Cell. Cardiol. 7: 91-103.

20. Vikert A, Sharov VG. 1976. Ultrastructure of rabbit heart outside ischemia zone of acute heart failure obtained against the background of experimental myocardial infarction. J. Mol. Cell. Cardiol. 8: 403-40

21. Dayton WR, Schollmyer JV. 1980. Isolation from porcine cardiac muscle of a Ca^{2+}-activated protease that partially degrades myofibrils. J. Mol. Cell. Cardiol. 12: 533-551.

THE ROLE OF ACUTE LIPID PEROXIDATION IN DOXORUBICIN CARDIOTOXICITY

M. E. SCHEULEN, H. MULIAWAN, AND H. KAPPUS

1. ABSTRACT

Ethane expiration, which indicates lipid peroxidation, was determined immediately, 1 day, and 2 days after i.p. injection of doxorubicin (20, 45, and 65 mg/kg) in rats in vivo. None of these doses caused a significant increase in ethane formation, except a small elevation on the 2nd day after 45/kg. Treatment with 65 mg/kg was lethal within 24 hours, although no increase in ethane production was measured during the first 6 hours after administration. These results suggest that acute lipid peroxidation may not occur during doxorubicin metabolism in the rat and may not be one of the primary reactions in doxorubicin cardiotoxicity. Thus, cardio-protection by α-tocopherol and other free radical scavengers may be due rather to the trap of free oxygen radicals than to the prevention of lipid peroxidation during doxorubicin metabolism.

2. INTRODUCTION

The clinical utility of the potent antineoplastic antibiotic doxorubicin is limited by its cumulative cardiotoxicity to 550 mg/m^2 (1) in man. Enzymic reduction of doxorubicin to the semiquinone radical causes the formation of superoxide anions in vitro (2-9). It has been suggested that the dose-related doxorubicin cardiomyopathy may be due to lipid peroxidation caused by superoxide anions or other reactive oxygen species subsequently formed (9-14). As doxorubicin cardiotoxicity could be ameliorated by pretreatment with the antioxidant α-tocopherol in animals in vivo (9, 15-17), the presumption that lipid peroxidation is involved in the biochemical mechanism of doxorubicin cardiotoxicity was further supported. However, lethality was not changed by α-tocopherol (18), and recent reports demonstrated its failure to protect against cardiotoxicity (14,19).

Doxorubicin-induced lipid peroxidation has been shown in rat liver microsomes in vitro (6). In contrast, the results on doxorubicin-induced lipid peroxidation in vivo so far presented (17, 20-21) are ambiguous for two reasons. 1) Generally, malondialdehyde is not accepted as a good indicator for lipid peroxidation in vivo (22-24). Therefore, the need for improved studies on doxorubicin-induced lipid peroxidation in vivo has been pointed out (9). 2) It cannot be excluded that lipid peroxidation may be a secondary effect due to doxorubicin-induced myocardiolysis in the course of subacute or chronic doxorubicin treatment in vivo.

To avoid these two limitations, we measured the ethane expiration of rats immediately, 1 day, and 2 days after i.p. injection of doxorubicin to determine the lipid peroxidation during doxorubicin metabolism in vivo.

3. MATERIALS AND METHODS

Male Wistar rats (180-200 g) received food (Altromin [R]) and tap water ad libitum, except during ethane sampling periods. Commercially available doxorubicin (Adriblastin [R]; Farmitalia Carlo Erba GmbH, Freiburg, Germany) was dissolved in saline and administered to the rats by i.p. injection. Animals of the control groups received instead an equal volume of saline i.p. Immediately after treatment, the rats were placed in special gas-tight desiccators, the air in the desiccators was sampled, and the amount of ethane expired by the animals was measured up to 6 hours (25). The rats were reexamined for their ethane expiration on the following 2 days exactly 24 hours and 48 hours after the injection without any further treatment. Between sampling periods, the animals were removed from the desiccators and were kept under normal conditions.

4. RESULTS

Table 1 shows the amount of ethane expired by the rats during a sampling period of 6 hours, immediately, 24 hours, and 48 hours after i.p. injection of 20 mg, 45 mg, and 65 mg doxorubicin/kg, respectively, in comparison with the controls.

After 20 mg doxorubicin/kg, all animals survived and expired the same amount of ethane as did the control animals.

After 45 mg doxorubicin/kg, three out of six animals died until the 3rd day. Except for a relatively small increase in ethane expired by the doxorubicin-treated rats on the 2nd day, before and after this second

Table 1. Ethane expiration of doxorubicin-treated rats

Treatment	nmoles ethane / kg body weight / 6 hours		
	1st day	2nd day	3rd day
Control	3.17 ± 0.50 (n = 4)	2.31 ± 0.89 (n = 4)	2.68 ± 0.40 (n = 4)
20 mg doxorubicin/kg	3.66 ± 0.66 (n = 6)	2.59 ± 0.45 (n = 6)	2.75 ± 0.84 (n = 6)
Control	2.93 ± 0.57 (n = 4)	2.84 ± 0.86 (n = 4)	2.53 ± 0.41 (n = 4)
45 mg doxorubicin/kg	3.24 ± 0.29 (n = 6)	5.11 ± 0.38 (n = 4)	3.89 ± 0.80 (n = 3)
Control	3.27 ± 0.70 (n = 3)	--	--
65 mg doxorubicin/kg	4.48 ± 0.24 (n = 3)	--	--

Note: Ethane expiration measured immediately (1st day), 24 hours (2nd day, and 48 hours (3rd day) after i.p. injection. Control animals received saline i.p. Mean values ± S.D. are shown.

sampling period ethane production rates were the same as in the controls. Figure 1 demonstrates in detail that no significant increase in ethane formation could be observed during the sampling period of 6 hours immediately after i.p. injection of 45 mg doxorubicin/kg.

After the very high dose of 65 mg doxorubicin/kg, all animals died before the 2nd day. Thus, the ethane expiration of these rats could be determined only immediately after doxorubicin application. In spite of the lethal doxorubicin dose, the acute ethane production of the treated rats was not increased in comparison to the control animals.

5. DISCUSSION

The determination of exhaled saturated short-chain alkanes is regarded as the best measure available for lipid peroxidation in vivo (22-24). Furthermore, this method offers the advantage that lipid peroxidation can be monitored continuously in vivo. Ethane probably originates from the disintegration of peroxidized ω-3-polyunsaturated fatty acids, whereas

162

pentane is formed from ω-6-polyunsaturated lipid hydroperoxides. Thus, patterns of the hydrocarbons exhaled by animals treated with toxic agents depended on the varying amounts of polyunsaturated fatty acids in their diets (24). Selenium or α-tocopherol deficiency provoked higher amounts of ethane and pentane expiration, which could be further increased by additional treatment with toxic compounds (24,26).

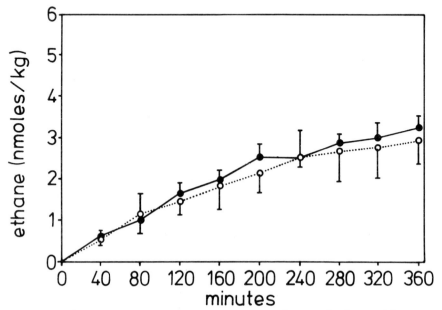

FIGURE 1. Time curves of ethane formation of rats during a 6-hour sampling period immediately (1st day) after a single injection of ● 45 mg doxorubicin/kg dissolved in saline i.p. (n = 6), O saline i.p. (n = 4). Mean values ± S.D. are shown.

Our investigations on the acute influence of doxorubicin on lipid peroxidation in rats in vivo demonstrate that none of the doxorubicin doses administered could induce immediate ethane formation, although doxorubicin is rapidly absorbed and shows high acute toxicity in rats after i.p. injection (11-12). Accordingly, in our series some of the rats died after treatment. It is unlikely that the comparatively low increase in ethane expiration observed in animals on the 2nd day after 45 mg doxorubicin/kg is responsible for the high acute toxicity of doxorubicin. With CCl$_4$ or other compounds inducing free radical reactions and lipid peroxidation in vivo, much higher amounts of ethane could be detected after the treatment of rats (22-25). Recently, a similarly small increase in ethane formation after treatment of rats with paraquat has been described and interpreted as not being causative for the acute paraquat toxicity in vivo (27-28). Like doxorubicin, paraquat has been shown to generate super-oxide anion radicals in vivo (22).

As no significant increase in ethane formation caused by doxorubicin was measured during the first 6-hour sampling periods, acute lipid peroxidation may not occur during doxorubicin metabolism in the rat in vivo, not even during reduction by cytochrome P-450 reductase in the liver, which starts immediately after treatment (3-5, 9). The semiquinone radical thus formed might spontaneously reduce molecular oxygen to the reactive super-oxide anion (3-8). Therefore, our results indicate that in vivo the super-oxide anion radical either is not formed during doxorubicin metabolism or is not able to provoke lipid peroxidation. In this respect, either the oxygen concentration or the detoxification reactions in the cells that metabolize doxorubicin could become crucial. Furthermore, acute lipid peroxidation may not be one of the primary reactions in doxorubicin cardiotoxicity. The cardioprotective effect of α-tocopherol has recently become a matter of controversy (9, 14-20) and may, according to our results, be due rather to the trap of free oxygen radicals than to the prevention of lipid peroxidation during doxorubicin metabolism.

On the other hand, it cannot be excluded that subacute or chronic treatment with low doses of doxorubicin results in higher lipid peroxidation rates than observed during acute doxorubicin dosage. Lipid peroxidation in the course of subacute or chronic doxorubicin treatment in vivo (17, 20-21) may be 1) a secondary effect due to doxorubicin-induced myo-cardiolysis or 2) an effect which becomes predominant after doxorubicin-dependent depletion of glutathione (29) and a subsequent decrease in gluta-thione peroxidase activity (30) or after doxorubicin-dependent inactivation or exhaustion of other detoxification reactions. This question will have to be answered to define the role of lipid peroxidation in doxorubicin cardiotoxicity.

6. ACKNOWLEDGMENT

We thank the Deutsche Forschungsgemeinschaft, Bonn-Bad Godesberg, Germany, for financial support (SFB 102, C4 and Ka 447/5).

REFERENCES

1. Lefrak EA, Pitha J, Rosenheim S, Gottlieb JA. 1973. Cancer 32: 302-314.
2. Handa K, Sato S. 1975. Gann 66: 43-47.
3. Bachur NR, Gordon SL, Gee MV. 1977. Mol. Pharmacol. 13: 901-910.
4. Bachur NR, Gordon SL, Gee MV. 1978. Cancer Res 38: 1745-1750.
5. Bachur NR, Gordon SL, Gee MV, Kon H. 1979. Proc. Natl. Acad. Sci. USA 76: 954-957.
6. Goodman J, Hochstein P. 1977. Biochem. Biophys. Res. Commun. 77: 797-803.
7. Sato S, Iwaizumi M, Handa K, Tamura Y. 1977. Gann 68: 603-608.
8. Thayer WS. 1977. Chem.-Biol. Interact. 19: 265-278.
9. Donehower RC, Myers CE, Chabner BA. 1979. Life Sci. 25: 1-14.
10. Carter SK. 1975. J. Natl. Cancer Inst. 55: 1265-1274.
11. Mettler FP, Young DM, Ward JM. 1977. Cancer Res. 37: 2705-2713.
12. Doroshow JH, Locker GY, Myers CE. 1979. Cancer Treat. Rep. 63: 855-860.
13. Von Hoff DD, Layard MW, Basa P, Davis HL, von Hoff AL, Rozencweig M, Muggia FM. 1979. Ann. Int. Med. 91: 710-717.
14. Van Vleet JF, Ferans VJ, Weirich WE. 1980. Amer. J. Pathol. 99: 13-42.
15. Myers CE, McGuire WP, Young RC. 1976. Cancer Treat. Rep. 60: 961-962.
16. Sonneveld P. 1978. Cancer Treat. Rep. 62: 1033-1036.
17. Yamanaka N, Kato T, Nishida K, Fujikawa T, Fukushima M, Ota K. 1979. Cancer Chemother. Pharmacol. 3: 223-227.
18. Mimnaugh EG, Siddik ZH, Drew R, Sikic BI, Gram TE. 1979. Toxicol. Appl. Pharmacol. 49: 119-126.
19. Breed JGS, Zimmerman ANE, Dormans JAMA, Pinedo HM. 1980. Cancer Res. 40: 2033-2038.
20. Myers CE, McGuire WP, Liss RH, Ifrim I, Grotzinger K, Young RC. 1977. Science 197: 165-167.
21. Stuart MJ, deAlarcon PA, Barvinchak MK. 1978. Amer. J. Hematol. 5: 297-303.
22. Bus JS, Gibson JE. 1979. In: Hodgson E, Bend JR, Philpot RM, eds. Reviews in biochemical toxicology, vol. 1. New York, Elsevier/North Holland, pp. 125-149.
23. Cohen G. 1979. In: Ciba Foundation Symposium 65 (new series). Oxygen free radicals and tissue damage. Amsterdam, Excerpta Medica, pp. 177-185.
24. Tappel AL. 1980. In: Pryor WA, ed. Free radicals in biology, vol. 4. New York, Academic Press, pp. 1-47.
25. Koster U, Albrecht D, Kappus H. 1977. Toxicol. Appl. Pharmacol. 41: 639-648.
26. Dillard CJ, Sagai M, Tappel AL. 1980. Toxicol. Lett. 6: 251-256.
27. Burk RF, Lawrence RA, Lane JM. 1980. J. Clin. Invest. 65: 1024-1031.
28. Steffen C, Muliawan H, Kappus H. 1980. Naunyn-Schmiedeberg's Arch. Pharmacol. 310: 241-243.
29. Doroshow JH, Locker GY, Baldinger J, Myers CE. 1979. Res. Commun. Chem. Pathol. Pharmacol. 26: 285-295.
30. Younes M, Siegers CP. 1980. Res. Commun. Chem. Pathol. Pharmacol. 27: 119-128.

THE PHYSICOCHEMICAL PROPERTIES AND TRANSMEMBRANEOUS TRANSPORT OF DOXORUBICIN

M. DALMARK

1. INTRODUCTION

Doxorubicin is one of our most widely used and potent drugs against human cancer. It is generally assumed that doxorubicin has to enter the cell across the plasma membrane in order to exert its therapeutic effect by interference with the function of the DNA in the cell nucleus through intercalation (1). The transport mechanism by which doxorubicin enters the cell across the rate-limiting barrier is still under debate. It has been proposed that doxorubicin is actively extruded from the cells, counteracting a facilitated diffusion transport process (a carrier-mediated transport) into the cells because 1) the cellular doxorubicin uptake increases in the presence of metabolic inhibitors, and 2) the doxorubicin transport shows saturation kinetics, self-inhibition, and substrate competition (2-4). However, a membrane-bound doxorubicin-activated ATP'ase has not yet been demonstrated. So far, doxorubicin has been demonstrated to be an inhibitor of the Na,K-activated membrane-bound ATP'ase (5). Furthermore, in order to understand the transmembraneous transport mechanism of a compound, one must demonstrate how the physicochemical characteristics of the compound in the water phases on both sides of the membrane are affected, for example, by the concentration of the compound itself, the concentration of other compounds, the temperature, and the pH. The purpose of the present paper is 1) to summarize data on some of the physicochemical properties of doxorubicin in aqueous solution, and 2) to describe how these properties apparently explain some of the features of doxorubicin transport across biological membranes. In the first section, some of the physicochemical properties of doxorubicin important to doxorubicin transport are described. In the next section, the experimental evidence for the perception of doxorubicin transport as a nonionic diffusion through the low dielectric domain of the cell membrane is summarized. In the third section, the deviations of the doxorubicin transport characteristics from those of a simple Fickian

diffusion transport process are discussed on the basis of the description
of the physicochemical properties of doxorubicin. It is concluded that
the doxorubicin transport mechanism might be a Fickian diffusion transport
process of the electroneutral doxorubicin molecule through the lipid domain
of the cell membrane like the transport mechanism of other lipophilic
compounds. The physicochemical properties of doxorubicin in aqueous solution
predict pH-dependence, saturation kinetics, substrate inhibition, and
nonlinear Arrhenius diagrams. The data indicate that one does not need to
assume existence of a carrier in order to explain the kinetic data. However,
the relationship between the metabolic status of the cell and the cellular
doxurubicin uptake is still not well understood.

2. THE PHYSICOCHEMICAL PROPERTIES OF DOXORUBICIN IN AQUEOUS SOLUTION

Doxorubicin is a glycosidic antibiotic constituted by a pigmented
aromatic aglycone linked to an aminosugar (6). The amino group is partly
ionized at physiological conditions, meaning that the doxorubicin monomer
exists as two physicochemical different species: 1) an unprotonized
electroneutral molecule, and 2) a protonized cation. The value of the pK
of the amino group given in the literature is not well defined with regard
to temperature and ionic strength (3,6), both of which are known to affect
the pK of the amino groups drastically (7,8). Furthermore, the determination
of the pK has been carried out by titration of rather concentrated doxorubicin solutions in water (1 m$\underline{M}$), a concentration range where carbon dioxide
present in the atmospheric air might be troublesome and special precautions
must be taken and explicitly stated. Finally, the pK of doxorubicin increases with doxorubicin concentration because doxorubicin self-associates
(9,10) simply for statistical reasons but, also, the intrinsic pK of the
amino group might change by electrostatic interaction. These factors are
probably the reason for the wide range of pK values given in the literature
(for example, cf. 11). The fraction of ionized doxorubicin is critical if
kinetic data are to be compared under various conditions. The data are
readily comparable with regard to the driving forces of the transport only
when the fraction of ionized doxorubicin is constant, for example, at
various temperatures (8). The unprotonized electroneutral doxorubicin
species is sparsely water soluble, in contrast to the doxorubicin cation.
Thus, it has been demonstrated that the doxorubicin partition between a lipid
and water phase at constant temperature and ionic strength is a sensitive

function of the pH in the water phase (9).

It was demonstrated more than 50 years ago in the German dye industry that aromatic dyes have peculiar physicochemical properties. It was demonstrated that dyes formed aggregates and changed light absorbance with concentration. Doxorubicin is an aromatic dye with four rings, of which three rings are aromatic and planar. It was observed that the light absorbance of doxorubicin as a function of concentration did not obey Lambert-Beer's law (12). In 1974 it was demonstrated that daunomycin self-associates in aqueous solution as a function of concentration and temperature (9). Later the self-association of doxorubicin was demonstrated (8,10,11). The doxorubicin molecules were apparently stacked together by hydrophobic forces through π-electron interaction. For electrostatic reasons, it is mainly electroneutral and sparsely water-soluble doxorubicin molecules that self-associate, but the complexes turn into more hydrophilic, positively charged aggregates by random association of the complexes with doxorubicin cations. This means that doxorubicin in aqueous solution appears as several physico-chemical different species ranging from monomers through dimers toward polymers, out of which some species are electroneutral and others carry one to several positive charges. The partition of the various species between a lipid phase and a water phase is greatly affected by the polymerization process with serious implications for the doxorubicin transport. The partition coefficient of doxorubicin is a function of concentration and temperature; this is also true in experimental situations where the heat of ionization of doxorubicin amino group has been taken into account (8). It appears that doxorubicin exists as a monomer in aqueous solution at concentrations below 10^{-5} $\underline{M}$ (37° C, pH 7.3, ionic strength 0.15) (8,10), because the lipid/water partition coefficient at lower concentration has been determined to be constant.

Anthracyclines form molecular associations--heteroassociations--with a broad range of compounds from very high molecular weight compounds to rather simple and low-molecular-weight molecules in aqueous solution. The ability of the anthracyclines to intercalate and form complexes with DNA is well known (1). Furthermore, anthracyclines interact with high-molecular-weight structures composed of negatively charged phospholipids (13-15), sulphated mucopolysaccharides (16), nonhistone protein from rat liver (17), and tubulin (18). Finally, anthracyclines interact with dinucleotides, nucleotides such as ATP, nucleosides, DNA-derived bases, as well as with a broad range of biologically active compounds such as tryptophan, propantheline, chloroquine, imipramine, propranolol, and caffeine (21; Dalmark and Johansen, unpublished), and flavin mononucleotide (19).

The ability of small heterocyclic compounds to increase the solubility of the sparsely water-soluble electroneutral doxorubicin molecule was in accordance with, for example, the solubilization of 3,4-benzpyrene in aqueous solution of caffeine and other nitrogeneous bases first described by Brock, Druckrey, and Hamperl in 1938 (20). The complex formation between doxorubicin and the low-molecular-weight compounds in aqueous solution was demonstrated by a decrease in the 1-octanol/water partition coefficient, meaning that the low-molecular-weight molecules increased the water solubility of doxorubicin by decreasing the apparent activity coefficient of doxorubicin in the water phase A decreased apparent activity coefficient of doxorubicin in the water phase close to the rate-limiting barrier of a cell membrane means that the doxorubicin driving force is smaller than would be expected from the doxorubicin concentration.

From a clinical point of view, the ability of plasma components such as human albumin to form complexes with doxorubicin is important. The apparent doxorubicin activity coefficient in plasma (37° C, pH 7.3) is approximately 0.15 the activity coefficient of doxorubicin in a salt solution at identical and therapeutical concentrations, indicating that 85 percent of doxorubicin in plasma is bound to plasma components (21).

The obvious interpretation of the binding forces of complex formation is short-range, hydrophobic forces assisted by long-range, electrostatic forces. All of the compounds contain planar aromatic ring systems which, when oriented in parallel with the aromatic chromophore of doxorubicin, interact with doxorubicin through π-electron interaction. Negatively charged compounds interact electrostatically with the doxorubicin cations.

3. THE LIPID PATHWAY OF DOXORUBICIN BY NONIONIC DIFFUSION

The doxorubicin transport across the Ehrlich ascites tumor cell membrane (4) and the human red blood cell membrane (22) increases with pH, demonstrating that the transported doxorubicin species is the electroneutral and hydrophobic species. This indicates that doxorubicin is transported in a fashion analogous to the transport of other titratable lipophilic compounds such as salicylic acid/salicylate (23). One would expect that highly lipophilic compounds that interact with the hydrophobic areas of the cell membran and increase the fluidity of the lipids accelerate the transmembraneous doxorubicin transport if the doxorubicin transport takes place through the low dielectric lipid domain of the cell membrane. This accelerative effect of lipophilic compounds such as aliphatic alcohols and local anesthetics (both positively and negatively charged) on doxorubicin transport has been demonstrated both in human red blood cells (22) and in Ehrlich ascites tumor cells (Dalmark and Hoffmann, unpublished) at concentrations of the compounds that did not affect the lipid/water partition of doxorubicin.

The interpretation of doxorubicin transport as a transport through the lipid domain of the cell membrane is supported by the observations that anthracyclines 1) reverse echinocytic red cells to biconcave disks (24), 2) increase the fluidity of membranes (25), 3) change the thermotropic properties of lipids (26), and 4) change their fluorescence spectrum in the presence of liposomes and cell membranes toward that observed in a low dielectric medium (26).

Comparison of the doxorubicin permeability in various cell types is not possible at present except for two cells. The permeability coefficients calculated from doxorubicin influx into human red blood cells and Ehrlich ascites tumor cells suspended in a Ringer's salt solution (37° C, pH 7.3) at 5 μM doxorubicin were 4×10^{-6} cm sec^{-1} and 2×10^{-5} cm sec^{-1}, respectively (21; Dalmark and Hoffmann, unpublished). These data do not support the perception of a different transport mechanism in the two-cell types in accordance with the effect of cell membrane modifiers on doxorubicin transport in the two-cell types.

The experimental data indicate that doxorubicin transport across biological membranes is a transport of the electroneutral doxorubicin species through the lipid domain of the cell membrane as a nonionic diffusion in a fashion similar to the transport of other lipophilic compounds. The present conclusion does not exclude the possibility of a doxorubicin adsorption to membrane proteins (which certainly takes place) but only claims that the major part of the transmembraneous transport of doxorubicin takes place through the lipid pathway of cell membranes.

4. APPARENT DEVIATIONS FROM THE PHENOMENOLOGY OF SIMPLE DIFFUSION

Doxorubicin transport shows saturation kinetics both in Ehrlich ascites tumor cells (2,4) and in human red blood cells (8,24). The observed half-saturation constant (approximately 80 μM) in human red blood cells correlated qualitatively and semiquantitatively with the half-maximal constant of the doxorubicin 1-octanol/water partition coefficient as a function of doxorubicin concentration. The observed half-saturation constant in ascites tumor cells was approximately one order of magnitude lower; however, one seldom, if ever, measures the concentration at the place where the permeability is highest. Furthermore, red cells and ascites tumor cells adsorb doxorubicin to a very different extent. The calculated surface concentration was approximately 5 μM in ascites cells suspended in a salt solution at 6 μM doxorubicin (Dalmark and Hoffmann, unpublished), in contrast to the absence of any signifi-cent adsorption to the red cell surface (21). So, the doxorubicin concentration at the rate-limiting barrier of the cell membrane in ascites tumor cells might be substantially higher than in the bulk water phase. Finally, it has been demonstrated that the amount of doxorubicin adsorbed to the cell surface in ascites tumor cells apparently saturates gradually at concentrations in the bulk phase above 20 μM (4).

The self-association of anthracyclines increases with decreasing tempera-ture (8,9). This means that the actual doxorubicin species increase their molecular weight and charge with decreasing temperature even at a constant intrinsic ionization of the doxorubicin amino group. The temperature-dependence of the doxorubicin is nonlinear and concentration-dependent in accordance with the shift in the physicochemical species of doxorubicin (7).

The importance of complex formation on doxorubicin transport and equili-brium distribution has been observed in various test systems. The doxorubicin influx (mol cm^{-2} sec^{-1}) into human red blood cells decreased to approximately 0.15 in cells suspended in autologous plasma compared with cells suspended in a Ringer's salt solution (37° C, pH 7.3) (21). The adenosine 5'-triphosphate and caffeine decreased doxorubicin influx at concentrations from 1-10 mM. The decreased doxorubicin influx markedly influenced the equilibrium distribution of doxorubicin between cells and medium both in human red blood cells (21) and in nucleated cells (27,28).

5. CONCLUSIONS

The physicochemical properties of the anthracyclines appear to have important consequences for the behavior of anthracyclines in biological systems. First of all, self-association and heteroassociation decrease the activity of doxorubicin to low values in aqueous solution compared with the total concentration. This decrease in activity affects the transport across the biological membranes, the equilibrium distribution across the cell membranes, and probably also the "reactivity" of doxorubicin with enzyme systems. The transmembraneous doxorubicin transport might be a simple diffusion transport process (nonionic diffusion) analogous to the transport of other lipophilic compounds.

6. ACKNOWLEDGMENT

This work has been supported by a grant from the Danish Cancer Society.

REFERENCES

1. Pigram, WJ, Fuller W, Hamilton LD. 1972. Stereochemistry of intercalation: Interaction of daunomycin with DNA. Nature (London), New Biol. 235: 17-19.
2. Danoe KJ. 1976. Experimentally developed resistance to daunomycin. Acta Path. Microbiol. Scand., suppl. 256.
3. Skovsgaard T. 1977. Transport and binding of daunomycin, adriamycin and rubidazone in Ehrlich ascites tumour cells. Biochem. Pharmacol. 26: 215-222.
4. Skovsgaard T. 1978. Carrier-mediated transport of daunomycin, adriamycin and rubidazone in Ehrlich ascites tumor cells. Biochem. Pharmacol. 27: 1221-1227.
5. Gosalves M, van Rossum GDV, Blanco MF. 1979. Inhibition of sodium-potassium-activated adenosine 5'-triphosphatase and ion transport by adriamycin. Cancer Res. 39: 257-261.
6. Arcamone F, Cassinelli G, Franceschi G, Penco S, Pol C, Redaelli S, Selva A. 1972. Structure and physicochemical properties of adriamycin (doxorubicin). In: Int. Symp. Adriamycin (Carter SK, Di Marco A, Ghione M, Krakoff IH, Mathé G, eds.). New York, Springer-Verlag, pp. 9-22.
7. Bates RG. 1973. Determination of pH. 2nd ed. New York, John Wiley, p. 90.
8. Dalmark M, Storm HH. In press. A Fickian diffusion transport process with features of transport catalysis: Doxorubicin transport in human red blood cells. J. Gen. Physiol.
9. Barthelemy-Clavey V, Maurizot J-C, Dimicoli J-L, Sicard P. 1974. Self-association of daunomycin. FEBS Lett. 46: 5-10.
10. Eksborg S. 1978. Extraction of daunomycin and doxorubicin and their hydroxyl metabolites: Self-association in aqueous solutions. J. Pharm. Sci. 67: 782-785.
11. Righetti PG, Menozzi M, Gianazza E, Valentini L. 1979. Protolytic equilibria of doxorubicin as determined by isoelectric focusing and "electrophoretic titration curves." FEBS Lett. 101: 51-55.
12. Bachur NR, Moore AL, Bernstein JG, Liu A. 1970. Tissue distribution and disposition of daunomycin in mice: Fluorometric and isotopic methods. Cancer Chemother. Rep. 54: 89-94.
13. Duarte-Karim M, Ruysschaert JM, Hildebrand J. 1976. Affinity of adriamycin to phospholipids: A possible explanation for cardiac mitochondrial lesions. Biochem. Biophys. Res. Commun. 71: 658-663.
14. Goormaghtigh E, Chatelain P, Caspers J, Ruysschaert JM. 1980. Evidence of a specific complex between Adriamycin and negatively charged

172

phosphlipids. Biochim. Biophys. Acta 597: 1-14.

15. Goormagtigh E, Chatelain P, Caspers J, Ruysschaert JM. 1980. Evidence of a complex between Adriamycin derivatives and cardiolipin: Possible role in cardiotoxicity. Biochem. Pharmacol. 29: 3003-3010.

16. Menozzi M, Arcamone F. 1978. Binding of adriamycin to sulphated mucopolysaccharides. Biochem. Biophys. Res. Commun. 80: 313-318.

17. Kikuchi H, Sato S. 1976. Binding of daunomycin to nonhistone proteins from rat liver. Biochim. Biophys. Acta 434: 509-512.

18. Chao Na, Timasheff SN. 1977. Physical-chemical study of daunomycin-tubulin interactions. Arch. Biochem. Biophys. 182: 147-154.

19. Kharasch ED, Novak RF. 1980. Ring current effect in Adriamycin-flavin mononucleotide complexation as observed by H FT NMR spectroscopy. Biochem. Biophys. Res. Commun. 92: 1320-1326.

20. Brock N, Druckrey H, Hamperl H. 1938. Zur Wirkungsweise carcinogener Substanzen. Arch. Exp. Pathol. Pharmakol. 189: 709-731.

21. Dalmark M, Johansen P. 1981. Regulations of doxorubicin (Adriamycin) transport across biological membranes by complex formation with nucleotides, nucleosides, and DNA-derived bases. Proc. Am. Assoc. Cancer Res. 22: 31.

22. Dalmark M. In press. Characteristics of doxorubicin transport in human red blood cells. Scand. J. Clin. Lab. Invest.

23. Dalmark M, Wieth JO. 1972. Temperature dependence of chloride, bromide, iodide, thiocyanate and salicylate transport in human red cells. J. Physiol. (London) 224: 583-610.

24. Mikkelsen RD, Peck-Sun L, Wallach DFH. 1977. Interaction of adriamycin with human red blood cells: A biochemical and morphological study. J. Mol. Med. 2: 33-40.

25. Tritton TR, Murphree SA, Sartorelli AC. 1978. Citation in Biochim. Biophys. Acta 512: 254-269. (See ref. 26.)

26. Goldman R, Facchinatti T, Bach D, Raz A, Shinitzky M. 1978. A differential interaction of daunomycin, adriamycin and their derivatives with human erythrocytes and phospholipids bilayers. Biochim. Biophys. Acta 512: 254-269.

27. Kessel D. 1979. Biologic properties of three anthracyclines as a function of lipophilicity. Biochem. Pharmacol. 28: 3028-3030.

28. Egorin MJ, Clawson RE, Ross LA, Bachur NR. 1980. Cellular pharmacology of N,N-dimethyl daunomycin and N,N-dimethyl Adriamycin. Cancer Res. 40: 1928-1933.

SECTION 3

DRUG DEVELOPMENT

INTRODUCTION

F. M. MUGGIA

The development of anticancer drugs has relied primarily on the identification of new structures showing efficacy against animal tumors. This
empirical research "trail" has contributed a greater number of compounds
than have efforts at synthetic development of drugs specifically and rationally directed against certain targets. A third route that is assuming an
increasingly greater importance is that of analog development, or what might
be dubbed the "modification trail." This particular route was thoroughly
exploited initially to improve the therapeutic index of alkylating agents.
We are now witnessing similar concentrated efforts with the anthracycline
antibiotics. Impressive therapeutic advances have been made in other biomedical research fields through this mixture of the empirical and rational
approaches. We shall point out highlights of this interplay which is
described in detail in the ensuing chapters.

The factors behind the antitumor selectivity of the anthracycline antibiotics are not known. However, structure-activity relationships may be
developed on a number of biochemical parameters which may then, in turn,
be examined for correlation with antitumor activity. Arcamone has summarized
the extensive investigations of his research team on a number of related
compounds. His classification of these compounds is based on their interaction with DNA, and he divides them into those with high, intermediate, and
low affinity. Within each one of these categories, drugs exhibit a spectrum
of antitumor efficacy in animal systems which may be considered the desired
biological parameter.

Other biological features such as cytotoxicity against human tumor
xenografts or human tumor colony-forming units will undoubtedly play an
increasingly greater role in the future in developing such structure-
activity relationships. The chemical moieties which modify DNA affinity
without destroying antitumor activity include 4'-epi-, 4-demethoxy-,
9-deacetyl, and -ol derivatives of doxorubicin and daunorubicin for the

high affinity compounds; 4'- sugar additions for intermediate affinity
compounds, and further sugar modifications, lypopilic side chains, and
acetylated daumosamine for the low affinity compounds.

Reactions other than that of DNA binding have captured the attention
of other researchers. Among these biochemical reactions one can list those
common to macromolecular binding and its consequences such as inhibition of
thymidine and uridine incorporation, inhibition of mitosis, and cytotoxicity.
In addition, drug interaction with cell surfaces, free radical activation
and lipid peroxidation, inhibition of calcium transport, and impairment of
mitochondrial function have received attention. Since the biochemical
reactions accounting for the antitumor selectivity of anthracyclines are
uncertain, these newer parameters may be as valid as the study of DNA binding.
Moreover, there are some lines of evidence pointing to the association of
certain biochemical reactions specific to toxicities. Thus, improvement on
the therapeutic index may also result from structure-activity studies focusing
on the elimination of certain toxic effects.

A major pathway of study has been the search for analogs with reduced
cardiotoxicity. Other toxic effects such as alopecia and wasting have
received lesser attention. Of more recent interest has been the elimination
of mutogenicity. Finally, drastic alterations in potency and pharmacology
may allow one to circumvent the intravenous route and its associated
toxicities such as phlebitis and extravasation.

Structure-activity studies in many of these biochemical parameters
have also emenated from laboratories in France and the United States. These
are summarized in the chapters by Mathé and Maral; Acton, Jensen, and Peters;
and Tihon and Issell. Workers in Japan are also contributing to the cooperative evaluation of anthracyclines including some of their own derivatives
such as aclacinomycin A (1) and THP-adriamycin. Other unique structures being
studied by workers other than the Italian group include nogalomycin derivative
such as 7-con-O-methylnogarol (2), dibenzyl derivitives requiring in vivo
activation described by Acton, Jensen, and Peters, and an entire family of
anthracyclines exhibiting potent inhibition of RNA synthesis (3).

The implications of free-radical activation on drug development are discussed by Pietronigro. Free-radical reactions are probably contributing to
cardiotoxicity, extravasation toxicity, mutagenicity, and cardiogenicity, as
well as acute lethal effects in animals. Study of quenchers of anthracycline
free-radical activation and the various drug free-radical species as well as

activated oxygen species is ongoing in his laboratory. The contribution of
these biochemical reactions to antitumor efficacy are currently largely
unknown.

An emerging new area of drug development is that of carriers that may
alter drug disposition and uptake by various tissues. Electrical charges
on liposomes may specifically alter drug concentration in cardiac tissue;
data dealing with toxic effects in animals lend support to the concept that
the therapeutic index of doxorubicin may be improved by encapsulation of the
drug in positively charged liposomes. DNA-anthracycline complexes have been
tested clinically (4) but practical considerations coupled with absent proof
of cardiotoxicity have delayed additional investigations with these materials.
A related area of study is the disposition and activity of leucyl-daunorubicin
by the same group of workers. This coupled compound requires lysosomal enzyme
hydrolysis to yield daunorubicin. Extension of this concept to coupling
anthracyclines with monoclonal antibodies is also under investigation.

Not unlike other fields of drug development, the antitumor selectivity
of doxorubicin has seldom been exceeded by analogs. The second generation
of analogs introduced clinically has not yet offered convincing evidence of
superiority over the parent compounds. Nevertheless, as the field progresses
and greater knowledge is amassed on the mechanism of antitumor action and
toxicity of these compounds, the next generation of analogs promises to
introduce properties that will render these compounds superior to doxorubicin
in specific situations. For example, it is likely that orally active anthracyclines will find a therapeutic role. Also, the up-to-now elusive goal of
attenuation of cardiotoxicity appears within reach, with many conceptual
advances to be covered in a subsequent section. Once this goal is achieved
it will enable one to use these compounds in clinical circumstances that are
currently being avoided because of the specter of causing long-term toxic
effects. Routine use in adjuvant treatment and in tumors of elderly patients
such as prostatic cancer are two prominent examples.

Lastly, the possibility of expanding the therapeutic spectrum of these
compounds is the most attractive result of drug development. Certain findings
hint to variable selectivity patterns among various anthracyclines, so that
some analogs exert greater antileukemic effects and others may have activity
even in tumors such as colon cancer that up to now have been notoriously
resistant to doxorubicin. A related aspect to these differences in therapeutic spectra among families of anthracyclines is the possible absence of

cross-resistance among two classes of these antibiotics. In fact, recent clinical studies described in the last section of this volume already indicate the possibility of such responses to one anthracycline after doxorubicin or daunorubicin therapy has failed or the tumors have relapsed. Clinical results undoubtedly will provide an increasingly important stimulus to drug development.

REFERENCES

1. Ogawa M. 1982. This volume.
2. Bhuyan BK, Neil GL, Li LH, McGovren JP, Wiley PF. 1980. Chemistry and biological activity of 7-con-O-methylnogarol (7-Con-OMEN). In: Anthracyclines: Current Status and new developments. (Crooke ST, Reich SD, eds.) New York, Academic Press, pp. 365-395.
3. DuVernay VH, Mong S, Crooke ST. 1980. Molecular pharmacology of anthracyclines: Demonstration of multiple mechanistic classes of anthracyclines. In: Anthracyclines: Current status and new developments. (Crooke ST, Reich SD, eds.). New York, Academic Press, pp. 61-12.
4. Trouet A. 1978. Increased selectivity of drugs by linking to carriers. Eurp. J. Cancer 14: 105-111.

DOXORUBICIN AND RELATED COMPOUNDS. II. STRUCTURE-ACTIVITY CONSIDERATIONS

F. ARCAMONE, A. CASAZZA, G. CASSINELLI, A. DI MARCO, AND S. PENCO

In the last ten years several anthracycline glycosides related to doxorubicin have been obtained by semisynthesis, partial synthesis, total synthesis, biosynthesis and tested for "in vitro" and "in vivo" antitumor activity
in our laboratories with the aim of developing new anticancer agents endowed
with higher antitumor activity, larger spectrum of activity and lower toxicity in respect to the parent compound. The establishment of structure-activity relationships is an essential part of such program. It is now possible to
operate a retrospective investigation on data collected in these investigations in order to perform deductions concerning the said relationships. In
part I of this study (1) the importance of DNA as the main cellular receptor
of the antitumor anthracyclines and some physico-chemical properties of the
intercalation complex formed in solution between these compounds and DNA have
been described . In particular, these properties have been used for the classification of thirty daunorubicin and doxorubicin analogues according to their
affinity for DNA. We shall now discuss the correlations of biological activity in different experimental systems with the chemical structure of these
analogues on the basis of the said classification. The experimental systems
used are the effect on the colony forming ability of HeLa cells "in vitro"
and that on mice bearing transplantable tumors such as the L 1210, P 388
and Gross leukemias. All activity data reported in this paper are derived
from internal reports concerning the experiments performed at Istituto Nazionale per lo Studio e la Cura dei Tumori, Milan, by A. Di Marco, A.M. Casazza and G. Pratesi.

Compounds belonging to the "high relative affinity" group
   The structures of compounds showing a DNA binding constant equal or higher
than 0.8 times that of doxorubicin (Ib) are presented in Ia, Ic and IIa, IIb,
IIc, IId .These compounds bear modifications compatible with a high relative
affinity for calf-thymus DNA, namely at C-4' (IIa-c) and on ring D (Ic). Two
analogues, 13-dihydrodoxorubicin (doxorubicinol) and 3',4'-diepidoxorubicin,

Ia: R^1 = H, R^2 = OMe

Ib: R^1 = OH, R^2 = OMe

Ic: R^1 = R^2 = H

IIa: R^1 = H, R^2 = OH

IIb: R^1 = R^2 = OH

IIc: R^1 = R^2 = H

IId: R^1 = OH, R^2 = H

whose effect on DNA viscosity was distinctly lower than that shown by other members of this group (1) are not included. This is also the case of 9-dea-cetyl-9-hydroxymethyl daunorubicin, a compound endowed with biological activity comparable with the other members of this group, because available activity data were obtained using a different test system (2).

Table 1 describes the inhibition exerted by these compounds on cultured HeLa cells and the maximal tolerated doses (MTD) in different mouse leukemias. It can be observed that daunorubicin and doxorubicin display identical ID_{50} values on HeLa cells. The other compounds were as effective as the parents in this "in vitro" system, or more effective, as was the case of Ic. It should be noted here that some of these analogues, tested on HeLa cell clone used in our laboratory some years ago, were found at that time more cytotoxic than it appeared in more recent experiments. For instance, 4-demethoxydaunorubicin had been reported to be 200 times more cytotoxic than daunorubicin (3) and 4'-deoxydoxorubicin 18 times more cytotoxic than doxorubicin itself (4). In vitro data reported in Table 1 for the said analogues were obtained using a different clone (5), the value of ID_{50} indicated for 4'-deoxy-daunorubicin being however still the one obtained with the older clone. The highest non toxic doses recorded in the three different experimental systems were in the range 2.0 ÷ 10.0 mg/Kg, with the exception of the 4-demethoxy analogue Ic whose toxicity is 5 to 8 times higher than that of the parent compound 1a.

Table 1. DNA binding constants (expressed as the ratio of K_{app} of the analogue over K_{app} of doxorubicin determined in identical conditions), concentrations inhibiting by 50% the viability of HeLa cells (ID_{50}), and maximal tolerated doses (MTD $\leq LD_{10}$) in mice bearing experimental leukemias of anthracycline glycosides belonging to the "high relative affinity" group.

Compound	$\dfrac{K_{anal}}{K_{dox}}$	ID_{50} (ng/ml)	MTD[a] (mg/Kg)		
			L 1210[b]	P 388[b]	Gross[c]
Daunorubicin ·(Ia)	1.22	9	3.2	4.3	6.0
4'-Deoxydoxorubicin (IId)	1.19	13	2.5	2.0	2.75
4'-Epidaunorubicin (IIa)	1.03	10	-(e)	5.0	3.0[d]
Doxorubicin (Ib)	1.00	9	5.3	7.0	5.5 (3.75[d])
4'-Epidoxorubicin (IIb)	0.97	9	5.0	10.0	6.5
4-Demethoxydaunorubicin (Ic)	0.95	3	0.6	0.5	0.75
4'-Deoxydaunorubicin (IIc)	0.84	2	4.0	-	2.0

(a) Daunorubicin and doxorubicin data are median values from experiments whose results are reported in tables 1 to 6. (b) Treatment ip on day 1. (c) IV dose administered on days 1,2,3 (unless otherwise stated). (d) Dose administered on days 1 to 5. (e) Not determined.

The antitumor efficacy of the "high relative affinity" compounds on murine experimental leukemias is presented in Table 2, where it is expressed as T/C% values (average survival time of treated mice expressed as per cent of untreated tumor bearing animals) at optimal dosage.

Table 2. Values of T/C% at optimal non toxic doses (OD)[a] of compounds belonging to the "high relative affinity" group.

Compound	T/C %		
	L 1210[b]	P 388[b]	Gross[c]
Daunorubicin (Ia)	160[d]	179[d]	171,185
", 4'-epi (IIa)	-(e)	150	163[f]
", 4'-deoxy (IIc)	162,187	-	128
", 4-demethoxy (Ic)	146	180	185
Doxorubicin (Ib)	152[d]	228[d]	175[f],196
", 4'-epi (IIb)	156[d]	>402	183
", 4'-deoxy (IId)	155	204	233

(a) OD $\leq LD_{10}$. (b),(c) See Table 1. (d) Median values of at least three experiments. (e) Not determined. (f) Treatment iv on days 1 to 5.

All compounds listed in Table 2 show comparable efficacy in the L 1210 test. However doxorubicin and its analogues appear to be more effective than daunorubicin and its analogues in prolonging survival of mice bearing P 388 lymphocytic leukemia, 4'-epidoxorubicin being endowed with particularly high efficacy in this system. On the other hand 4'-deoxydoxorubicin is the most effective compound in the Gross leukemia test.

Compounds belonging to the "intermediate relative affinity" group

The structures of compounds showing a DNA binding constant in the range of 0.5 ÷ 0.8 times that of doxorubicin (see part I of this study) are presented in IIIa, IIIb, IVa, IVb, Va, Vb, VI and VIIa. They include analogues bearing modifications in the sugar moiety (IIIa,b; IVa,b), in side chain substitution (Va,b) and in the aglycone moiety (VI, VIIa). Compound IVb was included in this group because of viscosity data (1).

IIIa: R = H
IIIb: R = OH

IVa: R = H
IVb: R = OH

Va: R = OCOCH$_2$OH
Vb: R = N⌒O

VI

VIIa: R = OH
VIIb: R = H

Table 3 describes the toxicity exerted by these compounds on HeLa cells and in tumor-bearing mice. Out of the eight compounds reported, five show a ID_{50} value higher than 50 ng/ml, that is almost 8 times the median value of ID_{50} exhibited by compounds of Table 1, whereas doxorubicin 14-glycolate and the two 4'-O-methyl analogues display inhibitory activity on cultured cells at the same concentration levels as the parent compounds. The maximal tolerated doses are scattered in the range 2.9 ÷ 100 mg/Kg and are correlated with the ID_{50} values. except for compound VI.

Table 3. DNA binding properties, ID50 and MTD values (see Table 1) of anthracycline glycosides belonging to the "intermediate relative affinity" group.

Compound	$\dfrac{K_{anal}}{K_{dox}}$	ID_{50} (ng/ml)	MTD (mg/Kg)		
			L 1210[a]	P 388[a]	Gross[b]
3',4'-Diepidaunorubicin (IIIa)	0.70	175	50	40	-(c)
4'-O-Methyldaunorubicin (IVa)	0.68	13	–	4.4	–
3',4'-Diepi-6'-hydroxy-daunorubicin (IIIb)	0.68	>50	>17	–	–
Doxorubicin-14-glycolate (Va)	0.59	5	10	–	>10
14-Morpholinodaunorubicin (Vb)	0.57	1000	100	–	>78
9,10-Anhydrodaunorubicin (VI)	0.55	420	6.6	–	–
11-Deoxydoxorubicin (VIIa)	0.51	105	–	66	–
4'-O-Methyldoxorubicin (IVb)	0.48	5	2.9	4.4	2.9

(a),(b),(c) see footnotes (b),(c),(e) in Table 1

The efficacy of compounds belonging to this group on experimental murine leukemias is presented in Table 4. At optimal doses the effect on survival of tumor-bearing animals was comparable to that of the parent drugs, endowed with higher DNA binding ability. An exception is represented by compound VI, also showing a different conformation of the A ring (2) and a low effect on DNA viscosity (1). Also within this group doxorubicin analogues are clearly more effective than the daunorubicin analogues, the efficacy of compound IVb on the somewhat naturally doxorubicin resistant L 1210 system and on Gross leukemia being noteworthy.

184

Table 4. Values of T/C % at optimal non toxic doses (OD)[a] of
compounds belonging to the "intermediate relative affinity" group.

Compound	T/C %		
	L 1210[b]	P 388[b]	Gross[c]
Daunorubicin, 3',4'-diepi (IIIa)	137	181	-(e)
", 4'-O-methyl (IVa)	135	156	-
", 3',4'-diepi-6'-hydroxy (IIIb)	150	-	-
", 14-morpholino (Vb)	155	-	133
", 9,10-anhydro (VI)	89,100	-	-
Doxorubicin, 14-glycolate (Va)	184[d]	-	183[f]
", 11-deoxy (VIIa)	-	223	216
", 4'-O-methyl (IVb)	287,213	200	258[f]
Daunorubicin (Ia)	142[d]	179[d]	-
Doxorubicin (Ib)	175[d]	233,254	208,233 183[f],250[f]

(a)-(e) see footnotes to Table 2. (f) Treatment iv on day 1

Compounds belonging to the "low relative affinity" group

The structures of compounds showing DNA binding constants lower than 0.5 times selected for this part of our study are presented in VIIb, and in VIII-XIII. These analogues bear modifica-

tion in the aglycone moiety (VIIb) and in the sugar moiety (VIII-XIII), two of the latter (XI and XII) being the β-anomers of IIa and of doxorubicin (Ib) respectively.

Compounds of this group show ID_{50} values on cultured HeLa cells higher than 38 ng/ml (Table 5). Also in this case, as with the group reported in Table 3, the 4'-O-methyl analogue (X) displays a higher cytotoxicity as compared with the other compounds with a similar affinity for DNA. The toxicity in tumor-bearing mice of all compounds listed in Table 5 was low, the only exception being the already mentioned X.

Table 5. DNA binding properties, ID_{50} and MTD values (see Table 1) of anthracycline glycosides belonging to the "low relative affinity" group

Compound	$\dfrac{K_{anal}}{K_{dox}}$	ID_{50} (ng/ml)	MTD (mg/Kg) L 1210[a]	P 388[a]
11-Deoxydaunorubicin (VIIb)	0.41	54	>15	44
3'-Epidaunorubicin (VIII)	0.35	90	≥33	- (b)
3',4'-Diepi-6'-hydroxydoxorubicin (IX)	0.32	>1000	-	-
4'-Epi-4'-O-methyldaunorubicin (X)	0.27	38	-	20
1',4'-Diepidaunorubicin (XI)	0.17	185	-	>20
1'-Epidoxorubicin (XII)	0.13	1000	-	>20
N-Acetyldoxorubicin (XIII)	0.04	635	200	100

(a),(b) see footnotes (b) and (e) to Table 1

The effect of low relative affinity compounds on survival of mice bearing L 1210 or P 388 leukemia is presented in Table 6. The L-xylo analogue VIII and β-anomers XI and XII exhibited no antitumor activity in these systems.

Table 6. Values of T/C% at optimal non toxic doses (OD)[a] of compounds belonging to the "low relative affinity" group

Compound	T/C % L 1210[b]	P 388[b]
Daunorubicin, 11-deoxy (VIIb)	122	190
", 3'-epi (VIII)	125	- (c)
", 4'-epi-4'-O-methyl (X)	-	174,180
", 1',4'-diepi (XI)	-	125
Doxorubicin, 1'-epi (XII)	-	130
", N-acetyl (XIII)	150,150	172
Daunorubicin (Ia)	140[d]	181[d]
Doxorubicin (Ib)	200	218,260

(a),(b),(c)(d) see footnotes (a),(b),(e) and (d) to Table 2.

The 11-deoxy analogue VIIb was effective in the P 388 test. Noticeable antitumor activity was shown by 4'-O-methyl derivative X and by amide XIII.

Discussion

It is deduced, from the data reported in Tables 1,3 and 5, that there is a general relationship between the ability of binding to DNA and cytotoxicity on "in vitro" cultured cells. Other mechanisms, in addition to the interaction with cell DNA, have been suggested as being possibly involved in anthracycline cytotoxicity. These are (a) interaction with membrane phospholipids with consequent modification of membrane fluidity (6) or calcium ion transport (7); (b) interference with redox reactions and formation of toxic radical species (8); (c) the inhibition of mitochondrial oxidations (9,10,11); (d) the inhibition of membrane bound (Na^+, K^+)ATPase (12); (e) the interaction with transfer RNA (13). It seems, however, that these other mechanisms, even if present, do not represent the primary locus of anthracycline cytotoxicity. It is interesting to observe that the ID_{50} values are also generally correlated with the maximal tolerated doses "in vivo", and therefore the results reported here suggest a direct relationship between the ability of binding to DNA and general toxicity in the animal models. The exceptions, represented by some compound like the 4'-O-methylanalogues that exhibit higher cytotoxicity and "in vivo" toxicity than what is expected from the DNA binding properties, will be discus sed below.

The better performance of doxorubicin analogues as compared with daunorubicin analogues in the murine systems considered in this study indicates a higher selectivity of the compounds bearing the hydroxyacetyl side chain for the inhibition of growth of these types of tumor cells "in vivo". This higher selectivity is always observed in the P 388 and Gross leukemias, but only exceptionally in the L 1210 system. The different analogues appear therefore to share the different antitumor efficacies of the parent drugs, daunorubicin an doxorubicin. This observation may be related with the lower ability of doxorubicin to act as a substrate of daunorubicin reductase in comparison to daunorubicin (14), with the lower rate of metabolization of doxorubicin as compare to daunorubicin in different tissues, including heart, of different animal sp cies (15), with the more rapid excretion of radioactivity following administra tion of $[^3H]$daunorubicin than following administration of $[^3H]$doxorubici in experimental animals (16) and higher tissue levels of tritium in the latte than in the former case (17,18). The half-life of doxorubicin in murine sarco ma 180 ascite cells was 12 hours, whereas that of daunorubicin was four hour (19), doxorubicin inducing a more marked inhibition of labelled uridine inco poration into cell RNA than daunorubicin. Finally, a differential effect of doxorubicin in respect to daunorubicin as regards the immunological reactions of the host has been documented (20-24).

Data presented in this study also show some diversity in the antitumor efficacy within the doxorubicin analogues. It is of interest to note the high efficacy of 4'-epidoxorubicin in the P 388 system as this appears related with the higher tolerability of this analogue in respect to the parent (25). An explanation of the different pharmacological properties of 4'-epidoxorubicin and doxorubicin should be found in the behavior of the drugs in the animal body as regards distribution, metabolic fate and pharmacokinetics. The availability of radiolabelled anthracyclines now allows qualitative and quantitative comparison studies of related compounds. A recent investigation performed in rats in our laboratory has shown that $/^{-14}C_/$4'-epidoxorubicin exhibits significantly higher initial concentration of radioactivity than $/^{-14}C\_/$doxorubicin in kidney, lung and bone marrow, but lower in blood and, at later times after administration, in heart tissue. In agreement with previous findings obtained by the use of the fluorescence assay method (25), a more rapid clearance of 4'-epidoxorubicin in comparison with doxorubicin has also been demonstrated.

The remarkable effectiveness of 4'-O-methyldoxorubicin in the L 1210 test system is of particular interest. For this compound a higher rate of uptake in comparison with doxorubicin has been demonstrated in Ehrlich tumor cells (26). The corresponding 4'--O-methyldaunorubicin displayed a very low efficacy in this system, confirming the general superiority of doxorubicin-derived analogues in these experimental models. However, the 4'-O-methyl analogues, as well as the 14-esters of doxorubicin, do show a biological activity, both in terms of toxicity as well as efficacy, superior to that which could be expected on the basis of the affinity for DNA. This observation is in agreement with the documented rapid hydrolysis of the ester bond "in vivo" (27), whereas for the 4'-O-methyl analogues a more profound effect on DNA conformation than expected from the K_{app} values is indicated by the viscosity measurements (1). Alternatively, or in addition, a demethylation at 4' would originate in the parent compounds in cell cultures and in the animal body. Also, the antitumor properties of 14- -morpholinodaunorubicin and of N-acetyldoxorubicin "in vivo" should be related with a metabolic conversion to doxorubicin by respectively deamination and deacetylation. The "in vivo" hydrolysis of the amide linkage in daunorubicin and doxorubicin derivatives has been demonstrated in the case of the N-leucyldaunorubicin (28 and of N-trifluoroacetyldoxorubicin-14-valerate (29).

In conclusion, our study indicates that (a) cytotoxicity on cultured HeLa cells and toxicity in mice are correlated with the DNA binding properties of the anthracycline glycosides, (b) although other mechanisms may play a role in determining the antitumor activity of anthracyclines, available biological data confirm DNA as the main site of action of this compounds, (c) superior efficacy of doxorubicin over daunorubicin analogues in some systems indicate the importance of the hydroxyl function at C-14 for the pharmacological behavior at the animal level, (d) pharmacokinetic properties and metabolism are likely the basis of pharmacological differentiation of the analogues, and (e) antitumor activity of derivatives showing lower DNA binding ability may be related with bioactivation reactions giving rise to the parent compounds.

REFERENCES

1. Arcamone F, Arlandini E, Menozzi M, Valentini L, Vannini E. Paper presented at the Symposium on Anthracycline Antibiotics in Cancer Therapy, New York, September 16-18, 1981.
2. Arcamone F. 1981. "Doxorubicin," Medicinal Chemistry Series Vol. 17, Academic Press, New York.
3. Supino R, Necco A, Dasdia T, Casazza AM, Di Marco A. 1977. Cancer Res., 37, 4523.
4. Di Marco A, Casazza AM, Dasdia T, Necco A, Pratesi G, Rivolta P, Velcich A, Zaccara A, Zunino F. 1977. Chem.Biol. Interactions, 19, 291.
5. Geroni C. Unpublished data.
6. Tritton TR, Murphree SA, Sartorelli AC. 1978. Biochem.Biophys. Res. Comm., 84, 802.
7. Anghileri LJ. 1977. Arzneim. Forsch., 27, 1177.
8. Bachur NR, Gordon SL, Gee MV. 1978. Cancer Res., 38, 1745.
9. Ferrero ME, Ferrero E, Gaja G, Bernelli-Zazzera A. 1976. Bioch.Pharm., 25, 125.

10. Gosalvez M, Blanco M, Hunter J, Miko M, Chance B. 1974. Europ. J. Cancer, $\underline{10}$, 567.
11. Mailer K, Petering DH. 1976. Biochem. Pharmacol., $\underline{25}$, 2085.
12. Gosalvez M, van Rossum GDV, Blanco M. 1979. Cancer Res., $\underline{39}$, 257.
13. Shafer RH. 1977. Biochem. Pharmacol., $\underline{26}$, 1729.
14. Felsted RL, Gee MV, Bachur NR. 1974. J. Biol. Chem., $\underline{249}$, 3672.
15. Loveless H, Arena P, Felsted RL, Bachur NR. 1978. Cancer Res., $\underline{38}$, 593.
16. Di Fronzo G, Gambetta RA, Lenaz L. 1971. Rev. Eur. Etudes Clin. Biol., $\underline{16}$, 572.
17. Lenaz L, Di Fronzo G. 1972. Tumori $\underline{58}$, 213.
18. Martini A, Donelli MG, Mantovani A, Pacciarini MA, Fogar-Ottaviano E, Morasca L, Garattini S, Spreafico F. 1977. Oncology $\underline{34}$, 173.
19. Wang JJ, Chervinsky DS, Rosen JM. 1972. Cancer Res., $\underline{32}$, 511.
20. Casazza AM, Di Marco A, Di Cuonzo G. 1971. Cancer Res., $\underline{31}$, 1971.
21. Schwartz HS, Grindey GB. 1973. Cancer Res., $\underline{33}$, 1837.
22. Schwartz HS, Kanter PM. 1975. Cancer Chemother. Rep., $\underline{6}$, 107.
23. Casazza AM, Isetta AM, Giuliani F, Di Marco A. 1975. pp 123-131 in "Adriamycin Review" (Staquat M et al. Eds), European Press Medikon, Ghent, Belgium.
24. Orsini F, Pavelic Z, Mihich E. 1977. Cancer Res., $\underline{37}$, 1719.
25. Arcamone F, Di Marco A, Casazza AM. 1978. pp 297-312 in "Advances in Cancer Chemotherapy" (Humezawa H et al. Eds), Japan Sci. Soc. Press, Tokyo, Univ. Park Press, Baltimore.
26. Di Marco A, Skoosgaard T, Casazza AM, Pratesi G, Nissen NI, Danø K. 1981. to be published.
27. Arcamone F, Franceschi G, Minghetti A, Penco S, Redaelli S, Di Marco A, Casazza AM, Dasdia T, Di Fronzo G, Giuliani F, Lenaz L, Necco A, Soranzo C. 1974. J. Med. Chem., $\underline{17}$, 335.
28. Masquelier M, Baurain R, Trouet A. 1980. J. Med. Chem., $\underline{23}$, 1166.
29. Israel M, et al., paper presented at the 12th International Congress of Chemotherapy, Florence, Italy, July 19-24, 1981 and unpublished results from Author's (Arcamone F) laboratory.

SECOND-GENERATION ANTHRACYCLINES

G. MATHÉ and R. MARAL

1. INTRODUCTION

Many hundreds of analogs of daunorubicin (DNR), doxorubicin (DXR or Adriamycin) and of other compounds of the anthracycline family /‾anthracycline: a name given by H. BROCKMANN_7 have been isolated from culture broth or synthesized during the last twenty years. The aim of research in this field is to find new compound or derivatives which have:
- a broader spectrum and higher antitumoral activity
- a lower toxicity, principally a less cardiotoxic effect
- advantageous pharmacokinetics
- possibly no cross-resistance with the parent compounds.

In short, we are interested in compounds possessing a clear-cut superiority in activity and in toxicity over the parent compounds. Indeed, we know that slight side-chain modification may result in:
- a better therapeutic index
- a broadening of the spectrum of activity
- changes in metabolism, in membrane transport and in immunologic depression.

The main anthracyclines of which clinical activity has been evaluated, some of which are candidates for clinical study, may be divided into four groups:

Group A: the two parent compounds, daunorubicin (DNR) and 14-hydroxy DNR or doxorubicin (DXR) or Adriamycin (Figure 1).

Group B: DNR and DXR derivatives resulting from substitution on various parts of the molecule (B,C or D ring, C_{13}-C_{14} side-chain, daunosamine (Figure 2).

Group C: the aglycone is pyrromycinone, at C7 a glycosidic chain (di or trisaccharidic), and a carmethoxy-group at C10.

Group A
Parent compounds

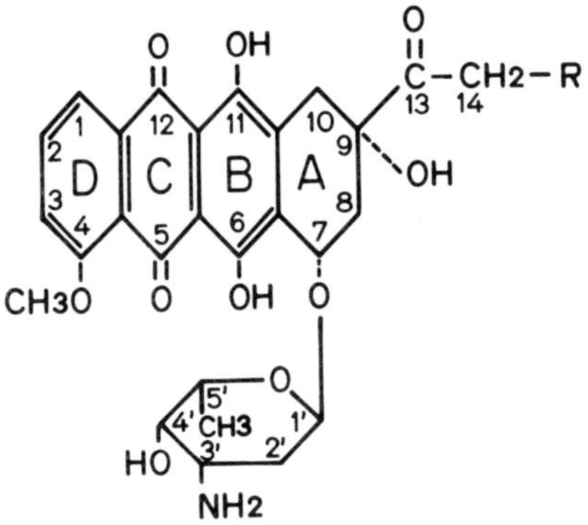

Compound	− R
Daunorubicin (DNR) (1963)	− H
14-hydroxy DNR (1967) or Doxorubicin (DXR)	
(Adriamycin)	− OH

Fig. 1

Group B
Main DNR or DXR derivatives

Derivatives	Substitutions on various parts of the molecule	
Reduction of ketogroup Daunorubicinol Doxorubicinol	C13	−CH2−
Carminomycin	C4 (DNR)	−OH
Demethoxy DNR	C4 (DNR)	−H
5-immo DNR	C5 (DNR)	−NH
Benzoylhydrazone derivative: zorubicin Rubidazone	C13−C14 (DNR)	CH3 −C=N-NH-CO- 
Diethoxyacetoxy DNR Detorubicin	C13−C14	−CO-CH2-O-CO-CH(OC2H5)2
N-trifluoracetyl-adriamycin-14-alkanoate AD-32 (14-valerate)	C13 C14 C'3	−CO-CH2-O-CO(CH2)3CH3 −NH.CO.CF3
AD-143 (14-O-hemi-adipate)	C13 C14 C'3	−CO-CH2-O-CO(CH2)4COOH −NH.CO.CF3
4'-epi-Adriamycin	C'4	OH C'4<
4'-deoxy Adriamycin	C'4	H2C'<
N-derivatives: N alkyl (N-acetyl or dimethyl) DNR or DXR	C'3 NH2	C'3 NH.CO.CH3 C'3N(CH3)2

Group B
Main DNR or DXR derivatives

Derivatives	Substitutions on various parts of the molecule	
N aryl (N-dibenzyl)	C'3NH2	C'3N(C6H5)2
N-Amino-acid and peptide derivatives of DNR or DXR N-L leu DNR	C'3NH2	C'3NH-CO-CH-CH2-CH2(CH3)2 NH2
Triferric derivatives: Quelamycin (DXR)	C11 C12	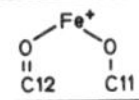 Fe⁺ O O C12 C11
Quelablastin (DNR)	C5 C6	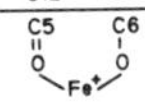 C5 C6 O O Fe⁺
	C'3 C'4	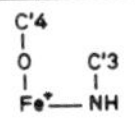 C'4 O C'3 Fe⁺ NH
4'-O-tetrahydro-pyranyl Adriamycin (b isomer) THP-Adria	C7	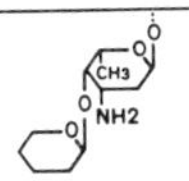 O CH3 O NH2
Aminocyclohexane Carboxylic ester of DNR Rubicyclamin (cis A,B)	C7	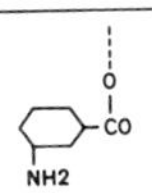 O CO NH2

Fig. 2

Among these compounds are: the aclacinomycins, marcellomycin (Figure 3).

Group D: the amino-sugar is linked to the D cycle (instead of A cycle). In this group are: nogalamycin and new interesting derivatives such as 7-con OMEN (Figure 4).

We will compare the activities of the main compounds of the different groups with those of the parent drugs DNR and DXR. Our knowledge of the compounds is very variable: some compounds have been under study for many years and others have only recently been made available for experimental and clinical study. It is interesting, if possible, to compare the experimental results with those available from the clinic to see if the experimental data are predictive for human therapeutics.

2. A MODEL FOR COMPARATIVE STUDY: EVALUATION AND COMPARISON OF THE PARENT COMPOUNDS DNR AND DXR

For many years, DNR and DXR have been extensively studied and a short comparative survey of the main available data is a good guide for the evaluation of new anthracyclines.

The following list shows the different fields in which such a comparative study is recommended, namely:
- cytotoxicity
- action on DNA and RNA synthesis
- pharmacokinetics at the cell level and subcellular localization
- distribution and metabolism in animals
- toxicological studies in animals
- cardiotoxicity in animals
- teratogenic activity
- genetic toxicity
- carcinogenic potential
- immunological activity
- experimental antitumor activity
- therapeutic activity in the clinic
- clinical toxicity
- resistance phenomenon

Group C

Pyrromycinone, glycosidic (di or trisaccharide)
side chain, carmethoxygroup at C10.
Aclacinomycins and compounds isolated from
the "bohemic complex" (anthracycline mixture)

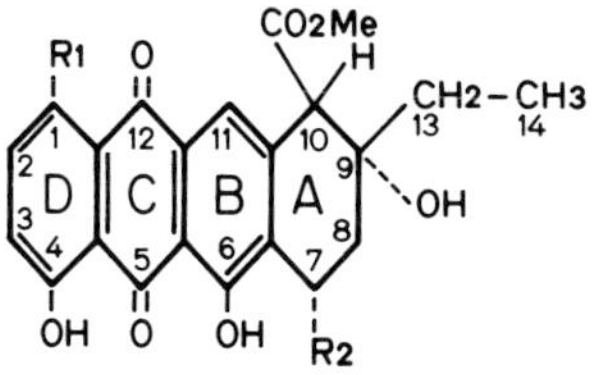

Fig. 3

	R1	R2 (∗)
Aclacinomycin A	–H	Rh–DF–Cin
Cinerubin A	–OH	Rh–DF–Cin
Rudolphomycin	–OH	Rh–DF–Red
Musettamycin	–OH	Rh–DF
Marcellomycin	–OH	Rh–DF–DF

(∗) rhodosamine (Rh)
2-deoxy-L-fucose (DF)
cinerubose (Cin)
rednose (Red)

Group D

Nogalamycin and derivatives
(aminosugar on D cycle, carmethoxy group at C10)

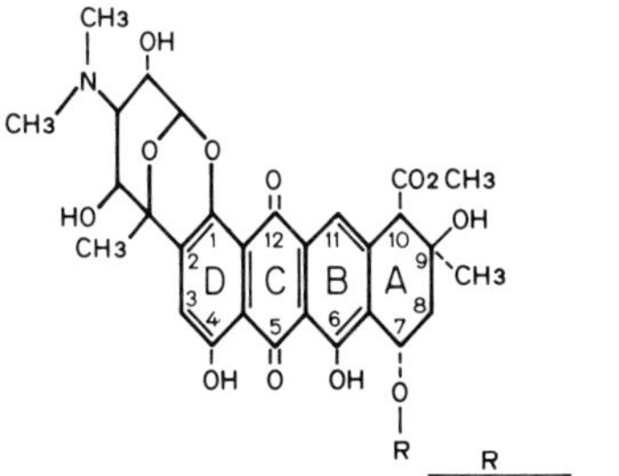

Fig. 4

Nogalamycin

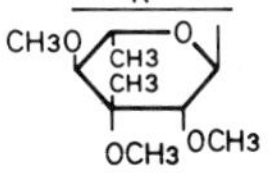

(Nogalose)

7-CON-O-methylnogarol
(7-CON-OMEN)

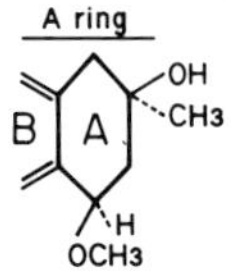

For DNR and DXR, which are DNA intercalating agents, the IC_{50} values corresponding to DNA synthesis, RNA synthesis, and nucleolar RNA synthesis, are not very different from each other (class 1 compounds) (1,2).

The free radical generation from the anthracycline molecules (catalyzed by NADPH and cytochrome P 450 reductase) may create disturbances in the respiratory chain electron transport. Oxygen radicals and peroxides may be at the origin of damage of bio-membrane and DNA. This is one general mechanism that probably contributes to the activity and to the toxicity of this drug family (3).

At the cell level, pharmacokinetic study shows a faster cellular input for DNA and a much slower disappearance of DXR from the cells (4). The enzymatic reduction of the Cl3 carbonyl group (aldoketoreductase) occurs more readily from DNR than from DXR (5). Not as much DXR is converted to DXR-ol as DNR is to DNR-ol, DXR being excreted more slowly. The tissue levels of DXR are therefore higher; this may explain differences in activity and in toxicity (6).

The study of the toxicity on different target organs shows some mild differences; for example, DNR is the more toxic by the IP route and DXR by the IV route.

For cardiac toxicity evaluation, various techniques (ECG, light electron microscopy) may be used in different systems and species (7): rabbit, rat, mouse, monkey, and hamster. Cardiac muscle cell cultures are also used (8). DXR is equitoxic to or a little more toxic than DNR; both drugs belong to the first group of DANTCHEV's classification (9) (Figure 5).

The hypotheses concerning the mechanism of cardiotoxicity are numerous: free radicals, lipid peroxidation, affinity to phospholipids and even immunological mechanisms.

Both compounds are teratogenic, mutagenic and carcinogenic.

DNR and DXR exert immunopharmacological activity; various results have been published that depend on dosage, schedule of treatments or nature of the test used.

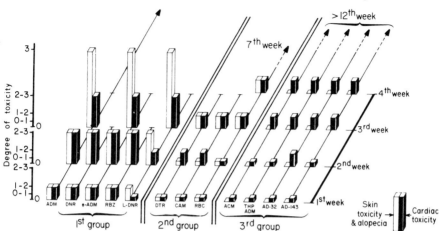

Fig. 5

On different murine tumors, DXR was frequently found to be more active than DNR (10,11). This difference could be due to the longer tissue exposure to DXR, secondary to slower excretion.

In the clinic, DNR and DXR are very useful antitumor antibiotics. DNR is effective in the treatment of acute leukemias. It would be of interest to have further trials of DNR in the solid tumor area (12). The activity of DXR has been established in leukemias and in various solid tumors.

Preclinical toxicological studies had a predictive value:

- bone-marrow is dose limiting

- cardiotoxicity is the main problem (cumulative toxic dose limits, for DNR: 600 mg/m2 and for DXR: 550 mg/m2; these figures may be examined again thanks to a new strategy in treatment schedules).

The phenomenon of resistance, very well documented in the laboratory, is an important problem in the clinic. We should point out the conflicting results concerning in vitro, in vivo and clinical cross-resistance, namely:

- the degree of cross-resistance between the anthracycline analogs,

- and the cross-resistance with compounds of other families.

3. COMPARATIVE STUDY OF COMPOUNDS OF THE SECOND GENERATION

For each anthracycline of interest in the second generation, taking into account our present knowledge, it is very rare that it is possible to give satisfactory answers concerning the preceding 14 items of the comparative list.

If we consider the comparative cytotoxicity on a weight basis (Table 1):

- carminomycin (13) and dm DNR or dm DXR (14) are more toxic than the parent compounds. On the contrary, rubidazone (15), detorubicin (16) and AD32 (17) are not so toxic; as for 4'-epi-DXR, it exerts a toxicity close to or less than DXR (18). Aclacinomycin A falls between DNR and DXR (19) and 7-con-OMEN is equally lethal in all phases of the cell cycle and less toxic than DXR (20).

The inhibiting activity on DNA and RNA synthesis is related t the chemical structure (1) (Table 1).

Group B compounds, like the parent compounds, belong to class I: the IC_{50} for DNA and RNA synthesis are not very different. But AD32 binds poorly to isolated DNA (21).

Group C compounds (Aclacinomycin A, marcellomycin, rudolfo-mycin) belong to the class II compounds of which IC_{50} for RNA synthesis is considerably lower than the IC_{50} for DNA synthesis (about 1/10), the difference for nucleolar RNA synthesis is even more marked (about 1/100) (19).

As for Group D, the compounds interact weakly with DNA and minimally inhibit DNA and RNA synthesis (22).

The subcellular localization of the drugs (Table 1) is mainl nuclear for compounds of Group B and C, except AD32, which is concentrated chiefly in the cytoplasm (23). 7-con-OMEN, of Grou D, is also localized in the cytoplasm (24).

Distribution and metabolism in animals (Table 2)

Carminomycinol (13-dihydro CMM) is a metabolite of carmino-mycin (25).

In blood and tissue, higher concentration levels are obtaine after IV or PO treatments with dm DNR or dm DXR; this is associated with a slower rate of the disappearance of the drugs (26).

Table 1

GROUP	COMPOUND	EXTENT OF CYTOTOXICITY	SYNTHESIS OF DNA AND RNA	PHARMACOKINETICS AND SUBCELLULAR LOCALIZATION AT CELL LEVEL :
	CARMINOMYCIN	MORE TOXIC THAN DNR OR DXR	CLASS 1 INHIBITION AT 2-3 FOLD LOWER CONCENTRATION THAN DNR	PRINCIPALLY NUCLEAR LOCALIZATION
	DM DAUNORUBICIN DOXORUBICIN	MORE TOXIC THAN PARENT COMPOUND (27 TO 100 TIMES)		
B	RUBIDAZONE	LESS TOXIC THAN DNR OR DXR	CLASS 1 SLOWER INHIBITION THAN THE PARENT COMPOUND	PRINCIPALLY NUCLEAR LOCALIZATION
	DETORUBICIN	NOT SO TOXIC AS DXR (1.5 TO 2 TIMES)	CLASS 1	PRINCIPALLY NUCLEAR LOCALIZATION
	AD - 32	LESS TOXIC THAN DXR (5 TIMES LESS)	BINDS POORLY TO ISOLATED DNA (DOES NOT APPEAR TO INTERCALATE DNA)	CONCENTRATED IN THE CYTOPLASM (NO OR POOR NUCLEAR FIXATION)
	4'-EPI-ADRIAMYCIN	CLOSE TO DXR	CLASS 1	PRINCIPALLY NUCLEAR LOCALIZATION. TAKEN IN GREATER AMOUNT BY CELL THAN DXR
C	ACLACINOMYCIN A	STRONGER THAN DNR WEAKER THAN DXR	CLASS 2 IC_{50} RNA 1/10 IC_{50} DNA IC_{50} NUCLEOLUS RNA VERY LOW	MAINLY CONCENTRATED IN THE NUCLEUS. LIPOPHILIC CHARACTER : GREATER SPEED OF CELL UPTAKE. FASTER RELEASE
	MARCELLOMYCIN		CLASS 2 AS ACLACINOMYCIN A	PRINCIPALLY IN THE NUCLEUS
D	7-CON-OMEN	EQUALLY LETHAL IN ALL PHASES OF CELL CYCLE	INTERACTS WEAKLY WITH DNA MINIMALLY INHIBITS DNA AND RNA SYNTHESIS	LOCALIZED IN THE CYTOPLASM

Table 2

GROUP	COMPOUND	DISTRIBUTION AND METABOLITES IN ANIMALS	TOXICOLOGICAL STUDIES IN ANIMALS	CARDIAC TOXICITY IN ANIMALS
	CARMINOMYCIN	METABOLITE : CARMINOMYCINOL (13-DIHYDRO CMM)	MORE TOXIC THAN DNR BONE-MARROW APLASIA	COMPARISON WITH DNR RAT = LESS TOXIC RABBIT = MORE TOXIC HAMSTER = TOXIC (2ND GROUP)
	DM DAUNORUBICIN DOXORUBICIN	DM DNR COMPARISON WITH DNR : HIGHER LEVEL (I.V. OR P.O. TREATMENTS) SLOWER RATE OF DISAPPEARANCE		LESS CARDIOTOXIC THAN THE PARENT COMPOUN
B	RUBIDAZONE	DNR PRODRUG, BUT LESS DNROL PRODUCED	LESS TOXIC THAN DNR AND DXR	ZBINDEN'S TECHNIQUE : 4,5 TIMES LESS CARDIOTOXIC THAN DNR AND DXR RABBIT = LESS CARDIOTOXIC HAMSTER = 1ST GROUP
	DETORUBICIN	DIFFERENCES WITH DXR : PRODRUG OF DXR WITH DISTINCT PHARMACOKINETICS	2 TIMES LESS TOXIC THAN DXR (I.V. TREATMENT)	HAMSTER = 2ND GROUP
	AD - 32	NOT A DXR PRODRUG. FASTER EXCRETION. NOT METABOLIZED IN DXR, BUT AD - 41, AD - 92	BONE MARROW TOXICITY LIKE DXR	HAMSTER = 3RD GROUP (VERY LOW TOXICITY)
	4'-EPI-ADRIAMYCIN	COMPARED WITH DXR : DIFFERENCES IN PHARMACOKINETICS	LESS TOXIC IN MICE THAN DXR (1,5)	COMPARISON WITH DXR RABBIT = SAME TOXICITY MICE = LESS TOXIC HAMSTER = 1ST GROUP
C	ACLACINOMYCIN A	AGLYCONE : AKLAVINONE AND GLYCOSIDIC METABOLITES I.V. AND ABSORBED BY THE G.I. TRACT (P.O. TREATMENT)	BONE-MARROW G.I. TRACT HEPATIC (TRANSAMINASE) DOSE : TWICE THAT OF DXR	RABBIT = SLIGHT AND REVERSIBLE HAMSTER = 3RD GROUP
	MARCELLOMYCIN	DOES NOT PRODUCE MYELOSUPPRESSION G.I. TOXICITY		RAT (CPK) = LESS THAN DXR MICE = CARDIOTOXIC
D	7-CON-OMEN		5 TO 12 TIMES DOSE OF DXR	RABBIT = 1/15 COMPARED TO DXR

Rubidazone is a DNR-prodrug, but, on a molar-basis, after administration of the analog, less DNR-ol is produced (27).

Detorubicin is a DXR pro-drug with distinct pharmacokinetics (28).

It has been shown that AD32 is not metabolized in DXR, and thus is not a pro-drug (29).

Differences in pharmacokinetics with the parent compound have been observed with 4'-epi-Adriamycin and the lower concentration in the cardiac tissue may correlate with the lower cardiotoxicity (18,30).

The metabolites of aclacinomycin A are the aglycone (aklavinone) and different glycosidic compounds. After PO treatment, aclacinomycin A is absorbed by the GI tract (19).

Toxicological studies in animals (Table 2)

Bone-marrow aplasia is one of the main toxic effects.

Group B compounds: many analogs are not so toxic as the parent compounds, for example: rubidazone (15), detorubicin (16) 4'-epi-adriamycin (30,31), AD32 (32). But carminomycin and dm DNR and DXR are more toxic than the parent compounds (31,33).

Group C compounds: Aclacinomycin A toxicity (bone-marrow and GI tract) is two times lower than DXR toxicity (19).

Marcellomycin does not produce important myelosuppression, but the problem is GI toxicity (34).

Group D compounds: on a weight basis, 7-con-OMEN is 5 to 12 times less toxic than DXR (22).

The evaluation of the cardiac toxicity in animals (Table 2) has given various results. For example, compared with DNR, carminomycin is less cardiotoxic in the rat (35), belongs to the 2nd group in the hamster test (9) and is more toxic in the rabbit (36). dm DNR and dm DXR are less toxic than the parent compounds (30). Rubidazone is 4 times less toxic than DNR or DXR according to ZBINDEN's technique (15); it is less toxic in the rabbit (37) but it belongs to the 1st group in the hamster test (9).

However, detorubicin, which belongs to the 2nd group in the hamster test (9), is as toxic as DXR in the rabbit (37).

AD32 exerts a very low cardiotoxicity (3rd group in the hamster test) (9).

4'-epi-Adriamycin, compared with DXR, is less cardiotoxic in the mouse and exerts a close or lesser cardiotoxicity in the rabbit (30), but belongs to the 1st group in the hamster test (9).

The cardiotoxicity of aclacinomycin A is slight and reversible in the rabbit (19) and in the hamster test is ranked in the 3rd group (9).

In the rat (CPK test), marcellomycin is less toxic than DXR, but is cardiotoxic in the mouse.

The cardiotoxicity of 7-con-OMEN is 1/15 compared to DXR (38).

Few results are at our disposal concerning the embryotoxicity and the teratogenic potential of these compounds. Carminomycin was found to be teratogenic (39) (Table 3).

Carminomycin (40), dm DNR and dm DXR (41), rubidazone (15), and detorubicin (16) were found more or less mutagenic than the parent compounds.

On the contrary, aclacinomycin A (42) and 7-con-OMEN (22) are not mutagenic in the same system (Table 3).

Generally, we lack extensive studies concerning the carcinogenic potential and the immunological activity of these various analogs (Table 3).

The experimental antitumor activities (Table 4) of the compounds are usually well documented. Carminomycin is more effective on L1210 leukemia and is active when taken orally (43).

dm DNR and dm DXR are more potent than the parent compounds, the chemotherapeutic indexes are better; the compounds are active when taken orally (44).

Rubidazone is as active as or more active than DNR and has a better chemotherapeutic index (15).

Detorubicin is equal or superior to DXR (45).

AD-32 is superior (32) or equal (46) to DXR.

4'-epi-DXR has a better chemotherapeutic index than DXR (30).

Aclacinomycin A, compared with DXR and DNR, is less active or has the same activity (19).

Marcellomycin is less active than DXR, but is as active as, or more so, than compounds of the C group, such as aclacinomycin A and musettamycin.

7-con-OMEN is as active as or more active than DXR (24).

Table 3

GROUP	COMPOUND	EMBRYOTOXICITY TERATOGENIC ACTIVITY	GENETIC TOXICITY	CARCINOGENIC POTENTIAL	IMMUNOLOGICAL ACTIVITY
B	CARMINOMYCIN	TERATOGENIC IN MICE	MORE MUTAGENIC THAN DNR		MORE DEPRESSIVE THAN DNR. ACTION ON B AND T CELLS
	DM DAUNORUBICIN DOXORUBICIN		MUTAGEN (TA 98)	CARCINOGENIC IN MICE	
	RUBIDAZONE		LESS MUTAGENIC THAN DNR OR DXR		
	DETORUBICIN		LESS MUTAGENIC THAN DXR		
	AD - 32				
	4'-EPI-ADRIAMYCIN				
C	ACLACINOMYCIN A		NON MUTAGENIC (TA 98)		
	MARCELLOMYCIN				
D	7-CON-OMEN		NON MUTAGENIC (AMES' TEST)		

Table 4

GROUP	COMPOUND	EXPERIMENTAL ANTITUMOR ACTIVITY	THERAPEUTIC ACTIVITY IN THE CLINIC	CLINICAL TOXICITY	RESISTANCE PHENOMENON
B	CARMINOMYCIN	L1210 = MORE EFFECTIVE THAN DNR ACTIVE P.O.	ACTIVITY IN LEUKEMIAS AND SOLID TUMORS (IN PROGRESS IN RUSSIA AND IN THE U.S.A)	ASSOCIATION WITH METHYL URACIL TO PREVENT CARDIOTOXICITY	CROSS-RESISTANCE WITH DNR AND DXR
	DM DAUNORUBICIN DOXORUBICIN	MORE POTENT THAN THE PARENT COMPOUNDS CHEMOTHERAPEUTIC INDEX BETTER ACTIVE P.O.	BEGINNING OF THE STUDY	MTD : I.V. : 18MG/M2 P.O. : 60MG/M2	
	RUBIDAZONE	AS ACTIVE AS OR MORE ACTIVE THAN DNR BETTER CHEMOTHERAPEUTIC INDEX	ACUTE LEUKEMIAS (ACUTE MONOBLASTIC) RESULTS IN SOLID TUMORS : NOT SO GOOD AS DXR	USUAL TOXICITY + FEVER, RASHES CUMULATIVE DOSE LIMITS = 3500MG/M2	CROSS-RESISTANCE WITH DNR AND DXR
	DETORUBICIN	EQUAL OR SUPERIOR TO DXR	SOLID TUMORS, SARCOMAS, MELANOMAS	MTD = 120MG/M2 I.V. (EVERY 3 W.) AS TOXIC AS DXR (SLIGHTLY LESS ALOPECIA)	CROSS-RESISTANCE WITH DNR AND DXR
	AD - 32	COMPARISON WITH DXR : CONFLICTING RESULTS : EQUAL OR SUPERIOR :	UNDER STUDY ACTIVITY	PROBLEMS OF ADMINISTRATION AND TOLERANCE	
	4'-EPI-ADRIAMYCIN	COMPARISON WITH DXR : BETTER CHEMOTHERAPEUTIC INDEX	COMPARISON WITH DXR : ACTIVITY SIMILAR HIGHER ELIMINATION RATE RESPONSES IN CASES REFRACTORY TO DXR	COMPARISON WITH DXR : LOWER GENERAL TOXICITY. LESS VOMITING, ALOPECIA, BONE-MARROW DEPRESSION	CROSS-RESISTANCE WITH DNR AND DXR BUT 4'-EPI-DEOXY-DXR IS ACTIVE ON DXR RESISTANT TUMORS GRAFTED IN NUDE MICE
C	ACLACINOMYCIN	COMPARISON WITH DNR AND DXR LESS ACTIVE OR SAME ACTIVITY	ACTIVE ON ACUTE LEUKEMIAS (AML, ALL AND LYMPHOSARCOMAS) MORE EFFECTIVE DAILY x 10 (THAN A SINGLE DOSE)	NO OR MILD ALOPECIA MILD CARDIOTOXICITY	MODERATELY ACTIVE ON A P388/DXR
	MARCELLOMYCIN	LESS ACTIVE THAN DXR AS ACTIVE AS OR MORE ACTIVE THAN ACLA-A, MUSETTAMYCIN			
D	7-CON-OMEN	AS ACTIVE AS OR MORE ACTIVE THAN DXR			

Therapeutic activity in the clinic (Table 4)

The study of carminomycin is in progress in the Soviet Union and the United States: it is active on leukemias and solid tumors (47).

The study of dm DNR and dm DXR is only just starting (Phase I).

Rubidazone is active on acute leukemia (48,49).

Detorubicin is active on solid tumors, sarcomas, melanoma. It is as toxic as DXR, but perhaps causing less alopecia (50,51).

AD32 is under study and is active, but problems of administration were encountered.

4'-epi-Adriamycin, compared with DXR is active and better tolerated (less vomiting, alopecia, bone-marrow depression)(52).

Aclacinomycin A is active in acute leukemias. No or mild alopecia and mild cardiotoxicity were encountered. The evaluation of its activity on solid tumors needs further study (53).

Drug resistance (Table 4)

Experimentally, in vivo, a cross-resistance between the various compounds is usually observed. Tapiero (54), using very high DNR or DXR resistant cell strains in vitro, observed no cross-resistance with aclacinomycin A. In the clinic, the cross-resistance is sometimes not clear and seems not to be present for aclacinomycin A. We should also mention that an analog, 4'-deoxy-DXR, is active on DXR-resistant tumors grafted in nude mice (55).

4. CONCLUDING REMARK

After about twenty years of international research in the anthracycline family, progress has been made with some offspring, but the parents are still thriving. We are now awaiting the arrival of the child prodigy.

REFERENCES

1. Crooke ST, Duvernay VH, Galvan L & Prestayko AW. 1978. Structure activity relationships of anthracyclines relative effects on macromolecular
   syntheses. Molecular Pharmacology 14, 290.
2. Duvernay VH, Mong S & Crooke ST. 1980. Molecular pharmacology of anthracyclines. p. 61 in "Anthracyclines : current status and new developments"
   (Crooke ST & Reich SD, eds). New York, Academic Press.
3. Bachur NR. 1979. Anthracycline antibiotic pharmacology and metabolism.
   Cancer Treatment Reports 63, 817.
4. Chervinsky D & Wang JJ. 1972. Uptake of adriamycin and daunomycin in
   L1210 leukemic cells. Proc. Amer. Assoc. Cancer Res. 13, 63.
5. Bachur NR, Steele M, Meriwether WD & Hildebrand RC. 1976. Cellular
   pharmacodynamics of several anthracycline antibiotics. J. Med. Chem.
   19, 651.
6. Bachur NR, Egorin MJ & Hildebrand RC. Daunorubicin and adriamycin metabolism in the Golden Syrian Hamster. Biochem. Med. 1973, 8, 352.
7. Doroshow JH, Locker GY & Myers CE. 1979. Experimental animal models of
   adriamycin cardiotoxicity. Cancer Treat. Rep. 63, 855.
8. Lampidis TJ, Johnson LV, Israel M & Canellos GP. 1980. Increased nuclear
   accumulation of adriamycin (ADR) and damage in cardiac muscle vs. cardiac
   non-muscle cells in culture. Proc. Amer. Assoc. Cancer Res. 21, 275.
9. Dantchev D, Slioussartchouk V, Paintrand M, Hayat M, Bourut C & Mathé G.
   1979. Electron microscopic studies of the heart and light microscopic
   studies of the skin after treatment of golden hamsters with adriamycin,
   detorubicin, AD32 and aclacinomycin. Cancer Treat. Rep. 63, 875.
10. Di Marco A, Gaetani M & Scarpinato B. 1969. Adriamycin (NSC-123.127):
    a new antibiotic with antitumor activity. Cancer Chemoth. Rep. 53, 33.
11. Sandberg JS, Howsden FL, Di Marco A & Goldin A. 1970. Comparison of
    the antileukemic effect on mice of adriamycin (NSC 123.127) with dauno-
    mycin (NSC 82.151). Cancer Chemoth. Rep. 54, 1.
12. Von Hoff DD, Rozencweig M & Slavik M. 1978. Daunomycin : an anthracy-
    cline antibiotic effective in acute leukemia. p. 1 in "Advances in
    Pharmacology and Chemotherapy". vol. 15, New York, Academic Press.
13. Duvernay VH, Pachter JA & Crooke ST. 1980. Molecular pharmacological
    differences between carminomycin, and its analog, carminomycin-11-methyl
    ether, and adriamycin. Cancer Res. 40, 387.
14. Arcamone F, Bernardi L, Giadino P et al. 1976. Synthesis and antitumor
    activity of 4-demethoxy-daunorubicin, 4-demethoxy-7,9-diepidaunomycin
    and their beta anomers. Cancer Treat. Rep. 60, 829.
15. Maral R. 1979. Biological activities of rubidazone. Cancer Chemoth.
    Pharmacol. 2, 31.
16. Maral R, Ducer JB, Farge D, Ronsinet G & Reisdorf D. 1978. Préparation
    et activité antitumorale expérimentale d'un nouvel antibiotique semi-
    synthétique : la diétoxyacétoxy)-14 daunorubicine (33.921 RP).
    C.R. Acad. Sci, Paris (D), 286, 443.
17. Azarus H, Yuan G, Tan E & Israel M. 1978. Comparative inhibitory effects
    of adriamycin, AD-32 and related compounds on in vitro cell growth and
    macromolecular synthesis. Proc. Amer. Assoc. Cancer Res. 19, 159.
18. Arcamone F, Pencos S, Vigevani A, Redaeli S, Franchi G et al. 1975.
    Synthesis and antitumor properties of new glycosides of daunomycinone
    and adriamycinone. J. Med. Chem. 18, 703.
19. Oki T. 1980. Aclacinomycin A. p. 323 in "Anthracyclines : current status
    and new developments" (Crooke ST & Reich SD, eds). New York, Academic
    Press.

20. Bhuyan BK, Blowers CL & Shugars KD. 1980. Lethality of nogalamycin, nogalamycin analogs, and adriamycin to cells in different cell cycle phases. Cancer Res., 40, 3437.

21. Krishan A, Dutt K, Israel M & Ganapathi R. 1981. Comparative effects of adriamycin and N-trifluoroacetyladriamycin-14-valerate on cell kinetics, chromosomal damage and macromolecular synthesis in vitro. Cancer Res., 41, 2745.

22. Adams EG & Bhuyan BK. 1980. Effects of 7-con-O-methylnogarol (7-OMEN) on cell progression of CHO and L1210 cells in vitro and L1210 cells in vivo. Proc. Amer. Assoc. Cancer Res. 21, 283.

23. Seeber S. 1980. Nuclear and cellular accumulation of aclacinomycin A, AD-32, carminomycin and marcellomycin in daunorubicin-sensitive (EAC-S) and resistant (EAC-DMM) Ehrlich ascites. Proc. Amer. Assoc. Cancer Res. 21, 272.

24. Bhuyan BK, Neil G, Li LH, Mc Govern JP & Wiley PF. 1980. Chemistry and biological activity of 7-con-O-methylnogarol (7-con-OMEN). p. 365 in "Anthracyclines : current status and new developments" (Crooke ST & Reich SD, eds). New York, Academic Press.

25. Pittman KA, Fandrich S, Rozencweig M, Baker LH, Lenaz L & Crooke ST. 1980. Clinical pharmacologic studies of carminomycin. Proc. Amer. Assoc. Cancer Res. 21, 180.

26. Formelli F, Casazza AM, Di Marco A, Mariani A & Pollini C. 1979. Fluorescence assay of tissue distribution of 4-demethoxy-daunorubicin and 4-demethoxydoxorubicin in mice bearing solid tumors. Cancer Chemoth. Pharmacol., 3, 261.

27. Baurain R, Deprez-de-Campeneere D & Trouet A. 1979. Distribution and metabolism of rubidazone and daunorubicin in mice. A comparative study. Cancer Chemoth. Pharmacol., 2, 37.

28. Deprez-de-Campeneere D, Baurain R & Trouet A. 1979. Pharmacokinetic, toxicologic and chemotherapeutic properties of detorubicin in mice : a comparative study with daunorubicin and adriamycin. Cancer Treat. Rep., 63, 861.

29. Israel M, Karkowsky M & Khetarpal VK. 1981. Distribution of radioactivity and anthracycline-fluorescence in tissues of mice one hour after (^{14}C)-labeled AD-32 administration. Cancer Chemoth. Pharmacol., 6, 25.

30. Casazza AM. et al. 1980. Effects of modifications in position 4 of the chromophore or in position 4' of the aminosugar on the antitumor activity and toxicity of daunorubicin and doxorubicin. p. 403 in "Anthracyclines: current status and new developments" (Crooke ST & Reich SD, eds). New York, Academic Press.

31. Casazza AM. et al. 1978. Antitumor activity, toxicity and pharmacological properties of 4'-epi-adriamycin. Curr. Chemoth., 2, 1257.

32. Israel M, Modest EJ & Frei E III. 1975. N-trifluoroacetyladriamycin, an analog with greater experimental antitumor activity and less toxicity than adriamycin. Cancer Res., 35, 1365.

33. Gause GF. 1978. Antitumor antibiotics from actinomycetes. Zbl. Bakteriol. Parasitenk. Infektionkr. Hyg. 1 abt. Orig A, Suppl.6n 345.

34. Bradner WT & Huftalen JB. 1978. Marcellomycin : an anthracycline without leukopenic effect in BDF1 mice. Proc. Amer. Assoc. Cancer Res. 19, 46.

35. Gause GF, Brazhnikova MG & Shorin VA. 1974. A new antitumor antibiotic carminomycin (NSC-180.024). Cancer Chemoth. Rep., 58, 255.

36. Kirchner E, Guettner J, Fritsch RS & Haertl A. 1981. Toxic effects of violamycin B1, carminomycin and daunorubicin on the myocardium of rabbits. Acta Pharmacol. Toxicol 48, 87.

204

37. Jaenke RS, Deprez-de-Campeneere D & Trouet A. 1980. Cardiotoxicity and comparative pharmacokinetics of six anthracyclines in the rabbit. Cancer Res., 40, 3530.
38. Mc Govern JP. et al. 1979. Chronic cardiotoxicity studies in rabbits with 7-con-O-methylnogarol, a new anthracycline antitumor agent. Cancer Res., 39, 4849.
39. Damjanov I & Celluzzi A. 1980. Embryotoxicity and teratogenicity of the anthracycline antibiotic carminomycin in mice. Research Comm. Chem. Pathol. & Pharmacol. 28, 497.
40. Kurlov OV, Koifman EK & Goldber ED. 1978. Comparative cytogenic effect of carminomycin and rubomycin antitumor antibiotics. Antibiotiki 23, 537.
41. Marquardt H, Philips FS, Marquardt H & Sternberg SS. 1979. Oncogenicity of 4-demethoxydaunomycin : lack of correlation among in vivo short-term tests and between in vitro and in vivo findings. Proc. Amer. Assoc. Cancer Res., 20, 45.
42. Umezawa K, Sawamura M, Matsushina T & Sugimura T. 1978. Mutagenicity of aclacinomycin A and daunomycin derivatives. Cancer Res., 38, 1782.
43. Gause GF, Sveshnikova MA, Ukholina RS, Gavrilina GV, Filicheva VA & Gladkikh EG. 1973. Production of antitumor antibiotic carminomycin by Actinomadura carminata Sp. Nov. Antibiotiki 18, 675.
44. Casazza AM, Bertazzoli C, Partesi G, Bellini O & Di Marco A. 1979. Antileukemic activity and cardiac toxicity of 4-demethoxydaunorubicin in mice. Proc. Amer. Assoc. Cancer Res., 20, 16.
45. Maral R. et al. 1980. Experimental and clinical activity of a new anthracycline derivative : detorubicine (14-diethoxyacetoxydaunorubicin). p. 172 in "Recent Results in Cancer Research" (Mathé G & Muggia FM,eds). vol. 74, Berlin-Heidelberg, Springer Verlag.
46. Giuliani FC. et al. 1981. Comparative antineoplastic activity of AD-32 and doxorubicin (DX) against human tumors xenografted in the athymic mouse. Intern. Congress Chemotherapy, Firenze, abstract 105.
47. Reich SD & Crooke ST. 1980. Carminomycin. p. 295 in "Anthracycline: current status and new developments" (Crooke ST & Reich SD, eds). New York, Academic Press.
48. Jacquillat C, Weil M, Gemon-Auclerc MF, Izrael V, Bussel A, Boiron M & Bernard J. 1976. Clinical study of rubidazone (20.050 RP), a new daunorubicin-derivative compound in 170 patients with acute leukemias and other malignancies. Cancer 37, 653.
49. Bickers J, Benjamin R, Wilson H, Eyre H, Hewlet J & Mc Credie K. 1981. Rubidazone in adults with previously treated acute leukemia and blast cell phase of chronic myelocytic leukemia: a Southwest Oncology Group Study. Cancer Treat. Rep. 65, 427.
50. Jacquillat C, Auclerc MF, Weil M, Maral J, Degos L, Auclerc G, Tobelem G, Schaison G & Bernard J. 1979. Clinical activity of detorubicin : a new anthracycline derivative. Cancer Treat. Rep., 63, 889.
51. Weil M. et al. 1981. Diethoxyacetoxy (detorubicin). in "Anthracyclines Symposium". In press. Masson, New York.
52. Bonfante V. 1981. Toxic and therapeutic activity of 4'-epi-doxorubicin. in "Anthracyclines Symposium". To be published by Masson, New York.
53. Mathé G. et al. 1981. Phase II clinical trial of aclacinomycin A in acute leukemia and leukemic lymphosarcoma. in "Anthracyclines Symposium". To be published by Masson, New York.
54. Tapiero H. et al. 1981. Comparative uptake of adriamycin, daunorubicin and aclacinomycin A in sensitive and resistant Friend leukemia cells. in "Anthracyclines Symposium". To be published by Masson, New York.
55. Giuliani FC & Kaplan NO. 1980. New doxorubicin analogs active against doxorubicin-resistant colon tumor xenografts in the nude mouse. Cancer Res. 40, 4682.

FACTORS IN SELECTION OF NEW ANTHRACYCLINES

E. M. ACTON, R. A. JENSEN, AND J. H. PETERS

1. INTRODUCTION*

In spite of the unique importance of doxorubicin (A) for the
treatment of cancer and the utility, though more limited, of
daunorubicin (D), better anthracyclines are needed that are more
active and less toxic (1). The design and selection of new analogs should now be possible on a better basis than ever before,
because of the background of information that has been built up
over the past 15 years. In addition to knowledge about the clinical applications and limitations of doxorubicin and a number of
analogs, there is now considerable information about the biochemical mechanisms and metabolic disposition of these agents,
as well as the structure-activity relationships observed from
the antitumor screening of numerous analogs--nearly 600 at the
NCI alone. Many of these analogs were synthesized at a time when
the best approach was the systematic chemical derivation of
accessible functional groups. Because a practical total synthesis
of anthracyclines is still lacking, semisynthesis continues to be
the best approach to new analogs, but the site of derivation and
the type of change can now be more rationally chosen. Our current
studies emphasize structural changes at the quinone and at the
sugar amine. We attempt, even in preliminary biological evaluation of the resultant analogs, to combine tests for antitumor
properties with tests for toxic side effects, mechanisms of
action, and metabolic changes.

These studies were supported by Cancer Research Emphasis grant
CA 25711 from the National Cancer Institute, DHHS. Results prior
to 1977 were obtained under contract NO1-CM-33742 from the NCI.

*Abbreviations used are A, doxorubicin; D, daunorubicin; Im,
imino; Bzl, benzyl; and diH, dihydro.

2. IMINO DERIVATIVES

The quinone is of interest because it appears to be a key site of biochemical action in the anthracyclines, as in numerous other quinone-bearing chemical structures with antitumor properties (2, 3). The redox properties of the quinone unit have received considerable attention, especially the reversible one-electron reduction that occurs in biological systems and leads to formation of semiquinone and oxygen-derived free radicals (2-5). Many investigators have associated this process with cardiotoxicity in the anthracycline series, but an involvement of free radicals in the antitumor effects can not be excluded. The pattern of effects might be altered by changes in chemical structure at the quinone site, but there has been almost no opportunity to test this possibility. In the entire anthracycline series so far the only change in quinone structure has been the conversion of daunorubicin and doxorubicin to the 5-imino derivatives (6, 7). This conversion did in fact produce significant changes in biological properties (8). 5-Iminodaunorubicin (ImD) appeared to be less cardiotoxic, whereas 5-iminodoxorubicin (ImA) showed a virtually unsurpassed increase in antitumor efficacy, albeit at high doses.

X = H, 5-iminodaunorubicin (ImD)

X = OH, 5-iminodoxorubicin (ImA)

The biological test data for ImD and ImA, compared with D and A, are given in Table 1. The first imino derivative was ImD. It was found to retain but not surpass the antitumor efficacy (T/C = 130%) of D against advanced mouse leukemia P388 (q4d 5,9,13). The potency of ImD at first appeared to be greater (lower optimum dose, 3 instead of 8 mg/kg), but a series of tests against various mouse tumors (unreported data from NCI) gave the overall impression of little change in either efficacy or potency *in vivo* by conversion of D to its quinone imine. Because of the importance assigned to mechanisms involving DNA, most of the *in vitro* tests in Table 1

Table 1. Comparison of Biological Properties of the 5-Imino Derivatives[a]

| compound | activity versus mouse leukemia P388 | | leukemia L1210 cells inhibn of synth ED$_{50}$, μM | | ΔT_m of isolated helical DNA in solution | microsomal O$_2$ consumption, stimulation relative to A |
	efficacy % T/C	optimum dose q4d 5,9,13 mg/kg	DNA	RNA	°C	%
ImD	130	3	1.6	1.3	6.2	8.2
ImA	217	100 (highest dose)	2.0	2.1	6.9	7.5
D	130	8	1.0	0.3	11.2	82, 109
A	160	8	1.5	0.7	13.4	100
	NCI		D.L. Taylor, SRI			J.H. Peters, G.R. Gordon, SRI

[a] The data are from ref. 7, except for the data on ImA versus P388, which are new and at a higher dose.

were for DNA interactive properties. Of perhaps greater interest are results from the test for enhanced consumption of oxygen when drug is added to liver microsomes. Both A and D strongly stimulate O$_2$ consumption over the endogenous level, and this can be used as a measure of the capacity of anthracyclines to generate free radicals (2, 3, 9, 10). ImD was far less effective, giving only 8.2% of the rate of O$_2$ consumption observed with an equal concentration of A. The diminished capacity of ImD to produce oxygen-derived radicals was independently observed in the diminished rate of cleavage of covalently closed circular DNA, presumably by radicals, following activation of ImD (compared to D) by chemical prereduction (11). In addition, electrochemical studies involving cyclic voltammetry showed that ImD was more difficult to reduce than D, and that the reduced form of ImD was nearly impossible to re-oxidize (11, 12).

These results can be compared with the diminished cardiotoxic potency of ImD, as measured by the increased doses required to produce chronic electrocardiographic changes in the rat. This test was developed by Zbinden, who measured ECG changes serially with repeated intraperitoneal doses of drug, and defined cardiotoxic potency as the minimum cumulative dose that produced presumably irreversible widening of the QRS complex

(13). Recently, we have achieved more sensitive measurement of the ECG waves by computerized averaging and recording. We have included prolongation of the QαT interval along with QRS in the observation, and we now define cardiotoxic potency from the cumulative dose to produce 10% prolongation based on additional criteria (14). Occurrence of the ECG changes has also been correlated with changes in electrical and mechanical properties of cardiac tissue from the treated rats. The results with A (Table 2) were based on treatment with multiple doses at levels of 1, 2, and 4 mg/kg (IP). Regardless of dose regimen, the lowest cumulative dose to produce 10% prolongation (i.e., the cardiotoxic endpoint) was the same, 8 mg/kg for QRS prolongation and 4 mg/kg for QαT. In contrast to this, the cardiotoxic endpoint for ImD after multiple doses of 4, 10, and 16 mg/kg (IP) varied with regimen. Only the results from the 4-mg level are given in Table 2, a total of 48 mg/kg to produce 10% QRS prolongation, and 36 mg/kg for QαT. This gives the most conservative estimate of the

Table 2. Cardiotoxic Potency in Rats: Total Dose to Cause Electrocardiographic Changes

compound	15% prolongation of QRS mg/kg	10% prolongation of QRS mg/kg	10% prolongation of QαT mg/kg
A	10-12	8[a]	4[a]
ImD	64	48[b]	36[b]
	G. Zbinden et al., ref. 13	R.A. Jensen, SRI, 1981	

[a]After multiple doses of 1, 2, or 4 mg/kg. The cumulative dose for 10% prolongation was thus independent of regimen. [b]After multiple doses of 4 mg/kg. After multiple doses of 10 or 16 mg/kg, higher cumulative doses (up to 80 mg/kg) were required for 10% prolongation, suggesting an even greater decrease in cardiotoxic potency. This variability with regimen has been observed only with ImD so far. Until it can be explained, we assume the low-dose results are more reliable and less subject to questions such as bioavailability.

decrease in cardiotoxic potency in going from A to ImD, i.e., a factor of from 6- to 9-fold. (The results at higher levels of ImD indicated higher cumulative doses could be obtained before 10% QRS or QαT prolongation was observed, i.e., that the cardiotoxic potency was even further reduced; studies are in progress to test whether the lesser effect at increased dose levels might be related to reduced bioavailability.) Earlier, Zbinden reported a 5-fold decrease (13). The advantage in diminished cardiotoxicity predicted for ImD would seem to be significant, even though neither antitumor efficacy nor antitumor potency was much affected.

Truly superior antitumor efficacy has been encountered however, upon converting the quinone unit of doxorubicin to the imine. At the highest dose tested so far, ImA (Table 1) recently produced a T/C of 217%. Such values are virtually unsurpassed against mouse leukemia P388 (q4d 5,9,13). Results with doses greater than 100 mg/kg are still to be obtained. Absence of any animal deaths at these unusually high doses suggests a general potency decrease. The *in vitro* test results in Table 1 showed no distinction between ImD and ImA. In the test for microsomal O_2 consumption, ImA showed as poor a capacity as ImD for the generation of radicals. However, the as-yet-undetermined cardiotoxic potency of ImA *in vivo*, relative to the antitumor potency, will be a critical factor for evaluating the potential of ImA. The importance in analog development of comparing the *in vivo* potencies of effects cannot be overemphasized.

3. N-BENZYL DERIVATIVES

The sugar amine is a biologically important functional group in anthracycline structure that can readily be subjected to various types of chemical derivation. For more than ten years, most investigators have assumed that the basic amine enhances the binding or complexation of anthracyclines with DNA through electrostatic binding with a DNA phosphate group, but a recent X-ray crystallographic study produced a new model with no role for the amino group in anthracycline-DNA binding (15). Generally, removal of the amino group from the anthracycline structure or blocking its basicity by N-acylation has proven to be a deactivation. However, a few exceptional analogs, e.g., AD32 (16) and 3'-deamino-3'-hydroxydoxorubicin (17), have shown superior efficacy, but even then potency was diminished and much higher doses were required.

We have found that a versatile method for introducing wide changes in chemical structure and yet producing active new analogs that retain basicity is the reductive N-alkylation of the anthracyclines with a variety of aldehydes or ketones and sodium cyanoborohydride (18). The formation of a series of active N-alkyl derivatives has been described (19). Because the N-alkylation is a reductive method, the by-products of 13-ketone reduction (13-dihydro analogs, or 13-diH) are commonly formed, usually in smaller amounts. Most of the N-alkyl compounds were not readily distinguished from A or D in the antitumor screen using mouse leukemia P388. Where outstanding activity was clearly observed was in the lipophilic N-benzyl (N-Bzl) series. With reduction of the 13-ketone, in addition to both mono- and di-benzylation, A and D each formed the two N-Bzl-13-diH derivatives listed in Table 3. In each series, there is a trend toward increase in efficacy and decrease in potency, in going from parent, to mono, to dibenzyl. In fact, the T/C values of 209% for N,N-diBzl-D and 210% for N,N-diBzl-13-diH-A are among the highest observed against P388 in the q4d 5,9,13 schedule. (N,N-DiBzl-A has not yet been tested at sufficiently high doses, because little of it was formed.) For further investigation, N,N-diBzl-D with an optimum dose of 38 mg/kg was

Table 3. Antitumor Properties of N-benzylation Products[a]

N-Benzyl derivatives	activity versus mouse leukemia P388	
	efficacy % T/C	optimum dose q4d 5,9,13 mg/kg
D	132	8
N-Bzl-D	184	19
N-Bzl-13-diH-D	168	19
N,N-diBzl-D[b]	209	38
N,N-diBzl-13-diH-D	184	25
A	160	8
N-Bzl-A	190	19
N-Bzl-13-diH-A	135	38
N,N-diBzl-A	active, incomplete test	
N,N-diBzl-13-diH-A	210	100

NCI

[a] Data from ref. 19. [b] Also superior to A versus mouse colon and mammary tumors, passed NCI Decision Network.

favored over the equally efficacious but less potent N,N–diBzl–13–diH–A with an optimum dose of 100 mg/kg.

N,N–Dibenzyldaunorubicin has been tested for cardiotoxic potency in rats by the serial measurement of ECG changes with multiple dosing (14). The results are shown in Table 4, in comparison with A. Table 4 also compares the antitumor potencies (from the mouse leukemia P388 screen) for N,N–diBzl–D and for A, so that a preliminary estimation of the therapeutic advantage of diBzl–D can be made. Rats were treated with N,N–diBzl–D in a series of doses at 10 mg/kg and at 20 mg/kg (IV, dosing IP has been abandoned as ineffective for any but the lowest levels of this compound, owing to its low solubility and precipitation in the peritoneal cavity). As with A, the cardiotoxic endpoint in terms of the lowest cumulative dose to produce 10% prolongation of the QRS (240–280 mg/kg) or QαT (170–180 mg/kg) complex was independent of the dose regimen. Table 4 shows that cardiotoxic potency decreased 30- to 45-fold in going from A to N,N–diBzl–D, whereas the antitumor potency decreased only 4.8-fold

Table 4. Comparison of Potencies of Effects

	in mice	in rats	
	Antitumor Potency	Cardiotoxic Potency	
		in electrocardiogram, total dose to cause 10% widening of	
	opt dose (q4d 5,9,13) vs P388	QRS complex	QαT complex
Compound	mg/kg	mg/kg	mg/kg
A	8	8 (irreversible)	4
N,N–diBzl–D	38	240–280 (reversible)	170–180
Ratio (decrease in potency for diBzl)	$\frac{1}{4.8}$	$\frac{1}{>30-35}$	$\frac{1}{>42-45}$
	NCI	R.A. Jensen, SRI, 1981	

$$\text{therapeutic advantage for N, N-diBzl} = \frac{\text{antitumor potency ratio}}{\text{cardiotoxic potency ratio}} \geqslant \frac{\frac{1}{4.8}}{\frac{1}{30-45}} \geqslant \frac{8}{1}$$

(simultaneously giving an increase in efficacy). Hence, approximately an 8-fold advantage can be calculated for N,N-diBzl-D over A, based on separation of antitumor and cardiotoxic effects. In fact, the separation of effects is probably greater than this calculation shows. After dosing with N,N-diBzl-D was stopped, the treated rats were kept and monitored for several months before being sacrificed, and the ECG changes were found to undergo reversal. This could be correlated with the apparent recovery, observed in different animals, of the hearts from microscopic tissue damage. On the other hand, no evidence of reversibility has ever been observed with A after the cardiotoxic endpoint is attained. It is possible that the cardiotoxic endpoint for N,N-diBzl-D might be irreversible at a higher cumulative dose than we have attained, but significantly higher doses appear infeasible by the IV route of administration we have used. Current studies (20) indicate oral dosing is nearly as effective as the previous IV dosing, but it is not yet certain whether the oral route will continue to be effecient at much higher doses.

When the commonly used *in vitro* tests were applied to N,N-diBzl-D, it was soon observed there was little or no activity in any *in vitro* system that was tried. Table 5 shows results from the entire series of N-Bzl derivatives (corresponding to those in Table 3) for binding to helical DNA (based on elevation of the T_m), inhibition of DNA/RNA synthesis in L1210 cells, bacterial mutagenicity in Ames tester strains TA98, and stimulation of microsomal O_2 consumption leading to free radical generation. Except for Ames mutagenicity, which is apparently absent in all N-alkyl derivatives, the loss of activity seems to be gradual in going from parent A or D, to mono, and finally to N,N-diBzl derivatives. Since the mono-N-Bzl compounds consistently retain appreciable activity, the break point seems to come between mono and diBzl. At first, the *in vitro* inactivity of N,N-diBzl-D seemed incompatible with the enhanced efficacy *in vivo*. We now think this is explained by the metabolic conversion of N,N-diBzl-D. Our recent measurements in tissue and plasma from treated rats show there is stepwise debenzylation at the amino N, in addition to the usual reduction of the 13-ketone (20). The major metabolites thus include the entire series of N-Bzl derivatives (Table 3) formed from D, as well as D itself. N,N-DiBzl-D may therefore be considered a prodrug, requiring *in vivo* activation, for any or all of these active analogs. It seems possible that the debenzylation-activation

Table 5. In Vitro Tests of N-Benzyl Series

compound	ΔT$_m$ of isolated helical DNA in solution °C	leukemia L1210 cells inhibn of synth ED$_{50}$, μM DNA	leukemia L1210 cells inhibn of synth ED$_{50}$, μM RNA	Ames mutagenicity revertant/nmol	stimulation of microsomal O$_2$ consumption, % rel to A	
D	11.2	0.66	0.33	100	109, 82	active
N-Bzl-D	10.2	1.6	0.17	0.5	8	
N-Bzl-13-diH-D	6.2	1.7	0.32	0.5	21	
N,N-diBzl-D	1.4	> 100	10	0.5	2	
N,N-diBzl-13-diH-D	0.0	220	8	0.5	4	~inactive
A .	13.4	1.5	0.58		100	active
N-Bzl-A	11.3	0.65	0.09			
N-Bzl-13-diH-A	7.6	1.4	0.29			
N,N-diBzl-A	-1.2	110	4.8			
N,N-diBzl-13-diH-A	insol	160	8.0			~inactive

D.L.Taylor, SRI   V. Simmon, SRI   J.H Peters, G.R. Gordon, SRI

process may involve some selectivity that accounts for the apparent separation of oncolytic and cardiotoxic effects. In further drug design, it may also be possible to use the metabolically cleavable N-benzyl group to create new prodrugs of other active analogs.

N,N-dibenzyldaunorubicin

3'-deamino—3'—(4-morpholinyl) daunorubicin

4. PIPERIDINO/MORPHOLINO ANALOGS

Most of the N-alkyl analogs have been synthesized simply by reductive alkylation of A or D with monoaldehydes or monoketones, but a distinct class has been generated by reductive alkylation with dialdehydes. For example, both aldehyde functions of the common 5-carbon dialdehyde, glutaraldehyde, gave reductive alkylation successively at a single amino group, constructing a new ring that incorporated the amino N (19). Test data for the resulting piperidino derivatives of A and D are shown in Table 6. These analogs attracted attention not only for their activity against mouse leukemia P388, but also for their potent and selective inhibition of RNA synthesis. The ED_{50} values in Table 6 show that the piperidino compounds were from 10 to 18 times more potent against RNA than DNA synthesis. Most other analogs, like A and D in Table 6, were only about 2 times more potent against RNA synthesis. A suggestion has been made that selective inhibition of RNA synthesis denotes a Class II of anthracyclines (21). This designation was based on inhibition of nucleolar RNA synthesis, where very striking increases in potency can be observed, so it is uncertain how relevant to this are the results in Table 6 for the whole cell. Structurally, with the piperidino derivatives, the addition of a new ring to the sugar may have some relevance to the fact that the Class II anthracyclines so far have all been disaccharides or trisaccharides.

Two types of changes in the piperidino structure were explored with the analogs in Table 7 (22). Introduction of a ring O was provided by the morpholino analog (synthesized by reductive alkylation of D with

2,2'-oxybisacetaldehyde). With the N-cyclohexyl derivative, the amino N was moved out of the piperidino ring. Both changes were combined in the N-(tetrahydro-4-pyranyl) derivative. It is immediately apparent that morpholino-D (T/C = 166%) retained the antitumor efficacy of A (T/C = 160%) against mouse leukemia P388, but exhibited the activity at a greatly decreased dose--0.2 mg/kg compared to 8 mg/kg for A (q4d 5,9,13). This 40-fold increase in potency is the greatest reported for any anthracycline so far. (A similar potency increase was observed for the 13-dihydro derivative of morpholino-D vs leukemia P388, and morpholino-D showed a 20-fold increase in potency vs B16 melanoma.) What this potency increase implies about the therapeutic potential of morpholino-D has yet to be investigated in further tests, but it seems possible that undesirable side effects may not be magnified in potency to the same degree and may be missing at the doses needed for cancer treatment with morpholino-D.

Almost as striking and even more unexpected is the complete absence of activity for N-cyclohexyl-D up to very high doses. The only apparent difference in structure between piperidino-D and N-cyclohexyl-D is an increase in conformational flexibility of the N-cyclohexyl ring relative to the piperidino ring. This seems hardly sufficient to account for a

Table 6. Piperidino Analogs and Comparison of Biological Results

compound	amino substit.	activity versus mouse leukemia P388[a]		leukemia L1210 cells inhibn of synth[a] ED_{50}, μM		ΔT_m of isolated helical DNA in solution[a]	microsomal O_2 consumption stimulation relative to A[b]
		efficacy % T/C	optimum dose q4d 5,9,13 mg/kg	DNA	RNA	°C	%
A	NH_2	160	8	1.5	0.58	13.4	100
D	NH_2	130	8	0.66	0.33	11.2	82, 109
piperidino A[c]	⌬N	158	9.4	0.70	0.04	15.4	
piperidino D[c]		177	6.2	0.50	0.05	16.8	87
		NCI		D.L. Taylor, SRI			J.H. Peters, G.R. Gordon, SRI

[a]Data from ref. 19. [b]Data from ref. 10. [c]The systematic names are 3'-deamino-3'-(1-piperidinyl) A and -D.

Table 7. Comparison With Morpholino and Cyclohexyl Analogs

compound	amino substit.	activity versus mouse leukemia P388		leukemia L1210 cells inhibn of synth ED_{50}, μM		ΔT_m of isolated helical DNA in solution $^\circ C$	microsomal O_2 consumption stimulation relative to A %
		efficacy % T/C	optimum dose q4d 5,9,13 mg/kg	DNA	RNA		
A	NH_2	160	8	1.5	0.58	13.4	100
piperidino D	(piperidino ring structure)	177	6.2	0.50	0.05	16.8	88
morpholino D[a]	(morpholino ring structure)	166	0.2	0.76	0.10	6.1	25
cyclohexyl D	(cyclohexyl-NH structure)	⩽108 (inact)	⩽200	64	16	0.6	57
tetra-H-pyranyl D[a]	(tetrahydropyranyl-NH structure)	136	100	2.0	0.61	4.0	68
		NCI		D.L. Taylor, SRI			J.H. Peters, G.R. Gordon, SRI

[a] The systematic names are 3'-deamino-3'-(4-morpholinyl)D and N-(tetrahydro-4-pyranyl)D.

deletion in activity, although structural rigidity often favors a specific interaction at a receptor site. Going from N-cyclohexyl to N-(tetrahydro-pyranyl) again shows the favorable effect of the ether oxygen at the 4-position. Moderate activity (T/C = 136%) against leukemia P388 was restored, but a very high dose (100 mg/kg) was required. Apparently the effect of starting with the cyclohexyl type of structure could not be overcome. We concluded at this stage that antitumor activity in this type of structure is optimized when the amino N is incorporated within the new ring, and when an ether O is present at or near the 4-position of the new ring. Presumably this ether O is at an interactive site not previously encountered with anthracycline activity.

Activity observed with additional substituted piperidino analogs is shown in Table 8. The important ether oxygen at the 4-position of the

Table 8. Extension of the Piperidino 4-Substituent

| compound | amino substit. | activity versus mouse leukemia P388 | | leukemia L1210 cells inhibn of synth ED$_{50}$, μM | | ΔT_m of isolated helical DNA in solution | microsomal O$_2$ consumption stimulation relative to A |
		efficacy % T/C	optimum dose q4d 5,9,13 mg/kg	DNA	RNA	°C	%
A	NH$_2$	160	8	1.5	0.58	13.4	100
piperidino D	(N-piperidine)	177	6.2	0.50	0.05	16.8	88
4-methoxy	(N-piperidine, OMe)	199	6.2	0.63	0.12	13.3	82
4-(methoxymethyl)	(N-piperidine, CH$_2$OMe)			0.61	0.08	16.3	84
4,4′-bis(methoxymethyl)	(N-piperidine, MeOCH$_2$ CH$_2$OMe)			1.3	0.05	9.2	50
		NCI		D.L. Taylor, SRI			J.H. Peters, G.R. Gordon, SRI

added ring was successfully moved into the side chain, as can be seen from
the improved antitumor efficacy (T/C = 199%) of the 4-methoxypiperidino
analog. Recent results on the 4,4-bis(methoxymethyl)piperidino analog
T/C = 212%) indicate that elaboration of the ether-bearing substituent
can produce still further increases in efficacy. So far, none of the
substituted-piperidino analogs has produced any potency increase. A new
derivative that combined the increased potency of the morpholino structure
with the efficacy increase of the methoxy-substituted morpholino structure
would be of great interest. Clearly, it is important to continue exploring
structural changes within this class of derivatives. Eventually, optimized
structures from different classes of derivatives might be combined to
produce a still higher degree of structure optimization.

The anthracyclines are complex, polyfunctional molecules, with access to multiple mechanisms of biological action, and an almost unlimited potential for structure modification and analog development. The examples that have been described illustrate that as the biological tools are developed for evaluating drug efficacy, side effects, and mechanism of action--as quantitatively as possible so that comparisons can be made--the possibilities for superior, selective agents become better than ever.

ACKNOWLEDGMENTS

Among the chemists cited in the references to analog synthesis, the authors are especially indebted to C. W. Mosher and G. L. Tong with regard to the present work. The authors are indebted to D. L. Taylor for *in vitro* assays. Detailed results on electrocardiographic measurement of cardiotoxicity (R.A.J.) and on metabolism and disposition and the oxygen cycling properties of numerous analogs (J.H.P. and coworkers) are quoted from manuscripts in preparation.

REFERENCES

1. Carter SK. 1980. *Cancer Chemother. Pharmacol. 4*, 5.
2. Bachur NR, Gordon SL, Gee MV. 1978. *Cancer Res. 38*, 1745.
3. Bachur NR, Gordon SL, Gee MV, Kon H. 1979. *Proc. Natl. Acad. Sci. USA 76*, 954.
4. Lown JW, Sim SK, Majumdar KC, Chang RY. 1977. *Biochem. Biophys. Res. Comm. 76*, 705.
5. Kalyanaraman B, Perez-Reyes E, Mason RP. 1980. *Biochim. Biophys. Acta 630*, 119.
6. Tong, GL, Henry DW, Acton EM. 1979. *J. Med. Chem. 22*, 36.
7. Acton EM, Tong GL. 1981. *J. Med. Chem. 24*, 669.
8. Peters JH, Evans MJ, Jensen RA, Acton EM. 1980. *Cancer Chemother. Pharmacol. 4*, 263.
9. Gordon GR, Peters JH, Acton EM. 25-28 Aug 1980. 2nd Chem. Congress, No. Amer. Continent, Amer. Chem. Soc., Las Vegas, NV. BIOL abstract #136.
10. Gordon GR, Kashiwase D. 1981. *Proc. Amer. Assn. Cancer Res. 22*, 256.
11. Lown JW, Chen H, Plambeck JA, Acton EM. 1979. *Biochem. Pharmacol. 28*, 2563.
12. Lown JW, Chen H, Plambeck JA, Acton EM. 1981, in press. *Biochem. Pharmacol.*
13. Zbinden G, Bachmann E, Holderegger C. 1978. *Antibiot. Chemother. 23*, 255.
14. Jensen RA. 1981. *Proc. Amer. Assn. Cancer Res. 22*, 269, and additional unpublished results.
15. Quigley GJ, Wang AH, Ughetto G, van der Marel G, van Boom JH, Rich A. 1980. *Proc. Natl. Acad. Sci. USA 77*, 7204.
16. Israel M, Modest EJ, Frei E. 1975. *Cancer Res. 35*, 1365.
17. Horton D, Priebe W, Turner WR. 1981. *Carbohyd. Res. 94*, 11.
18. Acton EM. 1980. *in* "Anthracyclines: Current Status and New Developments" (Crooke ST, Reich SD, eds.) p. 15. Academic Press, New York.

19. Tong GL, Wu HY, Smith TH, Henry DW. 1979. *J. Med. Chem. 22*, 912.
20. Peters JH, Kashiwase D, Gordon GR, Hunt CA, Acton EM. 1981. *Proc. Amer. Assn. Cancer Res. 22*, 256, and additional unpublished results.
21. Crooke ST, Duvernay VH, Galvan L, Prestayko AW. 1978. *Mol. Pharmacol. 14*, 290.
22. Mosher CW, Wu HY, Fujiwara AN, Acton EM. 1981, in press. *J. Med. Chem.*

IMPLICATIONS OF FREE RADICAL ACTIVATION FOR IMPROVED ANTHRACYCLINE THERAPY

D. D. PIETRONIGRO

1. INTRODUCTION

The anthracyclines are an effective new class of antitumor antibiotics. Adriamycin (ADM) is the most extensively investigated member of this class. In addition to its clinically advantageous tumor cell toxicity (TCT), it exhibits diverse biologic actions. These include unwanted side toxicities which limit its usefulness. The exact mechanisms by which ADM exerts both TCT and side toxicities remain to be elucidated. In the past three or four years, much interest has been generated concerning the possible involvement of ADM radicals (ADM·) in these toxicities. This interest has been fueled by the realizations that ADM is activated to ADM· throughout biologic system that ADM side toxicities can be inhibited by a number of antioxidants, and that ADM-stimulated radical formation produces DNA damage.

With the dual aim of identifying possible cellular sites of ADM· attack and direct ADM· quenchers, we have tested the direct reactivity of ADM· with a number of compounds. Coenzyme Q and tetrazolium salts are direct quencher of ADM·. The results suggest that coenzyme Q may be a site of ADM· attack. Direct ADM· quenchers may be used to

(1) test the involvement of ADM· in the many biologic actions of ADM;

(2) provide an approach towards specificity in modulating free radical reactions; and

(3) alter ADM toxicities to clinical advantage.

2. BIOLOGIC ACTIVATION OF ADRIAMYCIN TO FREE RADICALS

ADM is activated to free radicals throughout biologic systems (Table 1). The ability of ADM to spontaneously form ADM· and O_2^- at physiologic pH (1) suggests low level radical production at all sites harboring ADM at o above pH 7.0. Spontaneous ADM· formation is proportional to ADM concentrati (unpublished data) and therefore would be more pronounced in regions of higher ADM concentration. Radical generation increases with rising pH

over the range 7.0 to 8.8 (1,2) and proceeds in the presence of intact
L1210 cells (unpublished data).

Table 1. Adriamycin radical formation.

Activation Systems	
Spontaneous	Mitochondria
Microsomes	Ehrlich Ascites Tumor Cells
Nuclear Membrane	Red Blood Cells

The matrix side of the inner mitochondrial membrane, a region high in
pH, is a potential site of rapid spontaneous ADM· production. Mitochondrial
swelling, which occurs subsequent to ADM treatment, may facilitate penetration of ADM into the mitochondrial matrix.

Spontaneous ADM· production in the extracellular space may be particularly
damaging since this compartment is devoid of the substantial antioxidant
systems found in the intracellular environment (3). The external plasma
membrane surface would be vulnerable to direct radical attack. The cardioprotective effect of superoxide dismutase (SOD) plus catalase in animals
receiving ADM (4) may be due to extracellular radical scavenging since these
enzymes do not readily enter cardiac cells. Extravasation toxicity may also
depend partly upon extracellular ADM· formation (5).

In addition to spontaneous ADM· production, ADM is readily activated
at radical "hot spots" in membrane electron transport systems. These are
loci along the chain where electron leakage to O_2 or other suitable one-
electron acceptors results in free radical formation. NADPH cytochrome P-450
reductase represents a major radical-generating locus in the endoplasmic
reticulum and nuclear membrane, while NADH dehydrogenase and coenzyme Q
comprise radical "hot spots" in mitochondria.

Microsomes prepared from every tissue thus far examined activate ADM
and other anthracyclines to free radicals (6-8). The site of ADM· formation
is NADPH cytochrome P-450 reductase (9-11). It is well known that P-450
reductase provides a locus at which a wide range of antitumor chemicals,
carcinogens and other agents are activated to free radicals (6-13). In the
presence of O_2, microsomal activation of ADM· results in lipid peroxidation
with subsequent deterioration of membrane structure and function (9).

ADM· activation by nuclei (14) is probably dependent upon the NADPH
P-450 reductase of the nuclear envelope (15). The concept of nuclear

membrane activation is particularly enticing, since DNA-nuclear membrane complexes probably play a critical role in cell viability and may represent a target of radical attack. In this regard, it has been demonstrated that membrane-initiated free radical reactions destroy DNA (16).

Cardiac mitochondria activate ADM to ADM· with subsequent O_2^- formation in the presence of O_2. NADH dehydrogenase, a locus which generates radicals from a number of quinones (17), appears to be the major site of ADM· generatic (18,19).

High concentrations of intact Ehrlich ascites tumor cells generate a weak ADM· signal when incubated with ADM (6). The signal, which is difficult to reproduce (S. Sato, personal communication), may result from any one or a combination of the activation pathways outlined above.

Evidence of ADM· and daunomycin radical formation in intact red blood cells has been presented showing increased one-electron oxygen metabolism (20 Activation is dependent upon oxyhemoglobin and it was hypothesized that in an analogous manner, oxyhemoglobin may activate ADM· in cardiac cells. If correct, this hypothesis would help explain the cardiotoxic specificity of the anthracyclines. Others have suggested that the relative deficiency of antioxidant enzymes in the heart may explain this specificity (21), rather than differences in radical activation rates. This key question remains to b resolved.

It should be mentioned that ADM also affects plasma membrane electron transport (22) and this interaction probably results in ADM· generation. Plasma membrane redox systems are present in a wide variety of cell types and may exert control on a number of systems including maintenance of ionic gradients, cyclic nucleotide regulation and cell division. Many other anthracyclines and antitumor antibiotics also interfere with plasma membrane redox function (F.L. Crane, personal communication).

Anthracycline radical activity may therefore occur in virtually every subcellular environment. The magnitude of radical generation at a given site depends upon both the localization properties of the anthracycline in questic and its propensity to interact with the electron transport factors at that site. Anthracycline radicals may therefore produce toxicity at multiple subcellular sites.

3. BIOLOGIC TOXICITIES OF ADRIAMYCIN: ARE FREE RADICALS INVOLVED?

Free radicals are believed to mediate toxicities induced by a wide variety of agents and disease states. (For a review, see references 3, 23-25.) Although the subcellular sites of radical generation and the initial species formed may differ in each case, the subsequent formation of active oxygen species, i.e., O_2^-, $\cdot OH$, H_2O_2 and $^1O_2$, seems to be a common pathway in many of these situations. The high reactivity of some of the species formed makes virtually every cellular molecule and structure vulnerable to attack. The idea that cells are often presented with toxic free radicals is supported by the extensive interconnected system of free radical scavengers which exist in all cells (Table 2).

Table 2. Cellular antioxidant defenses.

α-Tocopherol	GSH Peroxidase
Ascorbic Acid	Superoxide Dismutases
GSH	Catalase

Evidence suggests that ADM free radical activation may play a role in some of the toxicities induced by Adriamycin. The evidence may be grouped into four categories: (1) antioxidant depletion in target tissues; (2) damage to molecules susceptible to free radicals; (3) inhibition of toxicity by exogenous antioxidants; and (4) increased toxicity in animals with deficient antioxidant defenses. Some of the major toxicities induced by ADM are listed in Table 3.

Table 3. Toxicities induced by ADM.

Acute Lethality	Mutagenicity
Cardiotoxicity	Carcinogenicity
Extravasation Toxicity	Tumor Cell Toxicity

Acute lethality produced in animals receiving high doses of ADM is accompanied by increased lipid peroxide and malondialdehyde levels (products of lipid free radical attack) in both serum and heart (26,27). Coadministration of α-tocopherol or coenzyme Q_{10} inhibits the increase in free radical products, as well as the lethality induced by ADM, but does not inhibit the lethality of 5-fluorouracil (26-29). Likewise, ADM-induced cardiotoxicity is inhibited by a number of antioxidants, including coenzyme Q_{10} (30-32), α-tocopherol (27,33-35), n-acetylcysteine (36), cysteamine (37) and superoxide dismutase plus catalase (4). Furthermore, decreases in GSH (37), GSH-peroxidase and selenium (21,38) occur in the hearts of ADM-treated animals, and animals with a nutritionally induced GSH-peroxidase deficiency (low selenium diet) exhibit increased ADM toxicity (21). Taken together, these experiments support the proposal that acute lethality and cardiotoxicity produced by ADM are mediated by ADM·.

Extravasation toxicity encountered during intravenous ADM infusion deserves increasing attention, since recent findings suggest the greater clinical efficacy of continuous infusion as opposed to bolus ADM doses. A recent report demonstrates that a combination of the free radical quenchers α-tocopherol and DMSO protect against ADM-induced skin ulceration (5); however, others have been unable to reproduce these results (R. Wolgemuth, personal communication).

The anthracyclines are both mutagenic (39-41) and carcinogenic (41-43). The hypothesis that free radicals may be involved in mutagenesis and carcinogenesis has been recently discussed (44). Briefly, many mutagens and carcinogens are themselves free radicals, are converted to active free radicals in vivo, stimulate the production of free radicals, or are the products of biological free radical reactions (44). Conversely, many antioxidants, including selenium, ascorbic acid, vitamin E and BHT, inhibit mutagenesis and carcinogenesis produced by a variety of agents (45-49). Furthermore, dietary intake of polyunsaturated fatty acids, stimulators of free radical reactions, increase the carcinogenic potential of 7,12-DMBA (50,51).

The possibility that these particularly alarming toxicities of the anthracyclines (i.e., mutagenicity and carcinogenicity) may be controlled by coadministration of free radical quenchers warrants thorough investigation A recent study suggests that cysteamine·HCl does not inhibit anthracycline-induced carcinogenicity (41).

The most important toxicity of ADM is its tumor cell toxicity (TCT). The mechanisms of this toxicity are unknown. ADM· may mediate ADM TCT via three possible pathways: (1) generation of active oxygen resulting in lipid peroxidation; (2) generation of active oxygen which may attack non-lipid cellular targets; or (3) direct attack on cellular targets.

Unlike the acute lethal and cardiotoxicities, ADM TCT is not inhibited by coenzyme Q_{10}, α-tocopherol or n-acetylcysteine (27,30,36). These in vivo studies were all performed on single cell tumors and should be repeated on solid tumors. With this qualification in mind, these results suggest that antioxidant administration may increase the therapeutic index of ADM. They

<u>cannot</u> however be taken as evidence suggesting the lack of involvement of active oxygen and lipid peroxidation in ADM TCT since it is unclear whether these antioxidants were actually incorporated into the tumor cells.

Since L1210 and P388 microsomes (8) as well as intact Ehrlich ascites tumor cells (6) activate ADM to ADM·, it has been suggested that ADM TCT may be mediated by direct attack of ADM· on cellular targets (8,52-54). The carbon centered C7 radical (C7·) may be capable of hydrogen abstraction or direct adduct formation. Cellular targets may include DNA, RNA, membranes and DNA-nuclear membrane complexes.

In addition to the anthracyclines (55,56) many other antitumor anti-biotics, including mitomycin C (57-59), bleomycin (60-62), streptonigrin (63) and actinomycin D (64), stimulate free radical activation and may damage DNA in the process. It is therefore tempting to propose free radical activation as a unifying mechanism of antitumor antibiotic action.

If ADM TCT <u>is</u> mediated directly by ADM·, O_2 may be expected to inhibit ADM TCT, i.e., ADM should be more toxic to hypoxic rather than oxygenated cells. Some workers have found this to be true while others have not (65-67). The reasons for these divergent results are unclear.

In summary, no available evidence directly argues either for or against the involvement of ADM· in TCT at clinically relevant ADM concentrations.

4. HYPOTHESIZED CENTRAL ROLE OF ADM· IN ADM TOXICITIES: CONCEPT OF DIRECT ADM· QUENCHERS

Based on the evidence discussed in Sections 2 and 3, ADM· are hypothe-sized to play a central role in ADM-induced toxicities (8,27,52)(see Figure 1). Activation of ADM to ADM· may be accomplished by both reductive and oxidative pathways. A number of distinct ADM· species may be generated (Section 5). The most extensively investigated reductive pathway of ADM· activation is that which results in the formation of the ring C semiquinone (ADMSQ·). In the absence of a suitable one-electron acceptor, this species spontaneously rearranges and sheds daunosamine, forming C7 radicals (C7·)(Figure 3). C7· are believed to abstract hydrogen atoms to form ADM 7-deoxyaglycones. The aglycones may then be further reduced in one-electron steps to aglycone radicals.

A major pathway of reactivity of ADM· will be via their interaction with O_2 resulting in the formation of active oxygen species, i.e., $O_2^{-\cdot}$, ·OH, H_2O_2 and $^1O_2$. These species induce cell damage by initiating lipid

226

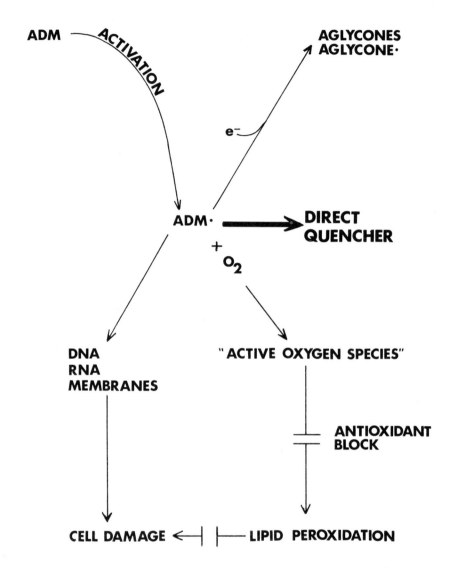

FIGURE 1. Hypothesized central role of ADM· in ADM toxicities. ADM· are
hypothesized to mediate ADM toxicity directly, by attacking critical
cellular targets, and indirectly by stimulating active oxygen formation.
Direct ADM· quenchers would alter both pathways, thus providing a broad
approach to manipulation of ADM· in biologic systems.

peroxidation in membranes. Antioxidants will block both the initiation (by scavenging active O_2 species) and propagation stages of lipid oxidation. Alternatively, active O_2 species may attack non-lipid targets, i.e., DNA, RNA (arrow not shown), and antioxidants may or may not inhibit this pathway, depending upon antioxidant delivery to the critical site. This oxygen-dependent radical pathway is probably involved in ADM induced acute lethality and cardiotoxicity, providing the basis of their inhibition with antioxidants (Section 3).

ADM· may also produce cell damage by direct attack on critical cellular targets. Targets may include DNA, RNA, membranes and DNA-nuclear membrane complexes. Antioxidants will not block this oxygen independent direct pathway.

Each of the ADM· reactions shown, i.e., aglycone formation, interaction with O_2, interaction with cellular targets, must be viewed as competing pathways. The preferred pathway in any instance will depend upon the initial ADM· species formed, O_2 availability, and proximity of cellular targets. In hypoxic regions of solid tumors, for instance, O_2 independent pathways would be favored.

Since ADM· are hypothesized to play the central role in ADM toxicities shown diagramatically in Figure 1, we have taken the approach of identifying direct quenchers of these species. Direct ADM· quenchers, i.e., compounds which eliminate ADM·, should alter those actions of ADM dependent upon ADM·. They therefore constitute probes to test the involvement of ADM· in the many actions of ADM. Direct ADM· quenchers may inhibit ADM-induced cell damage by eliminating toxic ADM· and/or by preventing the formation of active oxygen. Alternatively, the interaction between ADM· and quencher may result in the production of more highly toxic species causing enhancement of cell toxicity. ADM· quenching can be exerted in both hydrophobic and hydrophilic environments. Selectivity may be obtained with respect to O_2 tension. In this regard, ADM· quenchers unable to compete with O_2 for ADM· may alter ADM toxicities only in cells with low O_2 tension. Effects may therefore be produced in hypoxic-anoxic tumor cells without being produced in cardiac tissues. Direct ADM· quenchers therefore provide a broad approach to manipulation of ADM· in biologic systems.

5. ADRIAMYCIN RADICAL SIGNALS AND RADICAL STATES

Due to its structural complexity, ADM can be activated to a number of distinct radical states. The symbol ADM· therefore actually represents multiple distinct radical species. These species may have different reactivities and may be responsible for different actions of ADM.

We have generated radical signals from ADM using different methods of activation. Some of these signals are shown in Figure 2. Figure 2a shows the signals associated with ADM radicals which form spontaneously when ADM solutions are adjusted to physiologic pH (1). These radicals have a g value of 2.0041 and a peak-to-peak line width of 2.60 gauss, as determined by the method of Mason (68) using TEMPONE as a standard (2). It was earlier suggested that these radicals were semiquinone species formed by quinone-dihydroquinone electron transfer (1). Recent work in our laboratory shows the inability of daunomycin to form these radical species spontaneously, highlighting the importance of the C-14 hydroxyl in the spontaneous activation. The narrow line width and dependence upon the C-14 hydroxyl may suggest that these spontaneously formed radicals have lone electron density associated with the side chain rather than the anthraquinone π-cloud. However, their identity remains undetermined. Figure 2b shows the ADM radical signal obtained upon reduction with $NaBH_4$ at 0.5/1.0 mole $NaBH_4$: mole ADM. The signal has a g value of 2.0039 and a peak-to-peak line width of 3.70 gauss. Not only is this signal broader, but its line shape is gaussian compared to the lorentzian shape of the spontaneously formed radicals, suggesting that the radical species comprising these two distinct signals are probably different.

When $NaBH_4$ is added in larger proportion (6/1-$NaBH_4$:ADM), the signal shown in Figure 2c develops. The signal appears to have at least two components, i.e., a 33-line spectrum superimposed upon a singlet of about 3.70 gauss. The g value is 2.0039. The structure of the radicals activated by borohydride reduction and responsible for the signals shown in Figures 2b and 2c await rigorous determination.

Adriamycin radical signals similar to those shown in Figure 2 have also been generated in other laboratories. Activation methods have included $NaBH_4$ (54), microsomes (6,8), whole Ehrlich ascites tumor cells (6) and NADPH cytrochrome P-450 reductase (55). G values of 2.0035 (54), 2.004 (6) and 1.939 (55) have been reported. The value 1.939 is probably

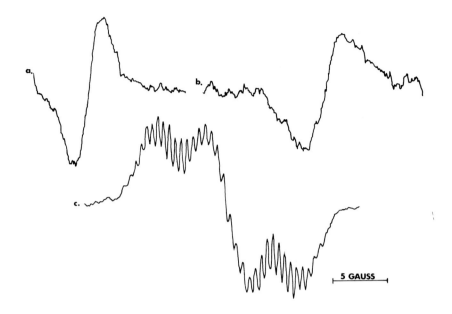

FIGURE 2. Adriamycin radical signals. Radical signals were generated from ADM by different hypoxic activation conditions and recorded on a Varian X-band E3 electron paramagnetic spectrometer. Conditions: a. 1.0 mg ADM in 1.0 ml Tris·HCl 50 mM, pH 8.0; b. 1.0 mg ADM in 1.0 ml sodium phosphate 5 mM, pH 7.0 activated by 0.87 μmole NaBH$_4$; c. 1.0 mg ADM in 0.5 ml H$_2$O activated by 10 μmole NaBH$_4$, pH 8.3. Machine parameters: field set 3390 gauss (a,b), 3395 gauss (c); scan range 50 gauss (a,b,c); microwave power 5 mW (a,b), 2 mW (c); time constant 3.0 sec (a), 10.0 sec (b,c); modulation amplitude 1.6 gauss (a,b), 0.25 gauss (c); scan time 8 min (a), 16 min (b), 0.5 hrs (c); receiver gain 10 X 10^5 (a), 2 X 10^6 (b), 8 X 10^5 (c).

inaccurate since true measurement requires comparison to standards and cannot be based upon calculation directly from machine parameters. In this regard, calculation of g values for the signals shown in Figure 2 based upon instrumental settings yield values close to 2.000 rather than the true values listed above.

Figure 3 shows some possible radical states of ADM·. One electron reduction of the quinone ring yields ADM semiquinone radicals (ADMSQ·). It has been suggested that this species is formed during activation by microsomes (7,8) and NaBH$_4$ (54), and is responsible for the signals in Figures 2b and 2c. In the absence of a suitable electron acceptor, ADMSQ· seem to undergo spontaneous rearrangement and scission leading to the

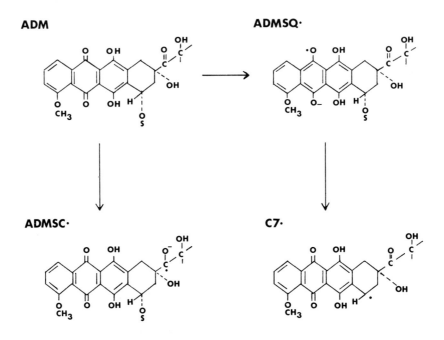

FIGURE 3. Adriamycin radical states.

formation of C7 radicals (C7·). Evidence for the existence of these carbon centered radicals (52) is the presence of 7-deoxyaglycones and 7-deoxyaglycone dimers (69,70). Another potential site of lone electron density is the α_1, α_2-diketol side chain structure of ADM (ADMSC·). Side chain radical formation would destabilize the side chain resulting in cleavage. The finding that C14-labeled ADM administered in vivo is not totally recovered and some of the C14 is found in $^{14}CO_2$ (52) suggests that side chain radical activation may be important in vivo.

The radicals shown in Figure 3 are all produced by one-electron reduction of ADM. It must be stressed that one electron oxidation of either the dihydroquinone structure or the C9 or C14-OH of the α_1, α_2-diketol side chain structure would also result in ADM· formation as would one-electron reduction of the aglycones. In this regard, we also have generated ADM· signals by oxidation of ADM (unpublished results). Evidence suggests that in an analogous manner, other anthracyclines including daunomycin, 5-iminodauno-mycin, carminomycin, rubidazone, nogalamycin, aclacinomycin A, aklavinone

and 1-deoxypyrromycin may also be activated to diverse radical states
(6,8,54,69,70, unpublished results). In summary, anthracyclines can be
activated to a number of distinct radical states which may possess different
reactivities and attack different targets.

6. DIRECT ADRIAMYCIN RADICAL QUENCHING ACTIVITY

The reactivity of adriamycin radicals was studied by electron
paramagnetic spectrometry (EPR)(Figure 4). ADM· activated both spontaneously
and by $NaBH_4$ were investigated.

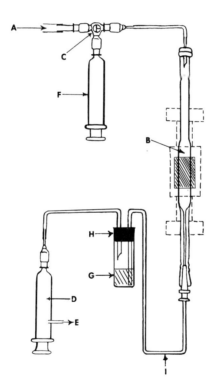

FIGURE 4. EPR delivery system. ADM is activated to radicals under anoxic
conditions in a septum fitted (H) glass vial (G). Quenchers, or vehicle
controls, are injected anoxically and the mixture is positioned (B) and
examined for the presence of radicals (1).

When radicals are activated by the addition of Tris·HCl, pH 7.9, the associated EPR signal increases for approximately 20 min at which time saturation is reached (Figure 5). Addition of 50 μl H_2O or 10 μl EtOH has no effect upon radical formation (5a), while 50 μl DMSO decreases radical yield by about 10% and prolongs saturation time to 26 minutes (5b). A signal height of 13.5 cm corresponds to a radical concentration of 1.4 μM, using TEMPONE as a standard (2). Once reaching saturation, radical concentration remains constant for at least one hour.

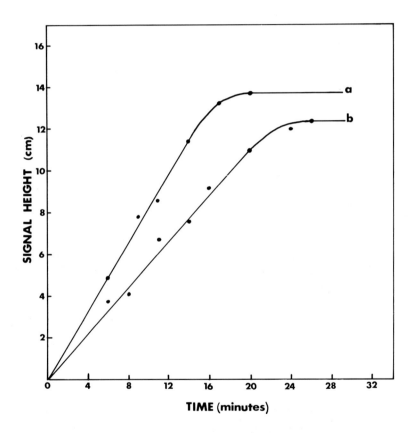

FIGURE 5. Spontaneous ADM radical generation. Tris·HCl 1 M, pH 7.9 (25 μl) was added to ADM (0.5 mg/0.45 ml H_2O) to initiate radical formation (t=0). Three minutes later, the following additions were made: (a) none; or 50 μl H_2O; or 10 μl EtOH. (b) 50 μl DMSO. Two minutes later the sample was positioned and examined for the presence of radicals. Machine parameters as in Figure 2a.

A number of antioxidants and other compounds were assayed for direct ADM· quenching activity (Table 4.)

Table 4. Adriamycin radical quenching activity.

	% Quenching
Antioxidants	
α-tocopherol 0.1, 0.5 mM	0
N-acetylcysteine 0.1, 0.5 mM	0
Ascorbic Acid 0.1, 0.5 mM	0
SOD 1 μg/ml	0
SOD + Catalase 1 μg/ml each	0
Coenzyme Q_{10} 0.1 mM	100
Tetrazolium Salts	
NBT 0.1 mM	100
MTT 0.1 mM	100
INT 0.1 mM	100
BSPT 0.04 mM	27.0 $\pm$ 4.2
Miscellaneous	
Fenamole 0.1 mM, 0.5 mM	0
Promethazine·HCl 0.1 mM	0
ICRF-159 0.07 mM	0

Quenching activity was assayed by the methodology and timing presented in Figures 4 and 5. Coenzyme Q_{10} and α-tocopherol were injected using both EtOH and DMSO vehicles; all other compounds used H_2O vehicle. Each compound was tested at least 3 times.

$$\% \text{ Quenching} = \left(1 - \frac{\text{ADM· signal height in presence of compound}}{\text{ADM· signal height in presence of vehicle}}\right) \times 100$$

Signal heights were measured at 30 minutes when H_2O or EtOH was the vehicle and 40 minutes when DMSO was the vehicle.

Coenzyme Q_{10} and tetrazolium salts are direct ADM∘ quenchers. Together, Q_{10} and the tetrazoliums provide hydrophilic and hydrophobic ADM· quenching potential. Q_{10} quenching is independent of vehicle (EtOH or DMSO). The antioxidants α-tocopherol, n-acetylcysteine and ascorbic acid are inactive even at 0.5 mM. Since a tetrazole ring is the active principal of electron transfer in the tetrazolium salts, we assayed fenamole, another tetrazole-containing compound. Fenamole however is inactive, as are promethazine·HCl and ICRF-159. SOD is inactive alone and in combination with catalase.

Figure 6 shows the EPR spectrum of ADM· generated by adding $NaBH_4$ to ADM. The signal reaches maximum height by the time of the first scan and maintains this height for at least 20 minutes. Addition of 20 µl H_2O or 20 µl EtOH subsequent to $NaBH_4$ has no effect on ADM· formation (6a). N-acetyl cysteine exhibits no direct interaction with these radicals (6a). On the other hand, Q_{10} effectively quenches these radicals as it does those generated spontaneously (6b).

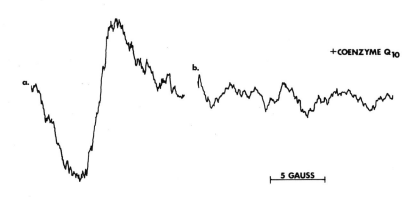

FIGURE 6. Coenzyme Q_{10} quenching of ADM·. $NaBH_4$, 2 mg/ml in 10 mM sodium phosphate, pH 7.0 (20 µl), was added to ADM (1 mg/1.0 ml 5 mM sodium phospha pH 7.0) in four 5 µl aliquots at 4-minute intervals. Four minutes following the last $NaBH_4$ injection, the following additions were made: (a) none; or 20 µl EtOH; or 20 µl H_2O; or 20 µl n-acetylcysteine (100 nmoles in H_2O). (b) 20 µl coenzyme Q_{10} (100 nmoles in EtOH). Four minutes later the sample was positioned and examined for the presence of radicals. Machine parameter are the same as in Figure 2b except receiver gain = 3.2×10^6.

The mechanism by which the tetrazolium salts quench ADM· has been studied (2). Quenching is the result of a direct ADM· scavenging, i.e.,

$$NBT_{ox} + ADM· \longrightarrow ADM + NBT·$$

The NBT radical (NBT·) rapidly disproportionates (71)

$$NBT· + NBT· \longrightarrow NBT_{ox} + NBT_{red}$$

eliminating all radicals from the system. The reactivity of NBT with ADM· is high enough so that even in the presence of O_2, direct electron transfer occurs between ADM· and NBT (2); that is, NBT and O_2 compete for ADM·.

The mechanism by which coenzyme Q_{10} exerts ADM· quenching activity is a present unknown. Coenzyme Q has long been suggested as a possible site of

ADM-induced damage. Mitochondrial perturbations involving Q_{10}-dependent enzymes have been reported (72,73), and it is well known that Q_{10} administration blocks ADM-induced acute lethal toxicity and cardiotoxicity (Section 3). The results presented above showing a direct interaction between ADM· and Q_{10} may, in part, be the basis of these effects. If Q_{10} is a specific site of ADM· attack, then ADM and Q_{10} given in combination may offer greater benefits than ADM in combination with other antioxidants.

7. CONCLUSIONS

1. Anthracycline radical activation may occur in virtually every subcellular environment. The magnitude of radical generation at a given site will depend upon both the localization properties of the anthracycline in question, as well as its propensity to interact with electron transport factors at that site. Anthracycline radicals may therefore produce toxicity at multiple subcellular sites.

2. Anthracyclines can be activated to a number of distinct radical states which may possess different reactivities and attack different targets.

3. Coenzyme Q may be a specific site of ADM· attack. ADM and Coenzyme Q_{10} given in combination may therefore offer a more superior clinical benefit than ADM in combination with other antioxidants.

4. Direct ADM· quenchers should be useful tools in determining which actions of ADM are mediated by ADM·.

ACKNOWLEDGMENTS

I wish to thank Erin Lawton, John Mignano and Janet Pomerantz for technical assistance; Michael Koren for helpful conversations; and Kinga Koreh and Janet Grana for helping to prepare this manuscript. This work was supported by grants from NIH (BRSG SO7RRO5399-19) and Pioneer Systems, Inc.

REFERENCES

1. Pietronigro DD, McGinness JE, Koren MJ, Crippa R, Seligman ML, Demopoulos HB. Spontaneous generation of adriamycin semiquinone radicals at physiologic pH. Physiol. Chem. Phys. 11: 405-414, 1979.
2. Pietronigro DD, Koren MJ, Demopoulos HB. Evidence for both direct and superoxide-mediated reduction of nitroblue tetrazolium by adriamycin radicals. Submitted for publication.

236

3. Del Maestro RF. An approach to free radicals in medicine and biology. Acta Physiol. Scand. Suppl. _492_: 153-168, 1980.
4. McGinness JE, Proctor PH, Demopoulos HB, Hokanson JA, Van NT. In vivo evidence for superoxide and peroxide production by adriamycin and cis platinum. In: Oxygen Induced Pathology, AP Autor (ed.). New York, Academic Press, 1982.
5. Svingen BA, Powis G, Appel PL, Scott M. Protection by α-tocopherol and dimethylsulfoxide (DMSO) against adriamycin induced skin ulcers in the rat. Res. Comm. Chem. Path. Pharm. _32_: 189-192, 1981.
6. Sato S, Iwaizumi M, Handa K, Tamura Y. Electron spin resonance study on the mode of generation of free radicals of daunomycin, adriamycin and carboquone in NAD(P)H-microsome system. Gann 68: 603-608. 1977.
7. Bachur NR, Gordon SL, Gee MV. Anthracycline antibiotic augmentation of microsomal electron transport and free radical formation. Mol. Pharm. _13_: 901-910, 1977.
8. Bachur NR, Gordon SL, Gee MV. A general mechanism for microsomal activation of quinone anticancer agents to free radicals. Ca Res. _38_: 1745-1750, 1978.
9. Goodman J, Hochstein P. Generation of free radicals and lipid peroxidation by redox cycling of adriamycin and daunomycin. Biochem. Biophys. Res. Comm. _77_: 797-803, 1977.
10. Oki T, Komiyama T, Tone H, Inui T, Takeuchi T, Umuzawa H. Reductive cleavage of anthracycline glycosides by microsomal NADPH-cytochrome c reductase. J. Antibiot. _30_: 613-615, 1977.
11. Handa K, Sato S. Stimulation of microsomal NADPH oxidation by quinone group-containing anticancer chemicals. Gann _67_: 523-528, 1976.
12. Lai CS, Grover TA, Piette LH. Hydroxyl radical production in a purified NADPH-cytochrome c (P-450) reductase system. Arch. Biochem. Biophys. _193_: 373-378, 1979.
13. Ohnishi K, Lieber CS. Respective role of superoxide and hydroxyl radical in the activity of the reconstituted microsomal ethanol-oxidizing system. Arch. Biochem. Biophys. _191_: 798-803, 1978.
14. Bachur NR, Gee MV. Microsomal reductive glycosidase. J. Pharmacol. Exp. Ther. _197_: 681-686, 1976.
15. Zimmerman JJ, Kasper CB. Immunological and biochemical characterization of nuclear envelope reduced nicotinamide adenine dinucleotide phosphate-cytochrome c oxidoreductase. Arch. Biochem. Biophys. _190_: 726-735, 1978.
16. Pietronigro DD, Jones WBG, Kalty K, Demopoulos HB. Interaction of DNA and liposomes as a model for membrane-mediated DNA damage. Nature _267_: 78-79, 1977.
17. Iyanagi T, Yamazaki I. One-electron-transfer reactions in biochemical systems. V. Difference in the mechanism of quinone reduction by the NADH dehydrogenase and the NAD(P)H dehydrogenase (DT-diaphorase). Biochim. Biophys. Acta _216_: 282-294, 1970.
18. Doroshow JH. Mitomycin C-enhanced superoxide and hydrogen peroxide formation in rat heart. J. Pharm. Exp. Therap. _218_: 206-211, 1981.
19. Thayer WS. Adriamycin stimulated superoxide formation in submitochondri particles. Chem. Biol. Interact. _19_: 265-278, 1977.
20. Henderson CA, Metz EN, Balcerzak SP, Sagone AL. Adriamycin and daunomyc generate reactive oxygen compounds in erythrocytes. Blood _52_: 878-885,
21. Doroshow JH, Locker GY, Myers CE. Enzymatic defenses of the mouse heart against reactive oxygen metabolites. Alterations produced by doxorubici J. Clin. Invest. _65_: 128-135, 1980.

22. Crane FL, MacKellar WC, Morre DJ, Ramasarma T, Goldenberg H, Grebing C, Löw H. Adriamycin affects plasma membrane redox functions. Biochem. Biophys. Res. Comm. 93: 746-754, 1980.
23. Slater TF. Free radical mechanisms in tissue injury. Pion Limited, London, 1972.
24. Fitzsimons DW (ed.). Oxygen free radicals and tissue damage. Ciba Foundation symposium 65, Excerpta Medica, New York, 1979.
25. Demopoulos HB. Control of free radicals in biologic systems. Fed. Proc. 32: 1903-1908, 1973.
26. Yamanaka N, Kato T, Nishida K, Fujikawa T, Fukushima M, Ota K. Elevation of serum lipid peroxide level associated with doxorubicin toxicity and its amelioration by (d)-α-tocopherol acetate or coenzyme Q_{10} in mouse. Ca. Chemother. Pharmacol. 3: 223-227, 1979.
27. Myers CE, McGuire WP, Liss RH, Ifrim I, Grotzinger K, Young RC. Adriamycin: The role of lipid peroxidation in cardiac toxicity and tumor response. Science 197: 165-167, 1977.
28. Myers CE, McGuire W, Young R. Adriamycin: Amelioration of toxicity by α-tocopherol. Ca. Treat. Rep. 60: 961-962, 1976.
29. Lubawy WC, Dallam RA, Hurley LH. Protection against anthramycin-induced toxicity in mice by coenzyme Q_{10}. J. Natl. Ca. Inst. 64: 105-109, 1980.
30. Bertazoli C, Ghione M. Adriamycin associated cardiotoxicity: Research on prevention with coenzyme Q. Pharm. Res. Comm. 9: 235-250, 1977.
31. Domae N, Sawada H, Matsuyama E, Konishi T, Uchino H. Cardiomyopathy and other chronic toxic effects induced in rabbits by doxorubicin and possible prevention by coenzyme Q_{10}. Ca. Treat. Rep. 65: 79-91, 1981.
32. Cortes EP, Gupta M, Chou C, Amin VC, Folkers K: Adriamycin cardiotoxicity: Early detection by systolic time interval and possible prevention by coenzyme Q_{10}. Ca. Treat. Rep. 62: 887-891, 1978.
33. Sonneveld P. Effect of α-tocopherol on the cardiotoxicity of adriamycin in the rat. Ca. Treat. Rep. 62: 1033-1036, 1978.
34. Van Vleet JF, Greenwood L, Ferrans VJ, Rebar AH. Effect of selenium-vitamin E on adriamycin-induced cardiomyopathy in rabbits. Am. J. Vet. Res. 39: 997-1010, 1978.
35. Van Vleet JF, Ferrans VJ. Evaluation of vitamin E and selenium protection against chronic adriamycin toxicity in rabbits. Ca. Treat. Rep. 64: 315-317, 1980.
36. Doroshow JH, Locker GY, Ifrim I, Myers CE. Prevention of doxorubicin cardiac toxicity in the mouse by n-acetylcysteine. J. Clin. Invest. 68: 1053-1064, 1981.
37. Olson RD, MacDonald JS, Harbison RD, Van Boxtel CJ, Boerth RC, Slonim AE, Oates JA. Altered myocardial glutathione levels: A possible mechanism of adriamycin toxicity. Fed. Proc. 36: 303, 1977.
38. Revis NW, Marusic N. Glutathione peroxidase activity and selenium concentration in the hearts of doxorubicin-treated rabbits. J. Mol. Cell. Card. 10: 945-951, 1978.
39. Umezawa K, Sawamura M, Matsushima T, Sugimura T. Mutagenicity of aclacinomycin A and daunomycin derivatives. Ca. Res. 38: 1782-1784, 1978.
40. Seino Y, Nagao M, Yahagi T, Hoshi A, Kawachi T, Sugimura T. Mutagenicity of several classes of antitumor agents to salmonella typhimurium TA98, TA100 and TA92. Ca. Res. 38: 2148-2156, 1978.
41. Marquardt H. This volume.

238

42. Marquardt H, Philips FS, Sternberg SS. Tumorigenicity in vivo and induction of malignant transformation and mutagenesis in cell cultures by adriamycin and daunomycin. Ca. Res. 36: 2065-2069, 1976.
43. Bertazzoli C, Chièli T, Solcia E. Different incidence of breast carcinomas or fibroadenomas in daunomycin or adriamycin treated rats. Experientia 27: 1209-1210, 1971.
44. Demopoulos HB, Pietronigro DD, Flamm ES, Seligman ML. The possible role of pathologic free radical reactions in carcinogenesis. J. Environ. Path. Tox. 3: 273-303, 1980.
45. Chan JT, Black HS. The mitigating effect of dietary antioxidants on chemically-induced carcinogenesis. Experientia 34: 110-111, 1978.
46. Daoud AH, Griffin AC. Effect of retinoic acid, butylated hydroxytoluene, selenium and sorbic acid on azo-dye hepatocarcinogenesis. Ca. Lett. 9: 299-304, 1980.
47. Shamberger RJ, Corlett CL, Beaman KD, Kasten BL. Antioxidants reduce the mutagenic effect of malondialdehyde and beta-propiolactone. Part IX, Antioxidants and cancer. Mut. Res. 66: 349-355, 1979.
48. Jacobs MM, Griffin AC. Effects of selenium on chemical carcinogenesis. Comparative effects of antioxidants. Biol. Trace Elem. Res. 1: 1-13, 1979.
49. Shamberger RJ, Beaman KD, Corlett CL, Kasten BL. Effect of selenium and other antioxidants on the mutagenicity of malonaldehyde. Fed. Proc. 37: 261, 1978.
50. Carroll KK. Lipids and carcinogenesis. J. Environ. Path. Tox. 3: 253-271, 1980.
51. King MM, Bailey DM, Gibson DD, Pitha JV, McCay PB. Incidence and growth of mammary tumors induced by 7,12-dimethylbenzanthracene as related to the dietary content of fat and antioxidant. J. Natl. Ca. Inst. 63: 657-663, 1979.
52. Bachur N. Antracycline antibiotic pharmacology and metabolism. Ca. Treat. Rep. 63: 817-820, 1979.
53. Sinha BK. Binding specificity of chemically and enzymatically activated anthracycline anticancer agents to nucleic acids. Chem.-Biol. Interact. 30: 66-77, 1980.
54. Sinha BK, Chignell CF. Binding mode of chemically activated semiquinone free radicals from quinone anticancer agents to DNA. Chem.-Biol. Interac. 28: 301-308, 1979.
55. Berlin V, Haseltine WA. Reduction of adriamycin to a semiquinone free radical by NADPH cytochrome P-450 reductase produces DNA cleavage in a reaction mediated by molecular oxygen. J. Biol. Chem. 256: 4747-4756, 1981.
56. Lown JW, Sim SK, Majumdar KC, Chang RY. Strand scission of DNA by bound adriamycin and daunorubicin in the presence of reducing agents. Biochem. Biophys. Res. Comm. 79: 705-710, 1977.
57. Tomasz M. H_2O_2 generation during the redox cycle of mitomycin C and DNA-bound mitomycin C. Chem. Biol. Interact. 13: 89-97, 1976.
58. Kalyanraman B, Perez-Reyes E, Mason RP. Spin trapping and direct electron spin resonance investigations of the redox metabolism of quinone anticancer drugs. Biochim. Biophys. Acta 630: 119-130, 1980.
59. Lown JW, Begleiter A, Johnson D, Morgan R. Studies related to antitumor antibiotics, Part V. Reaction of mitomycin C with DNA examined by ethidium fluorescence assay. Can. J. Biochem. 54: 110-119, 1976.
60. Lown JW, Sim SK. The mechanism of bleomycin-induced cleavage of DNA. Biochem. Biophys. Res. Comm. 77: 1150-1157, 1977.

61. Oberley LW, Buettner GR. The production of hydroxyl radical by bleomycin and iron (II). FEBS Lett. $\underline{97}$: 47-49, 1979.
62. Sugiura Y. Production of free radicals from phenol and tocopherol by bleomycin-iron (II) complex. Biochem. Biophys. Res. Comm. $\underline{87}$: 649-653, 1979.
63. Cone R, Hasan SK, Lown JW, Morgan AR. The mechanism of the degradation of DNA by streptonigrin. Can. J. Biochem. $\underline{54}$: 219-223, 1976.
64. Sinha BK, Cox.MG. Stimulation of superoxide formation by actinomycin D and its N^2-substituted spin-labeled derivatives. Mol. Pharm. $\underline{17}$: 432-434, 1980.
65. Teicher BA, Lazo JS, Sartorelli AC. Classification of antineoplastic agents by their selective toxicities towards oxygenated and hypoxic tumor cells. Ca. Res. $\underline{41}$: 73-81, 1981.
66. Smith E, Stratford IJ, Adams GE. The resistance of hypoxic mammalian cells to chemotherapeutic agents. Br. J. Can. $\underline{40}$: 316, 1979.
67. Harris JW, Shrieve DC. Effects of adriamycin and X-rays on euoxic and hypoxic EMT6 cells in vitro. Int. J. Radiat. Oncol. Biol. Phys. $\underline{5}$: 1245-1248, 1979.
68. Mason RP, Peterson FJ, Holtzman JL. The formation of an azo anion free radical metabolite during the microsomal azo reduction of sulfonazo III. Biochem. Biophys. Res. Comm. $\underline{75}$: 532-540, 1977.
69. Oki T, Komiyama T, Tone H, Inui T, Takcuchi T, Umezawa H. Reductive cleavage of anthracycline glycosides by microsomal NADPH-cytochrome c reductase. J. Antibiot. $\underline{30}$: 613-615, 1977.
70. Mason RP. Free radical metabolites of foreign compounds and their toxicological significance. In: Reviews in Biochemical Toxicology (Part I), E Hodgson, JR Bend, RM Philpot (eds.). Elsevier/North-Holland, 1979, pp. 151-200.
71. Bielski BJ, Shiue GG, Bajuk S. Reduction of nitroblue tetrazolium by CO_2^- and O_2^- radicals. J. Phys. Chem. $\underline{84}$: 830-833, 1980.
72. Iwamoto Y, Hansen IL, Porter TH, Folkers K. Inhibition of coenzyme Q_{10}-enzymes, succinoxidase and NADH-oxidase, by adriamycin and other quinones having antitumor activity. Biochem. Biophys. Res. Comm. $\underline{58}$: 633-638, 1974.
73. Kishi T, Watanabe T, Folkers K. Bioenergetics in clinical medicine: Prevention by forms of coenzyme Q of the inhibition by adriamycin of coenzyme Q_{10}-enzymes in mitochondria of the myocardium. Proc. Natl. Acad. Sci. $\underline{73}$: 4653-4656, 1976.

SCREENING FOR SECOND-GENERATION ANTHRACYCLINES IN A HUMAN TUMOR CLONING SYSTEM

D. D. VON HOFF

1. INTRODUCTION

The human tumor cloning system is an <u>in</u> <u>vitro</u> soft agar technique developed by Hamburger and Salmon (1,2). It allows growth of a variety of human malignancies. The cloning system has the potential for helping to select the most appropriate anticancer agent for a particular patient's tumor in much the same way the most appropriate antibiotic is selected for an individual patient's infection (3,4). In addition, the cloning system has shown promise for screening for antitumor activity of a variety of new anticancer agents (5,6,7).

In this paper, we present our experience with utilizing the cloning system for the detection of antitumor activity of a number of investigational as well as second-generation anthracycline antibiotics.

2. MATERIALS AND METHODS

Over the past 24 months, a total of 4916 patients have had their tumors sent to our laboratory for growth in the human tumor cloning system. All tumor specimens were obtained after informed consent had been obtained as part of routine diagnostic or therapeutic procedures. Solid tumor specimens or lymph node metastases were obtained at surgery, minced to 2-mm fragments under sterile conditions and immediately placed in McCoy's 5A + 10% heat-inactivated newborn calf serum + 1% penicillin and streptomycin. These solid tissues were minced with scissors and passed through decreasing sizes of wire mesh gauge from 50 mesh to 500 mesh. They were washed by centrifugation as previously described (1,2,8). Ascites, pleural, pericardial, and bone marrow samples were obtained by standard techniques. The fluid was placed in sterile containers containing 100 units of preservative-free heparin per milliliter of malignant fluid.

After being centrifuged at 150 x g for 10 minutes, the cells were harvested and washed twice in Hank's balanced salt solution with 10%

heat-inactivated newborn calf serum. The viability of cells in the single cell suspensions from solid tumors and effusions was determined in a hemocytometer with trypan blue.

The assay for tumor colony-forming cells was performed as described by Hamburger and Salmon (1,2) and will not be described here. The conditioned media utilized by Hamburger and Salmon has not been found to be useful in our studies (8).

After preparation of both bottom and top layers, the plates were examined under an inverted microscope to ensure the presence of a good single cell suspension. The plates were then incubated at 37° C in a 7% CO_2 humidified atmosphere.

Drug sensitivity studies were carried out with Adriamycin, daunomycin, and a variety of other anthracyclines (see Table 1).

Table 1. Anthracyclines studied in the cloning system

Adriamycin
Daunomycin
7-OMEN(7-con-0-methylnogarol)
N-N-Dibenzyl Daunorubicin
5-Iminodaunoribucin
5-Iminodoxorubicin
4'-Epiadriamycin
Discreet compound
Discreet compound

Stock solutions for these standard and investigational drugs were prepared in sterile buffered saline or water and stored at -70° C in aliquots sufficient for individual use. Subsequent dilutions were made in saline for incubation. Concentrations for in vitro tests with Adriamycin and daunomycin ranged from 0.04 to 4 µg/ml, whereas concentrations for the investigational anthracyclines ranged from 0.02 to 10 µg/ml. All drug incubations were performed for 1 hour as previously described (4,6).

Cultures were examined on day-14 with an FAS II colony counter (Bausch and Lomb). Aggregates of 50 or more cells were considered colonies. The number of colonies growing on drug-treated plates (done in triplicate) were compared with the number of colonies growing in triplicate control plates and a percent decrease in tumor colony-forming units (TCFUs) (if any) was calculated.

3. RESULTS

3.1. Experience with Adriamycin

A total of 4916 patients' tumors have been placed in culture over the past 2 years. In these patients' tumors, we have performed 4339 assays for Adriamycin activity. The number of successful assays (meaning that there were at least 30 colonies on control plates) was 2765 or 65% of the total Adriamycin tests performed.

Table 2 details experience with the use of Adriamycin against patients' tumors in vitro. None of these patients had received any prior chemotherapy. The in vitro response rate can be compared to the response rates in patients reported in the literature (9).

Table 2. In vitro responses to Adriamycin for patients who have not had prior chemotherapy

Tumor type	In vitro response rate[a]	Clinical response rate[b]
Breast	21	37
Lung		
Small cell	28	33
Adenocarcinoma	12	21
Lymphoma	36	32
Ovarian	22	16
Prostate	11	14
Sarcoma	18	27
Neuroblastoma	20	30
Testicular	25	20
Melanoma	0	0
Colorectal	7	13

a, $\geq 70\%$ decrease in tumor colony-forming units at a concentration of 0.04 µg/ml of Adriamycin.
b, From reference 9.

It is clear from Table 2 that the cloning assay would have detected activity for Adriamycin in breast cancer patients and in patients with small-cell lung cancer, lymphoma, ovarian cancer, etc. It is also clear from Table 2 that Adriamycin would not be active in patients with melanoma or colorectal cancer. This is certainly the clinical experience with Adriamycin.

3.2. Experience with other anthracyclines

As noted in Table 1, we have screened a large number of other anthracyclines in the human tumor cloning system. This experience represents
about 1100 in vitro drug tests. The most frequently cited example of one
anthracycline being superior to another is the alleged superiority of
Adriamycin over daunomycin. To determine the antitumor activity of both
compounds in vitro, we tested each drug against the same patient's tumor
at a concentration of 0.04 g/ml for 1 hour. Table 3 details these results.

Table 3. In vitro activity of Adriamycin versus daunomycin

Tumor type	Response to Adriamycin	Response to daunomycin[a]
Breast	21	18
Small-cell lung cancer	28	32
Sarcoma	13	15
Testicular	17	21
Colorectal	6	6

a, $\geq$70% decrease in TCFUs at 0.04 µg/ml.

From Table 3, it is clear that the in vitro response rates for Adriamycin
and daunomycin are indeed quite similar.

As an example of data obtained for other anthracycline analogs, Table 4
details results with the nogalomycin derivative 7-con-O-methylnogarol or 7-OMEN
(10).

Table 4. In vitro response rates[a] to Adriamycin versus 7-OMEN

Tumor type	% Response rates to Adriamycin[b]	% Response rates to 7-OMEN
Breast	18	15
Colorectal	10	10
Small-cell lung	21	19
Squamous cell lung	0	0

a, for >10 patients tested simultaneously.
b, $\geq$70% decrease in TCFUs.

It is clear from the data in Table 4 that 7-OMEN does not have clear-cut
advantage in terms of overall in vitro response over Adriamycin. There were
individual instances either where 7-OMEN was superior to Adriamycin or

244

vice versa, but the number of these instances is very small. The data are similar for the other anthracyclines listed in Table 1.

3.3. Other biologic studies

The human tumor cloning system can be utilized in the study of tumor cell biology, which is relevant to anthracyclines. Figure 1 shows dose response curves for in vitro studies with Adriamycin against human breast cancer.

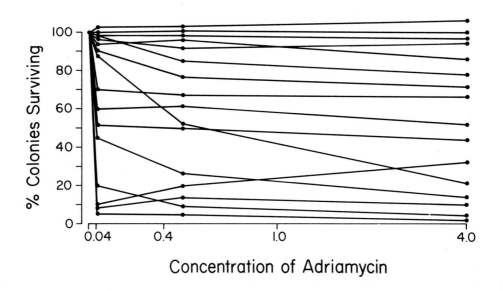

FIGURE 1. Effect of a 1-hour incubation with Adriamycin at a variety of dose levels on human breast cancer colony-forming units. Each point represents the average of three plates with a standard error of ±14%. (Adapted from reference 11 with permission.)

As can be seen in Figure 1, seven out of ten curves demonstrated a plateau with increasing concentrations of Adriamycin. This is in contrast to the dose response curves usually seen for cell lines. This plateau may represent population(s) of clonogenic cells resistant to Adriamycin.

4. DISCUSSION

There is no doubt that the human tumor cloning system can be utilized to screen for antitumor activity of conventional and investigational anthracycline antibiotics. To date, despite a rather extensive (and expensive) experience with eight analogs of Adriamycin, we have been unable to detect an advantage of one anthracycline over another (in terms of in vitro antitumor activity). The implications of this finding are numerous. For one thing, although it has been thought that Adriamycin has better clinical antitumor activity than does daunomycin, this is not what is seen in vitro. In reality, daunomycin has had very few trials in patients with solid tumors (1,2). Whenever daunomycin has been tested in patients with solid tumors, it has had comparable activity to what would be expected for Adriamycin (12). Recently reported clinical trials in patients with acute leukemia indicate that Adriamycin and daunomycin may have comparable antitumor activity (13). Thus, even the most frequently cited example of an advantage of one anthracycline (Adriamycin) over another (daunomycin) may be in question.

Overall, we have found that all the anthracyclines tested have similar in vitro activity. Only in a few selected patients is one analog superior to another. Without performing in vitro tests on each patient's tumor, we are unlikely to discern major differences in response rates in clinical trials with the anthracycline analogs we have studied.

The cloning system is a very good model for study of the mechanisms of resistance of tumors to the anthracyclines. The remarkable plateau in cell kill seen for 70% of patients' tumors with high doses of Adriamycin is of major interest. This information could be important for studies that utilize intraperitoneal or intravesicular Adriamycin where the object is to obtain high local levels of drug. From our data, we would predict that, overall, increasing local concentrations of Adriamycin will not give dramatic response rates. These intracavitary treatments might be better directed only to those few patients whose tumors show increasing clonogenic cell kill with increasing concentrations of Adriamycin.

Future work on the mechanisms of anthracycline resistance will utilize cell lines that are derived from colonies that survive treatment with Adriamycin. Some of these lines are being developed in San Antonio to determine the mechanisms of resistance to the anthracyclines.

REFERENCES

1. Hamburger, A. W., Salmon, S. E: Primary Bioassay of human tumor stem cell. Science 197:461–463,1977.
2. Hamburger, A. W., Salmon, S. E.: Primary Bioassay of human myeloma stem cells. J. Clin. Invest. 60:846–854, 1977.
3. Salmon, S. E., Hamburger, A.W., Soehnlen, B., Durie, B. G., Alberts, D. S., Moon, T. E.: Quantitation of differential sensitivity of human tumor stem cells to anticancer drugs. N. Engl. J. Med. 298:1321–1327, 1978.
4. Von Hoff, D. D., Casper, J., Bradley, E., Sandbach, J., Jones, D., Makuch, R. Association between human tumor colony forming assay results and response of an individual patient's tumor to chemotherapy. Am J. Med. 70:1027–1032, 1981.
5. Salmon, S. E., Alberts, D., Meyskens, F., Durie, B., Jones, S., Soehnlen, B., Young, C. A new concept: In vitro phase II trial with the human tumor stem cell assay (HTSCA). Proc Am Assoc Cancer Res/Asco 21:329, 1980.
6. Von Hoff, D. D., Coltman, C. A. Jr., Forseth, B. Activity of Mitoxantrone in a human tumor cloning system. Cancer Res. 41:1853–1855, 1981.
7. Von Hoff, D.D., Coltman, C. A. Jr., Forseth, B. Activity of 9-10 Anthracenedicarbo aldehyde bis ((4,5-dihydro-1H-imidazol-2-yl)hydrazone)dihydrochloride (C1216,942) in a human tumor cloning system: Leads for phase II trials in man. Cancer Chemother. Pharmacol 1981 in press.
8. Von Hoff, D.D., Casper, J., Bradley, E., Trent, J. M., Hodach, A., Reichert, C. Makuch, R., Altman, A. Direct cloning of human neuroblastoma cells in soft agar. Cancer Res. 42:3591–3597, 1980.
9. Blum, R., Carter, S., Adriamycin: A new antitumor drug with significant clinical activity. Ann Int. Med. 80:249–259, 1974.
10. Li, L. H., Kuentzel, S. L., Murch, L. L, Pshigoda, L. M., and Krueger, W. C. Comparative biological and biochemical effects of nogalamycin and its analogs on L1210 leukemia. Cancer Res 39:4816–4822, 1979.
11. Von Hoff, D.D., Sandbach, J., Osborne, C. K., Metelmann, C., Clark, G. M., O'Brien, M. Potential and Problems with growth of breast cancer in a human tumor cloning system. Breast Cancer Res. and Treat In press, 1981.
12. Von Hoff, D.D., Rozencweig, M., Slavik, M., Muggia, F. M. Activity of Daunomycin in Solid Tumors. JAMA 236:1693, 1976.
13. Yates, J. W., Glidewell, O., Wiernick, P., Holland, J. F. A study of daunorubicin vs Adriamycin induction and monthly vs bimonthly maintenance in acute myelocytic leukemia from CALGB. Proc Am Soc Chem Oncol 22:487, 1981.

ACTIVITY OF ANTHRACYCLINES ON HUMAN TUMORS IN VITRO

C. TIHON AND B.F. ISSELL

INTRODUCTION

The selection of new anticancer drugs for study in humans has classically required extensive preclinical testing in animal tumor models. Over 325,000 synthetic and naturally occurring compounds have been tested for antitumor activity between 1955 and 1975. Of these, 3,000-4,000 compounds have reached clinical trials in man resulting in approximately 30-40 useful compounds available commercially today (1). A reason for the large number of failures is the poor correlation between the animal antitumor data and human responses in clinical trials. Furthermore, the poor animal-human correlation may have resulted in some useful anticancer compounds in man being discarded because of poor animal antitumor activity.

The recent development of the human tumor cloning assay by Hamburger and Salmon has opened a new window for looking at anticancer compound development. The high correlation between in vitro assay results and clinical patient response has encouraged application of this in vitro assay to anticancer compound development. The ability to test several compounds and each at several concentrations further enhances the utility of this system.

We have previously used this assay to compare the activities of the podophyllotoxins (2) and the nitrosoureas (3) in order to determine if one analog may have a superior antitumor effect in a specific tumor type. The objective of this present study is to use the in vitro clonogenic assay to identify an anthracycline with human tumor cytotoxicity greater than Adriamycin.

MATERIALS AND METHODS

The anthracycline antibiotics used in the assay were Adriamycin, daunorubicin, carminomycin, carminomycinol, aclacinomycin, musettamycin, marcellomycin, and pyrromycin. All compounds were tested at 10^{-7}, 10^{-6}, 10^{-5}, and 10^{-4} M concentrations. Drug incubation was for 60 minutes in serum-free growth medium at 37°C before plating in agarose. Tumor specimens were acquired from the Tumor Procurement Service of Memorial Sloan-Kettering Institute. All specimens were from patients where surgery was the primary treatment modality and only two patients (both ovarian cancer) had received previous chemotherapy. One of these patients had received Adriamycin.

The assay system is basically that of Hamburger and Salmon (4) with the following modifications. Conditioned spleen cell medium was not used in the underlayer, and the top and/or bottom agar layers were replaced with Low Melting Point Agarose. Processing of solid tumors was done mechanically. Samples were counted at Day 0, Day 15, and Day 21-25. All assays were performed in triplicates except the control (without drug treatment), which was carried out in two sets of triplicates. All data presented here represent assays where at least 30 colonies were counted in the control culture dishes.

RESULTS

Specimens from surgically resected solid tumors of the following types were used in this study: three ovarian, two breast, two non-small-cell lung, one colon, endometrial, prostate, pancreatic, and mesothelioma. The results reported are from tumors which had evaluable control dishes and where there were sufficient specimens for the comparative testing of the majority of anthracyclines. Figure 1 compares the potencies of the anthracycline analogs. The assay results are expressed as the percent of colony number decrease in the drug treated dishes compared to the control untreated

dishes at varying drug concentrations. An increased reduction
in colony numbers was seen with increased drug concentrations
in all cases. Aclacinomycin, marcellomycin, and carminomycinol
were more effective than daunorubicin, Adriamycin, and musettamycin which in turn were more effective than carminomycin and
pyrromycin in inhibiting colony formation on an equal molar
concentration basis. 2.5×10^{-7} M of aclacinomycin inhibited
colony formation to the same extent as 2.5×10^{-6} M of Adriamycin
and 1×10^{-5} M of pyrromycin. Carminomycinol, a metabolite
of carminomycin appears more potent than the parent compound
in this system.

FIGURE 1:

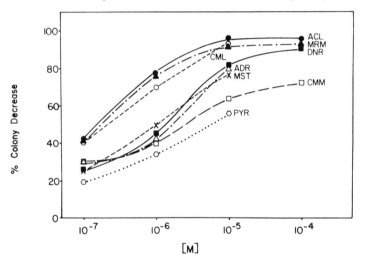

Anthracycline Activities in Human Tumor Cloning Assay

An arbitrary criterion of 70% colony number decrease from
the control dishes was chosen (5) to evaluate the activity
spectra of the analogs. Figure 2 displays these results.
Aclacinomycin and marcellomycin yielded more positive assays
in the tumors tested than the other analogs with carminomycin
and pyrromycin being the least active ones. It is of interest
to note the sharp increase in activity for Adriamycin from
10^{-6} M to 10^{-5} M.

250

FIGURE 2:

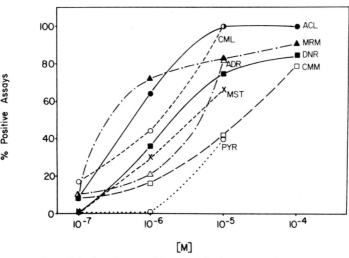

Positive Anthracycline Human Tumor Cloning Assays

In clinical studies, Adriamycin and aclacinomycin appear approximately equipotent on a patient tolerance basis. At 5×10^{-6} $\underline{M}$, which approximates peak Adriamycin serum concentration for patients (6), Adriamycin produces a 70% colony number decrease in half of the tumors studied, while aclacinomycin inhibited over 90% of tumors. At 5×10^{-7} $\underline{M}$, or one-tenth of the peak serum concentration, Adriamycin had a positive assay in less than 20%, while aclacinomycin had a positive effect in over 60% of the tumors studied.

Table 1 shows the different tumor activities of Adriamycin, aclacinomycin, marcellomycin, carminomycin, and carminomycinol at 10^{-6} $\underline{M}$ drug concentrations. Aclacinomycin showed positive inhibition in six tumors which appeared resistant to Adriamycin. In only one tumor specimen did Adriamycin have a positive assay while acalacinomycin yielded a negative result. Carminomycinol was superior to carminomycin in three different tumors.

TABLE 1

ACTIVITIES OF 10^{-6} M ANTHRACYCLINES
IN HUMAN TUMOR CLONING ASSAY

TUMOR	ADR	ACL	MCM	CMM	CML
Ovarian	-	-	-	-	o
Ovarian	-	+	+	-	-
Ovarian	-	+	+	-	+
Breast	+	+	+	+	o
Breast	-	-	o	-	o
Colon	-	+	-	-	o
Lung	+	+	+	-	-
Lung	-	+	+	-	o
Endometrial	-	+	+	-	o
Prostate	+	-	-	-	+
Mesothelioma	-	+	+	+	+
Pancreatic	-	+	+	-	+

(+) Represents a 70% decrease in colony number in drug-treated
samples; (-) Represents a less than 70% decrease; (o) Not
tested.

DISCUSSION

From these preliminary results, it appears that aclacinomycin exhibits superior antitumor activity to Adriamycin
in the tumors so far tested. Marcellomycin and carminomycinol,
the active metabolite of carminomycin, also appear superior
to Adriamycin, but unlike acalcinomycin, these compounds
also seem to be more toxic than Adriamycin in man based on
molar-tolerated dose considerations. It is important to
note that most of the tumors tested were from patients who
had not been previously exposed to chemotherapy. These
results could be quite different in patients who had been
previously exposed to chemotherapy where the induction or
selection of drug-resistant clones may have occurred.

The steep dose response relationship of Adriamycin
between 10^{-6} and 10^{-5} molar concentrations is interesting
and may suggest a special advantage for the use of this
compound in regional therapy where patients may tolerate
higher local tumor drug concentrations than with systemic
drug administration.

The ability to test several different compounds at different concentrations in the same tumor specimen makes the human clonogenic assay an attractive system for screening cytotoxic compounds. However, its potential can be realized only by an accurate knowledge of the intratumor concentrations of active drug species achievable in man _in vivo_. The refinement of this system must, therefore, go hand-in-hand with the refinement of our drug metabolism and pharmacokinetic capabilities. Validation from the results of clinical trials with compounds selected for study by this assay is eagerly awaited.

ACKNOWLEDGMENTS

The authors wish to thank Audrey Farwell and Julie Hustad for their technical assistance and Judi Brinck for preparation of this manuscript.

REFERENCES

1. Von Hoff, D.D., Rozencweig, M., Soper, W.M., Helman, L.J., Penta, J.S., Davis, H.L., and Muggia, F.M.: Whatever Happened to NSC _____ ? - An Analysis of Clinical Results of Discontinued Anticancer Agents. Cancer Treat. Rep. 61: 759-768 (1977).
2. Hamburger, A.W., and Salmon, S.E.: Primary Bioassay of Human Tumor Stem Cells. Science 197: 461-463 (1977).
3. Issell, B.F., Tihon, C., and Curry, M.E.: Etoposide (VP-16-213) and Teniposide (VM-26) Comparative _in vitro_ Activities in Human Tumors. Cancer Chemother. and Pharmacol. (In press, 1981).
4. Issell, B.F., Tihon, C., and Curry, M.E.: Activity of Nitrosoureas on Human Tumors _in vitro_. Nitrosoureas - Current Status and New Developments (Prestayko, A.W., Crooke, S.T., Baker, L., Carter, S., and Schein, P., eds.). Academic Press, New York, pp. 361-365 (1981).
5. Von Hoff, D.D., Casper, J., Bradley, E., Sandbach, J., Jones, D., and Makush, R.: Association between Human Tumor Colony-Forming Assay Results and Response of an Individual Patient's Tumor to Chemotherapy. Am. J. Med. 70: 1027-1032 (1981).

6. Chan, K.K., Cohen, J.L., Gross, J.F., Himmelstein, K.J., Bateman, J.R., Yeu, T.L., and Marlis, A.S.: Prediction of Adriamycin Disposition in Cancer Patients Using a Physiologic, Pharmacokinetic Model. <u>Cancer Treat. Rep.</u> <u>62</u>: 1161-1171 (1978).

PHARMACOLOGIC AND THERAPEUTIC CHARACTERISTICS OF ANTHRACYCLINE LIPOSOME
PREPARATION

A. RAHMAN, A. GOLDIN, AND P. SCHEIN

INTRODUCTION

Adriamycin, an anthracycline antibiotic, is an important antitumor
agent isolated from cultures of Streptomyces peucetius (1). Adriamycin
has demonstrated activity for a wide range of human malignancies including lymphomas (2,3,4), leukemia (3,4,5,6), and solid tumors including
gastric and pancreatic cancer (3,4,7,8). The mechanism of action is
the formation of complex with nuclear DNA by intercalating between base
pairs, thus causing steric obstruction to DNA-dependent RNA synthesis
(9,10). Adriamycin produces acute toxicity in the form of bone marrow
depression, alopecia, and oral ulceration (3,4,8). The principal treatment-
limiting toxicity of adriamycin is the product of delayed cardiotoxicity,
which is manifested in the form of refractory congestive heart failure
(11,12). This cumulative myocardial damage has been correlated with
doses in excess of 500 mg/m^2, or less in patients with prior mediastinal
irradiation.

Recently, attempts have been made to control the pharmacokinetics and
disposition of drugs by encapsulation into liposomes (13,14). Liposomes
are lipid vesicles consisting of one or more concentric phospholipid
bilayers alternating with aqueous compartment (15). Encapsulation of
drugs within liposomes offers a simple and potent means of modifying and
controlling the pharmacology of a variety of drugs. The encapsulation
procedure can alter the relationship between drug and host with respect
to tissue disposition, membrane permeation, and enzymatic modification.
Factors that may influence the clearance of liposomes from blood and uptake into tissue include liposomal surface charge and size (16,17) and
possibly the relative rate of endocytic activity of the respective
tissue (18,19). In this regard, heart tissue, in contrast to most neoplasms, has a relatively low endocytotic capacity (20). Our laboratories
have, therefore, studied extensively the pharmacology of liposomal

encapsulated adriamycin to selectively reduce the uptake of the drug in cardiac tissue, thereby reducing the cardiotoxicity while preserving the antitumor activity of the drug. The studies were undertaken to elucidate the role of liposomal charge and lipid composition in altering the pharmacokinetics of adriamycin.

Preparation of Liposomes

Liposomes were prepared by using phosphatidyl choline, cholesterol, stearyl amine or phosphatidyl serine. For the preparation of positive liposome 50.6 μmole of phosphatidyl choline, 20.7 μmole of cholesterol, 14.8 μmole of stearyl amine were mixed with 14.8 μmole of adriamycin (molar ratio of lipids 10:4:3). Similarly, the negative liposomes were prepared with 50.6 μmole of phosphatidyl choline, 20.7 μmole of cholesterol and 5.03 μmole of phosphatidyl serine with 14.8 μmole of adriamycin (molar ratio of lipids 10:4:1). The organic solvents were then evaporated gently under a stream of nitrogen so that a thin film of lipid was formed around the sides of the flasks. Ten ml of 0.01 $\underline{M}$ phosphate buffer with 0.85% NaCl (pH 7.4) were then added to the dried lipid and drug film, and the mixture was dispersed with a magnetic stirring bar, yielding multilamellar liposomes. After a half hour swelling period, these multilamellar liposomes were then sonicated for 20 minutes under a nitrogen atmosphere in a bath type sonicator (Heat System Model 220 F) at 35°C. The non-entrapped adriamycin was separated from liposomal encapsulated drug by extensive dialysis against 0.01 $\underline{M}$ phosphate buffered saline pH 7.4 at 4°C over a period of 30 hours with at least 3 changes of buffer solutions. The amount of adriamycin captured under these conditions was determined by fluorescence (21) after the completion of dialysis.

The amount of adriamycin encapsulated under these conditions was 55% in the specific negative liposomes and 35% in the positive liposomes of the total input dose. The higher efficiency of entrapment of drug into these liposomes suggests that adriamycin intercalates into the hydrocarbon region of the liposome membranes. Liposomes were used the same day and when required were diluted with 0.01 $\underline{M}$ phosphate buffer with 0.85% NaCl (pH 7.4) so as to administer equivalent doses of adriamycin in mice as either free or entrapped drug.

In Vivo Studies

Male DBA/2 mice weighing 18-25 gm were used to evaluate the influence
of liposomal encapsulation on plasma levels and physiologic disposition
of adriamycin. Free and entrapped adriamycin in either negative or
positive liposomes were administered intravenously via a lateral tail
vein at a dose of 4 mg/kg and at 2% of body weight. At 5,15,30,60,120,
240,360 and 480 min and at 24 hr, 4 mice in each group were bled from
the orbital sinus and blood was collected in heparinized tubes, centrifuged at 3000 rpm for 10 minutes and the plasma layer separated and
frozen. Mice were killed by cervical dislocation and the liver, kidney,
heart, spleen and lungs were rapidly excised and rinsed in normal saline
and stored at -20°C until assayed. Plasma and tissues were analyzed for
adriamycin fluorescent equivalents according to the method of Bachur et
al (21).

The respective plasma levels following a dose of adriamycin, 4 mg/kg,
as free drug or entrapped in liposomes is shown in Figure 1. The plasma
levels of adriamycin equivalents following free drug administration
remained at a concentration below 1 µg/ml, for all time periods. Encapsulation of the drug within liposomes markedly altered the plasma
clearance kinetics of adriamycin, effectively retarding the removal
of the drug from the circulation. The peak plasma concentration of drug
equivalents in mice receiving the liposomal form of adriamycin was at
least 10-fold higher with negative liposomes and 6-fold higher with
positive liposomes. The area under the plasma concentration time curve
(AUC) as shown in Table 1 indicates that i.v. administration of free
adriamycin is accompanied by a rapid decrease in plasma levels followed
by a large volume of distribution in agreement with previous studies
(22). However, the AUC values for adriamycin entrapped in negative liposomes were 12-fold higher and about 8-fold higher with positive liposomes than the values for free drug.

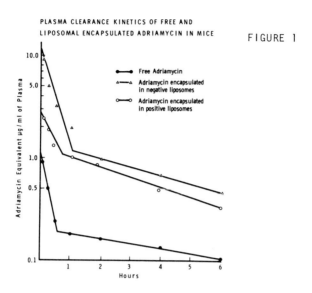

PLASMA CLEARANCE KINETICS OF FREE AND
LIPOSOMAL ENCAPSULATED ADRIAMYCIN IN MICE   FIGURE 1

Figure 2 represents the cardiac uptake of free and liposomal entrapped adriamycin when injected i.v. into DBA/2 mice at a dose of 4
mg/kg. The peak drug concentration in heart occurred in 30 minutes both
with the free drug and drug entrapped in negative liposomes; the values
were 8.3 and 9.1 µg/g wet weight respectively. In contrast, the peak
cardiac uptake with adriamycin encapsulated in positive liposomes
occurred at 5 minutes and the drug equivalents were only 4.6 µg/g. From
10 min to 2 hr the maximum cardiac concentrations of drug equivalents
with positive liposomes was one-third or less than that achieved after
administration of drug in negative liposomes or free adriamycin. It is
apparent that adriamycin administered entrapped in positive liposomes
results in a reduction of the in vivo uptake of this drug in murine
cardiac tissue. The tissue concentration x time (CXT) values for the
cardiac organ for the 24-hour period were 55.2 and 83.5 µg.hr.gm.$^{-1}$ for
free drug and drug entrapped in negative liposomes respectively: the
corresponding values for the drug entrapped in positive liposomes were
40.1 µg.hr.gm^{-1}. Hence, not only was the peak concentration of drug in
cardiac tissue reduced when adriamycin was administered in positive
liposomes, but also the total concentration of the drug to which the

tissue was exposed was decreased substantially as compared to free or drug entrapped in negative liposomes (Table 2).

TABLE 1

Influence of Liposomal Entrapment of Adriamycin

On Areas Under the Plasma Concentration - Time Curve[1,2,3]

	(AUC $0 \to 8$ HR.)
	µg hr. ml - 1
Free Adriamycin	0.723
Adriamycin Entrapped in Negative Liposomes	9.18
Adriamycin Entrapped in Positive Liposomes	5.46

[1]Male DBA-2 mice received 4 mg/kg adriamycin HCl I.V. alone or in the form of liposomal entrapped adriamycin. The method of preparation is described in "Methods."

[2]Blood was collected from an orbital sinus at selected intervals over eight hours.

[3]Adriamycin equivalents were measured fluorometrically after extraction of plasma with 3 volumes of 0.3 $\underline{N}$ HCl in 50% ETOH.

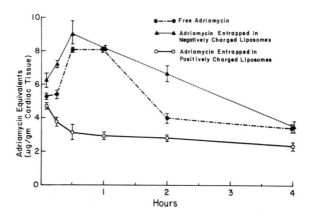

Figure 2:
Figure 2: Adriamycin disposition in mice heart following i.v. administration of free and liposomal entrapped drug. Bars S.D.

The organ selectivity of this phenomenon is evidenced by the increased concentration of adriamycin in other tissues of mice when administered entrapped in positive liposomes. Table 2 presents the tissue concentration x time (CxT) values for the 24-hour period of observation for selected organs. An increased uptake of liposome-entrapped adriamycin, as compared to free drug, was found in liver, spleen and lung. This is in agreement with other studies which have demonstrated that liposome-entrapped drugs can be targeted preferentially to the organs of the reticuloendothelial system (23,24,25). Liposome encapsulation not only enhanced the total amount of drug accumulated in these tissues but also altered the relative distribution. Liposomal adriamycin was concentrated 4-fold in liver and in spleen when compared with free drug. These studies suggest that liposomal charge can be used to achieve an altered disposition of this neoplastic agent, with a specific reduction in cardiac uptake.

TABLE 2

Effect of liposomal entrapment of Adriamycin on tissue CxT values[1]

$C \times T \ (\mu g.hr.g^{-1})$

	Heart	Lung	Liver	Kidney	Spleen
Free Adriamycin	55.15	60.67	88.62	115.1	101.71
Adriamycin entrapped in negative liposomes	83.37	59.58	211.2	119.13	174.27
Adriamycin entrapped in positive liposomes	40.10	104.32	408.21	141.07	394.7

1. C x T values are calculated from 5 min to 24 hours.

Antitumor Studies

To investigate the effectiveness of adriamycin encapsulated in liposomes against solid tumor, studies were conducted in Lewis Lung Carcinoma injected subcutaneously into the right flank of BDF_1 mice, with 10 mice per group (26). Following tumor implantation mice were injected intravenously on days 8,10, and 12 with adriamycin 4 mg/kg, either as free drug or entrapped in negative or positive liposomes. The mean tumor mass $(L \times W^2)$ was measured after tumor implantation as shown in Figure 3. With free adriamycin at day 16, the mean tumor size was reduced 48%, as compared to tumor-bearing controls receiving blank positive liposomes.

The same dose of adriamycin entrapped in positive liposomes and negative liposomes reduced the tumor mass 46% and 34%, respectively.

Cardiotoxicity Studies

Our studies have demonstrated that adriamycin-induced acute cardiotoxicity is significantly reduced when the drug is administered entrapped in positive liposomes (27); electron microscopic studies demonstrated that the myocytes and myofibrillar structure of cardiac muscle were markedly well preserved. The next series of studies was directed toward determining the chronic cardiotoxicity of free adriamycin and adriamycin entrapped in liposomes. Male DBA/2 mice weighing 22-25 g were randomly distributed in groups of six and maintained under standardized environment. Free adriamycin and adriamycin entrapped either in positive or negative liposomes were administered via a tail vein at a dose of 4 mg/kg at 2% of body weight. All mice were injected twice a week for a total of 7 treatments. After the fourth and sixth injection, treatment was discontinued for 2 weeks to allow for recovery of bone marrow function. One week following the last injection, the mice were killed by cervical dislocation and the hearts were immediately removed and placed in physiological saline. The apex of the left ventricle with part of the septum was fixed for light microscopy and electron microscopic evaluation.

Figure 4a presents a typical area of myocardial damage following treatment with free adriamycin, as seen by light microscopy, characterized by extensive vacuolation and loss and/or disorganization of contractile elements. In contrast, light microscopic sections of heart from mice treated with adriamycin entrapped in positively charged liposomes (Figure 4b) showed an overall appearance comparable to that of control tissue. Mice treated with drug entrapped in negative liposomes showed degenerative alterations of myocardium similar to those in free-drug-treated mice.

The results of electron microscopic examination of the heart tissue correlated well with the light microscopic findings. Administration of free adriamycin caused a pattern of cardiac damage characterized by loss of myofibular elements, mitochondrial damage, nuclear abnormalities, swollen and distended sacroplasmic reticulum leading to vacuolization and increasing myeloid body accumulation. These lesions were present in all cardiac samples examined. Figure 5 represents an atypical example of degenerative lesions of cardiac tissue treated with adriamycin, with a myocyte

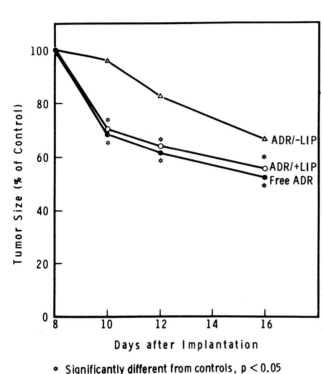

* Significantly different from controls, p < 0.05

Figure 3

Treatment of mice given implants of Lewis Lung carcinoma s.c. Adriamycin (4 mg/kg) was administered i.v. to mice on Days 8,10 and 12 after tumor implantation as free drug or drug entrapped in positive or negative liposomes. The percentage of reduction of tumor mass was assessed by measuring the largest perpendicular diameters of the primary tumor at serial time points after implantation (26). Free ADR/-LIP, Adriamycin entrapped in negatively charged liposomes; ADR/+LIP, Adriamycin entrapped in positively charged liposomes. *Significantly different from controls, p<0.05 (Student's test).

containing large accumulations of myeloid bodies, autophagic vacuoles, and other inclusion bodies of electron dense material. This corresponds to the most severe damage observed in these samples prior to absolute dissolution and myolysis of the cells. Free and pleomorphic-shaped mitochrondria are present even at this apparent late stage of toxicity. Myofilaments can be seen in short segments, haphazardly dispersed throughout the damaged cell, while some areas appear devoid of even remnants. Cardiac tissues of mice treated with adriamycin entrapped in negatively charged liposomes also demonstrated loss of filaments, enlarged mitochondria, disruptive loss of cristae and expanded nuclear membrane. However, electron microscopic examination of the cardiac muscles of mice treated with positive liposomes demonstrated a significant protection from drug-induced toxicity, with only minor loss of parallel fibrillar arrangement and myofilaments in limited focal areas. As shown in Figure 6 the majority of the tissue demonstrated normal vasculature and intercalation of myocytes as compared to control groups.

A statistical evaluation of the scoring of toxic lesion recorded in the cardiac ultrastructure of different groups of mice treated either with free or liposomal entrapped adriamycin is presented in table 3. The mean qualitative (extent) and quantitative (severity) score for free adriamycin and adriamycin entrapped in negative liposomes group is 2.7 and 2.23 respectively. However, the mean score for the group of mice treated with positive liposomes is substantially reduced; with a value of 1.12 ($p < 0.05$). There appears to be a better than two-fold scoring protection of both the extent and severity of cardiac lesions for the mice treated with adriamycin entrapped in positive liposomes as compared to the free drug.

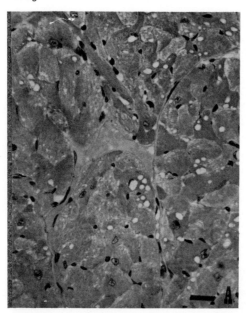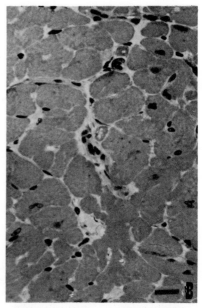

Figure 4   Light micrographs of 1μm methacrylate sections of DBA mouse cardiac tissue, hematoxylinemethylene blue-basic fuchsin stain, all x1000. Bar represents 10μm.

A.   Free adriamycin group, extensive vacuolization and loss of cellular elements and atrophic degeneration are pronounced.
B.   Positive liposome group, largely undamaged.

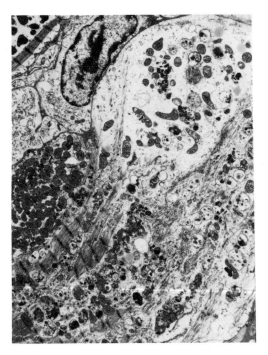

FIGURE 5

Electron micrographs of free
adriamycin group showing progression of cardiotoxic manifestations present simultaneously
in any one sample. Uranyl acetate
and lead citrate (UA/LC) stain.

Severe atrophic degenerative
state of myocyte showing replace-
ment of elements with electron
dense materials, autophagic
vacuoles and myelin figures.
Note bizarre and grouped mitochrondria. Score $\leq$ 4 x3,500.
bar=3μ.

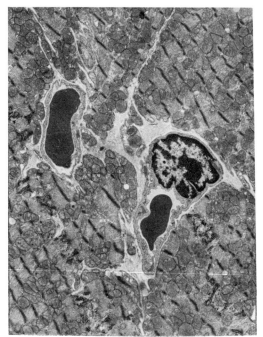

FIGURE 6

Electron micrographs of DBA cardiac
tissue. (UA/LC) stain.

Positive liposome group depicting
normal endothelium and surrounding myocyte structure. Note
uniformities of myofilaments,
banding patterns, arrangement
of mitochondria and intercalated
discs x3,000 bar represents 3μ.

TABLE 3

Electron Microscopic Evaluation of Adriamycin
Cardiotoxicity

Blocks	T_{Qual}	T_{Quant}	$T_{Q + Q}$	M_T	Average
*FA$_1$	23	37	60	3.00	
FA$_2$	31	31	62	3.10	
FA$_3$	17	28	45	2.25	2.70
FA$_4$	27	22	49	2.45	
-ve/lip$_1$	21	32	53	2.65	
-ve/lip$_2$	28	39	67	3.35	
-ve/lip$_3$	10	11	21	1.05	2.23
-ve/lip$_4$	23	30	53	2.65	
-ve/lip$_5$	13	16	29	1.45	
+ve/lip$_1$	9	12	21	1.05	
+ve/lip$_2$	11	18	29	1.45	
+ve/lip$_3$	16	20	36	1.80	
+ve/lip$_4$	5	7	12	0.60	1.12
+ve/lip$_5$	9	12	21	1.05	
+ve/lip$_6$	8	8	16	0.80	

*FA   - Free Adriamycin Group.

-ve/lip - Adriamycin Entrapped in Negative Liposomes.

+ve/lip - Adriamycin Entrapped in Positive Liposomes.

Influence of Liposomal Cholesterol Content on the Disposition of Adriamycin

The addition of cholesterol to the mixture of phospholipids has been
demonstrated to decrease membrane permeability at biologically relevant
temperatures (28). It was considered that positive and negative liposomes containing a high proportion of cholesterol might demonstrate a
more sustained in vivo plasma concentration of the entrapped drug.

To test this hypothesis, we prepared positive liposomes with entrapped
adriamycin consisting of a 10:10:3 molar ratio of phosphatidyl choline,
cholesterol and stearyl amine. The negative liposomes with entrapped
adriamycin were prepared to contain a 10:10:1 molar ratio of phosphatidyl
choline, cholesterol and phosphatidyl serine. The remaining experimental
procedures were similar to those described earlier (27).

Sprague-Dawley rats weighing 300-400 gm were used to perform the plasma
pharmacokinetic, biliary excretion and pharmacologic disposition of

adriamycin as free and liposomal entrapped drug. Rats were anesthetized with pentobarbital (45 mg/kg/ip) and the femoral artery was isolated and cannulated with PE10 tubing. The femoral vein was isolated and drug injections were performed at 4 mg/kg over a period of 2 minutes with free and entrapped adriamycin in positive and negative liposomes. Blood was drawn through the cannulated artery at 5,15,30,45,60,120 and 240 minutes after the drug administration in heparinized syringes and plasma was separated immediately and stored at -20°C. In each group of treatment 4 rats were used.

Four rats in each treatment group were utilized to perform the biliary excretion studies of adriamycin as free drug or entrapped in liposomes. Rats were anesthetized with pentobarbital (45 mg/kg) intraperitoneally and a midline incision was made. The common bile duct was isolated and cannulated with polyethylene tubing. Drug injections were performed through the right femoral vein. Bile was collected into iced preweighted tubes at specified time intervals. Six hous after injection, rats were killed and heart, liver, kidney, lungs, spleen, small intestine were excised quickly, rinsed in ice-cold saline and stored at -20°C until assayed.

Plasma Pharmacokinetic in Rats

The plasma pharmacokinetic o⁻ free and liposomal entrapped adriamycin in rats at a dose of 4 mg/kg is presented in figure 7. Following injection of free adriamycin, the peak plasma concentration achieved was 3.13 µg/ml at 5 minutes which fell to 0.58 µg/ml at 1/2 hour. The free drug cleared from the plasma very rapidly with a large volume of distribution. However, rats injected with adriamycin entrapped in positive liposomes and negative liposome at a dose of 4 mg/kg evidenced a 6 and 10 fold higher plasma levels of drug equivalents. The plasma half-life of the liposomal preparation increased 6 fold compared to free drug, with a concommittant 4 fold decrease in total clearance of the drug when administered entrapped in liposomes.

Biliary excretion studies of free drug and drug entrapped in positive and negative liposomes were carried out in cannulated rats at a dose of 4 mg/kg. With free adriamycin the peak drug excretion in bile was achieved in 15 minutes, the values being 480 ± 17.11 µg/ml. The peak bile concentration of drug equivalent following administration of adriamycin entrapped in positive liposomes was achieved in 30 minutes with a

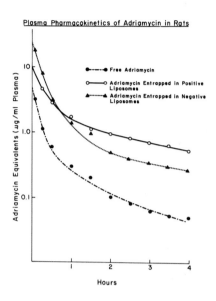

Plasma Pharmacokinetics of Adriamycin in Rats

● —·— ● Free Adriamycin

○——○ Adriamycin Entrapped in Positive Liposomes

▲·······▲ Adriamycin Entrapped in Negative Liposomes

FIGURE 7

Rats were injected with free or liposomal en-trapped adriamycin at a dose of 4 mg/kg i.v. Blood was collected at selected intervals and drug levels were mea-sured fluorometrically after extraction of plasma with 3 volumes of 0.3 NHCl in 50% ETOH.

FIGURE 8

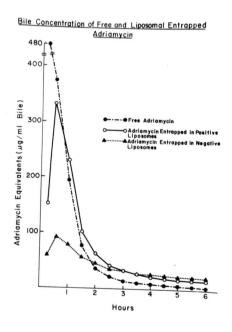

Bile Concentration of Free and Liposomal Entrapped Adriamycin

● —·— ● Free Adriamycin

○——○ Adriamycin Entrapped in Positive Liposomes

▲·······▲ Adriamycin Entrapped in Negative Liposomes

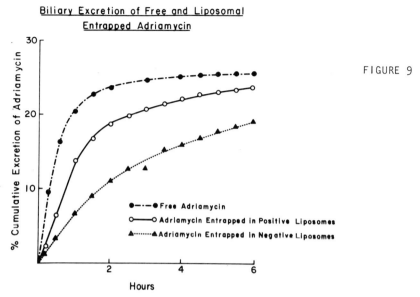

Biliary Excretion of Free and Liposomal Entrapped Adriamycin

FIGURE 9

value of 335 ± 36.0 μg/ml. Though the peak drug concentration in bile
with negative liposomes was also achieved at 30 minutes, the value of
drug equivalent was only 89.5 ± 12.4 μg/ml (Figure 8). The rates of
drug excretion in the bile with the three forms of drug administration
were quite different. After 30 minutes of free drug injection, about
15% of the administered drug was recovered in the bile whereas only 6% of
adriamycin in positive liposomes was recovered and about 3% with adriamycin entrapped in negative liposomes. However, by six hours, the percent excretion of the drug in the bile following the administration of
adriamycin in various forms approached equivalently; the values being
19-25%, of the injection dose (Figure 9).

The tissue distribution of free and liposomal entrapped adriamycin was
determined in rats 6 hours after drug administration. The level of adriamycin equivalents in cardiac tissue was 6.4 μg/gm following free drug
administration; this compared to a 3.2 and 2.7 μg/gm when adriamycin was
injected entrapped in positive and negative liposomes (Table 4). It
appears that administration of adriamycin in liposomes selectively regards
the uptake of the drug in the cardiac tissue. Adriamycin administered
entrapped in liposomes appear to be preferentially concentrated in the
tissues of reticuloendothelial system. The drug is concentrated 8 fold
in liver, 2 fold in spleen and 3 fold in lungs when administered in

liposomes, when compared to free drug.

Drug-lipid Interaction to Alter Pharmacodynamics

The role of liposome components in determining the disposition of adriamycin in cardiac tissue is an important consideration. It can be expected
that the intrinsic properties of the anthracycline drugs and liposome
components can be exploited to retard the uptake of the drugs in cardiac
tissue. Recently, using the membrane-model system, Gormaghtigh et al. studied
the interaction of adriamycin and cardiolipin (29), and adriamycin was shown to
have a marked specificity for adsorption into the cardiolipin monolayers.
This property was utilized in our studies to further retard the uptake of
adriamycin in cardiac tissue.

TABLE 4

Tissue Levels of Adriamycin Equivalents
in Rats 6 Hrs. After Administration of
free and Liposomal Entrapped Drug

μg/gm of tissue

Tissue	Free Adriamycin	Adriamycin Entrapped in positive liposomes	Adriamycin Entrapped in negative liposomes
Heart	6.4	3.3	2.70
Liver	4.53	29.2	34.45
Spleen	14.13	33.8	51.45
Lung	8.27	15.0	10.2
Kidney	10.06	4.8	5.35
Intestine	4.6	1.8	3.90

Adriamycin liposomes, with cardiolipin, were prepared as described
elsewhere (30). These liposomes were injected to DBA/2 mice at a dose
of 4 mg/kg i.v. and drug levels in cardiac tissue were followed for 24
hours as shown in Figure 10. The peak drug concentration is achieved
at 5 minutes with cardiolipin liposomes; the value being 3.4 μg/gm of
cardiac tissue compared to 8.3 μg/gm observed with free drug administration. By two hours the cardiac levels of adriamycin equivalents
with cardiolipin liposomes was only 1 μg/gm of tissue, whereas it was
more than 4 μg/gm during the same period with free drug delivery. The
tissue concentration x tissue (C x T) values for free adriamycin for the
24 hour period of observation was 55.1 $\mu g.hr.gm^{-1}$; the corresponding
values for the cardiolipin liposomes were only 7.8 $\mu g.hr.gm^{-1}$. These
studies clearly demonstrate that varying the lipid components of liposomes can specifically restrict the uptake of adriamycin into cardiac
tissue. The high affinity of adriamycin association with cardiolipin

imparts a more stable liposomal encapsulation which controls its uptake in heart.

Discussion

Recently, liposomes have been shown effective as carriers of drugs and other biologically active agents (27,31,32). Several systems have been described where liposomal encapsulation of antineoplastic agents has been achieved which potentiated their biological activity. We have demonstrated a reduced uptake of adriamycin in cardiac tissue of mice when the drug is injected entrapped in positive liposomes. Free adriamycin has been shown to enter cells via passive diffusion or carrier mediated transport (33), whereas liposomes have been demonstrated to enter either by membrane fusion or endocytosis (34). Endocytotic uptake leads to lysosomal localization (19,35) of liposomes and entrapped materials. Once within lysosomes, liposomes are disrupted (19) and liberate their contents, which can then act either locally or, after their escape from lysosomes, in other cellular compartments. Moreover, tissues vary in endocytotic capacity, with liver, spleen, and certain tumors having relatively higher activity compared to heart and kidney. Our in vivo studies in mice strongly suggest that the route of uptake of adriamycin entrapped in positive liposome is significantly altered with respect to cardiac tissue. The maximal drug concentration in cardiac tissue following administration

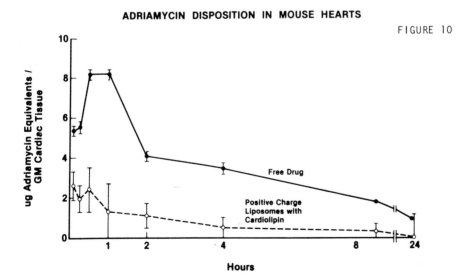

ADRIAMYCIN DISPOSITION IN MOUSE HEARTS

FIGURE 10

of adriamycin entrapped in positively charged liposomes was one-half that achieved after administration of free drug or entrapped in negative liposome (Figure 2). Not only was the peak concentration of drug in cardiac tissue reduced, but the total concentration of drug to which the tissue was exposed was reduced substantially (Table 2). The plasma clearance kinetics of liposome-encapsulated drug seems to be dictated by the behavior of the liposomes themselves. Upon administration of liposome entrapped adriamycin in mice or rats, six to ten fold higher plasma levels are achieved as opposed to the administration of free adriamycin (Figure 1 and Figure 7). Liposome encapsulation also markedly altered the relative disposition of drugs among various tissues and the absolute levels of drug accumulation by the tissues as indicated in Table 2 and 4.

Biliary excretion studies in rats have demonstrated an altered clearance of the drug from the body. Free adriamycin was excreted much faster with a peak concentration of drug equivalent of 480 μg/ml as compared to 335 μg/ml and 89.5 μg/ml of drug entrapped in positive liposome and negative liposomes respectively. This is contrary to the fact that liposomal entrapped adriamycin is preferentially concentrated about 4 to 8 fold in liver. This delayed excretion of liposomal encapsulated drug may represent a delayed release from the liposomes.

Our cardiotoxicity studies in mice have shown significantly reduced chronic cardiac damage when adriamycin is administered entrapped in positively charged liposome at a dose of 28 mg/kg. This degree of protection of the cardiac muscle of mice appears to be well correlated with the lowering of drug uptake in this organ (27). The morphologic alteration observed in the cardiac tissue after repeated intravenous administration of free adriamycin corresponds well with other investigations (36). However, as indicated in Table 3 there is a greater than two-fold protection in both the extent and severity of cardiac lesions with the positive liposome regimen.

The affinity of adriamycin association with cardiolipin and subsequent entrapment in liposomes demonstrates a pronounced effect on the uptake of drug in cardiac tissue. The cardiolipin liposomes appear to retard very effectively the uptake of adriamycin in mice heart as well as enhance its elimination from this organ. As indicated in Figure 9, there is hardly any drug left in cardiac tissue by 4 hours when adriamycin is administered in cardiolipin liposomes as opposed to free drug administration. It appears that this drug delivery system can be successfully exploited to achieve a reduced cardiotoxicity and better therapeutic index. The major treatment-limiting toxicity of adriamycin, aside from bone marrow depression, is cumulative and potentially irreversible cardiac damage. A drug delivery system which selectively reduces the cardiac uptake of drug while retaining full antitumor effectiveness may have potential clinical application.

Acknowledgements

The authors wish to express their deep appreciation to Ms. Karen O. Bivins for her assistance in the preparation of the manuscript.

REFERENCES

1.   DiMarco A, Gaetani M, Scarpinato B. 1969. Adriamycin (NSC-123127):
      A new antibiotic with antitumor activity. Cancer Chemother Rep
      53:33-37.
2.   Bonadonna G, DeLena MD, Monfardini S, et al. 1975. Combination
      chemotherapy with Adriamycin in malig nant lymphoma. In Adriamycin
      Review. Ghent, Belgium, European Press Medicon, pp. 200-215.
3.   Bonadonna G, Monfardini S, DeLena MD, Fossati-Bellani, F, Beretter,
      G. 1970. Phase I and preliminary Phase II evaluation of Adriamycin
      (NSC-123127). Cancer Res 30:2572-2582.
4.   Wang JJ, Cortes E, Sinks LF, Holland JF. 1971. Therapeutic effect
      and toxicity of Adriamycin in patients with neoplastic disease.
      Cancer 28:837-843.
5.   Haanen C, and Hillen G. 1975. Combination chemotherapy with doxo-
      rubicin in "bad risk" leukemia patients. In Adriamycin Review.
      Ghent, Belgium, European Press Medicon, pp 193-199.
6.   Oldham RK, and Pomeroy TC. 1972. Treatment of Ewing's sarcoma
      with Adriamycin (NSC-123127). Cancer Chemother Rep 56:635-639.
7.   Middleman E, Luce J, Frei E. 1971. Clinical trials with Adriamycin.
      Cancer 28:844-850.
8.   Philips FS, Gilladoga A, Marquardt H, Sternberg SS, Vidal PM. 1975.
      Some observations on the toxicity of Adriamycin (NSC-123127). Cancer
      Chemother Rep Part 3, Vol. 6 (2):177-181.
9.   DiMarco A, Zunino F, Silvestrini R, Gambarucci C, Gambetta RA. 1971.
      Interaction of some daunomycin derivatives with deoxyribonucleic
      acid and their biological activity. Biochem Pharmacol 20:1323-1328.
10.   Ward DC, Reich E, Goldberg IH. 1965. Base specificity in the inter-
      action of polynucleotides with antibiotic drugs. Science 149:1259.
11.   Lefrak EA, Pitha J, Rosenheim S, Gottlieb JA. 1973. A clinico-
      pathologic analysis of Adriamycin cardiotoxicity. Cancer 32:302-
      314.
12.   Rinehart JJ, Louis RP, Balcerzak SP. 1974. Adriamycin cardiotoxi-
      city in man. Ann Intern Med 81:475-478.
13.   Rahman YE, Kisieleski WE, Buess EM, Cerny EA. 1975. Liposomes con-
      taining ^{3}H-actinomycin D differential tissue distribution by
      varying the mode of drug incorporation. Eur J Cancer 11:883-889.
14.   Kimelberg, HK. 1976. Differential distribution of liposome-entrapped
      ^{3}H-methotrexate and labelled lipid after intravenous injection in
      a primate. Biochim Biophys Acta 448:531-550.
15.   Bangham AD, Standish MM and Watkins JC. 1965. Diffusion of uni-
      valent ions across the lamallae of swollen phospholipids. J Mol
      Biol 13:238-252.
16.   Juliano RL, Stamp D. 1978. Pharmacokinetic of liposome-encapsu-
      lated antitumor drugs. Biochem Pharmacol 27:21-27.
17.   Juliano, RL and Stamp D. 1975. The effect of particle size and
      charge on the clearance rates of liposomes and liposome encapsu-
      lated drugs. Biochem Biophys Res Commun 63:651-658.
18.   Gregoriadis G, Wills EJ, Swan CP, Tavill AS. 1974. Drug-carrier
      potential of liposomes in cancer chemotherapy. Lancet 1:1313-1316.
19.   Segal AW, Wills EJ, Richmond JE, Slavin G, Black CDV and Gregoriadis,
      G. 1974. Morphological observations on the cellular and sub-
      cellular destination of intravenously administered liposomes. Br
      J Exp Pathol 55:320-327.
20.   Trouet A, Deprez-de Campeneere D, deDuve C. 1972. Chemotherapy
      through lysosomes with a DNA-daunorubicin complex. Nat New Biol

239:110-112,

21. Bachur NR, Moore AL, Burnstein JG, Lio A. 1970. A tissue distribution and disposition of daunomycin in mice. Fluorometric and Isotopic Methods. Cancer Chemother Rep 54:89-94.

22. Yesair DW, Schwartzbach E, Shuck D, Denine EP, Asbell MA. 1972. Comparative pharmacokinetics of daunomycin and Adriamycin in several animal species. Cancer Res 32:1177-1183.

23. Rahman A, Kessler A, Macdonald J, Waravedkar V, Schein P. 1979. Liposomal delivery of Adriamycin. Proc Am Assoc Cancer Res 20:288.

24. Rahman A, Guiterraz P, Raschid S, Mhatre R, Schein PS. 1981. Pharmacokinetics of liposome-encapsulated doxorubicin. Fed Proceedings 40:685.

25. Gregoriadis G, Neerunjin D. 1974. Control of the rate of hepatic uptake and catabolism of liposome entrapped proteins injected into rats. Eur J Biochem 47:179-185.

26. Sikic BI, Collins JM, Mimnough EC, Gram TE. 1977. Improved therapeutic index of bleomycin when administered by continuous infusion in mice. Cancer Treat Rep 62:2071-2081.

27. Rahman A, Kessler A, More N, Sikic B, Rowden G, Woolley P, Schein P. 1980. Liposomal protection of adriamycin-induced cardiotoxicity in mice. Cancer Res 40:1532-1537.

28. deGier J, Mandersloot JC, Van Deenen LLM. 1968. Lipid composition and permeability of liposomes. Biochem Biophys Acta 150:666-675.

29. Goormaghtigh E, Chatelain P, Caspers J and Ruysschaert JM. 1980. Evidence of a specific complex between adriamycin and negatively charged phospholipids. Biochem Biophys Acta 597:1-14.

30. Rahman A, White G, More N, Pradham S, Schein PS. 1981. Protection of chronic cardiotoxicity of Adriamycin by liposomal delivery. Proc Am Assoc Cancer Res 22:269.

31. Mayhew E, Papahadjopoulos D, Rustum YM, Dave C. 1976. Inhibition of tumor cell growth in vitro and in vivo by 1-β-D-arabinofurano-sylcytosine entrapped within phospholipid vesicles. Cancer Res 36:4406-4411.

32. Poste G, Papahadjopoulos D. 1976. Drug containing lipid vesicles render drug-resistant cells sensitive to actinomycin D. Nature (Lond). 261:699-701.

33. Skorsgaard T. 1978. Carrier-mediated transport of daunorubicin, Adriamycin and rubidazone in Ehrlich ascites tumor cells. Biochem Pharmacol 27:1221-1227.

34. Poste G, Papahadjopoulos D. 1976. Lipid vesicles as carriers for introducing materials into cultured cells: Influence of vesicle lipid composition on mechanism(s) of vesicle incorporation into cells. Proc Natl Acad Sci USA 73:1603-1607.

35. Gregoriadis G. 1974. In Enzyme therapy in lysosomal storage disease (Tager JM, Houghwinkel GJM, and Daems WT, eds), p. 131 North-Holland Publ. Amsterdam.

36. Bertazzoli C, Bellisin O, Magrini U, Tosaner MG. 1979. Quantitative experimental evaluation of adriamycin cardiotoxicity in the mouse. Cancer Treatment Reports 63:1877,

N-L-LEUCYL DERIVATIVES OF ANTHRACYCLINES: TOXIC AND CHEMOTHERAPEUTIC PROPERTIES

A. TROUET, D. DEPREZ-DE CAMPENEERE, R. BAURAIN, M. MASQUELIER, AND R. JAENKE

Various N-aminoacids of daunorubicin (DNR) have been synthesized in an attempt to develop a method for linking DNR to protein carriers, which would enable DNR to be released intralysosomally after endocytosis of the drug-carrier conjugate by tumor cells (1,2,3). It rapidly became evident that these amino-acid derivatives could be interesting by themselves as potential prodrugs of DNR. It was assumed that these prodrugs could have proper pharmacokinetic properties and be activated into DNR either inside the tumor cells or in their vicinity by enzymatic hydrolysis.

Among the various DNR derivatives tested, N-L-leucyl-DNR (leu-DNR) was found to be the most interesting (2), and this inspired us to synthesize L-leucyl-doxorubicin (leu-DOX) and L-leucyl-detorubicin (leu-DET). The methods of synthesis are similar to those described for leu-DNR (1).

The affinity for DNA of leu-DNR and leu-DOX is about 3 to 4 times weaker than that of DNR and DOX, as determined by a spectrophotometric method and Scatchard plot (Table 1) (4).

These results suggest that the leucyl derivatives are probably inactive or very weakly active as such and need to be transformed into DNR, DOX, or DET in order to exert their chemotherapeutic activity.

When compared with their parent compounds, leu-DNR, leu-DOX, and leu-DET are about 4 times less toxic in terms of LD_{50} values (Table 2) as determined in mice after i.v. administration. The hematopoietic toxicity of the compounds was studied on C57Bl/6j mice. We determined the dose by reducing by 50% the bone-marrow pluripotent stem cells (CFU_s) and committed myeloid stem cells (CFU_c) as previously described (5). The results given in Table 3 confirm the overall toxicity data and indicate that the leucyl anthracyclines are about 3 times less toxic for both medullar stem cells.

The chronic cardiotoxicity of the leucyl anthracyclines was studied in rabbits as previously described (6). A maximal tolerated dose, defined as the maximal dose compatible with long-term survival (11 or 16 weeks) and

Table 1. DNA binding parameters

Drug	$Ka \ldots 10^{-6}$	n_{max}	n
DNR	.297 ± .026	.161 ± .014	5
DOX	.649 ± .058	.159 ± .005	6
DET	.849	.137	1
Leu-DNR	.094 ± .017	.187 ± .012	4
Leu-DOX	.181 ± .038	.207 ± .003	4
Leu-DET	–	–	–

The affinity constants (Ka) and the maximal number of binding sites (n_{max}) were determined by a spectrophotometric method at 22° C and pH 7.4 (4). Herring sperm were used as a source of DNA. $\underline{n}$ = number of assays.

Table 2. Comparative overall toxicity of N-L-leucyl derivatives of anthracycline after i.v. administration into mice

Drug	LD_{50}* (mg/kg per day)	
	mean	S.D.
DNR	16.8	1.2
DOX	14.4	2.3
DET	15.9	0.8
Leu-DNR	67.0	1.8
Leu-DOX	46.7	1.8
Leu-Det	71.6	1.6

*LD_{50} = dose which induces 50% lethality in mice after 30 days of observation. Mean and S.D. of at least two separate assays are given. Drugs were administered i.v. on 2 consecutive days into NMRI mice.

not limiting with regard to hematopoietic and gastrointestinal toxicity, was determined for each drug. The lowest dose after 16 weeks of twice-weekly injections was observed for DOX (1 mg/kg per injection) and DET (1.15 mg/kg). DNR was slightly less toxic (1.3 mg/kg) although leu-DNR, leu-DOX, and leu-DET were about three times less toxic with doses of 4.6, 3.0, and 3.5 mg/kg, respectively.

The hearts of the animals that had survived more than 60 days were examined histologically after 11 or 16 weeks of drug administration for the presence of cardiac lesions. Both the sacrificed animals and those dying

Table 3. Hematopoietic toxicity of N-L-leucyl derivatives of anthracyclines after single i.v. administrations into mice

Drug	CFU$_S$ assay ID$_{50}$* (mg/kg)	CFU$_C$ assay ID$_{50}$* (mg/kg)
DNR	3.4	3.8
DOX	3.2	2.5
DET	3.4	4.7
Leu-DNR	9.2	8.5
Leu-DOX	10.5	9.8
Leu-DET	–	13.6

*ID$_{50}$ = dose which induces 50% cytotoxicity toward bone-marrow pluri-
potent stem cells (CFU$_S$ assay) or committed myeloid stem cells
(CFU$_C$ assay), 24 hours after single i.v. injections into mice.

before the scheduled 11 and 16 weeks were examined carefully for signs of
congestive heart failure (CHF), such as hydrothorax, hydropericardium,
and/or abdominal ascites.

In Figure 1, we report for 11 and 16 weeks of treatment the percentage
of rabbits showing microscopical signs of cardiomyopathy and the percentage
displaying symptoms of CHF. The most striking reduction in cardiotoxicity
is observed with leu-DNR, since no animals displayed symptoms of CHF and only
40% showed histological signs of cardiomyopathy after 16 weeks.

The cardiotoxicity of leu-DET and leu-DOX was also reduced but to a
lesser extent; this being mainly expressed by the much decreased percentage
of CHF. These results are very well correlated by pharmacokinetic data
obtained in rabbits (6) and in mice (submitted for publication) with leu-DNR
and leu-DOX. Indeed, after an i.v. injection at equimolar doses, the
levels of total drug (intact drug + metabolites) as determined by high
performance liquid chromatography (HPLC) (7) reached in the heart are much
lower in the case of leu-DNR and leu-DOX than after DNR and DOX. The observation that leu-DNR is less toxic than leu-DOX can be explained by the
fact that the amount of DOX found in the heart after injection of leu-DOX
is greater than that of DNR after administration of leu-DNR. This is
probably related to a greater enzymatic hydrolysis of leu-DOX into DOX by
heart muscle enzymes as tested in vitro with heart homogenates.

The chemotherapeutic activity of the three leucyl anthracycline derivatives was studied after i.v. administration at equitoxic doses in DBA$_2$

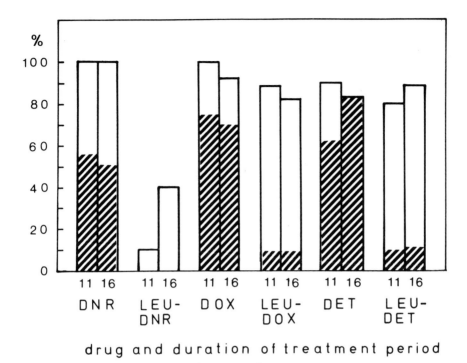

FIGURE 1. Anthracycline-induced cardiomyopathy in rabbits after chronic treatment. The percentage of rabbits surviving 60 days or more of anthracycline treatment and developing drug-induced myocardial lesions is shown. Hatched areas represent the percentage of animals that developed congestive heart failure.

mice inoculated with L1210 leukemic cells i.p., i.v., or s.c. (Table 4). The leucyl derivatives are slightly less active than are the parent compounds against the i.v. form of L1210 leukemia but are much more active on the i.p. and s.c. forms as shown by the very much increased ILS values; by the high percentage of long-term survivors; and, with the exception of leu-DOX, by a greater reduction of the s.c. tumor size.

Leu-DNR was shown to be more efficacious than was DNR on s.c.-implanted L1210 cells. This was demonstrated by administering intravenous equitoxic doses of leu-DNR and DNR and observing the effects on multiplication of L1210 cells enclosed in a Millipore diffusion chamber implanted subcutaneously. As illustrated in Figure 2, the cytoreduction was significantly higher and more prolonged after injection of leu-DNR. We think that the

Table 4. Chemotherapeutic activity of N-L-leucyl derivatives and of their
parent drugs on murinc Ll210 leukemia

Ll210 cells		Drug	Doses mg/kg per day	Increase in life span (%)	No. survivors on day 30/ total no. of mice	Average tumor diaméter (mm)	
Number	Route					day 8	day 12
10^4	i.p.	DNR	11	88	1/29	–	–
10^4	i.p.	DOX	6	120	2/10	–	–
10^4	i.p.	DET	9	92	1/ 8	–	–
10^4	i.p.	Leu-DNR	44	>247	13/19	–	–
10^4	i.p.	Leu-DOX	20	>233	5/ 9	–	–
10^4	i.p.	Leu-DET	40	>221	8/ 9	–	–
10^4	i.v.	DNR	11	66	0/37	–	–
10^4	i.v.	DOX	7	76	4/25	–	–
10^4	i.v.	DET	9	71	0/24	–	–
10^4	i.v.	Leu-DNR	44	39	0/ 7	–	–
10^4	i.v.	Leu-DOX	24	40	0/ 8	–	–
10^4	i.v.	Leu-DET	45	59	0/ 9	–	–
10^5	s.c.	DNR	11	67	3/27	0.4	2.9
10^5	s.c.	DOX	7	234	19/27	0	0
10^5	s.c.	DET	9	92	1/ 8	0	1.5
10^5	s.c.	Leu-DNR	44	215	14/25	0	0.1
10^5	s.c.	Leu-DOX	24	>228	20/29	0	0.1
10^5	s.c.	Leu-DET	45	>220	8/ 9	0	0

Note: Ll210 cells were inoculated on day 0 into DBA_2 mice. Drugs were
given i.v. on days 1 and 2 at equitoxic doses.

higher effect of the i.v.-administered drug on tumor cells residing subcutaneously or intraperitoneally could be the result of a better distribution
of the leucyl derivatives in these tissues or cavities, possibly in relation
to their greater lipophilicity.

This hypothesis is supported by the results obtained during an experiment
in which diffusion chambers were implanted s.c. and in which levels of DNR or
leu-DNR and their respective metabolites were determined by HPLC up to 20
hours after an i.v. injection of DNR and leu-DNR at equimolar doses (Figure
3). The total drug levels found in the diffusion chambers were higher after
injection of leu-DNR and most significantly so after 2 hours when the levels

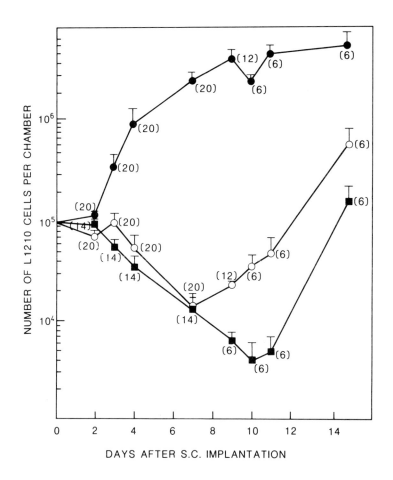

FIGURE 2. Cytotoxic effects of daunorubicin and leucyl-daunorubicin on L1210 cells growing in diffusion chambers implanted s.c. into DBA₂ mice. Two chambers were implanted s.c. on day 0 and drugs were given i.v. at equitoxic doses on days 1 and 2. (●), control animals without treatment; (O), animals treated with DNR at 11 mg/kg per day; (■), animals treated with leu-DNR at 44 mg/kg per day. Numbers between brackets indicate the number of diffusion chambers evaluated. Means ±S.D. are given.

obtained were about 3 times higher than those observed after administration of DNR.

In conclusion, leu-DNR, leu-DOX, and leu-DET seem to be prodrugs of DNR, DOX, and DET. The leucyl derivatives probably diffuse faster into the peritoneum and the subcutaneous tissues but are taken up to a lesser extent

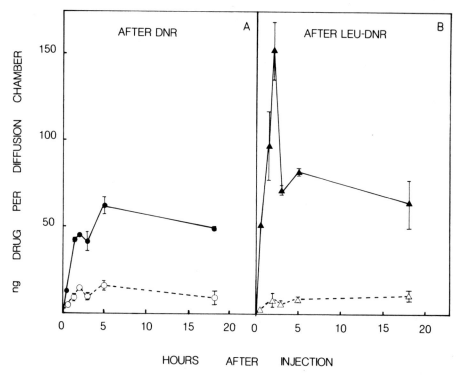

FIGURE 3. Drug accumulation and metabolism in subcutaneously implanted diffusion chambers after a single i.v. injection of leucyl-daunorubicin (leu-DNR) and daunorubicin (DNR) into mice. DBA$_2$ mice were loaded s.c. on day 0 with diffision chambers. Drugs were given i.v. on day 2 at equimolar doses corresponding to 25 mg/kg in DNR. Total drug (——) and DNR (---) were detected by HPLC and fluorometry and followed in the chambers after injection of DNR (A) or leu-DNR (B). Means ±S.D. of at least two separate assays (including an average of eight chambers per point) are given.

by tissues such as the heart and, probably, the hematopoietic system. They are probably prodrugs since, as such, their affinity for DNA is significantly reduced and they can be transformed enzymatically into their active parent compounds both intracellularly and extracellularly.

Leu-DNR, leu-DOX, and leu-DET are interesting compounds that deserve further studies on the basis of their very low experimental cardiotoxicity, their lower overall and hematopoietic toxicity, and their high chemotherapeutic activity on the i.p. and s.c. forms of L1210 leukemia.

ACKNOWLEDGMENTS

This work was supported by the Caisse Generale d'Epargne et de Retraite, Brussels, Belgium, and by Rhone-Poulenc, S.A., Paris, France.

REFERENCES

1. Masquelier, M., Baurain, R. & Trouet, A. 1980. Amino acid and dipeptide derivatives of daunorubicin. 1. Synthesis, physicochemical properties and lysosomal digestion. J. Med. Chem. 23, 1166-1170.
2. Baurain, R., Masquelier, M., Deprez-De Campeneere, D. & Trouet, A. 1980. Amino acid and dipeptide derivatives of daunorubicin. 2. Cellular pharmacology and antitumor activity on L_{1210} leukemic cells in vitro and in vivo. J. Med. Chem. 23, 1171-1174.
3. Trouet, A., Baurain, R., Deprez-De Campeneere, D., Layton, D. & Masquelier, M. 1980. DNA, liposomes and proteins as carriers for antitumoral drugs. In " Recent results in cancer research, vol.75 (G.Mathé & F.M.Muggia, eds)Springer Verlag, 229-235.
4. Schneider, Y.-J., Baurain, R., Zenebergh, A. & Trouet, A.1979. DNA-binding parameters of daunorubicin and doxorubicin in the conditions used for studying the interaction of anthracycline-DNA complexes with cells in vitro. Cancer Chemother. Pharmacol. 2, 7-10.
5. Huybrechts, M. & Trouet, A. 1980. Comparative toxicity of detorubicin and doxorubicin free and DNA-bound, for hemopoietic stem cells. Cancer Chemother. Pharmacol. 5, 79-82.
6. Jaenke, R.S., Deprez-De Campeneere, D. & Trouet, A. 1980. Cardiotoxicity and comparative pharmacokinetics of six anthracyclines in the rabbit. Cancer Res. 40, 3530-3536.
7. Baurain, R., Deprez-De Campeneere, D. & Trouet, A. 1979. Determination of daunorubicin, doxorubicin and their fluorescent metabolites by high pressure liquid chromatography : plasma levels in DBA_2 mice. Cancer Chemother. Pharmacol. 2 , 11-14.

ALTERNATIVE METHODS OF DRUG DELIVERY

K. E. ROGERS, E. A. FORSSEN, AND Z. A. TÖKLÈS*

1. INTRODUCTION

Research in our laboratory has focused on new methods for improving the therapeutic efficacy of anthracyclines by overcoming host toxicities and increasing their action against sensitive and resistant tumor types. We now summarize our findings from two novel methods of drug delivery. The first approach utilized liposome-concealed Adriamycin (ADR), which delivers the drug by mechanisms other than those normally used. The second method provides multiple drug-binding sites by covalently coupling ADR to a polymer support.

2. MATERIALS AND METHODS

2.1. Preparation of liposomes

Methods for preparing ADR liposomes have been described in earlier reports (1,2). Briefly, a complex of phosphatidylcholine (PC) and ADR is formed by addition of a solution of the drug in 0.077 $\underline{M}$ NaCl to the dried lipid in a 2:1 molar ratio (PC:ADR). After sonication, this mixture is then added to a dried mixture of PC:phosphatidylserine:cholesterol at a molar ratio of 0.6:0.2:0.3 per mole of ADR. Following further sonication, liposome-entrapped ADR is separated from free drug by gel filtration on Sephadex G-50. Electron micrographs were produced following the negative staining procedure of Enoch and Strittmatter (3). One drop of liposome suspension was placed on a Formvar coated grid. Thirty seconds later, one drop of staining solution (1% uranil acetate, pH 5) was added and left to stand 1 minute. The solution was drained off and the grids air-dried prior to examination on the electron microscope.

---

*Author to whom correspondence should be directed.

2.2. Preparation of polyglutaraldehyde microspheres (PGLs)

The methods of Margel and Rembaum (4) were used to prepare unbound PGLs. After extensive washing to remove unreacted glutaraldehyde, the PGLs were passed through a 1.2-micron Millipore filter disc. The filtrate was collected, resuspended in 20% bovine serum albumin, and centrifuged at 88 x g for 10 minutes. The pelleted microspheres were resuspended in double distilled water and evaluated for size distribution using laser flow cytometry and scanning electron microscopy.

2.3. Coupling of Adriamycin

A solution of Adriamycin-hydrochloride was prepared by dissolving 6 mg of the drug in 5 ml of double distilled water adjusted to pH 6.5 with 0.01 N hydrochloric acid. One hundred mg of unbound PGLs were added and allowed to react with the drug for 2 hours at room temperature. The reaction was stopped by centrifuging the microspheres at 9500 x g for 30 minutes, and the pellet was washed with distilled water until spectrophotometric analysis demonstrated that no additional free ADR could be removed. Coupled microspheres (ADR-PGLs) were then treated with 0.5% NP-40 for 2 hours. After the detergent had been removed, ADR-PGLs were treated for 1 hour with liposomes containing phosphatidylserine, phosphatidylcholine, and cholesterol in a 2:6:3 molar ratio. Covalently bound ADR was quantitated by difference after the concentration of unbound ADR remaining in the reaction solution and in each subsequent wash had been determined.

3. RESULTS

3.1. Liposome-entrapped Adriamycin

Following the administration of free or entrapped ADR, levels of the drug and its fluorescent metabolites were determined for plasma and cardiac tissue as shown in Tables 1 and 2. Despite the increased plasma levels of ADR-equivalents produced by liposome-mediated delivery, the cardiac tissue of animals treated with ADR-liposomes accumulated less fluorescent material than did the tissue of those animals treated with equal amounts of the free drug. However, because of the high initial rate of drug uptake, the peak level of fluorescence was greater in heart tissue exposed to free ADR. At 24 hours, the cardiac tissue from both treatment groups was nearly equivalent to the background fluorescence of untreated tissue samples.

The antitumor activities of free and encapsulated Adriamycin were compared

Table 1. Plasma levels of ADR fluorescent equivalents for free and liposome-entrapped drug

Time following injection (hours)	Plasma concentration (microgram/ml ± SEM) [a]	
	Free ADR	Liposome ADR
0.5	1.06 + .03	5.09 + .75
1.0	0.55 ± .01	3.10 ± .07
2.0	0.56 ± .02	1.45 ± .08
4.0	0.36 ± .01	0.60 ± .03
8.0	0.26 ± .01	0.48 ± .04
24.0	0.06 ± .00	0.11 ± .02

a. Plasma levels of ADR fluorescent equivalents in mice following intravenous injection of the drug either in free or liposome-entrapped form at a dose of 5 mg/kg. Each point indicates the average value for duplicate determinations from four animals. Values are in ADR equivalents.

Table 2. Cardiac tissue levels of ADR fluorescent equivalents for free and liposome-entrapped drug .

Time following injection (hours)	Cardiac tissue concentration (ng/mg ± SEM) [a]	
	Free ADR	Liposome ADR
0.5	7.53 + .73	5.63 + .59
1.0	8.83 + 1.09	5.10 + .54
4.0	4.72 + .89	1.66 + .25
8.0	2.40 + .24	1.24 + .27
12.0	1.22 + .54	0.39 + .24
24.0	1.1 + .60	0.29 + .14

a. Cardiac tissue levels of ADR fluorescent equivalents in mice following intravenous injection of 5 mg/kg ADR either in the free or liposome-entrapped form. Each point represents the average value from four animals. Values are in terms of ADR equivalents.

for their ability to suppress the growth of solid sarcoma-180 as shown in Table 3. Three intravenous treatments were given at 1-week intervals in Swiss Webster mice bearing the tumors as subcutaneous implants. At 24 days postimplantation, liposome-entrapped ADR appeared equally effective as free drug. ADR-liposomes limited tumor growth to the same extent as did the free drug, 33% of the untreated control values. Free drug mixed with empty

Table 3. Activity of free and liposomal ADR against sarcoma-180 tumor

| Days after tumor implantation | Tumor volume (mm^3) $\pm$ SEM[a] | | |
	Saline controls	Free ADR	Liposome ADR
9	655 + 190	522 + 53	429 + 72
17	1347 + 503	872 + 99	745 + 185
23	1495 + 541	560 + 141	632 + 318

a. Antitumor activities of free and liposomal ADR were compared using solid sarcoma-180 tumor. Swiss Webster mice received three courses of intravenous ADR therapy (5 mg/kg) at 1-week intervals beginning 7 days after subcutaneous tumor implantation. Both the free and entrapped ADR demonstrated significant activity over that of the saline controls (P = <0.05).

liposomes was less effective than either entrapped or free drug alone and was able to limit tumor growth to only 71% of control.

The in vivo activities of free and entrapped ADR against Lewis lung solid tumor are compared in Table 4. ADR-liposomes demonstrated much greater anti-tumor activity than did the free drug. In terms of volume, the tumors in the ADR-liposome treatment group were inhibited to 33% and 43% of controls at 20 and 23 days, respectively. Free ADR, on the other hand, was able to limit tumor growth to only 52% and 63%. Equivalent treatment with free drug plus empty liposomes demonstrated very little inhibitory activity. Tumor growth in this group was not significantly different from that of controls (P >0.2).

Control mice immunized with hRBCs and receiving only normal saline were able to produce a marked titer of hemagglutinating antibodies as indicated in Table 5. Administration of free ADR, 5 mg/kg at 24 and 48 hours after each immunization significantly reduced the levels of circulating antibodies (P <.002). In contrast, the administration of an identical regimen of liposome-entrapped drug produced no significant loss in humoral response (P >0.1).

3.2. Polymer-coupled Adriamycin

Synthesis of PGLs yielded a population of microspheres with diameters ranging from 2.1 x 10^3 Å to approximately 1.2 x 10^4 Å. Low-speed centri-fugation through 20% bovine serum albumin allowed PGLs smaller than 2.5 x 10^3 Å to be removed. The mean diameter of the remaining PGLs was estimated by laser flow cytometry to be 4500 Å, and this size was confirmed

Table 4. Activity of free and liposomal ADR against Lewis lung carcinoma

Days after tumor implantation	Tumor volume $(mm^2) \pm SEM$[a]		
	Saline	Free ADR	Liposome ADR
8	78 + 39	91 + 38	14 + 7
15	78 + 224	602 + 89	411 + 122
20	2341 + 598	1236 + 217	745 + 158
23	2719 + 586	1722 + 259	1162 + 273

a. C57Bl/6 mice received three i.p. doses of ADR (5 mg/kg) at 7-day intervals beginning at 2 days postimplantation.

Table 5. Titers of hemagglutinating antibody measuring Adriamycin suppression of immune responses

Mode of treatment	Maximum serum dilution able to cause hemagglutination $\pm$ SEM[a]
Free ADR	1: 1.33 + 0.41
Liposomal ADR	1: 146 + 38
Saline controls	1: 214 + 70

a. Swiss Webster mice were tested for their ability to form hemagglutinating antibodies to xenogeneic red blood cells following ADR therapy. Mice receive 0.1 ml of a 10% red blood cell suspension in PBS as a subcutaneous injection. Mice were then treated at 24 and 48 hours later with 5 mg/kg of free liposome-entrapped ADR of saline. One week later, the immunization and drug treatments were repeated. Titers are the greatest serum dilutions capable of the complete agglutination of a 2% suspension of red blood cells.

by scanning electron microscopy.

Following fractionation, the PGLs were used for ADR coupling. Initial binding efficiency was 101 nmol ADR/l mg PGL. Noncovalently bound ADR was removed by the subsequent detergent and liposome washes. The final coupling efficiency of the covalently bound ADR was 43 ± 7 nmol ADR/l mg PGL. This figure represents approximately 9.7×10^6 molecules of ADR bound to a microsphere with an average diameter of 4500 Å.

Cells incubated with ADR-PGLs, equivalent to 1 μM ADR, released less than 0.08% of the covalently bound drug over a 24-hour period. Increasing the time of incubation to 96 hours did not increase the amount of ADR releas. Control studies demonstrated that 100% of the free ADR can be recovered with the extraction techniques used.

Cytostatic activities of the free drug and ADR-PGLs were evaluated by IC$_{50}$ determinations. Five cell lines were used to test for the cytostatic activity (Table 6). Cytostatic activity of covalently coupled ADR was at least equal to that of the free drug using the sensitive cell lines CCRF-CEM, L1210, and S-180. The ADR-PGLs were approximately 10 times more active than was free ADR for the resistant cell lines CCRF-CEM/Vbl 100 and CCRF-CEM/Vbl 500.

Table 6. Cytostatic activity of free ADR and ADR-PGLs

Cell lines	IC$_{50}$ (μM) free ADR	IC$_{50}$ (μM) PGL-ADR
L1210	0.028	0.015
S-180	0.023	0.056
CCRF-CEM	0.011	0.012
CCRF-CEM/Vbl 500	0.32	0.020
CCRF-CEM/Vbl 100	0.39	0.020

Note: The IC$_{50}$ values represent the average of three determinations ± .1% S.D.

4. DISCUSSION

The first set of experiments utilized ADR entrapped in artificial lipid vesicles. The administration of these ADR vesicles was shown to produce an increase in the plasma levels of the drug and/or its fluorescent metabolites. The greatest difference in plasma levels occurred in the first 4 hours after injection during the distribution phase. This difference was probably due to an increased half-life in circulation. It could also have occurred if the entrapped material were metabolized to fluorescent compounds to a greater extent than was the free drug. Beyond 4 hours, the plasma fluorescence began to decline at the same rate for both free and entrapped ADR. The same observation could be obtained if the liposomes became leaky in circulation and lost the entrapped material. Earlier experiments (1) indicated that ADR liposomes would lose only about 11% of the entrapped material over a 4-hour period when incubated in plasma at 37° C; however, they may actually be less stable under in vivo conditions. Although liposome entrapment did appear to eliminate most heart toxicity for even high doses (2), cardiac tissue continued to be associated with significant, though lower, levels of drug. This may be due to uptake by cells other than cardiac myocytes such as

capillary endothelial cells. It could also be caused by a different subcellular localization of the entrapped drug at sites not associated with
toxicity.

An earlier investigation compared free ADR and entrapped ADR for antitumor activity against ascitic leukemias using intraperitoneal injections (2).
This represented a situation where liposomes were administered directly to the
tumor cells. For further evaluation of antineoplastic activity, ADR-liposomes
were used in treatment of sarcoma-180 and Lewis lung solid tumors. The
sarcoma-180 tumor normally responds well to intravenous ADR therapy (5). At
equal dosage levels, liposome-entrapped drug displayed the full antineoplastic
activity of free ADR. When tested against Lewis lung tumor, ADR-liposomes
demonstrated greater activity than did the free drug. This is significant
since the Lewis lung carcinoma responds only poorly to free ADR, thus indicating that liposome-entrapped ADR may be superior to free drug for
treatment of some resistant tumors (6).

Adriamycin exerts its greatest suppressive effect on antibody formation
when it is administered after antigenic challenge, indicating that it may be
acting on lymphoid cells in their proliferative state (7). This study
demonstrated that the encapsulation of ADR in anionic liposomes clearly prevents suppression of antibody production. The mechanism for this effect is
not clear.

In an earlier study (1), no distinct difference in spleen drug levels
could be seen at 1 hour. By 4 hours, however, animals treated with liposome-
entrapped ADR did show a significant decrease in spleen levels. Only total
drug was estimated; thus, any metabolic differences caused by liopsome entrapment were not quantitated. Elevated drug levels in bone marrow and
lymphoid tissues do not necessarily correlate with immune toxicity. Studies
with actinomycin-D liposomes revealed that aqueous phase vesicles protected
both bone marrow and spleen without reducing the amount of drug in these
tissues (8); thus, liposomes may spare the immune system by a mechanism
other than that of the reduction of tissue drug levels. Subcellular distribution and metabolism of the entrapped drug may contribute to the observed differences in toxicity.

The subcellular site or sites of action for Adriamycin have not been
conclusively determined (9). Although binding to DNA has been indicated
as a principle site (10), others may include membrane phospholipids (11) and
mitochondrial enzymes (12). Our experiments have indicated that it is pos-

sible to separate the immune toxic and cardiotoxic effects of ADR from its antitumor activity. This finding suggests that different cellular sites, such as plasma membranes, may exist for these responses. Future studies on the subcellular distribution and/or metabolism of free and entrapped drug may reveal important differences that can be used in the design of new anthracycline analogs with increased therapeutic benefit.

The second system of drug delivery utilized Adriamycin covalently bound to a solid phase support. This system was chosen to study effects of the drug on plasma membranes of tumor cells. Theoretically, the action of a drug coupled to a support would be limited to cell-surface interactions, thus eliminating intracellular effects. Polyglutaraldehyde microspheres were chosen as the drug carrier because they are easily synthesized in a variety of diameters. In addition, PGLs possess functional aldehyde groups which provide a coupling site for ADR. The release studies demonstrated that viable cells cannot remove a significant amount of the covalently bound ADR from microspheres. These studies, joined with the fact that the ADR-PGLs are too large to enter the nucleus through the nuclear pore (13), lead to the conclusion that the coupled drug must act at a site other than DNA. The site proposed for the pharmacological action of ADR-PGLs is the plasma membrane. Supportive evidence includes scanning electron microscopy, which visualizes changes in the cell surface. The most striking change is blebbing, which occurs within 24 hours after exposure to the ADR-PGLs. Blebbing is the result of separation of the microfilamentous cortex from the cell's periphery (14). Since the assembly of microtubules and microfilaments are required for endocytosis of large particles, blebbing significantly reduces the possibility of internalized microspheres and increases the probability that the coupled microspheres must act at the cell surface. In addition, preliminary fluorescence microscopy studies indicate that the microspheres are localized predominantly at the cell surface.

It is significant that ADR coupled to PGL retains its full activity in the cytostatic assays with sensitive cell lines. More notable is the fact that resistant cell lines are at least 10 times more sensitive to the polymer-bound drug than they are to free ADR. Since the drug is attached to a solid support, the actual number of ADR molecules which is available for binding to the plasma membrane is less than the concentration values suggest. This is a direct result of steric effects and implies that the cytostatic activity of covalently bound ADR is even greater than the IC_{50} values indicate. There are two mechanisms to account for the increased activity. First, free ADR undergoes metabolic degradation and inactivation in subcellular compartments subsequent to internalization. Assuming that the ADR-PGLs are localized entirely at the cell surface, the covalently bound drug would not be subject to this type of degradation. Also, it is conceivable that if ADR-PGLs are internalized, the polymer bound drug would not be available to the sub-cellular compartments in the identical manner of the free drug. The final result would be a decreased rate of metabolic breakdown and continuous perturbation of the cell surface.

Finally, this mode of drug delivery provides multiple and repetitious sites for drug-cell interactions. Evidence suggests that one type of ADR resistance may be the result of a decreased affinity for the drug (15). The repetitious interactions of ADR-PGLs would be able to overcome that type of resistance. Results obtained with the resistant cell lines are consistent with this interpretation. Initial studies with ADR-PGLs are promising in terms of the cytostatic activity that can be obtained with the drug-microsphere complexes. It is noteworthy that the multiple interactions of ADR-PGL may be able to overcome various types of drug resistance. Future studies wil localize the site of action of the ADR-PGLs and investigate their cytotoxic activity and activity in vitro and in vivo.

5. ACKNOWLEDGMENT

The authors wish to express their appreciation to the Weingart Foundation for its generous support.

REFERENCES

1. Forssen EA, Tökès ZA. 1979. In vitro and in vivo studies with adriamyc: liposomes. Biochem. Biophys. Res. Commun. 91: 1295-1301.
2. Forssen EA, Tökès ZA. 1981. Use of anionic liposomes for the reduction chronic doxorubicin induced cardiotoxicity. 1981. Proc. Nat. Acad. Sc: USA 78: 1873-1877.
3. Enoch HG, Strittmatter P. 1979. Formation and properties of 1000 Å diameter, single bilayer phospholipid vesicles. Proc. Nat. Acad. Sci. USA 76: 145-149.
4. Margel S, Zisblatt S, Rembaum A. 1979. Polyglutaraldehyde: A new re-agent for coupling proteins to microspheres and for labeling cell-surfac receptors. II. Simplified labeling method by means of non-magnetic and magnetic polyglutaraldehyde microspheres. J. Immunol. Methods 28: 341-353.
5. Casazza AM. 1979. Experimental evaluation of anthracycline analogs. Cancer Treat. Rep. 63: 835-844.
6. Carter SK. 1980. Clinical evaluation of analogs. III. Anthracyclines

Cancer Chemother. Pharmacol. 4: 5-10.

7. Vecchi A, Mantovani A, Tagliablue A, Spreafico F. 1976. A characterization of the immunosuppressive activity of adriamycin and daunomycin on
humoral antibody production and tumor allograft rejection. Cancer Res.
36: 1222-1227.

8. Rahman YE, Hanson WR, Bharucha J, Ainsworth EJ, Jaroslow BN. 1978.
Mechanisms of reduction of antitumor drug toxicity by liposome encapsulation. Ann. NY Acad. Sci. 308: 325-342.

9. Di Marco A. 1975. Adriamycin: mode and mechanism of action. Cancer
Chemother. Rep., part 3, 6: 91-106.

10. Nakata Y, Hopfinger AJ. 1980. Predicted mode of intercalation of
doxorubicin with dinucleotide dimers. Biochem. Biophys. Res. Comm.
95: 583-588.

11. Goormaghtigh E, Chatelan P, Caspers J, Ruysschaert JM. 1980. Evidence
of a complex between Adriamycin derivatives and cardiolipin: Possible
role in cardiotoxicity. Biochem. Pharmacol. 29: 3003-3010.

12. Thayer WS. 1977. Adriamycin stimulated superoxide formation in submitochondrial particles. Chem. Biol. Interact. 19: 265-278.

13. Flickenger CD, Brown JC, Kutchai HC, Ogilvie J. 1979. Medical cell
biology. Philadelphia, W. B. Saunders Co.

14. Condeelis J. 1979. Isolation of concanavalin A caps during various
stages of formation and their association; ith actin and myosin. J.
Cell. Biol. 80: 751-754.

15. Gaudio LA, Yesair DW, Taylor RF. 1980. Cancer chemotherapeutic drug
binding to macromolecular lipids from L1210 leukemia cells and to known
lipids. Proc. Amer. Assoc. Cancer Res. 21: 18.

SECTION 4

CARDIOTOXICITY

INTRODUCTION

C. E. MYERS

This section is devoted to the mechanism of cardiac toxicity and to its clinical assessment. Because of the constraints of time and resources, I have made no attempt to present the complete spectrum of opinion on this issue but, rather, have focused on recent investigations which seem to have far-reaching implications.

In terms of mechanisms, this section focuses almost entirely on the free radical hypothesis. Some justification for this emphasis should be provided. Although the mechanism of the cardiac toxicity is far from settled, the free radical hypothesis has stimulated much discussion and research. As a result, over the past 2 years, a significant proportion of the papers published on the mechanism of cardiac toxicity has focused positively or negatively on this hypothesis. Thus, the chapters in this section are merely reflecting the intense activity in this area. There are, however, other schools of thought about the mechanism of cardiac toxicity that warrant comment.

Many of the anthracyclines, including doxorubicin and daunorubicin, bind avidly to cell membranes. Duarte-Karim et al. (1), Tritton et al. (2), Goormaghtigh et al. (3), and Mikkelsen et al. (4) have studied this process in some detail. It is now known that doxorubicin will bind to cardiolipin, one of the phospholipids in cell membranes. Tritton has pointed out that cardiolipin content is high in the membranes of transformed cells and cardiac mitochondria. This has led Tritton (2) to propose that tumor response and cardiac toxicity result from this cardiolipin binding. This proposal is very attractive for a number of reasons. First, altered membrane function could

well explain many of the observations which have been made
about the cardiac toxicity. For example, doxorubicin causes
alterations in sodium and calcium distribution in cardiac
tissue. This phenomenon could well be secondary to altered
membrane function. Second, there are certain anthracyclines
that bind poorly to DNA, yet are toxic for tumor cells. AD32
is an example. Cell killing through a membrane-dependent
mechanism could well explain the action of drugs such as this.
The major problem posed by this hypothesis is that of explaining
why doxorubicin membrane binding might be toxic for the cell.

The other hypothesis of considerable merit is that of Folkers
and coworkers (5,6) that doxorubicin affects ubiquinone function.
Ubiquinone plays a major role in cardiac mitochondrial ATP
generation and is an important cofactor for a number of enzymes.
Folkers and coworkers have demonstrated a competitive relationship between doxorubicin and ubiquinone for these enzymes.
Further, Bertazzoli et al. (7) have demonstrated that ubiquinone administration lessens the cardiac toxicity of doxorubicin
in rabbits. A clinical trial is proceeding based upon these
observations, the results of which will be of interest.

As a final comment, it is important to point out that none
of the current hypotheses fully explains all of the properties
of doxorubicin cardiomyopathy, and much work remains before
a full understanding of this phenomenon is achieved.

REFERENCES
1. Duarte-Karin M, Ruysschaert, JM, and Hildebrand J.
    1976. Biochem. Biophys. Res. Comm. 71: 658.
2. Tritton TQ, Murphree, GA, and Sartorelli, AC. 1978.
    Biochem. Biophys. Res. Comm. 84: 802.
3. Goormaghtigh E, Chatelain P, Caspers J, and Ruzsschaert
    JM. 1980. Biochem. Biophys. Acta 597: 1.
4. Mikkelsen, QB, Lin PS, Wallach DF. 1977. J. Mol.
    Med. 2: 33.
5. Folkers K, Liu M, Watanabe T, Porter TH. 1977. Biochem.
    Biophys. Res. Comm. 77: 1536.
6. Folkers K, Choe JV, and Combs AB. 1978. Proc. Nat.
    Acad. Sci. 75: 5178.
7. Bertazzoli C, Sala L, Solica E, and Ghione M. 1975.
    IRCS Med. Sci.: Biochem; Cancer; Cardiovasic; Hematol.
    Pharmacol. 3: 468.

THE ROLE OF FREE RADICAL DAMAGE IN THE GENESIS OF DOXORUBICIN CARDIAC TOXICITY

C. E. MYERS

1. HISTORICAL

Between 1975 and 1977, Sato and coworkers (1-3) published a series
of papers that documented the conversion of daunorubicin and doxorubicin
to semiquinone radicals by the microsomal enzyme P450 reductase. In
addition, these workers showed that these semiquinone radicals could, in
turn, reduce oxygen to superoxide radicals. In 1977, we put forth the
hypothesis that the cardiac toxicity of these agents might be the result
of oxygen-radical generation in cardiac tissue (4). In that same year,
Thayer (5) showed that doxorubicin stimulated superoxide production
from submitochondrial particles from cardiac mitochondria, and Bachur (6)
showed oxygen-radical production from cardiac sarcosomes. In the years
that have followed, these observations have been extended and the free
radical hypothesis now stands as the one that most nearly accounts for
the characteristics of this cardiomyopathy. The chemistry of anthracycline
free radicals will be discussed in other chapters of this book. Briefly,
however, the semiquinone radicals will react rapidly with oxygen to yield
superoxide radicals. When oxygen availability is limited, these radicals
can undergo a rearrangement (halftime of 1 second) to an aglycone free
radical that appears to be capable of alkylating (7,8) both proteins
and DNA. Therefore, in considering tissue damage from anthracycline
radicals, one must consider not only the damage caused by superoxide
and its reaction products, but also that which results directly
from the reactivity of the drug radical.

2. SOURCES OF CARDIAC SEMIQUINONE FREE RADICAL GENERATION

There are multiple sites for anthracycline radical generation
in cardiac tissue. First, there is a background rate of spontaneous

radical generation which occurs with doxorubicin in aqueous solution
(9). Cardiac mitochondria probably represent the major site of enzymatic
radical generation. The cardiac mitochondria represent approximately
50% of the heart muscle by weight and volume. Thayer (5), Bachur (6), and
most recently Doroshow (10) have shown that doxorubicin will cause a
five fold increase in cardiac mitochondrial superoxide production.
Doroshow (11) and Bachur (6) have also shown that sarcosomes, derived
from the sarcoplasmic reticulum, also produce superoxide upon exposure
to doxorubicin. Finally, Pan et al. (12) have shown that pig heart
NADH-cytochrome C reductase produces superoxide in the presence of
doxorubicin.

Although these enzymatic sites of radical formation have been
demonstrated, direct proof of radical formation in the intact heart
is lacking. The nearest approach to this has been the recent
demonstration of oxygen-radical generation in heart tissue slices (13).
In a less direct fashion, we (4) and others (14,15) have detected evidence
of oxygen-radical-mediated damage to cardiac lipids in animals and man.

3. CARDIAC DEFENSE AGAINST FREE RADICAL ATTACK

The enzymes known to be able to convert doxorubicin to a free
radical include not only those mentioned above, but also xanthine
oxidase. Thus, the liver, which possess mitochondria, xanthine
oxidase and microsomal P450 reductase in abundance, is richly endowed
with the capacity to form anthracycline free radicals. In spite of
this, heart but not liver is damaged by doxorubicin. Why is the
heart damaged but not the liver after doxorubicin exposure? Results
from our laboratory and others suggest that this difference may be
explained by the ability of the two tissues to defend themselves against
free radical attack. Superoxide radicals are detoxified in a two-step
process in which they are first converted to hydrogen peroxide and
then to water. Superoxide dismutase is responsible for the conversion
of superoxide to hydrogen peroxide. Both catalase and glutathione
peroxidase convert hydrogen peroxide to water. We and others (16, 5)
have shown that hearts of mice, rats and rabbits essentially lack
catalase; whereas liver represents a rich source of this enzyme.
Superoxide dimutase content of heart is between one-half and one-
fourth that of liver.

The other major enzyme in this series is glutathione peroxidase. This enzyme uses reduced glutathione to reduce hydrogen peroxide and lipid peroxides to water and lipid alcohols, respectively. There are two forms of this enzyme. Gluthathione peroxidase I is a selenium-containing enzyme found in the cytosol of cells and in the mitochondrial matrix of liver cells (17). Glutathione peroxidase II is an enzyme discovered by us in the process of examining cardiac tissue radical defenses (18). It differs from glutathione peroxidase I in that it is localized to the mitochondrial membrane and is not dependent upon selenium. In examining the subcellular distribution of glutathione peroxidase I and II in heart and liver, we (18) have discovered striking differences. Mitochondrial matrix glutathione peroxidase I is present in high concentration in liver mitochondria but completely absent from cardiac mitochondria. The mitochondrial membrane glutathione peroxidase II is equivalent in the two tissues. These differences take on added significance when one considers the importance of mitochondria as a source for doxorubicin-induced oxygen radicals. Finally, the cytosolic glutathione peroxidase I activity is equal in the two tissues. However, we have found that doxorubicin leads to a rapid decline in the activity of the cytosolic glutathione peroxidase I (16). Revis and Marusic (19) have shown that this decline in glutathione peroxidase I becomes persistent in the rabbit chronic cardiac toxicity model. Thus, after doxorubicin, cardiac tissue is left with superoxide dismutase and the membrane glutathione peroxidase II as the only mechanisms of oxygen radical detoxification. Are these changes in glutathione peroxidase I significant? There is circumstantial evidence that suggests that these changes may be critical for the heart. As mentioned above, glutathione peroxidase I is selenium dependent. Indeed, the activity of this enzyme in mammalian cells in general, and in the heart specifically (20), is strictly dependent upon the selenium content of the diet. In this regard, it is interesting to note that one of the consistent manifestations of selenium deficiency is cardiomyopathy (21), presumably because hydrogen peroxide is a normal byproduct of cardiac metabolism (22). From this, one might also expect that selenium deficiency might result in increased sensitivity to doxorubicin. We have shown that that is the case (16). Thus, the evidence suggests that doxorubicin increases myocardial superoxide and hydrogen peroxide generation at a time when it also abrogates a major intracelluar defense against free radical attack. These results also suggest that the selective cardiac toxicity of the anthracycline results from three factors: (1) the ability of anthracyclines to elicit oxygen radical production from cardiac mitochondria and sarcoplasmic reticulum; (2) the absence in cardiac tissue of catalase and mitochondrial matrix glutathione peroxidase I and (3) the ability of doxorubicin to decrease the activity of cardiac cytosolic glutathione peroxidase I.

4. RELATIONSHIP BETWEEN FREE RADICAL PRODUCTION AND THE PATHOPHYSIOLOGY OF DOXORUBICIN CARDIAC TOXICITY.

How well does the free radical hypothesis account for the specific characteristics of the anthracycline cardiomyopathy? The cardiomyopathy is characterized by destruction of the actin—myosin complex, dilation of the sarcoplasmic reticulum and abnormalities in the myocardial calcium pools. The dilation of the sarcoplasmic reticulum can be easily explained by damage to this membraneous structure caused by anthracycline—stimulated radical production at this site (11). The alterations in calcium pool handling are to be expected because the two most important sites for regulation of myocardial calcium pools are the sarcoplasmic reticulum and the mitochondria, both sites of anthracycline—induced radical formation. The elevated calcium concentration seen in doxorubicin—treated hearts (23) may also in turn have pathologic consequences. Heart tissue contains proteases which are activated by calcium (24) and which might then lead to increased destruction of the actin—myosin complex.

One of the interesting aspects of this cardiac toxicity is that it is cumulative in nature and that the incidence of cardiomyopathy increases as a geometric rather than linear function of total cumulative dose administered. In this regard, the observation of Revis and Marusic (19) that the depression in glutathione peroxidase I is chronic may be relevant. A chronic progressive decline may lead to greater sensitivity of the heart to oxygen-radical-mediated damage as the cumulative total dose increases.

If the scenario outlined above is correct, then anthracyclines that do not act as good substrates for the free radical generating enzymes should be less cardiotoxic. In this regard, it is interesting to note that aclacinomycin A and 5-imino-daunorubicin are relatively inactive as substrates for the free radical generating enzymes and are much less cardiotoxic than doxorubicin (25-27).

5. USE OF FREE RADICAL SCAVENGERS

The foregoing discussion provides the rationale to attempt to prevent cardiac toxicity by the use of substances which scavenge free radicals. Before reviewing this use of specific free radical scavengers, I believe it important to point out that such substances are not all equivalent They differ significantly in the specific radicals scavenged, in their pharmacology and tissue distribution and thus should not all be expected to be of equal effectiveness.

5.1 TOCOPHEROL

Historically, this was the first free radical scavenger with reported activity. In our initial paper proposing the free radical hypothesis, we noted that tocopherol lessened the acute cardiac damage seen in mice after doxorubicin (4). This activity of tocopherol in the acute models of cardiac damage has since been repeatedly confirmed (28-33). However, repeated attempts to test tocopherol in the chronic models of doxorubicin cardiac toxicity have revealed little or no protective effect (34-36).

In vitro, tocopherol has been shown (6) to affect dramatically anthracycline-stimulated oxygen consumption in the P450 reductase system. In addition, tocopherol has been shown to block doxorubicin induced peroxidation in human platelets. From this, one can infer that the less than optimal activity of tocopherol in vivo is not because it lacks chemical reactivity with the radicals produced. The problem may well lie in other characteristics of this vitamin. First, it is a lipid soluble substance with essentially no solubility in aqueous medium. In the body, it resides almost entirely in cell membranes and appears to exert its action selectively within those membranes.

It is not clear what activity, if any, might be anticipated against radicals generated in the aqueous phase of the cell. Also, it is not clear how much access tocopherol has to the sarcoplasmic reticulum and mitochondria of heart muscle, the two known sites of radical generation.

5.2 THIOLS

Gamma radiation is probably the best studied example of free-radical-mediated tissue injury, and a large number of radioprotective compounds have been produced that are thought to act as radical scavengers. Although radioprotective compounds may belong to general classes, by far and away the largest number of active compounds are thiols (37). As opposed to tocopherol, these compounds are water soluble. In addition, thiols might be expected to scavenge drug-free radicals either through the formation of drug-thiol adducts or through thiol donation of a hydride cap to the drug radical. Thus, thiols prevent hepatic necrosis in acetaminophen overdose via formation of drug-thiol adducts (38).

For all of these reasons, thiols have been examined for their ability to prevent doxorubicin-induced cardiac damage. This work has been performed both by our laboratory and Oates's group (39-43). It has been shown that thiols such as N-acetyl-cysteine lessen whole animal toxicity in acute and chronic toxicity models and completely prevent any acute cardiac damage. These agents have no effect on the antitumor efficacy of doxorubicin. The basis for this cardioprotective action seems to be a selective uptake of N-acetyl-cysteine by heart muscle as opposed to other tissues such as liver. The only controversy in this area at present is whether doxorubicin depresses cardiac reduced glutathione pools. Wang et al. (30) and Olson et al. (40) both report drops in cardiac-reduced glutathione after doxorubicin. However, our group (44) and Boor (45) have found that cardiac-reduced glutathione pools show a marked diurnal variation and that, when this is taken into consideration, doxorubicin does not significantly alter the reduced glutathione pools.

At NCI, we have elected to initiate a clinical trial testing the effect of N-acetyl-cysteine on the cardiac toxicity of doxorubicin.

The trial involves a randomization between doxorubicin alone and N-acetyl-cysteine plus doxorubicin with the cardiac toxicity monitored via radionuclide cineangiography. At present, close to 40 patients have been randomized on the trial. Unfortunately, less than a third of the patients have responded to doxorubicin. As a result, only 12 patients are evaluable at greater than 300 mg/m^2 total dose, 6 in each arm. At present there is no statistically significant difference between the two groups, but the results are promising. Patients in the doxorubicin-only group have lost their capacity to increase ejection fraction with exercise. In contrast, the group receiving doxorubicin plus N-acetyl-cysteine have preserved the normal increase in ejection fraction with exercise.

5.3   ICRF 159 AND 187

Herman et al.(46-48) have shown that these relatively nonpolar derivatives of EDTA lessen the cardiac toxicity of doxorubicin and daunorubicin. Wang et al.(49) have also shown that ICRF187 affects gastrointestinal toxicity of daunomycin. As an added benefit, ICRF 159 and 187 appear to enhance the antitumor efficacy of this compound (50). At first, these observations seemed unrelated to the free radical mechanisms discussed above. Recently, however, we (51) have demonstrated that doxorubicin-iron chelate has the capacity to bind to the surface of cell membranes and there catalyze the reduction of oxygen to superoxide radicals by glutathione. The result is rapid membrane destruction. ICRF 187 can abstract iron from the doxorubicin iron complex and prevent this course of events. In a related study, Kappus et al.(52) have shown that coadministration of iron and doxorubicin leads to far more lipid peroxidation than either iron or doxorubicin alone. Taken together, these results suggest that doxorubicin-iron complexes do form in vivo with toxic consequences which can be prevented by ICRF 187 and perhaps ICRF 159. One of the major questions now will be to try to determine which of the many mechanisms of anthracycline-induced radical formation are relevant in vivo.

304

REFERENCES

1. Handa K, Sato S. 1975, Gann 66: 43.
2. Handa K, Sato S. 1976, Gann 67: 523.
3. Sato S, Iwaizumi M, Handa K, Tamura Y. 1977, Gann 68, 603
4. Myers CE, Liss RH, Ifrim J. 1977, Science 197: 165.
5. Thayer WS. 1977, Chem-Biol Interactions 19: 265.
6. Bachur NR, Gordon SL, Gee MV. 1977, Mol Pharmacol 13: 901.
7. Sinha BK. 1980, Chem-Biol Interactions 30: 67.
8. Ghezzi P, Donelli MG, Pantarotto C, Fachinetti T, Garattini S. 1981, 30: 175.
9. Petronigro DP, McGinness JE, Koren MJ, et al. 1974, Physiol Chem Phys 11: 405.
10. Doroshow JH, Reeves J. 1980, Proc Am Assoc Cancer Res. 21: 1067.
11. Doroshow JH, Reeves J. 1981, Biochem Pharm 30: 259.
12. Pan SS, Pedersen L, Bachur NR. 1981, Mol Pharmcol 19: 184.
13. Burton GM, Henderson CA, Balcerzak SP et al. 1979, Int J Rad Oncol Biol Phys 5: 1287.
14. Lantz B, Adolfsson J, Langenlof B et al. 1979, Cancer Chemother Pharmacol 2: 95.
15. Poggi A, Delaini F, Donati MB. In Internal Medicine, Part I, Excerpta Medica, International Congress Series 502, p 386.
16. Doroshow JH, Locker GY, Myers CE. 1980, J Clin Invest 65: 128.
17. Flohe L, Gunzler WA, Schock HH. 1973, FEBS Lett 32: 132.
18. Katki AG, Myers CE. 1980, Biochem Biophys Res Comm 96: 85.
19. Revis NW, Marusic N. 1978, J Mol Cell Cardiol 10: 945.
20. Locker GY, Doroshow JH, Baldinger JC, Myers CE. 1979, Nutrition Rep Intern 19: 671.
21. Ganther HE, Hafeman DG, Lawrence RA et al. 1976, In Trace Elements in Human Health and Disease, Vol.2 p. 165.
22. Chance B, Spies H, Boveris A. 1979, Physiol Rev 59: 527.
23. Olson HM, Young DM, Prieur DJ et al. 1974, Ann J Path 77: 439.
24. Toyo-Oka T, Masaki T. 1979, J Molec Cell Cardiol 11: 769.
25. Oki T. 1977, Jap J Antibiotics 30: S-70.
26. Tong GL, Henry DW, Acton EM. 1979, J Med Chem 22: 34.
27. Lown JW, Chen HH, Plambeck JA. et al. 1979, Biochem Pharmacol 28: 2563.
28. Sonneveld P. 1978, Cancer Treat Rep 62: 1033.
29. Minnaugh EG, Siddik ZH, Drew R, Sikic BT and Gram TE. 1979, Tox and App Pharm 49: 119.
30. Wang YM, Madanat FF, Kimball JC et al. 1980, Cancer Res 40: 1022.
31. Weiner L, Averbach S and Singer O. 1979, Fed Proc 38: 3998.
32. Matsamura L et al. 1980, Fed Proc 39: 33.
33. Ogura R, Toyama H, Shimada T, Murakami M. 1979, J Applied Biochem 1: 325.
34. Breed JGS, Zimmerman ANE, Dormans JAMA et al. 1980, Cancer Res 40: 2033.
35. VanVleet J, Ferrans VJ. 1980, Ann J Vet Res 41: 691.
36. VanVleet J, Greenwood L, Ferrans VJ et al. 1978, Ann J Vet Res 39: 977.
37. Bacq ZM. 1965. Protection against Ionizing Radiation. Published by CC Thomas.
38. Mitchell JR, Thorgeirsson SS, Potter WZ, Jallow DJ, Keiser H. 1974. Clin Pharmacol Ther 16: 676.
39. Wells PG, Boerth RC, Oates JA, Harbison RD. 1980, Tox App Pharm 54: 197.

40. Olson RD, MacDonald JC, VanBoxtel JC et al. 1977, Fed Proc 36: 303.
41. Freeman RW, MacDonald JS, Olson RD et al. 1980, Tox App Pharm 54: 168.
42. Doroshow JH, Locker GY, Myers CE. 1979, Proc. Ann Assoc Cancer Res. 20: 253.
43. Doroshow JH, Locker GY, Myers CE. 1981, J Clin Invest 66. In press.
44. Doroshow JH, Locker GY, Baldinger J, Myers CE. 1979, Res Comm Chem Path Pharm 26: 285.
45. Boor PJ. 1979, Res Comm Chem Pathol Pharmacol 24: 27.
46. Herman E, Ardalan B, Bier C, Warandekar V, Krop S. 1979, Cancer Treat Rep 63: 89.
47. Herman E, Mhatre R, Chadwick D. 1974, Toxicol Appl Pharmacol 27. 517.
48. Herman EH, Ferrans VJ, Jordan W. 1981, Res Comm Chem Path Pharm 31: 85.
49. Wang G, Finch MD, Trevan D, Hellman K. 1981, Brit J Cancer 43: 871.
50. Woodman RJ, Cyszk RL, Kline J, Gang M. Venditti JM. 1975, Cancer Chemother Rep 59:689.
51. Myers C, Simone C, Gianni L et al. 1981, Proc. Assoc. Cancer Res 22: 112.
52. Kappus H. Muliawan H, Scheulen ME. In Mechanisms of Toxicity and Hazard Evaluation, p 635, Holmstedt B, Lauwerys R, Merceer M, Roberfroid M, eds. Elsevier/North-Holland Biomedical Press.

SCREENING FOR CARDIOTOXIC PROPERTIES

C. BERTAZZOLI, U. SAMMARTINI, M. G. TOSANA, L. BALLERINI, AND O. BELLINI

Since the first papers by Maral (1) and Serpick (2) in 1967 concerning
the toxicity and cardiotoxicity of rubidomycin and daunomycin (DNR), an
enormous amount of work has been done in practically all laboratory animal
species to induce and study the cardiotoxic effects of the anthracycline
antibiotics. Researchers have used in vitro and in vivo toxicological,
pharmacological, and biochemical methods. Here, therefore, only the main
aspects most closely related to the problems of screening anthracycline
antibiotics for cardiotoxicity will be discussed. I apologize to anyone
whose contributions are inadvertently omitted or if some topics are considered
in haste. Many authors have proposed experimental models to assess the
cardiotoxicity of these drugs; selected items from some of these models and
from other published data are listed in Table 1.

Important general toxicological considerations emerge from this com-
pendium. Single or repeated doses of anthracyclines induce, in all the
species used, clinical or functional symptoms of cardiac damage or cardiac
morphological alterations. These tend to manifest themselves slowly and
to worsen severely for a long time after discontinuation of treatment;
they appear practically irreversible.

Laboratory animals behave, therefore, like patients, not only in
showing the same cardiopathy (3) but also in the kinetics of damage (4,5).

The irreversibility and the toxic accumulation are probably linked
to the inability of the static tissues (6) (such as myocardium) to renew
irreparably damaged cells or subcellular structures.

Delayed and irreversible accumulation is, therefore, the first toxicological topic to be studied for this class of drugs, and data available to
date clearly suggest that an in vivo screening model should be used with
repeated treatment. For precise assessment of cardiotoxicity, it is also
important to know the time required for the lesion to stabilize and the

Table 1. Evidence of cumulative and delayed doxorubicin (DX) and
          daunoribicin (DNR) cardiotoxicity from some recent toxicological
          experimental in vivo models or studies.

Drug	Route	Dose range[a]	Sche.[b]	Kinetics of early appear. (days)	Heart alterat. worsening (+) during treatments	after	Ref. no.
			m o u s e				
DX	ip	10-20	S	2		+	7,8
DX	iv	10	S	1		+	9
DX	iv	20	S	56		+	10
DX	iv	5-10	R	56	+	+	10,11
			r a t				
DNR-DX	iv	5-25	S			+	12-14
DNR-DX	ip	1-4	R	3	+	+	15
DX	IV	1-10	R	21		+	5,14,16
			h a m s t e r				
DNR-DX	ip	3	R	7	+		18
			r a b b i t				
DNR-DX	iv	0.7-2.5	R	7	+	+	19-24
			d o g				
DX	iv	0.8-2	R	21	+		25-27
			m o n k e y				
DX	iv	1-6	R		+	+	28,29

a, mg/kg.
b, S, single doses; R, repeated intermittent doses.

correlation between the damage and the dose used in repeated treatment.

To acquire more information on these topics, we performed studies in
our laboratories in rats and mice that were treated with single or
repeated doses of doxorubicin (DX). Some of the findings are presented
in the following figures.

Figure 1 shows some cardiac parameters in groups of rats that had been
injected iv with single doses of 0.75, 1.5, 3, and 6 mg of DX/kg b.w. and
observed for 22 weeks with periodic EKG and investigation of myocardial

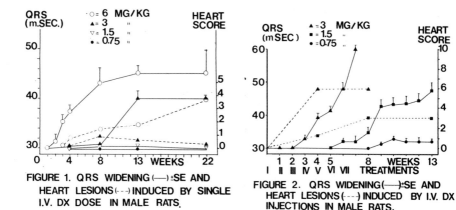

FIGURE 1. QRS WIDENING (——)±SE AND HEART LESIONS (---) INDUCED BY SINGLE I.V. DX DOSE IN MALE RATS.

FIGURE 2. QRS WIDENING(——)±SE AND HEART LESIONS (---) INDUCED BY I.V. DX INJECTIONS IN MALE RATS.

morphology in some killed subjects. The two lower doses never induced a widening of the QRS complex (according to Zbinden methods /15/), whereas 3 and 6 mg proportionally reduced conduction time. The alteration becomes detectable 8 weeks after 3 mg DX, reaches the maximum value after 13 weeks, and then remains constant. After 6 mg, the increase starts at the 2nd week, but the lesion becomes stable in about the same time.

From a morphological point of view, only the two larger doses induced histological heart degeneration, more evident with 6 mg. It is noteworthy that the cellular lesions appear 4-8 weeks after the injection but, with 6 mg are still increasing at the end of the observation time. EKG alterations behave differently from histological ones. No EKG or histological alterations were observed in control rats.

Groups of rats injected weekly with 0.75, 1.5, and 3 mg of DX iv for 7 weeks and monitored for 13 weeks as in the previous experiment (Fig. 2) showed earlier and greater QRS widening and earlier, more severe heart lesions than did the rats treated with equal single doses. In these conditions, too, initial EKG and histological alterations appear some weeks after the beginning of the treatment and stabilization is very late, depending on the dose or the parameter. No EKG or histological alterations were observed in control and 0.75-mg-treated rats. All rats treated with 3 mg died within 8 weeks, several with subcutaneous edema and ascites.

Similar results were observed in mice given single or repeated iv injections of DX (Fig. 3). A single injection of 4 mg was tolerated, but 10 mg induced moderate cardiomyopathy beginning 4 weeks after the injection, reaching the maximum value 8 weeks later, and not progressing thereafter.

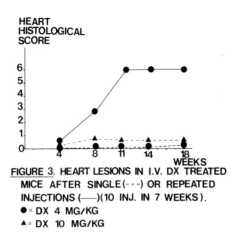

FIGURE 3. HEART LESIONS IN I.V. DX TREATED
MICE AFTER SINGLE(- - -) OR REPEATED
INJECTIONS (——)(10 INJ. IN 7 WEEKS).
● = DX 4 MG/KG
▲ = DX 10 MG/KG

When 4 mg were administered repeatedly, cardiac lesions appeared at the
same time; the damage was much more evident but stabilization was reached
4 weeks after interruption of treatment. Also in this experiment, no
histological lesions were observed in control mice.

These data confirm the high degree of accumulation of cardiotoxic
effects induced by repeated anthracycline doses and define the length of
time required for the initial appearance and stabilization of the damage
in these experimental conditions. There was no linear regression in rats
and mice between the extent of the histological lesions and the doses,
because larger doses accumulate more than do smaller ones. All these
findings mean 1) that the same lesion can be obtained with different
single doses, depending on the number of treatments and the observation
times and 2) that the cumulative dose must be used with caution, especially
when one is transferring results from one experiment to another but using
different schedules.

In screening anthracyclines, one must define, first of all, the duration
of the observation period, to ensure complete and stable expression of the
damage. For DX, 4 weeks of observations suffice to provide stable myocardial
damage in mice, at least at doses not too toxic for other tissues.

Of course, other extrinsic variables can indirectly interfere with
the cardiotoxicity of anthracyclines. These include animal species, strain,
sex, age, route of drug administration, diet, interaction of toxic damage
to other tissues, and so on. The most relevant factors are discussed here.

As regards the choice of animal species to be used, Doroshow (3) has
recently made an exhaustive review of the subject, which covers my opinions.

310

One can only add that in the rat and rabbit the cardiotoxic effects induced by anthracyclines develop simultaneously with a severe hyperlipidemic nephropathy (30), and that dogs and monkeys are too expensive for screening tests.

Conversely nephrotoxic effects are less important in the mouse (31). As Doroshow (3) pointed out, the mouse is available in inbred strains, is the least expensive of the species considered in terms of experimental cost, and is one of the most widely used animals for screening drugs for activity on transplantable tumors.

The administration route used should, as a general rule, be the same as in humans; this may be iv or, occasionally, oral; ip or sc injections are excluded because of the severe tissue reactions (32) and because anthracyclines are more toxic systemically on ip than they are on iv administration (33).

Another important point in the screening test is the choice of method one uses to demonstrate the cardiotoxic effect. At different times, clinical determination of myocardial enzymes in blood, such as CPK, LDH, etc. (13, 14, 16, 20, 22, 23, 34), EKG patterns (15, 17, 25, 35, 36), or more sophisticated noninvasive cardiac function tests (36,37) have been used to investigate myocardial impairment, when possible in the early stages of chronic intoxication.

The opinions of authors in this field are discordant (30), however, and in our experience correlations between functional data and morphological cardiac damage, in the same subject, are not always evident.

Probably the utility of these methods is limited to large animals and higher dosages. In large animals, as in humans, there is now a propensity to use biopsy methods, when possible (26).

A functional test widely used for screening purposes is that of the evaluation of QRS widening in rats proposed by Zbinden et al. (15). In our opinion, morphological heart examination is the preferable method, because it directly indicates the specific effect on the tissue involved.

In accordance with all the above considerations and the general criteria for pharmacotoxicological methods, we have developed a standardized and reproducible test in the mouse (31) based on the main features as listed in Table 2.

The histological lesion rating (Table 3) is based upon empirical evaluation of the severity and the extent of cell damage; the product of these two parameters gives the score (from 0 to 10) for each heart, and,

Table 2. General criteria adopted in our screening cardiotoxic test
in the mouse

1. Histological evaluation of the myocardial damage by light microscopy, on a semithin frontal median section of the whole heart.

2. Semiquantitative score of myocyte lesions.

3. Intravenous administration of the drug for 10 doses (in 7 weeks),
followed by 4 weeks of observations.

4. Use of three or more dose levels, starting from about one-third of
of the iv LD_{50}, calculated in the mouse, to obtain a dose-effect
regression line and to permit statistical analysis of the data.

Table 3. Morphologic evaluation of cardiac lesions

Degree	Definition
	Severity
1.	Sarcoplasmic microvacuolizations and/or inclusions and interstitial or cellular edema.
2.	Same as 1, plus sarcoplasmic macrovacuolizations or atrophia, necrosis, fibrosis, endocardial lesions, and thrombi.
	Extension
0.	No lesions.
0.5.	Fewer than 10 single altered myocytes in the whole heart section.
1.	Scattered single altered myocytes.
2.	Scattered small groups of altered myocytes.
3.	Widely spread small groups of altered myocytes.
4.	Confluent groups of altered myocytes.
5.	Most cells damaged.

using a nonparametric method, one can use this score for statistical
analysis.

For example, the next figures show the histological patterns observed
in DX-treated mice.

Figure 4 shows the typical morphology of a normal control heart; Figure
5 shows a heart with initial cell degeneration corresponding to a score of
0.5; and Figure 6 shows a heart with much more advanced damage, scored as 6.

Figure 7 shows the regression line obtained with DX at doses of 5, 10,
20, and 40 mg/kg b.w. from which a median cumulative cardiotoxic dose of
36.4 mg/kg was calculated.

We used this method to examine the cardiotoxic potency of some DX and

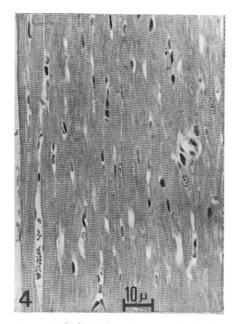 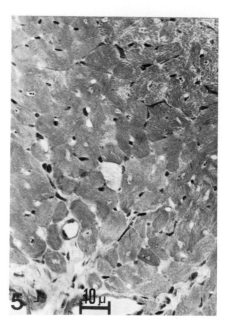

FIGURE 4 (left). Left ventricular myocardium from a control mouse.

FIGURE 5 (right). Left ventricular myocardium from a mouse given DX at a cumulative iv dose of 10 mg/kg. One cell exhibits fine cytoplasmic vacuolization. Score = 0.5.

DNR analogs, and the results are reported in Table 4, where the following data are given for each drug: the iv LD_{50} values in the mouse (all doses are expressed in mg of substance per kg b.w.), the maximal tolerated dose, the minimal cardiotoxic dose (the dose inducing a score of 0.5 for cardiac lesions), and the median cardiotoxic dose (the dose inducing a score of 5 obtained in the screening. All these doses are expressed as cumulative amounts and were obtained by extrapolation from the dose-response lines.

For some drugs, it was impossible to reach the median cardiotoxic dose, or even the minimal cardiotoxic dose, because these drugs are virtually noncardiotoxic, even at the highest injectable dose, or because the animals died from toxic effects on other tissues (such as intestine or bone marrow), as for 4-demethoxy-DX, 4'-deoxy-DX, 4'-O-methyl-DX, and 4-demethoxy-DNR.

This is the main difficulty in any test intended to show a chronic irreversible effect simultaneously with a chronic reversible one, when a drug is more potent from the latter aspect. The problem can easily be overcome, however, by spacing the treatments more widely, because the

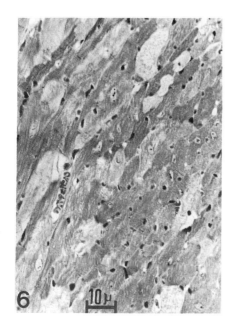

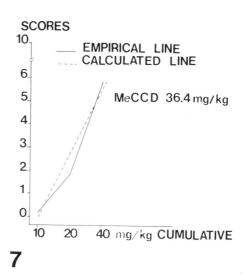

FIGURE 6 (left). Left ventricular myocardium from a mouse given DX at an iv cumulative dose of 40 mg/kg. Several cells exhibit vacuolization and myolysis. Score = 6.

FIGURE 7 (right) Regression line of cardiotoxicity scores after 10 doses of doxorubicin.

dose-response correlation for an irreversible effect is practically a fixed phenomenon linked to the cumulative dosage and not to time, provided that stable damage is achieved.

For the purpose of the test, however, determination of the maximum tolerated dose is sufficient.

The experimental predictivity of the test is demonstrated in the other columns, which show the same parameters of DX, 4'-epi-DX (38), 4-demethoxy-DX, 4'-deoxy-DX, DNR, and 4-demethoxy-DNR (37) obtained in chronic experiments in other animal species. Rats and dogs were given 39 iv doses in 13 weeks, rabbits 18 iv doses in 6 weeks.

The cumulative doses in the mouse, where available, are comparable with those for other animals within the limits of experimental variability.

The compounds examined up to now with the cardiotoxic screening are too few to permit any hypothesis about the structure-cardiotoxic potency relationship. It is interesting to note, however, that demethoxylation in position 4' on the aminosugar reduces the cardiotoxic potency.

Table 4. Acute toxicity and maximal tolerated (T), minimal (Mi), and median (Me) cardiotoxic doses deduced from cardiotoxic screening and chronic toxicological experiments with DX, DNR, and some analogs

Compound	Single iv tox. LD_{50} Mouse	Dose[a]	Repeated iv screening (10 doses) Mouse	Toxicity chronic experiments (39 D) Rat	(18 D) Rabbit	(39 D) Dog
Doxorubicin (DX)	10.2	T	12	11.7	7.2	7.8
		Mi	13	13.6	8.1	11.7[b]
		Me	36	29.2	18	tox.[b]
4'-Epi-DX	16	T	17		9.9	13.6
		Mi	19		11.7	15.6
		Me	47		25.2	tox.
4-Demethoxy-DX	2.9	T	3	1.9		
		Mi	6	4.6		
		Me	tox.	tox.		
4'-Deoxy-DX	10.2	T	>26		>5.4	>9.75
		Mi	tox.		tox.	tox.
		Me	–		–	–
2,3-Dimethyl-4-demethoxy-DX	18	T	9			
		Mi	11			
		Me	Ne[c]			
4'-O-methyl-DX	4.3	T	10			
		Mi	20			
		Me	tox.			
Daunorubicin (DNR)	18	T	17		13.5	
		Mi	20		14.4	
		Me	59		29.7	
4-Demethoxy-DNR	4.8	T	6.5	7.8	4.5	>4.68
		Mi	7.2	9.7	5.4	tox.
		Me	tox.	tox.	tox.	–
3',4'-Diepi-DNR	100	T	12			
		Mi	75			
		Me	Ne			

a, Doses extrapolated graphically (mg/kg).
b, tox., not evaluated because of toxic effects on proliferating tissues.
c, Ne, not evaluated due to technical difficulties.

This effect appears interesting for 4'-epi-DX and 4'-deoxy-DX; both compounds show similar or higher tolerated and cardiotoxic doses than does DX but, nevertheless, show higher activity on proliferating tissues.

In conclusion, we feel that the cardiotoxic screening of anthracyclines should be performed in vivo with repeated iv doses at intervals and should be based on the morphologic evaluation of stabilized cardiac damage.

The mouse test appears suitable for this purpose because it satisfies the basic requirements of a toxic screening: it gives semiquantitative direct evaluation of the specific effect on the target; it is predictive as regards other more extended studies and it permits comparison, in the same animal, with the activity data, within an acceptable experimental cost.

REFERENCES

1. Maral R, Bourat G, Ducrot R, Fournel J, Ganter P, Julou L, Koenig F, Myon J, Pascal S, Pasquet J, Populaire P, De Ratuld Y, Werner GH. 1967. Pathol. Biol. 15: 903.
2. Serpick AA, Henderson ES. 1967. Pathol. Biol. 15: 909.
3. Doroshow JH, Locker GY, Myers CE. 1979. Canter Treat. Rep. 63: 855.
4. Von Hoff DD, Layard HW, Basa P, Davis HL, Von Hoff AL, Rozencweig M, Muggia FM. 1979. Ann. Intern. Med. 91: 710.
5. Young RC, Ozols RF, Myers CE. 1981. N. Engl. J. Med. 305: 139.
6. Miquel J, Economos AC, Bensch KG, Atlan H, Johnson Jr. JE. 1979. Age 2: 78.
7. Rosenoff SH, Olson HM, Young DM, Bostick F, Young RC. 1975. J. Natl. Cancer Inst. 55: 191.
8. Young RC, Rosenoff S, Olson HM. 1975. In: Proceedings of the 2nd EORTC International Symposium (Adriamycin Review, Brussels, Belgium, May 16-18, 1974), Ghent, Belgium, European Press.-Medikon.: 149.
9. Lambertenghi-Deliliers G, Zanon PL, Possoli EF, Bellini O. 1976. Tumori 62: 517.
10. Lenaz L, Sternberg SS, Dellarven E, Vidal PM, Philips FS. 1978. Proc. Am. Assoc. Cancer Res. and Asco.: 19: 213.
11. Forssen EA, Tökès ZA. 1981. Proc. Natl. Acad. Sci. USA 78: 1873.
12. Chalcroft SCW, Gavin JB, Herdson PB. 1973. Pathology 5: 99.
13. Olson HM, Capen CC. 1977. Lab. Invest. 37: 386.
14. Olson HM, Capen CC. 1978. Toxicol. Appl. Pharmacol. 44: 605.
15. Zbinden G, Brändle E. 1975. Cancer Chemother. Rep. 59: 707.
16. Mettler FP, Young DM, Ward JM. 1977. Cancer Res. 37: 2705.
17. Sonneveld P. 1978. Cancer Treat. Rep. 62: 1033.
18. Dantchev D, Slioussartchouk V, Paintrand M, Bourut C, Hayat M, Mathé G. 1979. C.R. Séanc. Soc. Biol. 173: 394.
19. Jaenke RS. 1974. Lab. Invest. 30: 292.
20. Jaenke RS. 1976. Cancer Res. 36: 2958.
21. Young DM, Fioravanti JL. 1975. Proc. Am. Assoc. Cancer Res. and Asco. 16: 73.
22. Olson HM, Young DM, Prieur DJ, Leroy AF, Reagan RL. 1974. Am. J. Pathol. 77: 439.
23. Suzuki T, Kanda H, Kawai Y, Tominaga K, Murata K. 1979. Jpn. Cir. J. 43: 1000.
24. Jaenke RS, Deprez-DeCampeneere D, Trout A. 1980. Cancer Res. 40: 3530.
25. Gralla EJ, Fleischman RW, Luthra YK, Stadnicki SW. 1979. Toxicology 13: 263.
26. Bristow MR, Scott Sageman W, Scott RH, Billingham ME, Bowden RE, Kernoff RS, Snidow GH, aniels JR. 1980. J. Cardiovas. Pharmacol. 2: 287.
27. Keohe R, Singer DH, Trapani A, Billingham M, Levandowski R, Elson J. 1978. Cancer Treat. Rep. 62: 963.
28. Denine EP, Schmidt LH. 1975. Toxicol. Appl. Pharmacol. 33: 162.
29. Sieber SM, Correa P, Young DM, Dalgard DW, Adamson RH. 1980. Pharmacology 20: 9.
30. Young DM. 1975. Cancer Chemother. Rep. 6: 159.
31. Bertazzoli C, Bellini O, Magrini U, Tosana MG. 1979. Cancer Treat.

Rep. 63: 1877.

32. Dorr RT, Alberts DS, Hsiao-Sheng GC. 1980. J. Pharmacol. Methods **4**: 237
33. Schaeffer J, El Mahdi, AM. 1977. Proc. Am. Assoc. Cancer Res. and Asco. 18: 23.
34. Bradner WT, Schurig JE, Huftale JB, Doyle GJ. 1980. Cancer Chem. Pharmacol. 4: 95.
35. Soldani G, Del Tacca M, Giovannini L, Bertelli A. 1981. Drugs Exptl. Clin. Res. 8: 31.
36. Long HJ III, Zeidner SR, Burningham RA. 1976. Proc.Am. Assoc. Cancer Res. and Asco. 17: 67.
37. Breed JGS, Zimmerman ANE, Meyler FL, Pinedo HM. 1979. Cancer Treat. Rep. 63: 869.
38. Casazza AM, Di Marco A, Bonadonna G, Bonfante V, Bertazzoli C, Bellini O, Pratesi G, Sala L, Ballerini L. 1980. Anthracyclines: Current status and new developments. Proc. Workshop on anthracyclines, Norfolk, Virginia, June 14-15, 1979. Crooke ST, Reich SD, eds. New York, Academic Press, 403 pp.

ROLE OF OXYGEN RADICAL FORMATION IN ANTHRACYCLINE CARDIAC TOXICITY

J. H. DOROSHOW AND G. Y. LOCKER

INTRODUCTION

Because of the clinical usefulness of the anthracycline antibiotics
(1), the dose-limiting myocardial toxicity of these antitumor agents remains
a major problem in oncologic pharmacology. Although the mechanism of
anthracycline cardiac toxicity is not yet completely defined, recent studies
have suggested that it may be due to unrestrained, drug-induced, cardiac
oxygen radical metabolism (2-5).

It is now clear that several flavin-containing enzymes will support
the one-electron reduction of the anthracycline quinone to its semiquinone
free radical in vitro (6,7). Since the anthracycline semiquinone appears
to be relatively long-lived (8), covalent binding of this drug intermediate
could produce enzyme or membrane damage directly (9). However, under
aerobic conditions, as in the myocardial cell, it appears to be more likely
that the cyclical oxidation and reduction of the anthracycline radical
would catalyze electron flow from reduced pyridine nucleotides to molecular
oxygen leading to the formation of superoxide anion, hydrogen peroxide, and
other reactive oxygen metabolites (10,11).

Oxygen radicals formed as a consequence of redox cycling by quinone-
containing antibiotics could have a deleterious effect on both membrane and
nucleic acid integrity as well as on cellular energy metabolism (12,13).
Thus, drug-stimulated oxygen radical formation might explain a wide variety
of biochemical effects on heart muscle previously shown to be produced by

anthracycline treatment under experimental conditions (14). In the studies presented here, we have examined the extent of cardiac reactive oxygen formation by anthracycline antibiotics in vitro; we have also examined the mechanism(s) of oxygen radical detoxification by cardiac muscle in an attempt to explain the apparently enhanced sensitivity of the heart to drug-induced free radicals. Our results indicate that free radical formation in vitro seems to occur at the same intracellular sites characteristically damaged by anthracycline administration in vivo (15). Furthermore, free radical production may itself interfere with a major myocardial defense against free radical attack.

METHODS

Experimental animals. For these experiments, male Sprague-Dawley rats weighing 180 to 200 grams were purchased from Mission Laboratory Supply Co., Rosemead, California. From the time of weaning, these animals were maintained on a diet of Wayne Lab-Blox rat pellets with water available ad libitum. Male CDF_1 mice at weaning were obtained from Dominion Laboratories, Dublin, Virginia; were housed in a constant (22°C) temperature environment; and were raised on defined diets as previously described (5). These animals were used after 6 weeks of maturation.

Materials. Doxorubicin hydrochloride of clinical grade was purchased from Adria Laboratories, Inc., Columbus, Ohio. Daunorubicin hydrochloride was obtained from the Investigational Drug Branch, Division of Cancer Treatment, National Cancer Institute, Bethesda, Maryland. NADPH type III, $NADP^+$, NADH grade III, histidine, EDTA, cytochrome c (type VI from horse heart), bovine erythrocyte superoxide dismutase (SOD), L-epinephrine, xanthine, xanthine oxidase (grade I), glutathione (reduced form, GSH; and oxidized form, GSSG), NADH dehydrogenase type I, 5,5'-dithiobis-(2-nitro-benzoic acid), glutathione reductase, o-phthalaldehyde, n-acetylcysteine, and D-α-tocopherol were obtained from Sigma Chemical Co., St. Louis, Missouri. Sodium acetate, acetic anhydride, metaphosphoric acid, and hydrogen peroxide were purchased from Fisher Scientific Co., Fair Lawn, New Jersey.

Preparation of tissue fractions. Experimental animals were killed by cervical dislocation, cardiac ventricles or left hepatic lobes were excised, trimmed of connective tissue, blotted dry and then minced while kept on melted ice. After homogenization of the minced tissue with a Brinkmann model PCU-2-110 Polytron, rat cardiac sarcoplasmic reticulum and mitochondria were prepared by differential ultracentrifugation as described previously (16). The mitochondrial fraction was frozen and thawed 3 times over a dry ice-methanol mixture to ensure membrane disruption before use. Cytosol from mouse heart and liver was obtained by centrifugation of the crude tissue homogenate for 60 min at 105,000 g and 5°C in a Beckman Model L5-50 ultra-centrifuge. Each sample of heart cytosol was obtained from the pooled ventricular tissue of 3 mice; a single left hepatic lobe was used to prepare liver cytosol. At the end of ultracentrifugation, the supernate was decanted and then used directly to determine enzyme activities in the respective tissue cytosols.

Oxygen radical formation in heart fractions. Superoxide anion production in heart fractions was determined by the rate of superoxide dismutase-inhibitable acetylated cytochrome c reduction. Cytochrome c was acetylated before use to eliminate interfering reactions by cytochrome c oxidases or reductases in the heart fractions (17). The initial rate of acetylated cytochrome c reduction in the presence and absence of superoxide dismutase was determined spectrophotometrically at 550 nm and 37°C in a Gilford Model 250 recording spectrophotometer equipped with a circulating water bath. As described previously (16), superoxide formation was calculated from the rate of acetylated cytochrome c reduction that was inhibited by superoxide dismutase using an extinction coefficient for cytochrome $\underline{c}$ (reduced minus oxidized) of 19.6 m$\underline{M}^{-1}$cm^{-1} (18). The effect of anthracycline treatment on the rate of NADPH oxidation in heart sarcosomes was examined at 340 nm and 37°C in a 1-ml reaction mixture containing 100 nmol NADPH, 200 µg sarcosomal protein, and various concentrations of anthracycline drug. Oxygen consumption in heart sarcosomes was measured at 37°C with a YSI model 53 oxygen monitoring system (11).

Enzyme assays. Glutathione peroxidase, superoxide dismutase, and catalase activities were measured in heart and liver fractions by previously described techniques (5). Tissue levels of reduced and oxidized glutathione were examined by the method of Hissin and Hilf (19).

Morphological studies. Light and electron microscopic studies of the tissue toxicity of doxorubicin were performed 96 hours after drug administration (20); cardiac morphological alterations were assessed blindly using the 0-3 scale described by Bristow et al. (21).

Protein determination. Protein concentrations were determined by the method of Lowry et al. using crystalline bovine albumin as the standard (22).

Statistics. Data were analyzed with the two-tailed $\underline{t}$ test for independent means (NS, not significant, $\underline{P} < 0.05$).

RESULTS

Effect of anthracycline drugs on cardiac oxygen radical formation. Anthracycline cardiac toxicity is characterized by vacuolation of the sarcoplasmic reticulum and disorganization of mitochondrial membranes (15); thus, we examined these cardiac organelles for their ability to catalyze anthracycline free radical formation. In heart sarcosomes, a limited amount of superoxide was formed after the addition of NADPH; however, in the presence of daunorubicin, superoxide dismutase-inhibitable acetylated cytochrome $\underline{c}$ reduction was substantially increased (Fig. 1). Treatment of

DAUNORUBICIN-STIMULATED CYTOCHROME c
REDUCTION IN CARDIAC SARCOSOMES

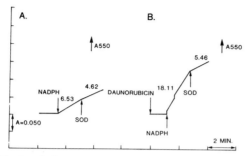

FIGURE 1. Effect of daunorubicin on acetylated cytochrome $\underline{c}$ reduction by cardiac sarcosomes. The sequential addition of NADPH (1 µmol), daunorubicin (135 nmol), or superoxide dismutase (10 µg) have each been indicated by an arrow. The numbers above these tracings represent the rate of acetylated cytochrome $\underline{c}$ reduction in nanomoles per minute per milligram protein. (Reprinted by permission from Doroshow and Reeves 1981, copyright 1981 by Pergamon Press Ltd., Oxford, England.)

heart sarcosomes with daunorubicin led to a dose-dependent increase in superoxide formation that was significantly higher than control levels for each drug dose tested (Fig. 2). Drug-induced superoxide production occurred only in the presence of NADPH (not NADH), was decreased by over 65% ($\underline{P}$<0.01) by the addition of excess NADP^{+}, and was abolished after denaturation of the sarcosomal protein by heat (data from reference 11). Furthermore, daunorubicin-stimulated superoxide production in heart sarcosomes was accompanied by a dose-related increase in sarcosomal NADPH oxidation as well as an increase in sarcosomal oxygen consumption from (mean ± S.E.) the control rate of 11.38 ± 0.32 nmoles/ min/mg (n=6) to 13.81 ± 0.40 nmoles/ min/mg (n=8) in the presence of 135 µM daunorubicin (11). The release of oxygen by the addition of catalase (3000 U/ml) to drug-treated sarcosomes indicated that hydrogen peroxide formation had also been stimulated by daunorubicin (data not shown). In related experiments, we have found that at equimolar concentrations, superoxide formation by doxorubicin was not significantly different from that produced by daunorubicin and that doxorubicin-

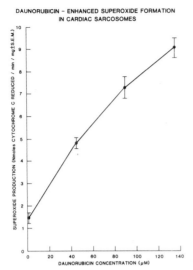

FIGURE 2. Effect of daunorubicin concentration on superoxide formation in heart sarcosomes. Data represent the mean ± S.E. of at least three experiments at every dose. For each drug concentration used, superoxide formation was significantly higher than in control samples, P<0.01.

enhanced superoxide formation occurred despite an intrinsic superoxide dismutase concentration in heart sarcosomes of (mean ± S.E.) 2.88 ± 0.42 μg SOD/mg protein (23).

We have also investigated the effect of anthracycline treatment on superoxide production in cardiac mitochondria. At a concentration of 135 μM doxorubicin increased mitochondrial superoxide production 6-fold, from a control rate (mean ± S.E.) of 2.86 ± 0.71 nmoles/min/mg (n=3) to 17.14 ± 2.14 nmoles/min/mg (n=4), P<0.01. Mitochondrial oxygen radical formation was NADH- and protein-dependent and rotenone-insensitive, suggesting that the mitochondrial NADH dehydrogenase complex was the enzymatic site for the mitochondrial reduction of doxorubicin (16). To evaluate that possibility further, we examined the ability of NADH dehydrogenase itself to support anthracycline-enhanced oxygen radical production. We found that doxorubici (135 μM) increased superoxide formation by NADH dehydrogenase nearly 20-fol from (mean ± S.E.) 0.06 ± 0.01 nmoles/min (n=6) to 1.15 ± 0.02 nmoles/min (n=3) using 5.4 µg enzyme protein (16).

Effect of anthracycline antibiotics on myocardial defenses against free radical attack. It has been demonstrated previously that the enzymes superoxide dismutase (EC 1.15.1.1), catalase (EC 1.11.1.6), and glutathione peroxidase (EC 1.11.1.9) act in concert to convert superoxide anion, hydrogen peroxide, and lipid hydroperoxides to nontoxic lipid alcohols or water (24). These enzymes and the cellular reducing equivalents provided by reduced glutathione and ascorbate allow most mammalian cells to detoxify completely the byproducts of reactive oxygen metabolism. However, alterations in the intracellular concentration of these protective enzymes and reducing equivalents can enhance tissue toxicity from drug-induced free radical production (25). Thus, we investigated the mechanisms by which heart muscle could detoxify oxygen radicals formed after treatment with doxorubicin. We found that liver catalase activity (mean ± S.E.) was 173.3 ± 10.5 U; the cardiac catalase level was 1.1 ± 0.4 U, or less than 0.6% of the activity found in the liver, P<0.001 (Fig. 3). Superoxide dismutase activity in heart muscle cytosol

DISTRIBUTION OF ENDOGENOUS DEFENSES AGAINST FREE RADICALS

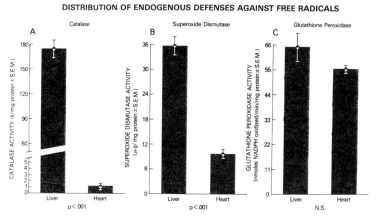

FIGURE 3. Comparison of cardiac and hepatic catalase, superoxide dismutase, and glutathione peroxidase activities. Heart and liver from experimental animals were assayed for catalase, superoxide dismutase, and glutathione peroxidase activities as described in Methods. Data represent the mean ± S.E. of at least three experiments for superoxide dismutase and glutathione peroxidase and the mean ± S.E. of five experiments for cardiac and hepatic catalase.

324

(mean ± S.E.; 9.7 ± 0.9 μg/mg) was also significantly lower than that in

liver (35.8 ± 2.3 μg/mg), P<0.001. However, the cardiac glutathione peroxidase

level (mean ± S.E.; 55.6 ± 1.2 nmole NADPH oxidized/min/mg) was not signifi-

cantly different from the hepatic enzyme activity (64.4 ± 6.7 nmole NADPH

oxidized/min/mg), NS. Thus, in comparison to liver, the heart has signifi-

cantly lower levels of two of the three enzymes that are involved in the

detoxification of oxygen radical metabolites (5).

We have also found that a single dose of doxorubicin caused an acute

depression in cardiac glutathione peroxidase activity (Fig. 4). Twenty-

four hours after drug treatment, cardiac enzyme levels were less than 45%

of control values, P<0.01; and significantly diminished enzyme activity

persisted for 72 hours after doxorubicin administration (5). At the time

of maximal inhibition of cardiac glutathione peroxidase, hepatic enzyme

activity was not changed (data not shown). Furthermore, treatment with

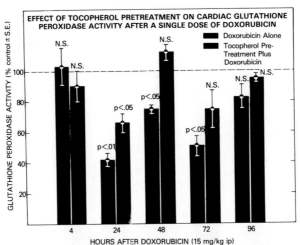

FIGURE 4. Effect of doxorubicin on cardiac glutathione peroxidase. In
these experiments, cardiac glutathione peroxidase activity in animals
treated with doxorubicin has been compared to simultaneously treated control
receiving physiologic saline. For each time point, bar on the left represent
animals receiving doxorubicin alone and the bar on the right represents
animals pretreated with 85 international units of D-α-tocopherol 24 hours
before therapy with doxorubicin. Data represent the percent control ± S.E.
for a minimum of three experimental and three control samples per time
point for each of the two experiments.

doxorubicin did not alter either cardiac or hepatic superoxide dismutase levels up to 96 hours after drug therapy (5). Although the mechanism of this drop in cardiac glutathione peroxidase activity is unknown, tocopherol pretreatment substantially ameliorated the degree and duration of glutathione peroxidase inhibition produced by doxorubicin (Fig. 4). Since it has been shown previously that glutathione peroxidase activity may be decreased by exposure to superoxide anion (26), it is possible that doxorubicin-enhanced cardiac oxygen radical production (blunted in part by a pharmacologic dose of α-tocopherol) may itself be responsible for the inhibition of glutathione peroxidase activity in the heart.

In addition to glutathione peroxidase inhibition, treatment with doxorubicin produces a significant alteration in myocardial glutathione content (Fig. 5). Twelve hours after drug administration, both reduced and oxidized cardiac glutathione levels were significantly decreased compared to simultaneously injected animals receiving saline (27). Decreased cardiac glutathione content after anthracycline administration has now been confirmed

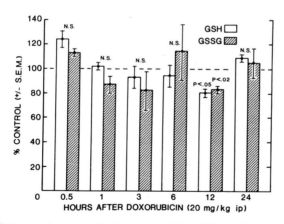

FIGURE 5. Effect of doxorubicin on cardiac GSH and GSSG. For every time point, cardiac glutathione content in animals treated with doxorubicin has been compared to that in simultaneously treated animals receiving physiological saline. Data represent the percent control ± S.E. for three experimental and three control samples per time period. (Reprinted by permission from Doroshow et al. 1979; copyright 1979 by PJD Publications Ltd., Westbury, New York.)

by two different groups (28,29); it appears to precede the change in gluta-thione peroxidase activity previously described, and could be a reflection of drug-enhanced myocardial oxygen radical formation in vivo.

Our studies on the mechanism of the formation and detoxification of oxygen radical metabolites by the anthracycline antibiotics suggested that augmentation of cardiac antioxidant defenses might ameliorate anthracycline-induced cardiomyopathy. We investigated the possibility that a sulfhydryl-containing compound might provide sufficient reducing capacity to prevent heart damage from doxorubicin (20). We found that the administration of pharmacologic concentrations of the cysteine analog n-acetylcysteine to mice receiving a lethal dose of doxorubicin decreased long-term mortality from nearly 100% to under 40% (Fig. 6). Furthermore, pretreatment of experimental animals with n-acetylcysteine when doxorubicin was administered

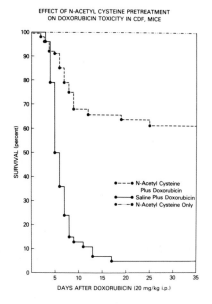

EFFECT OF N-ACETYL CYSTEINE PRETREATMENT
ON DOXORUBICIN TOXICITY IN CDF, MICE

FIGURE 6. Effect of n-acetylcysteine on doxorubicin toxicity. Animals received saline or n-acetylcysteine (2000 mg/kg p.o.) one hour before treatment with doxorubicin (20 mg/kg i.p.). N=15 for the group treated with physiological saline alone; N=60 for the group receiving doxorubicin after saline pretreatment; and N=53 for the group pretreated with n-acetyl-cysteine before doxorubicin administration.

on a multidose schedule also significantly prevented doxorubicin toxicity (data not shown). Finally, when cardiac electron micrographs from groups of mice receiving doxorubicin with or without n-acetylcysteine pretreatment were compared after being scored in a blinded fashion, we found that thiol administration produced a significant decrease in doxorubicin cardiac toxicity. In fact, in that study, electron microscopic features of heart damage were essentially eliminated by n-acetylcysteine pretreatment (20).

DISCUSSION

There is an increasing body of experimental evidence indicating that the cardiomyopathic effects of the anthracycline antibiotics result from drug-induced oxidative tissue injury (2-5). In particular, anthracycline-related reactive oxygen metabolism may overwhelm the limited capacity of cardiac muscle to detoxify free radicals resulting in extensive damage to myocardial membranes and other intracellular constituents.

We have shown that the anthracycline antibiotics enhance superoxide and hydrogen peroxide formation in cardiac mitochondria and sarcoplasmic reticulum in vitro. As predicted by Thayer (3), the mitochondrial reduction of the anthracyclines probably involves oxidation-reduction cycling catalyzed by the NADH dehydrogenase complex. On the other hand, superoxide production by the anthracyclines in heart sarcoplasmic reticulum consumed NADPH and was inhibited by $NADP^+$, suggesting that NADPH cytochrome P-450 reductase was responsible for quinone reduction in this fraction. It should be emphasized that under the conditions of these experiments, we have measured oxygen radical metabolism in excess of the organelle's capacity for detoxification. It is tempting to speculate that a similar phenomenon might occur in vivo, resulting in an outpouring of reactive oxygen species from at least two intramyocardial sites.

328

We have also found that cardiac muscle has limited enzymatic defenses against the toxic effects of peroxides, especially in comparison to liver, an organ that is also known to activate anthracyclines to their free radical metabolites. Furthermore, the activity of cardiac glutathione peroxidase, which provides a major pathway for the removal of active oxygen radicals from the heart, is depressed for 72 hours after a single dose of doxorubicin. The ameliorating effect of α-tocopherol on the inhibition of cardiac gluta- thione peroxidase by doxorubicin suggests that drug-induced free radicals may themselves impair the activity of this important antioxidant enzyme. •An alteration in cardiac reduced glutathione pools also may potentiate the effect of doxorubicin on the oxidation state of the selenocysteine molecule at the active site of glutathione peroxidase (30). In any case, drug-induced reactive oxygen formation occurring in the face of a prolonged depression of cardiac glutathione peroxidase activity might lead to intracellular peroxide accumulation; and a hydrogen or lipid peroxide concentration could be reached that would exceed the detoxifying capacity of the myocardial cell (3). Furthermore, because heart cells are so rich in heme-containing proteins that may undergo auto-oxidation, it is likely that the presence of excess intracellular peroxide in the anthracycline-treated heart would establish an extraordinarily favorable milieu for the formation of highly reactive hydroxyl and peroxy radicals with a proven capacity to produce membrane peroxidation.

Our pharmacological attempt to alter the deleterious effects of myocardial peroxide has focused on the administration of reduced sulfhydryl compounds to experimental animals receiving anthracycline antibiotics. The use of n- acetylcysteine provides the heart with a temporary, alternate source of reducing equivalents that may limit the adverse effects of doxorubicin- induced oxygen radical species. The potent hydroxyl radical scavenging activity of n-acetylcysteine may enhance its cardioprotective action further.

In summary, we suggest that reactive oxygen metabolism by the anthracycline antibiotics could be uniquely damaging to the heart because the organ's limited antioxidant defenses may allow a drug-initiated free radical chain reaction to produce an overwhelming oxidant stress on the myocardial cell.

Abbreviations used in the text: SOD, superoxide dismutase (EC 1.15.1.1); GSH, reduced glutathione; GSSG, oxidized glutathione.

REFERENCES

1. Carter SK. Adriamycin - a review. J. Natl. Cancer Inst. 1975; 55: 1265-1274.
2. Bachur NR, Gordon SL and Gee MV. A general mechanism for microsomal activation of quinone anticancer agents to free radicals. Cancer Res. 1978; 38: 1745-1750.
3. Thayer WS. Adriamycin stimulated superoxide formation in submitochondrial particles. Chem. Biol. Interact. 1977; 19: 265-278.
4. Sonneveld P. Effect of α-tocopherol on the cardiotoxicity of adriamycin in the rat. Cancer Treat. Rep. 1978; 62: 1033-1036.
5. Doroshow JH, Locker GY and Myers CE. Enzymatic defenses of the mouse heart against reactive oxygen metabolites. Alterations produced by doxorubicin. J. Clin. Invest. 1980; 65: 128-135.
6. Komiyama T, Oki T and Inui T. A proposed reaction mechanism for the enzymatic reductive cleavage of glycosidic bond in anthracycline antibiotics. J. Antibiotics. 1979; 32: 1219-1222.
7. Pan S and Bachur NR. Xanthine oxidase catalyzed reductive cleavage of anthracycline antibiotics and free radical formation. Molec. Pharmacol. 1980; 17: 95-99.
8. Sato S, Iwaizumi M, Handa K and Tamura Y. Electron spin resonance study on the mode of generation of free radicals of daunomycin, adriamycin, and carboquone in NAD(P)H-microsomal system. Gann. 1977; 68: 603-608.
9. Ghezzi P, Donelli M, Pantarotto C et al. Evidence for covalent binding of adriamycin to rat liver microsomal proteins. Biochem. Pharmacol. 1981; 30: 175-177.
10. Kalyanaraman B, Perez-Reyes E and Mason RP. Spin-trapping and direct electron spin resonance investigations of the redox metabolism of quinone anticancer drugs. Biochim. Biophys. Acta. 1980; 630: 119-130.
11. Doroshow JH and Reeves J. Daunorubicin-stimulated reactive oxygen metabolism in cardiac sarcosomes. Biochem. Pharmacol. 1981; 30: 259-262.
12. Goodman J and Hochstein P. Generation of free radicals and lipid peroxidation by redox cycling of adriamycin and daunomycin. Biochem. Biophys. Res. Commun. 1977; 77: 797-803.

13. Berlin V and Haseltine WA. Reduction of adriamycin to a semiquinone-free radical by NADPH cytochrome P-450 reductase produces DNA cleavage in a reaction mediated by molecular oxygen. J. Biol. Chem. 1981; 256: 4747-4756.

14. Lenaz L and Page JA. Cardiotoxicity of adriamycin and related anthracyclines. Cancer Treat. Rev. 1976; 3: 111-120.

15. Ferrans V. Overview of cardiac pathology in relation to anthracycline cardiotoxicity. Cancer Treat. Rep. 1978; 62: 955-961.

16. Doroshow JH. Mitomycin C-enhanced superoxide and hydrogen peroxide formation in rat heart. J. Pharmacol. Exp. Ther. 1981; 218: 206-211.

17. Azzi A, Montecucco C and Richter C. The use of acetylated ferricytochrome c for the detection of superoxide radicals produced in biological membranes. Biochem. Biophys. Res. Commun. 1975; 65: 597-603.

18. Yonetani T and Ray GS. Studies on cytochrome c peroxidase: Purification and some properties. J. Biol. Chem. 1965; 240; 4503-4508.

19. Hissin PJ and Hilf R. A fluorometric method for determination of oxidized and reduced glutathione in tissues. Anal. Biochem. 1976; 74: 214-226.

20. Doroshow JH, Locker GY, Ifrim I and Myers C. Prevention of doxorubicin cardiac toxicity in the mouse by n-acetylcysteine. J. Clin. Invest. 1981; in press.

21. Bristow MR, Thompson PD, Martin RP et al. Early anthracycline cardiotoxicity. Am. J. Med. 1978; 65: 823-832.

22. Lowry O, Rosebrough NJ, Farr A and Randall RJ. Protein measurement with the folin phenol reagent. J. Biol. Chem. 1951; 193: 265-275.

23. Doroshow JH and Reeves J. Anthracycline-enhanced oxygen radical formation in the heart. Proc. Am. Assoc. Cancer Res. 1980; 21: 266.

24. Fridovich I. The biology of oxygen radicals. Science (Wash. D.C.). 1978; 201: 875-880.

25. Omaye ST, Reddy KA and Cross CE. Enhanced lung toxicity of paraquat in selenium-deficient rats. Toxicol. Appl. Pharmacol. 1978; 43: 237-247.

26. Rister M and Baehner RL. The alteration of superoxide dismutase, catalase, glutathione peroxidase, and NAD(P)H cytochrome c reductase in guinea pig polymorphonuclear leukocytes and alveolar macrophages during hyperoxia. J. Clin. Invest. 1976; 58: 1174-1184.

27. Doroshow JH, Locker GY, Baldinger J and Myers CE. The effect of doxorubicin on hepatic and cardiac glutathione. Res. Commun. Chem. Path. Pharmacol. 1979; 26: 285-295.

28. Wang Y, Madanat F, Kimball JC et al. Effect of vitamin e against adriamycin-induced toxicity in rabbits. Cancer Res. 1980; 40: 1022-1027.

29. Olson RD, MacDonald JS, van Boxtel CJ et al. Regulatory role of glutathione and soluble sulfhydryl groups in the toxicity of adriamycin. J. Pharmacol. Exp. Ther. 1980; 215: 450-454.

30. Tappel AL, Forstrom J, Zakowski DE et al. The catalytic site of rat liver glutathione peroxidase as selenocysteine and selenocysteine in rat liver. Fed. Proc. 1978; 37: 706.

ACKNOWLEDGEMENTS

This work was supported by Public Health Service grant 29463-01 awarded by the National Cancer Institute, Department of Health and Human Services; by grant 622-G2-2 from the American Heart Association - Greater Los Angeles affiliate; and by a Special Fellowship awarded to Dr. Doroshow by the Leukemia Society of America. We wish to express our thanks to Dr. C.E. Myers of the Clinical Pharmacology Branch, National Cancer Institute, in whose laboratory our study of cardiac antioxidant defenses was begun; we also wish to thank Ms. Jill Reeves for her excellent technical assistance.

MORPHOLOGIC ASSESSMENT OF CARDIAC LESIONS CAUSED BY ANTHRACYCLINES

V. J. FERRANS

The clinical use of daunorubicin and doxorubicin, two anti-neoplastic drugs of the anthracycline family, has been limited by the development of cardiotoxic effects. These can be subdivided into acute, subacute and chronic depending upon their temporal relationship to the administration of the drugs. The acute effects consist of hypotension, tachycardia and various arrhythmias, which develop within minutes after intravenous administration. The subacute effects are characterized by fibrinous pericarditis or myocardial dysfunction, which occur within four weeks of the first or second dose of the drug. The chronic effects develop only after several weeks or months of treatment, sometimes after the course of therapy has been completed, and are manifested by the insidious onset of severe, often fatal congestive heart failure.

In reviewing the cardiac morphologic changes produced by anthra-cyclines, it is important to try to relate such changes to the biochemical effects that these agents induce in myocardium. This is difficult because of the multiplicity and complexity of the biochemical changes involved (some of which may be inevitable secondary consequences of other changes). Among these alterations are: 1) binding of anthracyclines (intercalation) to nuclear and mitochondrial DNA, leading to inhibition of DNA, RNA and protein synthesis, to fragmentation of DNA and to inhibition of DNA repair; 2) binding of anthracyclines to membranes, resulting in inter-ference with various functions of membranes, including Na-K-dependent

ATPase activity, calcium transport and intracellular electrolyte balance; 3) inhibition of reactions utilizing coenzyme Q; 4) chelation of divalent cations, including calcium, iron and copper; 5) decrease in the activity of glutathione peroxidase, and 6) promotion of complex peroxidative phenomena by means of reactions mediated by free radicals (1).

Acute cardiotoxicity of anthracyclines. The peripheral vascular effects of anthracyclines are consequences of histamine release, which in turn causes a secondary release of catecholamines. This concept is supported by the results of studies showing that the intravenous injection of doxorubicin or daunorubicin increases the plasma levels of histamine and catecholamines (2,3), that the hypotension caused by these agents can be almost completely prevented by pretreatment with compound 48/80, which releases histamine by degranulating mast cells (2), and that rat peritoneal mast cells are rapidly degranulated by exposure to doxorubicin (4). Morphologic changes related to the acute arrhythmias remain to be determined, although it is known that in chronic anthracycline toxicity, the specialized cardiac conducting cells of the rabbit, pig and dog show lesions similar to those in ordinary working myocardium (5,6). The only cardiac morphologic change that has been found to occur very shortly after administration of doxorubicin is fragmentation of the nucleolonema, with subsequent development of nucleolar segregation, which takes place in mouse myocardium as early as 10 minutes after a single injection of 10 mg/kg (7). Nucleolar segregation also occurs in mouse and rat hepatocytes and in rat ventricular myocardium after the administration of large, single doses of doxorubicin (8) and in Novikoff hepatoma cells treated with doxorubicin, carminomycin or marcellomycin (9). This change is also produced by other drugs, such as actinomycin D, which bind to DNA (10). Doxorubicin and daunorubicin penetrate rapidly into nuclei, to which they

impart a reddish fluorescence (11,12). Thus, these observations show
that anthracyclines produce acute, toxic effects on nuclei. The long-term
significance of nucleolar segregation is unclear, because the morphology
of nucleoli returns to normal by 14 hours after administration of doxorubicin (7).

Nuclear lesions have been observed only in a small percentage of
cardiac muscle cells in patients dying of chronic anthracycline toxicity
(11,13). These lesions consist of various degrees of unraveling of
chromatin fibers into fine fibrils and filaments. These changes are not
specific for anthracycline toxicity (13). We have not consistently
observed these changes in experimental animals given anthracyclines in
vivo, although we have reproduced them in monkey myocardium incubated
in vitro with anthracycline-containing solutions (13).

The observations just cited suggest that cumulative damage to DNA
in cardiac muscle cells (which are not capable of reproducing themselves,
thereby diluting the damage to the genetic material) can result from the
administration of repeated doses of anthracyclines, and that such damage
(including breaks in DNA) may not be properly repaired by cardiac muscle
cells, thus leading to severe interference with protein synthetic processes.
This is also shown by the fact that treatment with anthracyclines causes
an acute, considerable decrease in cardiac weight in experimental animals.
In our experience, this acute decrease in cardiac weight is not accompanied
by qualitative changes in the morphology of the myocytes. Since the half-
life of contractile proteins in cardiac muscle is in the range of one to
two weeks, these effects may be of crucial importance in the pathogenesis
of anthracycline-induced cardiomyopathy.

Subacute cardiotoxicity of anthracyclines. Bristow et al. (14)
described eight patients in whom cardiac dysfunction developed within four

weeks of receiving their first or second course of daunorubicin or doxorubicin. Four patients presented with pericarditis; three of these also had evidence of myocardial dysfunction. Cardiac morphologic findings in one of these patients consisted of: chronic anthracycline-type lesions (see below), focal myocardial necroses (the patient died in cardiogenic shock), fibrinous pericarditis, and infiltration of the epicardium with lymphocytes and polymorphonuclear leukocytes. The latter finding was in contrast with the more chronic lesions produced by anthracyclines, in which an inflammatory reaction is usually absent. An additional four patients presented with signs and symptoms of congestive heart failure. These patients either were elderly or had evidence of previous heart disease. One of these patients suffered a myocardial infarction 24 hours after receiving 60 mg/m^2 of daunorubicin; earlier doses in the same course had been associated with evidence of myocardial ischemia. Necropsy study in this patient showed no morphologic evidence of anthracycline cardiotoxicity. Bristow et al. (14) concluded that anthracyclines may manifest clinically significant cardiotoxicity at total cumulative doses much lower than those which have been associated with chronic cardiomyopathy.

Chronic cardiotoxicity of anthracyclines. The morphologic changes (Figs. 1-4) observed in chronic cardiotoxicity of anthracyclines (11,13-23) consist of: 1) cardiac dilatation and, occasionally, mural thrombosis; 2) degeneration and atrophy of cardiac myocytes, and 3) interstitial edema and fibrosis. Valvular and vascular lesions are not present. The cardiac dilatation and mural thrombosis are similar to those seen in patients with idiopathic congestive or ventricular-dilated cardiomyopathy. The degeneration of cardiac muscle cells assumes two forms: the first is characterized by myofibrillar loss, so that by light microscopy the affected cells appear pale-staining but nonvacuolated; the second type is manifested by marked

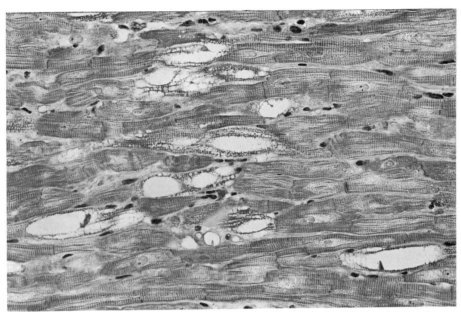

Figure 1. Light micrograph of one-micron-thick plastic section of myocardium of dog given 16 mg/kg of doxorubicin, showing typical vacuolization of cytoplasm. Alkaline toluidine blue stain, X 500.

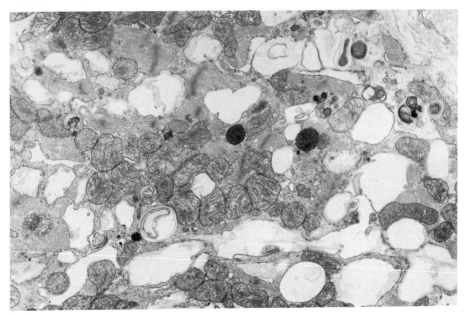

Figure 2. Electron micrograph showing dilated tubules of sarcoplasmic
reticulum and electron-dense lamellae in damaged cardiac muscle cell of
rabbit given 17 mg/kg of doxorubicin. X 13,000.

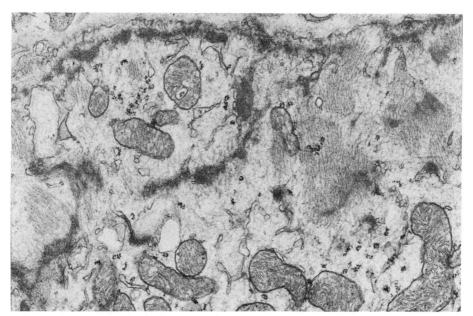

Figure 3. Marked loss of myofibrils in cardiac muscle cell of rabbit given 20 mg/kg doxorubicin. Remnants of myofibrils are seen in the form of electron-dense Z bands and disorganized myofilaments. X 25,000.

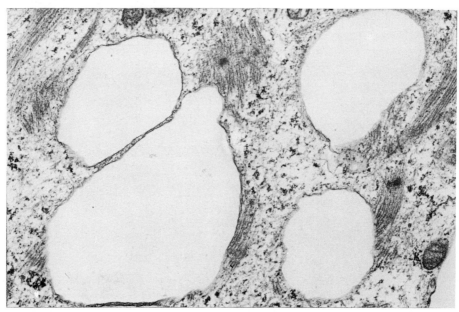

Figure 4. Marked dilatation of tubules of sarcoplasmic reticulum in Purkinje fiber in heart of pig given 13 mg/kg doxorubicin. X 35,000.

cytoplasmic vacuolization, usually associated with myofibrillar loss.
The reasons for these variations in the response of individual cells to
the same stimulus remain unknown.

In histologic preparations the cytoplasmic vacuolization is detected
more easily than the myofibrillar loss, particularly when the tissue has
undergone postmortem autolytic changes. One-micron-thick sections of
tissues embedded in glycolmethacrylate resin and stained with hematoxylin-
eosin or toluidine blue offer considerable greater histologic detail than
do sections of paraffin-embedded tissues and provide a practical alternative
to the use of electron microscopy for the morphologic evaluation of
anthracycline toxicity.

Electron microscopic studies (11,13,22-27) have shown that the
degeneration of cardiac muscle cells in chronic anthracycline toxicity is
a complex phenomenon that involves the myofibrils, the nuclei, the mitochondria and the membrane systems of the T-tubules, the sarcoplasmic
reticulum and the intercellular junctions. These alterations are
illustrated in figures 1-4. The myofibrils show disruption, with lysis
of the myofilaments. These changes account for at least part of the
cellular atrophy.

The cytoplasmic vacuolization is due mainly to pronounced swelling
of the tubules and cisterns of sarcoplasmic reticulum. Accumulation of
lipid and dilatation of tubules of the T-system also can contribute to
the vacuolated appearance. Dilated T-tubules are recognized by their
lining layer of basal lamina material. This layer is absent from dilated
tubules of sarcoplasmic reticulum, which have clear lumina and peculiarly
dense membranes. Dilatation of the sarcoplasmic reticulum is a nonspecific
change that occurs in a number of conditions in which cardiac myocytes
become edematous (28). It should be pointed out, however, that the most

vacuolated myocytes in chronic anthracycline toxicity do not show diffuse cytoplasmic swelling; in such cells the distension of the sarcoplasmic reticulum is a sharply localized phenomenon.

The intercellular junctions of damaged myocytes undergo dissociation, with formation of hemidesmosomes, intracytoplasmic junctions and spherical microparticles. None of these changes is specific. The hemidesmosomes are derived from the dissociation of desmosomes (29). The intracytoplasmic junctions are formed by the specialized apposition of two parts of the plasma membrane of the same cell, and probably result from the rearrangement of remnants of specialized components of previously present intercellular junctions (29). The spherical microparticles are related to the remodeling of plasma membranes, especially in areas of cellular dissociation (30).

The mitochondria show a variety of changes, including pleomorphism, decrease in overall size, alterations in matrix density, and formation of electron-dense concentric lamellae. Mitochondrial inclusions have been observed in human myocardium obtained at necropsy; however, such inclusions are of the amorphous density or flocculent type and are related to post-mortem autolysis (11). Calcific inclusions have not been demonstrated in mitochondria of anthracycline-treated animals. Some of the dense, concentric lamellae are associated with dense bodies which probably are derived from lysosomes. Mitochondrial changes are more prominent in acute than in chronic toxicity; the reverse is true of alterations in sarcoplasmic reticulum.

The finding of interstitial edema is in accord with observations showing that cardiac tissues in anthracycline toxicity have an increased content of calcium, sodium and water (27). Edema in anthracycline toxicity probably results from increased permeability of damaged membranes, with subsequent calcium overload and increases in the tissue content of sodium and water. The inhibition of Na-K-dependent ATPase may be important in this respect (31). The interstitial fibrosis is difficult to evaluate because the edema and the cellular atrophy exaggerate the prominence of the interstitial connective tissue. Endothelial damage has been observed in some animal species (24), but is not considered to be a feature of the toxicity in humans (22).

The features just described are basically the same in humans and in the rat (24), mouse (7,25), dog (32), pig (33) and rabbit (26) models of anthracycline toxicity. These changes are related to the total cumulative dose and to the time scheduling of individual doses. For a given cumulative dose, they tend to be less marked when the drug is given in smaller individual doses (1). Such changes can begin to develop, at least in mouse myocardium, within 24 hours after the administration of a large, single dose of doxorubicin (7). When smaller, repeated doses are given, the changes may take several weeks or months to develop. Three facts need to be emphasized with respect to the dose-cardiotoxicity relationships. The first is that the main target organs in very acute toxicity are the gastrointestinal tract and the bone marrow, in which lesions form that can cause death before the typical cardiac morphologic changes develop. The second is that there is significant variation in the severity of morphologic changes demonstrated by different patients or experimental animals in response to a given dose level, and the third is that the early lesions are focal, becoming more diffuse as their severity increases.

The relation between total cumulative dose of anthracyclines, the development of cardiac morphologic changes and the occurrence of congestive heart failure is of great clinical interest. Bristow el al. (34) have shown that the morphologic findings in endomyocardial biopsy can be used to guide additional therapy in patients in whom either the clinical findings or the total cumulative dose suggest a high risk of the development of anthracycline cardiomyopathy.

Isner et al.(35) evaluated the relationship between clinical evidence and histologic signs of anthracycline toxicity by reviewing the clinical and pathologic findings in 64 patients studied at necropsy, all of whom had received doxorubicin or daunorubicin chemotherapy. Twenty (31%) of the 64 patients had documented clinical toxicity consisting of impaired left ventricular systolic performance: in 7 (35%) of these 20 patients, histologic signs of toxicity were absent. In the remaining 13 patients, histologic signs of toxicity ranged from mild to severe. Of the 44 (69%) patients witnout clinical signs of drug toxicity, 21 (48%) had no histologic signs of cardiotoxicity; however, in 23 (52%) of the patients without clinical toxicity, morphologic signs of toxicity were present, mild in most patients, but extensive in four. Signs of severe histologic toxicity, found in 19 (30%) of the 64 patients, were associated with large doses (over 450 mg/m^2) of drug, mediastinal irradiation, and age over 70 years. The results of this study suggest that attempts to monitor cardiotoxicity by the evaluation of cardiac morphologic changes in patients undergoing anthracycline therapy may be limited by the fact that clinical evidence of cardiotoxicity may be present without accompanying histologic changes; likewise, histologic changes of anthracycline toxicity may be present without clinical evidence of toxicity.

Pathogenesis of cardiac morphologic changes induced by anthracyclines.

The pathogenesis of the changes enumerated above has not been fully elucidated, but it seems likely that several different drugs' effects are important. We believe that the myofibrillar loss results mainly from interference with protein synthesis; the nuclear changes, from the binding

of the drugs to nuclear DNA, and the changes involving the membrane systems
(sarcoplasmic reticulum and plasma membranes) from peroxidative phenomena.
It seems likely that calcium overloading contributes to the development
of anthracycline-induced lesions, as it does in other types of cellular
damage; however, treatment with calcium antagonists fails to protect
against this cardiotoxicity (3). The possibility that the lesions in
chronic anthracycline cardiotoxicity are due to release of histamine
and catecholamines has been suggested by studies showing that pharmacologic
blocking of catecholamine and histamine receptors (α, β, H_1 and H_2
receptors) reduces the severity of chronic anthracycline-induced lesions
(3). The mechanisms by which this protection is exerted are not clear,
as the doses of blocking agents used in this study were rather high;
however, the cardiac lesions produced by catecholamines (36,37) and
histamine (38) consist of focal necroses which differ considerably from
the chronic lesions produced by anthracyclines. Thus, we believe that
histamine and catecholamines have only a contributory role in the
pathogenesis of anthracycline cardiomyopathy.

Anthracyclines can initiate peroxidative phenomena by facilitating
the transfer of electrons from endogenous compounds such as NADPH to
oxygen, resulting in the formation of superoxides that can decompose
to hydroxy radicals, peroxy radicals and hydrogen peroxide. These in
turn can oxidize unsaturated fatty acids and other constituents of
membranes (1). A number of studies, the results of which are summarized
below, suggest that the morphologic features of the toxicity produced by
peroxidative and free radical phenomena vary according to the nature,
mechanism of formation and site of release of the offending compounds.
These observations also suggest that differences in the ability to provide
metabolic defenses against free radical damage may be the cause of

variations in the sensitivity response of individual patients to the cardiotoxic effects of anthracyclines.

Two observations by Myers et al. indicate that lipid peroxidation plays a role in the pathogenesis of anthracycline toxicity: the first is that the administration of very large doses of α-tocopherol, (vitamin E, a free radical scavenger) reduces significantly the acute toxicity and mortality produced by large doses of doxorubicin in mice, and the second is that malondialdehyde, a product of peroxidation and decomposition of unsaturated fatty acids, is readily detectable in the hearts of mice for two to six days after administration of doxorubicin, but not in the hearts of control mice or mice treated with both doxorubicin and α-tocopherol (39,40). Nevertheless, several studies from different laboratories have shown that α-tocopherol provides only very modest protection against the chronic cardiotoxicity of doxorubicin in several species of animals (41-45). In none of these species has it been possible to show that α-tocopherol induces a dramatic qualitative or quantitative change in the morphology of the cardiac lesions.

Ubiquinone, which acts as a free radical scavenger and as an antagonist to the inhibitory effects of anthracyclines on reactions mediated by coenzyme Q, also has been reported to ameliorate the acute and chronic toxicity of doxorubicin (46), again suggesting that such a toxicity is related to peroxidative phenomena. It is of interest to note that animals exposed to high concentrations of oxygen develop skeletal and cardiac muscle lesions which in several ways (including dilatation of sarcoplasmic reticulum) resemble those produced by anthracyclines (47). It is possible that such lesions are mediated by peroxidative changes.

In contrast to their similarity to changes produced by oxygen toxicity, the changes produced by anthracyclines differ from those occurring in radiation injury and in deficiency of selenium and vitamin E (Se-E), two conditions in which cardiac damage is known to be mediated by peroxidative and free radical phenomena. In radiation injury to the heart (48), the initial damage is most prominent in capillary endothelial cells, which become edematous or necrotic; platelet and fibrin thrombi are frequent. In later stages there is severe interstitial fibrosis; however, at no time do the cardiac myocytes show changes similar to those in anthracycline cardiotoxicity. The combined administration of doxorubicin and radiation to rabbits results in the superimposition of lesions typical of each of these two agents and in significant enhancement of the cardiotoxicity of doxorubicin (49,50). This enhancement (and a "recall phenomenon" for previous radiation) also has been demonstrated in humans (51).

Comparisons of the pathologic changes produced by anthracyclines and by Se-E deficiency are of interest because selenium and vitamin E, in conjunction with glutathione peroxidase, form an antioxidant system which prevents the peroxidation of membrane lipids and other cellular constituents. Cardiac lesions in Se-E deficiency have been best characterized in the pig (52, 53) and consist of: 1) multiple foci of necrosis, with hyalinization or with hypercontraction bands and mitochondrial swelling, disruption and calcification; 2) intramyocardial hemorrhage ("mulberry heart"); 3) fibrinoid necrosis of small intramural coronary arteries; and 4) capillary microthrombi composed of fibrin and platelets. The alterations cited above differ clearly from those in anthracycline toxicity, which in the pig induce (33) changes similar to those in humans and in other species.

Recent observations suggest that the role of α-tocopherol and selenium in the chronic cardiotoxicity of anthracyclines is secondary rather than primary. As discussed above, the administration of large doses

of selenium and vitamin E provides only modest protection against chronic
anthracycline cardiotoxicity (41-45). Furthermore, it has been shown
(54) that ferric or ferrous ions can form with doxorubicin a complex
which catalyzes the reduction of oxygen by both cysteine and glutathione,
producing superoxide and hydrogen peroxide. This complex also binds in
vitro to human erythrocyte ghost membranes and causes them to be
destroyed in the presence of glutathione. These results may provide
an explanation for the findings of Herman et al., who showed that ICRF
187 (razoxane), probably acting as an iron chelator, markedly reduces
the chronic cardiotoxicity of doxorubicin or daunorubicin in
experimental animals (55). Although this remains unproven at the
present time, it seems likely that the peroxidative damage which
mediates part of the chronic cardiotoxicity of anthracyclines is
catalyzed by this iron complex. Studies of this complex should provide
a new approach to the pharmacological prevention of chronic anthracycline
cardiotoxicity and its consequences.

REFERENCES

1. Young RC, Ozols RF, Myers CE. The anthracycline antineoplastic drugs. N Engl J Med 305:139, 1981.
2. Herman E, Young R, Krop S. Doxorubicin-induced hypotension in the Beagle dog. Agents Actions 8:551, 1978.
3. Bristow MR, Minobe WA, Billingham ME, Marmor JB, Johnson GA, Ishimoto BM, Sageman WS, Daniels JR. Anthracycline-associated cardiac and renal damage in rabbits: evidence for mediation by vasoactive substances. Lab Invest 45:157, 1981.
4. Regal E, Kaliner M, El-Hage A, Ferrans VJ, Kawanami O, Herman EH. Anthracycline-induced histamine release from rat mast cells. Agents Actions (in press).
5. Gandolfi A. Cardiotossicita cronica da adriamicina: studio morfologico ultrastrutturale sul miocardio ventricolare e sul sistema di conduzione del cuore di coniglio. Ateneo Parmense [Acta Biomed] 47:69, 1976.
6. Herman EH, Ferrans VJ. Unpublished observations.
7. Lambertenghi-Deliliers G, Zanon PL, Pozzoli EF, Bellini O. Myocardial injury induced by a single dose of adriamycin: an electron microscopic study. Tumori 62:517, 1976.
8. Merski A, Daskal I, Busch H. Effects of adriamycin on ultrastructure of nucleoli in the heart and liver cells of the rat. Cancer Res 36:1580, 1976.
9. Daskal Y, Woodard C, Crooke ST, Busch H. Comparative ultrastructural studies of nucleoli of tumor cells treated with Adriamycin and the newer anthracyclines, Carminomycin and Marcellomycin. Cancer Res 38:467, 1978.
10. Unuma T, Senda R, Muramatsu M. Mechanism of nucleolar segregation-differences in effects of actinomycin D and cycloheximide on nucleoli of rat liver cells. J Electron Microsc (Tokyo) 22:205, 1973.
11. Buja LM, Ferrans VJ, Mayer RJ, Roberts WC, Henderson ES. Cardiac ultrastructural changes induced by daunorubicin therapy. Cancer 32:771, 1973.
12. Egorin MJ, Hildebrand RC, Cimino EF, Bachur NR. Cytofluorescence localization of adriamycin and daunorubicin. Cancer Res 34:2243, 1974.
13. Buja LM, Ferrans VJ, Rabson AS. Letter: Unusual nuclear alterations. Lancet 1:402, 1974.
14. Bristow MR, Thompson PD, Martin RP, Mason JW, Billingham ME, Harrison DC. Early anthracycline cardiotoxicity. Am J Med 65:823, 1978.
15. Lefrak EA, Pitha J, Rosenheim S, Gottlieb J. A clinicopathologic analysis of adriamycin cardiotoxicity. Cancer 32:302, 1973.
16. Cortes EP, Lutman G, Wanka J, Wang JJ, Pickren J, Wallace J, Holland JF. Adriamycin (NSC-123127) cardiotoxicity. A clinico-pathologic correlation. Cancer Treat Rep 6:215, 1975.
17. Gilladoga AC, Manuel C, Tan CC, Wollner N, Murphy ML. Cardio-toxicity of adriamycin (NSC-123127) in children. Cancer Treat Rep 6:209, 1975.
18. Minow RA, Benjamin RS, Lee ET, Gottlieb JA. Adriamycin cardio-myopathy-risk factors. Cancer 39:1397, 1977.
19. Halazun JF, Wagner HR, Gaeta JF, Sinks LF. Daunorubicin cardiac toxicity in children with acute lymphocytic leukemia. Cancer 33:545, 1974.

20. Gilladoga AC, Manuel C, Tan C, Wollner N, Sternberg SS, Murphy ML. The cardiotoxicity of adriamycin and daunomycin in children. Cancer 37:1070, 1976.

21. Von Hoff DD, Rozencweig M, Layard M, Slavik M, Muggia FM. Daunomycin-induced cardiotoxicity in children and adults. A review of 110 cases. Am J Med 62:200, 1977.

22. Billingham ME, Mason JW, Bristow MR, Daniels JR. Anthracycline cardiomyopathy monitored by morphologic changes. Cancer Treat Rep 62:865, 1978.

23. Ferrans VJ. Overview of cardiac pathology in relation to anthracycline cardiotoxicity. Cancer Treat Rep 62:955, 1978.

24. Chalcroft SCW, Gavin JB, Herdson PB. Fine structural changes in rat myocardium induced by daunorubicin. Pathology 5:99, 1973.

25. Rosenoff SH, Olson HM, Young DM, Bostick F, Young RC. Adriamycin-induced cardiac damage in the mouse. A small animal model of cardiotoxicity. JNCI 55:191, 1975.

26. Jaenke RS. An anthracycline antibiotic-induced cardiomyopathy in rabbits. Lab Invest 30:292, 1974.

27. Olson HM, Young DM, Prieur DJ, Le Roy AF, Reagan RL. Electrolyte and morphologic alterations of myocardium in adriamycin-treated rabbits. Am J Pathol 77:439, 1974.

28. Ferrans VJ, Buja LM, Levitsky S, Williams WH, McIntosh CL, Roberts WC. Cardiac preservation: a morphologic study. Recent Adv Stud Cardiac Struct Metab 1:351, 1972.

29. Buja LM, Ferrans VJ, Maron BJ. Intracytoplasmic junctions in cardiac muscle cells. Am J Pathol 74:613, 1974.

30. Ferrans VJ, Thiedemann K-U, Maron BJ, Roberts WC. Spherical microparticles in human myocardium. An ultrastructural study. Lab Invest 35:349, 1976.

31. Gosalvez M, van Rossum GDV, Blanco MF. Inhibition of sodium-potassium-activated adenosine 5'-triphosphatase and ion transport by Adriamycin. Cancer Res 39:257, 1979.

32. Van Vleet JF, Ferrans VJ, Weirich WE. Cardiac disease induced by chronic adriamycin administration in dogs and an evaluation of vitamin E and selenium as cardioprotectants. Am J Pathol 99:13, 1980.

33. Van Vleet JF, Greenwood LA, Ferrans VJ. Pathologic features of adriamycin toxicosis in young pigs: nonskeletal lesions. Am J Vet Res 40:1537, 1979.

34. Bristow MR, Mason JW, Billingham ME, Daniels JR. Doxorubicin cardiomyopathy. Evaluation by phonocardiography, endomyocardial biopsy, and cardiac catheterization. Ann Intern Med 88:168, 1978.

35. Isner JM, Ferrans VJ, Cohen SR, Witkind BG, Virmani R, Gottdiener JS, Roberts WC. Variability of cardiac histologic toxicity in patients treated with anthracycline chemotherapy. Am J Cardiol 45:396, 1980.

36. Ferrans VJ, Hibbs RG, Weily HS, Weilbaecher DG, Walsh JJ, Burch GE. A histochemical and electron microscopic study of epinephrine-induced myocardial necrosis. J Mol Cell Cardiol 1:11, 1970.

37. Ferrans VJ, Hibbs RG, Walsh JJ, Burch GE. Histochemical and electron microscopical studies on the cardiac necroses produced by sympatho-mimetic agents. Ann NY Acad Sci 156:309, 1969.

38. Franco-Browder S, Guerrero M, Gorodezky M, Bravo LM, Aceves S. Lesiones miocárdicas producidas por liberadores de histamina en ratas. Arch Inst Cardiol Mex 30:720, 1960.

39. Myers CE, McGuire WP, Liss RH, Ifrim I, Grotzinger K, Young RC. Adriamycin: the role of lipid peroxidation in cardiac toxicity and tumor response. Science 197:165, 1977.
40. Myers CE, McGuire WP, Young RC. Adriamycin: amelioration of toxicity by α-tocopherol. Cancer Treat Rep 60:961, 1976.
41. Wang Y, Madanat FF, Kimball JC, Gleiser CA, Ali MK, Kaufman MW, Van Eys J. Effect of vitamin E against adriamycin-induced toxicity in rabbits. Cancer Res 40:1022, 1980.
42. Breed JGS, Zimmerman ANE, Dormans JAM, Pinedo HM. Failure of the antioxidant vitamin E to protect against adriamycin-induced cardiotoxicity in the rabbit. Cancer Res 40:2033, 1980.
43. Van Vleet JF, Greenwood L, Ferrans VJ, Rebar AH. Effect of selenium-vitamin E on adriamycin-induced cardiomyopathy in rabbits. Am J Vet Res 39:997, 1978.
44. Van Vleet JF, Ferrans VJ. Cutaneous lesions and hematologic alterations in chronic adriamycin intoxication in dogs with and without vitamin E and selenium supplementation. Am J Vet Res 41: 691, 1980.
45. Van Vleet JF, Ferrans VJ. Evaluation of vitamin E and selenium protection against chronic adriamycin toxicity in rabbits. Cancer Treat Rep 64:315, 1980.
46. Bertazzoli C, Sala L, Solcia E, Ghione M. Experimental adriamycin cardiotoxicity prevented by ubiquinone in vivo in rabbits. Int Res Commun Sys Med Sci 3:468, 1975.
47. Caulfield JB, Shelton RW, Burke JF. Cytotoxic effects of oxygen on striated muscle. Arch Pathol 94:127, 1972.
48. Fajardo LF, Stewart JR. Pathogenesis of radiation-induced myocardial fibrosis. Lab Invest 29:244, 1973.
49. Fajardo LF, Eltringham JR, Stewart JR. Combined cardiotoxicity of Adriamycin and X-radiation. Lab Invest 34:86, 1976.
50. Eltringham JR, Fajardo LF, Stewart R. Adriamycin cardiomyopathy: enhanced cardiac damage in rabbits with combined drug and cardiac irradiation. Radiology 115:471, 1975.
51. Billingham ME, Bristow MR, Glatstein E, Mason JW, Masek MA, Daniels JR. Adriamycin cardiotoxicity: endomyocardial biopsy evidence of enhancement by irradiation. Am J Surg Pathol 1:17, 1977.
52. Van Vleet JF, Ferrans VJ, Ruth GR. Ultrastructural alterations in nutritional cardiomyopathy of selenium-vitamin E deficient swine. I. Fiber lesions. Lab Invest 37:188, 1977.
53. Van Vleet JF, Ferrans VJ, Ruth GR. Ultrastructural alterations in nutritional cardiomyopathy of selenium-vitamin E deficient swine. II. Vascular lesions. Lab Invest 37:201, 1977.
54. Myers CE, Gianni L, Simone CB, Hendrickson M, Klecker R, Greene R. Oxidative destruction of erythrocyte ghost membranes catalyzed by the doxorubicin-iron complex. Biochemistry (submitted).
55. Herman EH, Ferrans VJ. Reduction of chronic doxorubicin cardiotoxicity in dogs by pretreatment with (±)-1,2-bis(3,5-dioxopiperazinyl-1-yl)propane (ICRF-187). Cancer Res 41: 3436, 1981.

CARDIAC MONITORING OF PATIENTS RECEIVING ANTHRACYCLINES

M. R. BRISTOW

In this chapter, I will briefly summarize the Stanford experience in the development of cardiac monitoring strategies for patients receiving anthracyclines.

1. TYPES OF MONITORING

Two general types of cardiac monitoring are available to the clinician administering a cardiotoxic anthracycline. The first method, a technique developed by our group, is direct assessment of anthracycline-type myocardial tissue damage. The tissue samples are obtained by right ventricular endomyocardial biopsy, a safe, reliable technique in the hands of experienced operators (1-3). The method for quantifying the degree of anthracycline damage is electron microscopic analysis of affected myocardial cells according to the system developed by Billingham (4-6). As a single test, this method yields maximal specificity and sensitivity for detecting anthracycline change and has been successfully used to identify individuals prospectively at risk for developing heart failure and to administer doxorubicin safely in excess of empiric dose limits (7).

The second type of cardiac monitoring is by serial measurement of cardiac function. The only noninvasive method possessing adequate sensitivity and specificity is serial radionuclide ejection fractions (8). Sensitivity of this method may be improved by performing stress testing, but this is accompanied by some loss of specificity (9). Other noninvasive methods of measuring myocardial performance, including M-mode echocardiograms and systolic time intervals, have not proven effective in most investigators' experience.

2. WHO SHOULD BE MONITORED?

Our experience is that only patients with risk factors
need cardiac monitoring (7). If patients without previous
mediastinal radiation, age >70, underlying heart disease,
history of hypertension, or previous receipt of $\geq$450 mg/m^2
of an anthracycline are excluded, the incidence of heart
failure during anthracycline treatment is negligible (7).
Cardiac monitoring should therefore be confined to risk-
patients, since monitoring is expensive, time-consuming, and
places unwanted constraints on drug administration. As defined
by the above criteria, in the absence of cardiac monitoring the
at-risk population has a heart failure risk of approximately
15-20% (7).

3. MONITORING BY DIRECT MORPHOLOGIC ASSESSMENT

Most observers now recognize the superiority of endomyocardial biopsy in the detection of anthracycline cardiotoxicity
(10-13). The method and its practical implementation are well
described (1,4-7) and need no further elucidation. The basis
for the reliability of the endomyocardial biopsy technique
is that it is both highly sensitive and specific for detection
of the anthracycline lesion. Its relatively superior sensitivity
is a product of the dose-effect and structure-function
relationships in anthracycline cardiomyopathy (11). These
relationships dictate that myocardial damage is nearly linearly
related to dose, while performance deterioration does not occur
until an advanced degree of damage is reached (11). As a
single test endomyocardial biopsy thus has considerably better
predictive value than performance measurements.

The basis for the high degree of specificity of endomyocardial
biopsy is that the EM-identified lesion is specific for
anthracycline effects, while performance abnormalities may
result from any type of myocardial insult.

3. MONITORING BY SERIAL PERFORMANCE MEASUREMENTS

Despite the limitations of the anthracycline structure-function relationship and the high incidence of background "nonspecific" performance abnormalities found in this patient population (11), it is possible to utilize noninvasive methods of measuring myocardial performance to monitor anthracycline cardiotoxicity. As first described by Alexander et al.(8), serial rest radionuclide ejection fractions can be used to identify patients at-risk for anthracycline-associated heart failure. Baseline studies are necessary to improve specificity (8,14),and serial studies are required to attain satisfactory sensitivity. Rest radionuclide ejection fractions are not satisfactory as single tests, but exercise ejection fractions do possess the sensitivity to be used as single tests (9). Because of the nonlinear, parabolic shape of the anthracycline cardiomyopathy structure-function relationship (11), it is imperative that radionuclide ejection fractions be performed quite frequently, i.e., every 50-60 mg/m^2 for rest studies and every 100-200 mg/m^2 if stress tests are included.

4. SUMMARY

After several years of investigation, two satisfactory methods of monitoring anthracycline cardiotoxicity have emerged. The choice of which to employ is largely a matter of what is available at individual institutions. Endomyocardial biopsy does have the advantage of better specificity and does not require previous baseline tests for comparison. Also, because the morphologic lesion does not appear to regress, the test retains its validity for months or years after drug administration. Radionuclide ejection fractions are more widely available and easier to administer. The cost of either strategy is not insignificant, and for this reason alone monitoring should be confined to at-risk patients.

REFERENCES

1. Mason J. 1978. Techniques for right and left ventricular endomyocardial biopsy. Am J Cardiol 41:887.
2. Bristow MR, Mason JW, Billingham ME, Daniels JR. 1978. Doxorubicin cardiomyopathy: evaluation by phonocardiography, endomyocardial biopsy, and cardiac catheterization. Ann Intern Med 88:168.
3. Bristow MR, Billingham ME, Mason JW, Daniels JR. 1978. Clinical spectrum of anthracycline antibiotic cardiotoxicity, Cancer Treat Rep 62:873.
4. Billingham ME, Bristow MR, Glatstein E, Mason JW, Masek M, Daniels JR. 1977. Adriamycin cardiotoxicity: endomyocardial biopsy evidence of enhancement by irradiation. Am J Surg Pathol 1:17.
5. Billingham ME, Mason JW, Bristow MR, Daniels JR. 1978. Anthracycline cardiomyopathy monitored by morphologic changes. Cancer Treat Rep 62:865.
6. Billingham ME, Bristow MR. In press. Endomyocardial biopsy for cardiac monitoring of patients receiving anthracycline. In Endomyocardial biopsy: techniques and applications. Fenoglio J , ed. C.R.C. Press.
7. Bristow MR, Lopez MB, Mason JW, Billingham ME, Winchester MA. In press. Efficacy and cost of cardiac monitoring in patients receiving doxorubicin. Cancer.
8. Alexander J, Dainiak N, Berger HJ et al. 1979. Serial assessment of doxorubicin cardiotoxicity with quantitative radionuclide angiocardiography. New Engl J Med 300:278.
9. Bristow M, Lopez M, McKillop J. 1980. Specificity and sensitivity of radionuclide ejection fractions in doxorubicin cardiomyopathy. Proc AACR/ASCO 21:154.
10. Mason JW, Bristow MR, Billingham ME, Daniels JR. 1978. Invasive and noninvasive methods of assessing adriamycin cardiotoxic effects in man: superiority of histopathologic assessment using endomyocardial biopsy. Cancer Treat Rep 62:857.
11. Bristow MR, Mason JW, Billingham ME, Daniels JR. 1981, in press. Dose-effect and structure-function relationships in doxorubicin cardiomyopathy. Am Heart J.
12. Henderson IC, Frei E. 1980. Adriamycin cardiotoxicity. Am Heart J 99:671.
13. Young RC, Ozols RF, Myers CE. 1981. The anthracycline antineoplastic drugs. New Engl J Med 305:139.
14. Choi W, Berger H, Alexander J et al. 1981. Serial radionuclide assessment of doxorubicin cardiotoxicity in cancer patients with abnormal baseline resting left ventricular performance. Am J Cardiol 47:474.

REDUCTION OF ADRIAMYCIN CARDIAC TOXICITY BY SCHEDULE MANIPULATION

R. S. BENJAMIN, S. S. LEGHA, M. VALDIVIEŠO, M. S. EWER, B. MACKAY, AND S. WALLACE

The concept of altering the therapeutic index of a chemotherapeutic agent by schedule manipulation is in no way new. Schedule dependency of an antitumor agent is defined in experimental studies by increased survival of tumor-bearing animals treated on one schedule rather than on another. Such an effect implies, of course, increased toxicity to the tumor on the more effective schedule. If increased host toxicity occurred to the same extent, however, there would be no net gain in survival. Thus, schedule dependency implies a greater increase in effectiveness than toxicity with schedule manipulation, that is, an increased therapeutic index. Most attempts at schedule manipulation deal with acute toxicity. For adriamycin, there is an easily demonstrable decrease in mucositis when the drug is given as a single dose compared with a 3-day or chronic schedule (1). It is unusual, however, for schedule dependency to be manifested by alterations in chronic toxicity.

The first suggestion that adriamycin cardiac toxicity might be schedule-dependent was the report of Weiss and his associates from the Central Oncology Group that weekly adriamycin administration was associated with minimal or no cardiac toxicity (2). This was confirmed by Chlebowski from the Western Cancer Study Group (3). The comparative cardiotoxic effects of the weekly regimens with the more commonly used single-dose or 3-day schedules repeated every 3-4 weeks is best seen in the retrospective review of Von Hoff et al. (4). By plotting the dose-related incidence of congestive heart failure versus cumulative dose, one can appreciate that the curve for the weekly schedule is shifted to the right so that a 10% risk of heart failure occurs at about 750 mg/m^2 rather than 550 mg/m^2.

Why then is adriamycin not routinely administered in a weekly schedule? We would assume that there are a number of reasons. First, the number of patients treated on that schedule is small compared with the single dose every 3 weeks. Relative antitumor activity per unit dose is not well defined for the various schedules. Weekly drug administration is cumbersome, requiring weekly patient visits to the physician and weekly decision making regarding chemotherapy dose. Patients are continually under the effects of weekly adriamycin chemotherapy, and they have not yet achieved the maximal toxic effects of one dose when the next is administered. Finally, although the cardiotoxicity data look convincing, they are based on subjective evaluation by the physician that a patient did or did not have congestive heart failure caused by adriamycin rather than on objective quantifiable data.

Quantitative study of the cardiotoxic effects of the anthracyclines was hampered in the past by lack of a sensitive, reproducible, direct measurement system for evaluating the degree of cardiotoxicity. Endomyocardial biopsy as developed by Drs Billingham, Bristow, and collaborators at Stanford University provides such a system since toxic effects can be quantified at the level of the target organ (5). The procedure is relatively simple and has been well described (6,7). There have been no deaths related to the biopsy procedure in approximately 1500 cases at Stanford (not all to assess adriamycin toxicity) and 400 in our own experience.

Cumulative adriamycin dose is the single most important factor for predicting the development of cardiac toxicity (4,8-10). We were struck by the initial demonstration from the Stanford group of the excellent correlation of cardiac biopsy grade according to the Billingham system with cumulative dose. The biopsy was sensitive enough to detect changes in the majority of patients at clinically safe doses, and mean biopsy grade at the 500 mg/m^2 level was just under 2. We reasoned, therefore, that treatment to a biopsy grade of 2, regardless of cumulative dose, would be safe. Dr. Mackay, our pathologist, exchanged all initial biopsy specimens with Dr. Billigham until they agreed on grading. He then modified the grading procedure into a more quantitative and therefore more easily reproducible system (11). When we compared biopsy score versus cumulative dose in our own patients treated with standard, single-dose, 3-4 weekly adriamycin administration with the results from the Stanford series, the agreement was remarkable. Particularly at cumulative dose levels below 500 mg/m^2, our biopsy grades differed from theirs by less than 1/10 of a point.

Our first study was an attempt to confirm the decreased cardiac toxicity of weekly adriamycin therapy. Patients with squamous lung cancer were randomized between two combination chemotherapy programs containing adriamycin at a dose of 60 mg/m^2/course. One group received the entire adriamycin dose as a single rapid infusion every 3 weeks while the other group received one-third of the dose weekly. Both groups received otherwise identical chemotherapy. Cardiac biopsy scores were significantly lower at each dose level for patients receiving weekly adriamycin compared with 3-weekly adriamycin. The response rate to the combination was slightly higher in the group receiving weekly adriamycin administration although the differences were not statistically significant; however, in this situation, weekly adriamycin administration was definitely no less effective than every-3-week administrations.

We reasoned that if weekly adriamycin indeed was less cardiotoxic, the most likely explanation was the low peak levels from the low weekly doses. The most effective way of decreasing peak levels is simply by prolonging infusion duration. We initiated studies, therefore, with progressive increases in infusion duration from 24 to 48 to 96 hours while retaining an intermittent 3-4 week treatment schedule (12). Clinical results of those studies are noted elsewhere in the chapter by Dr. Legha and others. Suffice it to say here, there was no decrease in the antitumor activity of adriamycin by decreasing peak levels. If anything, there may be a suggestion of enhanced antitumor activity. Acute toxic effects are quite similar to those seen with rapid infusion; however, nausea and vomiting are markedly diminished, and stomatitis is slightly increased.

The major obstacles to continuous infusion therapy are fear of extravasation and shortage of in-patient facilities. Both of these were overcome prior to initiation of our studies. Indwelling, silastic, central-venous catheters are used routinely for all infusions with position checked prior to each drug administration to assure that the catheter remains in the superior vena cava. We use the Centrasil or Intrasil catheters from Travenol Labs which are placed percutaneously, and a Seldinger technique is used rather than one requiring surgically placed Hickman catheters. Our catheters have been left in place for as long as 2 years, and the incidence of infectious complications during chemotherapy is no higher for patients with catheters than for those without.

Increasing infusion duration from 5 minutes to 24 hours results in a decrease in peak plasma levels of 5.5-fold (13). Prolonging the infusion to 96 hr results in a 13.5-fold decrease over that obtained with rapid infusion and a 2.4-fold decrease over levels obtained with 24 hr infusion.

In order to compare cardiac toxicity of patients treated with continuous infusion therapy versus those treated by rapid infusion, we chose a control group of 30 patients who had undergone 33 biopsies during the usual rapid infusion schedule (13). For the lower doses, these were the patients on the weekly versus 3-weekly study previously noted. For the higher doses, any patient receiving adriamycin who had reached a cumulative dose of approximately 450 mg/m^2 was considered eligible to continue therapy unless he or she developed a grade 2 biopsy. Thus, patients were chosen for biopsy by the random combination of events of responding to their chemotherapy and reaching a cumulative adriamycin dose of 450 mg/m^2 without clinical suspicion of congestive heart failure and when further adriamycin chemotherapy was desired by the treating physician. The control group was well matched with the continuous infusion group with regard to known risk factors for development of cardiac toxicity, particularly age, cardiac radiation, and prior history of hypertension or heart disease. Twenty-one patients treated with continuous infusion therapy were studied with 35 endomyocardial biopsies. The greater number of biopsies reflects the fact that these patients received and continued to receive higher adriamycin doses than the control group. Biopsies were repeated at least every 4 courses, or earlier, if noninvasive studies showed decreased cardiac function.

Median cumulative dose for the continuous infusion group was 600 mg/m^2 which is higher than the 465 mg/m^2 for the rapid infusion patients. When only the highest biopsy grades were studied for each patient, the mean for the continuous infusion patients was 0.9 compared with 1.6 for the rapid infusion group. When the distribution of biopsy changes was studied, patients with continuous infusion had a lower biopsy grade at each cumulative dose range. Fifty-one percent of the biopsies on the continuous infusion patients were normal or showed only minor changes of less than grade 1 magnitude compared with only 12% of those in the standard rapid infusion group. Conversely, only 10% of the biopsies on the continuous infusion group fell into the grade 2 or 3 category requiring drug discontinuation compared with 46% of those on

the standard schedule. These differences are all statistically significant.

Of interest, is the fact that both high grade biopsies on the
continuous infusion schedule occurred in patients with prior cardiac
radiation and with 48-hr rather than 96-hr infusions. We currently
estimate that cumulative dose can probably be doubled in the majority
of patients receiving 96-hr infusion. Further studies are under way
in patients receiving the 24-hr and 48-hr infusion schedules.

Key questions to be answered in future studies regard the duration
of infusion necessary for optimal drug usage. It is unlikely that continued therapy beyond a certain point will be effective, and studies
trying to determine the appropriate duration of adriamycin therapy without
consideration for a 450-500 mg/m^2 dose limitation are certainly warranted
for a number of tumors. These, coupled with studies of cumulative dose
requirements for varying infusion durations, will lead to revised recom-
mendations for optimal drug schedule and duration for future patients.

REFERENCES

1. Benjamin RS, Weirnik PH, and Bachur NR. 1974. Adriamycin chemotherapy-
    efficacy safety and pharmacology basis of an intermittent single high-
    dosage schedule. Cancer 33, pp 19-27.
2. Weiss AJ, Metter GE, Fletcher WA, et al. 1976. Studies on adriamycin
    using a weekly regimen demonstrating its clinical effectiveness and
    lack of cardiac toxicity. Cancer Treat. Rep. 60, pp 813-822.
3. Chlebowski RT, Paroly WS, Pugh RP, et al. 1980. Adriamcyin given as
    weekly schedule without a loading course. Clinically effective with
    a reduced incidence of cardiotoxicity. Cancer Treat. Rep. 64, pp 47-51.
4. Von Hoff DD, Layard MW, Basa P, et al. 1979. Risk factors for doxo-
    rubicin-induced congestive heart failure. Ann. Intern Med. 91, pp 710-71
5. Billingham ME, Bristow MR, Glatstein E, et al. 1977. Adriamycin
    cardiotoxicity: Endomyocardial biopsy evidence of enhancement by
    irradiation. Am. J. Surg. Path. 1, pp 17-23.
6. Mason JW. 1978. Techniques for right and left ventricular endomyocardial
    biopsy. Am. J. Cardiol. 41, pp 887-892.
7. Ewer MS, and Ali MK. 1981. Cardiac biopsy: A review of the procedure,
    complications and indications. Practial Cardiology 7, pp 143-154.
8. Gottlieb JA, Lefrak EA, O'Bryan RM, et al. 1973. Adriamcyin cardiomyo-
    pathy: Prevention by dose limitation. Proc. Am. Assoc. Cancer Research
    14, pp 88.
9. Lefrak EA, Pitha J, Rosenheim S, et al. 1973. A clinicopathologic
    analysis of adriamycin cardiotoxicity. Cancer 32, pp 302-314.
10. Minow RA, Benjamin RS, Lee ET, et al. 1977. Adriamycin cardiomyopathy -
    Risk factor. Cancer 39, pp 1397-1402.
11. Mackay B, Keyes LM, Benjamin RS, et al. 1981. Cardiac biopsy. Texas
    Society for Electron Microscopy 11, pp 7-15.
12. Legha SS, Benjamin RS, Mackay B, et al. 1981. In press. Adriamycin
    therapy by continuous intravenous infusion in patients with metastatic
    breast cancer. Cancer.

13. Benjamin RS, Legha SS, Mackay B, et al. 1981. Reduction of adriamycin cardiac toxicity using a prolonged continuous intravenous infusion. Proc. Am. Assoc. Cancer Research 22, pp 179.

RATIONALE AND DESIGN OF A TRIAL TO EVALUATE THE CARDIOTOXOCITY OF WEEKLY
SCHEDULES OF ADRIAMYCIN, WITH ENDOMYOCARDIAL BIOPSY USED AS AN END POINT

F. M. TORTI, B. LUM, M. R. BRISTOW, F. E. STOCKDALE, M. KOHLER,
M. E. BILLINGHAM, AND S. K. CARTER

1. INTRODUCTION

The use of Adriamycin in clinical oncology has been limited, at least
in certain settings, by a dose-dependent cardiotoxicity. For some patients
treated palliatively for advanced breast cancer, sarcomas, and other malignancies, Adriamycin must be withdrawn during a clinical response to prevent
cardiac toxicity. Furthermore, the recent introduction of Adriamycin into
adjuvant trials (1) as well as its use in curable cancers (2,3) has raised
concern about potential long-term effects of subclinical cardiac damage,
as the treated population with Hodgkin's disease and breast cancer ages. Thu
there is a need to diminish the cardiotoxicity in treating patients with palliative intent, as well as to limit subclinical toxicity in a younger population treated adjuvantly or with curative intent. To date, the major approach
to this problem have been 1) analog development, with the aim of equal antitumor efficacy with ameliorated cardiac toxicity; 2) cardioprotectors used in
concert with Adriamycin; and 3) scheduling alterations in the administration
of Adriamycin. This paper will deal with the use of the endomyocardial biops
to evaluate the cardiotoxicity of Adriamycin given on a weekly schedule.

2. RATIONALE FOR WEEKLY ADRIAMYCIN SCHEDULE

Two clinical trial groups used weekly schedules of Adriamycin shortly
after the phase I studies of Adriamycin had been completed. The Central Oncology Group first suggested in 1976 that weekly Adriamycin might be less
cardiotoxic. Weiss et al. reported on 442 patients treated with Adriamycin
a weekly schedule (4). They administered between 0.4 to 0.6 mg/kg/wk, with
loading dose of 0.4 mg/kg on days 1, 3, 8, and 10. Nine patients received
550-600 mg/m^2 Adriamycin; 28, between 600-1000; and 22, between 1000-2500.
Six patients developed clinical cardiac dysfunction; however, four of these
patients had had preexisting cardiac disease. In all cases, the authors

concluded that factors other than Adriamycin played a major role in the cardiotoxicity. Even if all of these cases of cardiac dysfunction were ascribed to Adriamycin, the incidence of congestive heart failure was less than that expected for conventional scheduling (see Table 1).

Table 1. Summary of studies of weekly dose schedules of Adriamycin

| Study | Schedule | Number of patients | Number of patients receiving a total dose (mg/m^2) of | | | No. of patients with CHF | Cardiac monitoring |
			450-6000	600-1000	>1000		
Weiss	weekly	442	9	28	22	0	clinical EKG
Weiss	weekly	207	--	36	27	2	clinical EKG
Chlebowski	weekly	336	21	10	--	0	clinical EKG
TOTAL		985	30	74	49	2	

Subsequently, Adriamycin in combination with other chemotherapeutic agents was evaluated by the Central Oncology Group (5). Again, minimal cardiotoxicity was noted. Sixty-three patients received between 600-1000 mg/m^2, and 36 patients received >1000 mg/m^2. Weekly schedules of Adriamycin without a loading course were evaluated by Chlebowski et al. (6). Sixteen patients received between 450-550 mg/m^2 Adriamycin; 5, between 550-600 mg/m^2; 10, >600 mg/m^2. There was no clinical congestive heart failure noted.

In these studies of the Central Oncology Group and the Western Cancer Study Group, 935 patients have received weekly Adriamycin. No differences were observed in response rates from the expected results with three weekly Adriamycin for the tumor types tested. However, none of these studies randomized between Adriamycin scheduling. Small differences in response rates among schedules, which would be missed in these retrospective comparisons, might well exist.

3. DESIGN OF CLINICAL TRIAL

The large experience with endomyocardial biopsy at Stanford has provided a large base of patients against which to compare the biopsy results of the weekly protocol. This comparison is facilitated by the high degree of specificity of the endomyocardial lesion identified by Billingham et al. for Adriamycin toxicity in this patient population (7).

Patients with a variety of malignancies sensitive to Adriamycin are

entered on one of the weekly Adriamycin regimens listed in Figure 1. The
vincristine is administered every other week in the Adriamycin-vincristine
regimen. Patients who remain in clinical response at empiric dose limitations
of Adriamycin undergo cardiac catheterization and endomyocardial biopsy.
Patients with minimal cardiac abnormalities receive further Adriamycin, the
exact dose dependent both on the catheterization and endomyocardial biopsy
results. By this method, some patients in clinical response can receive substantially more Adriamycin than empiric dose limitations would allow.

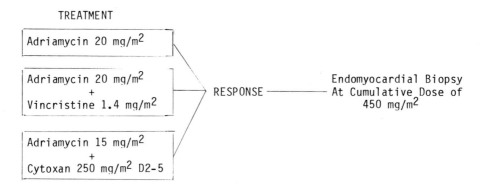

FIGURE 1. Chemotherapeutic regimens utilizing weekly Adriamycin--Northern
California Oncology Group protocol 1B81, adenocarcinoma: breast, unknown
primary, other sites.

4. PROPOSED METHODS OF ANALYSIS

The analysis of the trial will be performed with paired and unpaired
analyses. Figure 2 demonstrates one approach of unpaired analysis, where the
percentage of normal or near normal biopsy scores at 450 mg/m^2 is compared
for the approximately 180 patients biopsied with conventional scheduling of
Adriamycin versus those patients under a weekly schedule. An estimate of
the number of weekly Adriamycin biopsies required to reach statistical signif
icance is indicated. It is dependent upon the magnitude of the difference
in biopsy scores of the weekly and conventional dose schedules.

Paired analyses will match on patient age, status of prior cardiac
irradiation, dose of Adriamycin delivered, and concommitantly administered
drugs such as cyclophosphamide.

Any respective analysis is a compromise on a prospective comparison of
randomized schedules; small differences may be artifactual. However, this
retrospective analysis has particular strength since the end point is patho-

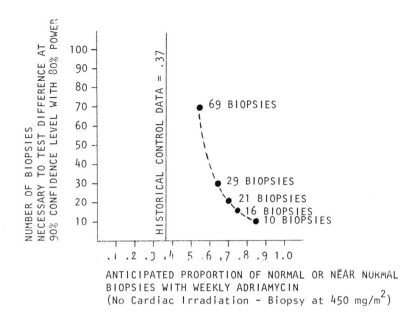

FIGURE 2. Design of nonpaired analysis: comparative endomyocardial biopsy results, weekly versus conventional scheduling of Adriamycin.

logical rather than clinical. Further, the pathological end point is not commonly seen in other types of cardiac damage but appears relatively specific for Adriamycin cardiomyopathy.

This study will undergo a preliminary analysis when approximately 10 to 20 patients have been biopsied at empiric dose limits of Adriamycin. If the trend of this early analysis appears to confirm the clinical experience of reduced cardiotoxicity of Adriamycin, more patients will be tested.

REFERENCES

1. Wendt AG, Jones SE, Salmon SE, Giordano GF, Jackson RA, Miller RS, Heusinkveld RS, Moon ET. 1979. Adriamycin-cyclophosphamide with or without radiation therapy. In: Adjuvant therapy of cancer II (E. Jones and SE Salmon, eds.). New York, Grune & Stratton, pp. 285-293.
2. Bonadonna G, Zucali R, Monfardini S, De Lena M, Uslengthi C. 1975. Combination chemotherapy of Hodgkin's disease with adriamycin, bleomycin, vinblastine, and imidazole carboxamide versus MOPP. Cancer 36: 252-259.
3. Einhorn LH, Williams SD. 1980. Chemotherapy of disseminated testicular cancer: A random prospective study. Cancer 46: 1339-1344.
4. Weiss AJ, Metter GE, Fletcher WS, Wilson WL, Grage TB, Ramirez G. 1976. Studies on adriamycin using a weekly regimen demonstrating its clinical effectiveness and lack of cardiac toxicity. Cancer Treat. Rep. 60:

813-822.

5. Weiss AJ, Manthel RW. 1977. Experience with the use of adriamycin in combination with other anticancer agents using a weekly schedule, with particular reference to lack of cardiac toxicity. Cancer 40: 2046-2052.

6. Chlebowski RT, Paroly WS, Pugh RP, Hueser J, Jacobs EM, Pajak TF, Bateman JR. 1980. Adriamycin given as a weekly schedule without a loading course: clinically effective with reduced incidence of cardiotoxicity. Cancer Treat. Rep. 64: 4751.

7. Billingham ME, Bristow MR, Glatstein E, Mason JW, Masek MA, Daliels JR. 1977. Adriamycin cardiotoxicity: Endomyocardial biopsy evidence of enhancement by irradiation. Am. J. Surg. Path. 1: 17-23.

ANTHRACYCLINES IN CANCER CHEMOTHERAPY

A. DI MARCO

HISTORICAL REMARKS

The discovery by Waksman (1) that a substance isolated by a soil actinomycetes and therefore called actinomycin had, besides antibacterial activity,
antitumor activity was the starting point for the programs aimed at the
isolation of substances produced by microorganisms endowed with inhibitory
activity on animal and human tissues. In 1951 in the Farmitalia laboratories,
I started a program for the investigation of the cytotoxic activity of crude
broths from cultures of newly isolated streptomycetes on tissue-cultured cells
and in parallel on the Lettré line of Ehrlich ascites tumors. In 1957 a team
of soil microbiologists from our laboratories isolated from a soil sample
obtained from Puglia a red-pigment-producing colony, named *Streptomyces
peucetius* (2). In preliminary trials we observed that the crude broth of the
cultured microorganisms produced a significant inhibition of growth of the
intraperitoneally inoculated tumor cells and an increase in life span. It was
therefore decided to proceed, with the cooperation of the chemists Arcamone,
Cassinelli and Orezzi, with the isolation of the pure substance responsible
for the antitumor activity and the identification of the structure. The first
report on this product appeared in 1963 (3) and the cytotoxic and antineoplastic activities were confirmed in subsequent reports (4-6).

The interest in daunomycin (DNR) as a therapeutic agent in cancer was
aroused from the pioneer work of the team of Dr. Karnofsky at the Sloan-
Kettering Memorial Hospital in New York, with their demonstration of an
activity in childhood leukemia as a remission inducer (7) and by the subsequent
extensive trial on the treatment of acute leukemia with rubidomycin reported
later by Bernard et al. (8). Following the demonstration of the antitumor
activity of DNR, an effort was made to obtain better drugs, modifying through
mutations the metabolic pattern of the producing organism. This was rewarded
by a preliminary demonstration of a superior inhibitory antitumor effect of
relatively crude products isolated from the culture of the organism

S. peucetius variety *caesius* (Gaetani et al., unpublished results). It took time, however, to get the pure products in reasonable amounts and to demonstrate its strict chemical resemblance to DNR (9-11) and its truly superior antitumor activity in experimental tumors (12) and clinical use.

Multiple cellular targets were soon identified such as the nucleus, and in the nucleus, the chromatin, or the chromosomes, and the nucleolus. Subsequentl modifications at the level of the cell membrane were observed (13). Severe chromosomal aberrations, such as chromosomal fragments, ring chromosomes, and endo-reduplicated cells, were observed in tissue-cultured cells exposed to DNR or doxorubicin (6, 14-16) as well as on human leukocytes (17).

UPTAKE AND RESISTANCE

Even if DNA is the ultimate target for this group of drugs the processes of cellular transport and accumulation are of crucial importance for the biological activity. Due to the relative lack of selectivity for the interaction with DNA of the presently known anthracyclines, changes in the ability to cross the cell membrane may cause a selective effect on cancer cells depending on the peculiarities of the cell surface structure.

Recent studies have also shown that a change in the process of cellular transport underlies the acquisition of the specific resistance to these drugs (22, 23). The fluorescence of DNR and doxorubicin shows that after penetration into the cell, these drugs are quickly fixed by nuclear structures, such as chromatin, mostly in perinucleolar areas. Autoradiography confirms that a large part of the drugs that enters the cells is taken up by the nucleus. After extraction nearly all of the antibiotic may be found (18) in the nucleoprotein fraction extracted with 2 $\underline{M}$ NaCl. In synchronized cultures of rat fibroblasts it was observed that the uptake of ^{3}H-DNR occurs throughout the regenerative cycle, but it reaches its maximum during DNA duplication (19). The accumulation of doxorubicin in the cells is remarkably lower than for DNR (20). An investigation of the intracellular distribution of DNR and doxorubicin showed that it is very similar to that of N-acetyl-β-glucosaminidase (marker enzyme of lysosomes). This lysosomal concentration seems to be more effective for DNR than for doxorubicin (21).

From in vitro studies it has been shown that DNR and doxorubicin cross the cell membrane easily and accumulate in the cells against a gradient. The rate of uptake in Ehrlich ascites tumor cells is proportional to the drug concentration in the medium (22), and the linear rate-concentration observed is compatible with a nonsaturated carrier-facilitated transport. This theory is in agreement with the striking influence of the pH of the incubation medium on the rate of cellular uptake and steady state level of DNR observed by Skovsgaard (24). From an investigation on the cellular accumulation of different anthracyclines an increase in the uptake with an increase in the partition coefficient lipids/water was observed (23). A reduced uptake was observed for N-acetyl-DNR in which the basic character of the group was obliterated. It has been suggested (25) that this may be understood on the basis of the Eisenman electrostatic model for ion exchange (26, 27) supposing the formation of an electrostatic bond between the protonated amino group and an anionic surface component. The membrane permeability should be proportional, following this model, to the solubility in lipids of the electrically neutral complex formed by the interaction with anionic component of the membrane (Fig. 1).

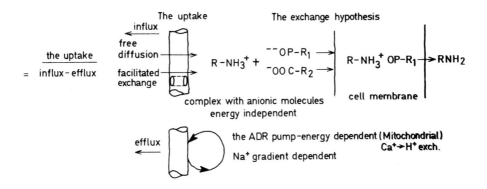

FIGURE 1.

Relevant anionic sites at the cell surface are a) mucopolysaccharides known to form complexes with adriamycin (28) and b) phospholipids such as cardiolipidic and phosphatidic acids (29). While the rate of uptake depends on the affinity of the drug for the carrier molecule, the amount of the drug bound to DNA will depend on the difference of the affinity to the carrier and to DNA. This is illustrated by a comparison of the uptake of DNR and doxorubicin; the more polar doxorubicin is, in fact, less quickly taken up by the cell, but has the same effect on DNA synthesis.

Danø (22) has provided evidence for an active efflux of DNR from Ehrlich ascites tumor cells that are resistant to this drug. The net uptake of the drug in these cells is considered as the difference at the steady state between the influx and the efflux. While the uptake in isolated nuclei from resistant cells is consistently lower than that of nuclei obtained from sensitive cells, the difference was much smaller than that between resistant and wild-type intact cells. The most important changes appear, therefore, to be at the level of membrane transport. A similar efflux mechanism was observed by Skovsgaard (24) in sensitive Ehrlich ascites tumor cells; the efflux was inhibited by the use of the inhibitor of oxidative phosphorylation NaN3, and the inhibition was counteracted by the addition of glucose to the incubation medium.

The physiological basis for this extrusion mechanism remains to be elucidated. The efflux of DNR could be coupled with the active extrusion of Na ions from the cell by the sodium pump. However, this is not supported by the fact that ouabain has no relevant effect on the uptake of DNR at steady state (22, 30). A strong increase in uptake was observed when resistant cells were incubated in a medium where sodium ions had been replaced by potassium ions (22). This could be explained by a dependence of the extrusion mechanism from the Na+ gradient. The extrusion of anthracyclines could depend on the Ca^{++}, H^+ exchange at the mitochondrial membrane, a process that requires ongoing electron transport and that is inhibited by uncoupling agents such as NaN3, or inhibitors of electron transport, such as antimycin and rotenone (31). This view is in agreement with the relevant increase in doxorubicin uptake verified in MEF cells treated with the antibiotic in the presence of the chelating agent EDTA (Supino, unpublished results).

BIOCHEMICAL EFFECTS AND MECHANISM OF ACTION

The main biochemical effect of the anthracyclines is related to nucleic aci synthesis, which has been observed in cell cultures (32, 33) and in tumor and different normal tissues of experimental animals (20, 34-36) (Fig. 2). From the studies of Kim and Kim (37) on synchronized cultures of HeLa cells, the cell-killing effect of DNA and doxorubicin is at a maximum when cells are exposed during the synthetic S phase. A high reduction in surviving fraction was observed also in mitotic cells, and to a lesser degree in cells in G_1 and G_2 phase (38). However, doxorubicin exerts a strong influence on the biochemical events that precede entering the cycle of normal quiescent cells, such as conditioned mice embryo cells (MEF) (39, 40). These cells are arrested in G_1 or G_0 phase, and active DNA synthesis and multiplication are initiated by

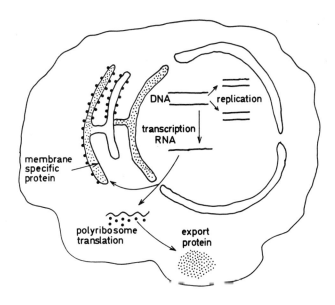

FIGURE 2.   Biochemical effects of anthracyclines.

simple addition of fresh serum containing the limiting factors.   We have
observed that the inhibiting effect of doxorubicin on MEF cells is the highest
when the drug is administered during the first 8 hr after serum addition (41)
when thymidine incorporation into DNA has not yet begun (Fig. 3).

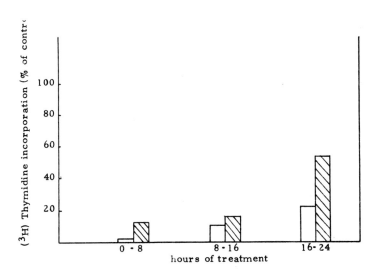

FIGURE 3.   Activity of doxorubicin on thymidine incorporation in serum-
stimulated MEF cells.   ☐, 0.5 µg/ml;   ◩, 0.05 µg/ml.

RNA synthesis is stimulated by serum and reduced, after half an hour, by doxorubicin (41) (Fig. 4).

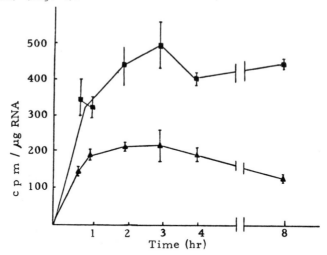

FIGURE 4. Activity of doxorubicin on uridine incorporation in serum-stimulated MEF cells. ■, Control; ▲, doxorubicin, 0.5 μg/ml.

The very nature of this early RNA synthesis has not been analyzed; however, we may suppose that it can be identified with the synthesis of heterogeneous, pre-rRNA, which is known to be highly sensitive to anthracyclines.

Protein synthesis is not primarily affected by DNR or doxorubicin (34, 37, 42, 43). The inhibition of leucine incorporation into proteins, which appears as a delayed effect at high concentrations of the drug, may be considered as a consequence of the failure of rRNA synthesis, as well as an inhibitory effect on mRNA synthesis (44). However, DNA and doxorubicin are able to complex with tRNA. The remarkable effect observed on DNA and RNA synthesis may be related to the in vitro observed inhibiting activity on DNA and RNA polymerase reactions. The activity of some enzymes related to DNA synthesis such as thymidine kinase, deoxycytidine-monophosphate deaminase, increases and DNA polymerase is not reduced after treatment of HeLa cells with DNR (34); this indicates that the drug does not act on the formation of these enzymes but on the availability of the template to the polymerases as a result of the interaction with DNA. In a study of RNA synthesis reaction catalyzed by *E. coli* RNA polymerase it was observed, in fact, that the DNR-induced inhibition may be overcome by an increase in the concentration of DNA, but it is unaffected by an increase in the concentration of the enzyme, which is consistent with an inactivation of the template function of DNA in the polymerase reaction (45).

Physico-chemical studies (46, 47) have shown that anthracyclines have a strong affinity to double helix native DNA. From studies on x-ray diffraction on DNA fibers a model of the drug-DNA complex has been proposed (48). The drug is supposed to be intercalated between adjacent base pairs into the B-structure of the double-strand DNA with the daunosamine ring situated in the large groove of the double helix. The charged nitrogen atom at C-3' is in close contact with a phosphate oxygen atom two residues away from the inter-calation site, and a hydrogen bond between the C-9 hydroxy group of DNR and the first phosphate is also possible.

Consistent with the intercalation model proposed by Pigram et al. (48) are the equilibrium measurements and the viscosity data. Experiments in which DNR was found to cause the uncoiling of the supercoiled structure of closed circular DNA in the same qualitative fashion of other drugs believed to inter-calate are also consistent with this model (49). Differences in the quantita-tive values of the apparent binding constant between DNR and doxorubicin, and of the dependence of K_{app} on the ionic strength may be explained by additional hydrogen bonds between the C-14 hydroxyl and doxorubicin and the phosphate group at the intercalation site.

A very different model has been proposed on the basis of recent studies on the crystalline complex between DNR and the complementary deoxyhexanucleotide d(CpGpTpApCpG) (50). Following this model the amino sugar lies in the minor groove of the double helix, without binding to DNA, and the aglycone chromo-phore at right angles to the long dimension of the DNA base pairs. The cyclohexene ring rests in the minor groove. Substituents on the ring have hydrogen binding interactions to the base pairs above and below the intercala-tion site. It should be noted that this model does not account for the strong influence of the unsubstituted amino group on the association constant of the complex with DNA, or for the salt effect on the dissociation of the complex (18, 51). The modalities of anthracycline binding to DNA may be strongly influenced, in vivo, by histones and acidic nuclear proteins, as well as by low-molecular-weight components. The apparent lack of selectivity for specific base sequences in DNA may be emendated in the future by a more extensive knowledge of the interaction with native chromatin.

An analysis of the structure-activity relationship between DNA binding and effects on DNA synthesis and cell viability in a series of anthracyclines has shown (9, 52, 53) that these are strictly related (54-56). Looking to the model the presence of the intercalation complex may impair the traveling of the RNA polymerase along the double helix. On the other hand, the complex could hamper the local melting of the double helix required for the duplication process. The question may be raised as to whether an inhibitory effect on RNA or DNA synthesis may have lethal effects on the cells or if the cell killing may be ascribed to some unreversible effect, related to the binding of the drug to DNA during the replicative phase.

According to some experimental data the lethal event responsible for cell death may be related to irreversible damage to the DNA structure rather than to a quantitative reduction in the amount of DNA synthesized in the cell. DNA damage has been demonstrated by sucrose sedimentation as DNA breaks in P388 ascite tumor cells in mice treated with DNR and doxorubicin (57). Single strand breaks as a consequence of exposure to doxorubicin have also been observed in different cell lines (58, 59). These authors also found evidence of a concentration-dependent induction of DNA double strand breaks after exposure of cells to low concentrations of doxorubicin for a period approaching the cell cycle duration. While the great majority of x-ray-induced single strand breaks are repaired by mammalian cells, it is generally agreed that double strand breaks are lethal events.

In a study of alkaline labile or strand scission produced in leukemia cells treated with different DNR or doxorubicin derivatives, Kanter and Schwartz (60, 61) found a strict correlation between the potency of 9 of 10 compounds (with the exception of doxorubicin octanoate) and parameters such as inhibition of thymidine incorporation (I), number of breaks per unit of molecular weight (n) and drug retention (r), i.e.,

$$P = (I \times n/r)$$

In some cases n may be a sufficient parameter to determine the potency. This analysis is compatible with the view that the inhibitory effect on nucleic acid synthesis and breaks are separate consequences of a common event, i.e., intercalation. Arguments in favor of this hypothesis are the absence of breaks formation in vivo and the lack of a stringent coupling between inhibition on DNA synthesis and lethal effect. Furthermore, it should be noted that very low concentrations of doxorubicin (1 — 10 ng), which enhance DNA synthesis of growing mice embryonic fibroblasts, cause transformation of these cells, which is compatible with the change at the genome level (Di Marco et al., unpublished results). As regards the in vivo situation, it should be noted that the potency is not strictly related to efficacy, i.e., doxorubicin is less potent than DNR or demethoxydaunorubicin but far more efficient on different tumors. The relationship $P = (I \times n/r)$ therefore appears adequate to evaluate the in vitro cytotoxicity, or the in vitro and in vivo ratio of potency for different drugs, but not for the evaluation of the antitumor efficacy.

The structural damage to DNA caused by these drugs may not be an immediate consequence of the intercalation in the DNA double helix but rather follow chemical or biologic events. The breaks may be a consequence of nuclease activation due to the distortion in DNA structure caused by intercalation, as reported by Paoletti et al. (62) for ethidium bromide. It has been suggested that distortion of the DNA helix induced by intercalators leads to strand scission by a nuclease, possibly a DNA repair enzyme of the nick-closure type, which could be identified with the protein that remains linked to DNA strands and is associated with DNA breaks (81). In this regard our observation is relevant that reduction in the number of living cells (as expressed by reduction in ^{3}H-thymidine or colony forming efficiency) induced by doxorubicin on MS$_2$T cells is related to the calcium ions concentration in the medium of the function:

$$y = b \times^{-m}$$

It might be therefore that calcium ions are required for the formation of the complex DNA-nucleolytic enzyme, which is essential to the production of the breaks. The release of nucleolytic enzymes could ensue from a specific destabilization of the lysosomal membranes by a Ca^{++}-dependent process. Relevant to this is the finding that a Ca^{++} sequestering agent such as ICRF-159 can considerably reduce the toxicity of DNR, which is accumulated in the lysosomes (21), but not of doxorubicin, which has a different intracellular distribution, preferentially nuclear (63-65). The secondary origin of DNA lesions is suggested by the observation that neither DNA nor doxorubicin provokes breaks in DNA, as analyzed by neutral or alkaline sucrose gradient, on isolated nuclei of Morris hepatomas or host liver; however, doxorubicin was observed to inhibit ^{3}H-TTP incorporation, preferentially in hepatoma nuclei (66)

A free radical mechanism for strand scission of DNA by bound doxorubicin and DNR has been recently proposed (67). Bachur et al. (68) observed an NADPH-dependent enzymatic activity in microsomes of various normal tissues and L1210 and P388 mouse tumors, which may catalytically activate the quinone rings of DNR and doxorubicin to free radicals. The intracellular activation to a free radical state and the site-specific association of these radicals with macromolecules would be responsible for the damage to cellular structures and

the cytotoxicity. Recent studies on the structure activity relationship
of some new anthracyclines are compatible with this hypothesis. Modifications
of the quinone ring by introduction of methyl groups in position 6, 11 may
greatly influence the electronic and steric structure of the chromophore and
therefore the ability to react with macromolecules, as well as the ability to
give rise to free radicals. The 6, 11 methyl 4'DNR, or doxorubicin analogues
have, in fact. very reduced binding ability and biologic activity (69). The
main objection to the free radical mechanism is the lack of evidence of the
formation of covalent bonds between anthracyclines and nucleic acids in
ordinary conditions in vitro or in vivo.

OTHER BIOCHEMICAL EFFECTS

Since anthracyclines may interact with molecules such as phospholipids
(29, 70) and mucopolysaccharides (28) associated with cell membranes, it has
been suggested (71) that some specific toxic effects may be related to drug-
induced change at the membrane level. An irreversible change in the membrane
phospholipids could result from the association with DNR or doxorubicin,
directly or as a consequence of the formation of free radicals by redox
agents (72).

A change in cell permeability is documented by the increase in cell volume
of HeLa cells exposed for relatively long periods to the antibiotic and by
the changes in intracellular concentration (i.c.) of Na^+ and Ca^{++} (Table 1).

Table 1. The sodium and potassium content and $K^+:Na^+$ ratio of HeLa cells
treated with doxorubicin for 3 h.

| Doxorubicin | Intracellular ion concentration [a] | | $K^+:Na^+$ [c] |
	Na^+ (mEq/liter cell water) [b]	K^+	
0	24.93 ± 5.25	133.41 ± 14.77	5.53
10^{-7} M	41.87 ± 3.04 [d]	142.57 ± 9.66	3.42

[a]
[b] Values are mean ± S.E. (n = 3).
  Cellular water content, mean value = 82.25 ± 1.02 ml/100 g.
[c] Extracellular space, mean value = 25.00 ± 3.82 ml/100 g wet weight.
[d] F < 0.05 using analysis of variance.
  P < 0.05, from a comparison of these values with the corresponding control
  value using Student's t test.

Since the increase in Na^+ i.c. is not balanced by a parallel decrease in
intracellular K^+, it cannot be ascribed to an inhibitory effect of doxorubicin

on the activity of Na^+/K^+ ATPase. The change in i.c. concentration of Na^+ and Ca^{++} (Table 2) should therefore be ascribed to an interference with a mechanism of regulation of the permeability to these cations, or with an extrusion mechanism of Na^+ ions that are ouabain insensitive.

Table 2. Calcium concentration of HeLa cells after 3 h of incubation in the presence of 10^{-7} M doxorubicin, obtained by chemical analysis and tracer kinetics.

| | Chemical analysis | | Kinetic analysis | |
	Control	Doxorubicin	Control	Doxorubicin
Cell Ca^{++} (nmol/10^6 cells)	14.319	26.825	10.259	16.828

Other experimental findings are related to an impairment of the calcium ion transport. Anghileri (73) observed an inhibition of Ca^{++} transport in a bi-phasic model system, as well as in the mitochondrial Ca^{++} incorporation. Moore et al. (74) have observed that doxorubicin and DNR are able to inhibit the energy-dependent Ca^{++} transport activity of cardiac mitochondria. Both antibiotics have a negligible effect on Ca^{++} uptake of microsomal preparations. The results suggest that doxorubicin and DNR inhibit mitochondrial Ca^{++} transport and have an inhibitory effect on the efflux of accumulated calcium. Caroni et al. (82) have recently shown that doxorubicin specifically inhibits the ouabain-insensitive Na^+/Ca^{++} exchange which takes place at the plasma membrane level of myocardial vesicles. This may be considered an auxiliary mechanism to keep the intracellular calcium low. In fact, it was observed that rabbits that developed doxorubicin-induced heart failure had markedly elevated levels of myocardial calcium compared to those animals that did not develop heart failure. The increased levels of calcium were stated as correlating well with ultrastructural evidence of increased intramitochondrial calcium (75). Mitochondrial membrane damages after DNR or doxorubicin admini-stration in the heart have been reported (78). However, these lesions appear many hours after drug administration and may be secondary consequences of the drug action at different molecular levels.

From a kinetic analysis of Ca^{++} flux in cultured, spontaneously beating, cardiac cells (76), it results that doxorubicin is able to suppress the early phase of exchangeable calcium pool and increases the rate constant and the Ca^{++} efflux from the two phases of slow exchangeable Ca^{++}, which represents the intracellular Ca^{++} pool. The interference with the mechanism of Ca^{++}

transport may be related in the experimental model with the effect on the contractable functions (77).

The demonstration of two almost distinct mechanisms underlying the anti-tumor or the cardiotoxicity of anthracyclines may direct the synthesis of analogues with different degrees of these properties. In effect some analogues, such as 4-demethoxy, or 4'-deoxy, present a different ratio of optimal antitumor dose/minimal cardiotoxic dose, but it is presumed that a more thorough knowledge of structure-activity relationship may lead to the synthesis of more effective or less toxic derivatives.

One can pose the question if the inhibitory activity of DNR and doxorubicin on the mechanism regulating the initiation of DNA synthesis may cause in vivo a differential activity on normal and neoplastic cells. In fact, in normal tissues a large number of stem cells is maintained out of the cycle by regulatory mechanisms such as calcium concentration (79), cAMP, cGMP, level and hormone concentrations. In tumor cells the dependence of growth initiation on calcium concentration (79) has become less stringent and may permit entering into the replicative phase at calcium concentrations that are too low to permit initiation for normal cells. A similar consideration should be given to the dependence of normal cells on cAMP for induction of proliferative activity (80).

It should therefore be possible to enhance the selective effect of cyto-toxic agents on tumor cells by modulating the work of these regulatory mechanisms. As an example of this approach to rational chemotherapy, I will mention here the studies we have in progress on the combination of doxorubicin with drugs such as glucagon and aminophylline (Pratesi, manuscript in preparation), which enhance cAMP level.

ACKNOWLEDGMENTS

I wish here to thank all the research people from Farmitalia Carlo Erba, the Istituto Nazionale per lo Studio e la Cura dei Tumori of Milan as well as foreign institutions who have made a substantial contribution to the work I have tried to summarize here. A special thanks to Mrs. Teresa Dasdia and Ms. Betty Johnston for their help in editing the manuscript.

REFERENCES

1. Waksman SA, Woodruff HB. 1940. Bacteriostatic and bactericidal substances produced by a soil actinomyces. Proc Soc Exp Biol Med 45:609.
2. Grein A, Spalla C, Di Marco A, et al. 1963. Descrizione e classificazione di un actinomecete (*Streptomyces peucetius* sp. *nova*) produttore du una sostanza ad attività antitumorale: la daunomicina. Giorn Microbiol 11:109.
3. Di Marco A, Gaetani M, Orezzi P, et al. 1963. Antitumor activity of a new antibiotic: daunomycin. Commun. 3rd Int. Cong. Chemistry, Stuttgart, July 22-27, 1963.
4. Di Marco A, Gaetani M, Dorigotti L, et al. 1964. Daunomycin: a new antibiotic with antitumor activity. Cancer Chemother Rep 38:31.
5. Di Marco A, Gaetani M, Orezzi P, et al. 1964. Daunomycin: a new antibiotic of the rhodomycin group. Nature 201:706.
6. Di Marco A, Soldati M, Fioretti A, Dasdia T. 1964. Activity of daunomycin, a new antitumor antibiotic, on normal and neoplastic cells grown in vitro. Cancer Chemother Rep 38:39.
7. Tan C, Kou-Ping Y, Murphy ML, Karnofsky DA. 1967. Daunomycin as antitumor antibiotic, in the treatment of neoplastic disease. Clinical evaluation with special reference to childhood leukemia. Cancer 20:333.
8. Bernard J, Boiron M, Jacquillat CL, et al. 1967. Traitement des leucémies aiguës lymphoblastiques de première atteinte pare une association de prednisone-vincristine-rubicomycine. Pathol Biol 16:919
9. Arcamone F, Cassinelli G, Fantini G, et al. 1969. Adriamycin, 14-hydroxydaunomycin, a new antitumor antibiotic from *S. peucetius* var. *caesius*. Biotecnol Bioeng 11:1101.
10. Arcamone F, Franceschi G, Penco S. 1969. Substances antibiotiques et procéde pour leur preparation. Belg Patent 732:968.
11. Arcamone F, Franceschi G, Penco S, et al. 1969. Adriamycin (14-hydroxydaunomycin), a novel antitumor antibiotic. Tetrahedron Lett 13:1007.
12. Di Marco A, Gaetani M, Scarpinato B. 1969. Adriamycin (NSC-123127) a new antibiotic with antitumor activity. Cancer Chemother Rep 53:33.
13. Murphree SA, Tritton TR, Sartorelli AC. 1977. Differential effects of adriamycin on fluidity and fusion characteristic of cardiolipin containing cytosomes. Fed Proc 36:303.
14. Massimo I, Dagna-Bricarelli F, Cherchi MG. 1972. Effects of adriamycin on blastogenesis and chromosomes of blood lymphocytes: in vitro and in vivo studies. In: International Symposium on Adriamycin, Eds. Carter SK, Di Marco A, Ghione M, Krakoff IH, Mathé G. New York, Springer-Verlag, p 36.
15. Vig BK, Kontras SB, Aubele A. 1969. Sensitivity of G_1 phase of mitotic cell cycle to chromosome aberrations induced by daunomycin. Mutat Res 7:91.
16. Vig BK, Samuels LD, Kontras S. 1970. Specificity of daunomycin in causing chromosome aberrations in human leukocytes. Chromosoma 29:62.
17. Vig BK. 1971. Chromosome aberrations induced in human leukocytes by the antileukemic antibiotic adriamycin. Cancer Res 31:32.
18. Calendi E, Di Marco A, Reggiani M, et al. 1965. On physicochemical interactions between daunomycin and nucleic acids. Biochim. Biophys. Acta 103:25.
19. Silvestrini R, Di Marco A, Dasdia T. 1970. Interference of daunomycin with metabolic events of the cell cycle in synchronized cultures of rat fibroblasts. Cancer Res 30:966.
20. Meriwether WD, Bachur NR. 1972. Inhibition of DNA and RNA metabolism by daunorubicin and adriamycin in L1210 mouse leukemia. Cancer Res 32:1137.

376

21. Noel G, Trouet A, Senebergh A, Tulkens P. 1975. Comparative cell pharmaco-kinetics of daunorubicin and adriamycin. Adriamycin Review Part II, p 99-105. Ghent, European Press Medikon.
22. Danø K. 1976. Experimentally developed cellular resistance to daunomycin: Cross resistance between anthracyclines and vinca alkaloids: Development of resistance to vincristine and vinblastine. Acta Pathol Microbiol Scand 256 (Suppl):3-80.
23. Di Marco A. 1978. Mechanism of action and mechanism of resistance to antineoplastic agents that bind to DNA. Antibiot Chemother 23:216-227
24. Skovsgaard T. 1977. Transport binding of daunorubicin, adriamycin and rubidazone in Ehrlich ascites tumor cells. Biochem Pharmacol 26:215-222.
25. Arcamone F, Bernardi L, Giardino P, Patelli B, Di Marco A, Casazza AM, Pratesi G, Reggiani P. 1976. Synthesis and antitumor activity of 4-demeth-oxydaunorubicin, 4-demethoxy-7,9-diepidaunorubicin and their anomers. Cancer Treat Rep 60:829-834.
26. Eisenman G. 1962. Cation-selective glass electrodes and their mode of operation. Biophys J 2:259-324.
27. Eisenman G. 1969. Ion-selective electrodes. In: Drust Special Publ. 314, p 1-56. Washington, NATO Bureau of Standards.
28. Menozzi M, Arcamone F. 1978. Binding of adriamycin to sulphated muco-polysaccharides. Biochem Biophys Res Commun 80:313-318.
29. Duarte-Karim M, Ruysschaert JM, Hildebrand J. 1976. Affinity of adriamycin to phospholipids: a possible explanation for cardiac mitochondrial lesions. Biochem Biophys Res Commun 71:658-663.
30. Dasdia T, Necco A, Di Marco A. 1976. Studies on the interference of ouabain on the cytotoxic activity of adriamycin. 24th Annu. Meeting European Tissue Culture Society Arhus.

31. Lehninger AL. 1970. Mitochondria and calcium ion transport. Biochem J 119:129-138.
32. Rusconi A, Calendi E. 1966. Action of daunomycin on nucleic acid metabo-lism. Biochem Biophys Acta 119:113.
33. Rusconi A, Di Marco A. 1969. Inhibition of nucleic acid synthesis by daunomycin and its relationship to the uptake of the drug in HeLa cells. Cancer Res 29:1509.
34. Kim KH, Gelbard AS, Djordjevic B, et al. 1968. Action of daunomycin on the nucleic acid metabolism and viability of HeLa cells. Cancer Res 28:2437.
35. Kitaura K, Imai R, Ishihara Y, et al. 1972. Mode of action of adriamycin on HeLa 5-3 cells "in vitro." J Antibiot 25:509.
36. Theologides A, Yarbro JM, Kennedy BJ. 1968. Daunomycin inhibition of DNA and RNA synthesis. Cancer 21:16.
37. Kim SH, Kim JH. 1972. Lethal effect of adriamycin on the division of HeLa cells. Cancer Res 32:323.
38. Barranco SC. 1975. Review of the survival and cell kinetic effects of adriamycin (NSC-123127) on mammalian cells. Cancer Chemother Rep 6:147.
39. Holley RW. 1972. A unifying hypothesis concerning the nature of malignant growth. Proc Natl Acad Sci USA 69:2840-2841.
40. Todaro GJ, Lasar GK, Green H. 1965. The initiation of cell division in a contact inhibited mammalian cell line. J Cell Comp Physiol 66:325-333.
41. Supino R, Casazza AM, Di Marco A. 1977. Effect of daunorubicin and adriamycin on nucleic acid synthesis of serum-stimulated mouse embryo fibroblasts. Tumori 63:31-42.
42. Di Marco A. 1967. Daunomycin and related antibiotics. In: Antibiotics. Vol. I. Eds. Gottlieb D, Shaw C. Heidelberg, Springer-Verlag.
43. Wang JJ, Chervinsky DS, Rosen FM. 1972. Comparative biochemical studies of adriamycin and daunomycin in leukemic cells. Cancer Res 32:511.

44. Crook LE, Rees KR, Cohen A. 1972. Effect of daunomycin on HeLa cell nucleic acid synthesis. Biochem Pharmacol 21:281.

45. Zunino F, Gambetta RA, Di Marco A, et al. 1975. A comparison of the effects of daunomycin and adriamycin on various DNA polymerases. Cancer Res 35:754.

46. Di Marco A, Arcamone F, Zunino F. 1975. DNA-complexing antibiotics: daunomycin, adriamycin and their derivatives. Arzneim Forsh Drug Res 25:368-375.

47. Neidle S. 1979. The molecular basis for the action of some DNA-binding drugs. Prog Med Chem 16:151-221.

48. Pigram WJ, Fuller W, Hamilton LD. 1972. Stereochemistry of intercalation: Interaction of daunomycin with DNA. Nature New Biol 235:17.

49. Waring MJ. 1970. Variation of the supercaloids in closed circular DNA by binding of antibiotics and drugs: Evidence for molecular models involving intercalation. J Mol Biol 54:247.

50. Quigley GJ, Wang AHJ, Ughetto G, van der Marel G, van Boom JH, Rich A. 1980. Molecular structure of an anticancer drug-DNA complex: Daunomycin plus d(CpGpTpApCpG). Proc Natl Acad Sci USA 77:7204-7208.

51. Zunino F, Di Marco A, Velcich A. 1977. Steric influence of the orientation of the primary amino group at position 3 of the sugar moiety of anthracycline antibiotics in DNA binding properties. Cancer Lett 2:271.

52. Andreina C. 1974. Attività antimitocondriale dell'adriamicina e della daunomicina su *Saccharomyces cerevisiae*. Doctoral Thesis.

53. Gottlieb JA, Hill CS Jr. 1975. Adriamycin (NSC-123127) therapy in thyroid carcinoma. Cancer Chemother Rep 6:283.

54. Benjamin RS, Wiernik PH, Bachur NR. 1974. Adriamycin chemotherapy. Efficacy, safety, and pharmacologic basis of an intermittent single high-dosage schedule. Cancer 33:19.

55. Bernard J, Paul R, Boiron M, Jacquillat Cl, Maral R. 1969. Rubidomycin. A New Agent Against Cancer. New York, Springer-Verlag, p. 46.

56. Di Marco A, Boretti G, Rusconi A. 1967. Trasformazione metabolica della daunomicina da parte di estratti di tessuti. Farmaco 7:535.

57. Schwartz HS. 1975. DNA breaks in P388 tumor cells in mice after treatment with daunorubycin and adriamycin. Res Commun Chem Pathol 10:51-64.

58. Byfield JE. 1977. Adriamycin cardiac toxicity: A different hypothesis. Cancer Treat Rep 61:497-498.

59. Cook PR, Brazell IA. 1977. Detection and repair of single strand breaks in nuclear DNA. Nature 263:679-682.

60. Kanter PM, Schwartz HS. 1979. Adriamycin-induced DNA damage in human leukemia cells. Leukem Res 4:001.

61. Kanter PM, Schwartz HS. 1980. Quantitative models for growth inhibition of human leukemia cells by antitumor anthracycline derivatives. Cancer Res in press.

62. Paoletti G, Couder H, Guerineau M. 1972. A yeast mitochondrial deoxyribonuclease stimulated by ethidium bromide. Biochem Biophys Res Commun 48:950-958.

63. Giuliani F, Di Marco A, Savi G. 1978. Activity of some antitumor drugs on lung metastases formation in mice bearing the MS-2 sarcoma. XII Int. Cancer Congress, Buenos Aires (Abstract 3, 20).

64. Woodman RJ. 1973. Enhancement of antitumor effectiveness of ICRF-159 (NSC-129943) against early Ll210 leukemia by combination with cis-diamine dichloroplatinum (NSC-119875) or daunomycin (NSC-82151). Cancer Chemother Rep 4:45-52.

378

65. Woodman RJ, Cysyk RL, Kline I, Gang M, Venditti JM. 1975. Enhancement of the effectiveness of daunorubycin (NSC-82151) or adriamycin (NSC-123127) against early mouse Ll210 leukemia with ICRF-159 (NSC-129943). Cancer Chemother Rep 59:689-695.

66. 66. Coetzee ML, Sartiano GP, Klein K, Ove P. 1977. The effect of several antitumor agents on 3H-TTP incorporation in host liver and hepatoma nuclei. Oncology 34:68-73.

67. Lown JW, Sirne S, Majumdar KC, Chang R. 1977. Strand scission of DNA by bound adriamycin and daunorubycin in the presence of reducing agents. Biochem Biophys Res Commun 76:705-710.

68. Bachur NB, Gordon S, Gee M. 1978. Enzymatic of quinone anticancer agents to free radicals. Fed Proc 37:1832.

69. Zunino F, Casazza AM, Pratesi G, Formelli F, Di Marco A. 1981. Effect of the methylation of aglycone hydroxyl groups on the biological and biochemical properties of daunorubicin. Biochem Pharmacol 30: in press.

70. Kanter PM, Kanter PM, Schwartz HS. 1978. Uptake of adriamycin (AM) by brain tissue after intracarotid administration. Proc Am Assoc Cancer Res 19:85.

71. Schwartz HS. 1976. Mechanism and selectivity of anthracycline amino-glycosides and other intercalating agents. Biomedicine 24:317-323.

72. Honda K, Sato S. 1975. Generation of free radicals of quinone growth-containing anticancer chemicals in nadph microsome system as evidenced by initiation of sulfite oxidation. Gann 66:43-47.

73. Anghileri LJ. 1977. Ca-2+-Transport inhibition by antitumor agents adriamycin and daunomycin. Arzneim Forsch Drug Res 27:1177-1180.

74. Moore L, Landon EJ, Cooney DA. 1977. Inhibition of the cardiac mito-chondrial calcium pump by adriamycin in vitro. Biochem Med 18:131-138.

75. Hammar SP, Krous H. 1977. Myocardial mitochondrial calcification in Reye's syndrome. Hum Pathol 8:95-98.

76. Dasdia T, Necco A, Minghetti A, Di Marco A. 1978. The effect of adriamycin on cAMP level and on calcium fluxes of cultured myocardial cells. ETCS, Glasgow.

77. Necco A, Dasdia T, Cozzi S, Ferraguti M. 1976. Ultrastructural changes produced in cultured, adriamycin-treated myocardial cells. Tumori 62: 537-543.

78. Lambertenghi-Deliliers G, Zanon PL, Pozzoli EF, Bellini O, Praga C. 1978. Ultrastructural alterations of atrial myocardium induced by adriamycin in chronically treated animals. Tumori 64:15-24.

79. Whitfield JF, Boyton AL, McManus JP, et al. 1980. The roles of calcium and cyclic AMP in cell proliferation. Ann N Y Acad Sci 339:216-240.

80. Di Marco A. 1979. Perspectives on the research of new anticancer agents. Bristol Myers Cancer Symposia, vol. 1:491-505.

81. Ross WE, Glaubiger D, Kohn KW. 1979. Qualitative and quantitative aspect of intercalator-induced DNA strand breaks. Biochim Biophys Acta 562:41-5

82. Caroni P, Villani F, Carafoli E. 1981. The cardiotoxic antibiotic doxo-rubicin inhibits the Na^+/Ca^{++} exchange of dog heart sarcolemmal vesicles FEBS Lett in press.

SECTION 5

DOXORUBICIN:
NEW CLINICAL INVESTIGATIONS

INTRODUCTION

F. M. MUGGIA

The successful clinical application of doxorubicin in the treatment
of human malignancy has been extensively covered in comprehensive reviews
(1-3). This volume does not intend to be comprehensive, but focuses
instead on new clinical applications. Studies of particular interest
are covered in detail in the ensuing chapters. These fall within the
following areas:

1. New disease targets. It is surprising that new targets for study
are still appearing more than one decade after the beginning of widespread
use of doxorubicin. However, even at this date, expanding
horizons are still becoming apparent as chemotherapeutic expertise is
disseminated to new areas of the world. For example, in Latin America
and in China, treatment of gastric cancer and of nasopharyngeal and
esophageal carcinomas with doxorubicin is now being evaluated. In our
midst, the definition of its role in Kaposi's sarcoma is being sought
as epidemics of the disseminated form of this malignancy arise among
immunosuppressed individuals. Because of its unique antitumor activity,
doxorubicin will continue to be a major candidate for study in any malignancy where the value and type of chemotherapy remain to be defined.

2. Dose-schedule alterations. Clues taken from clinical experience
indicated that the risk of cardiotoxicity could be minimized by more
frequent administration of the drug or by reduction of peak levels, achieved
by bolus administration. Evolving technology has allowed exploration
of continuous infusion schedules and safe documentation of cardiac effects
prior to any clinical damage. Preliminary data spanning 6 hours (New
York University studies) to 96 hours (M. D. Anderson Hospital studies) are
available. Researchers at M. D. Anderson already claim to have achieved
lowered cardiotoxic potential with equal or superior therapeutic effects (4).
We at NYU have also initiated studies evaluating the cardiotoxic potential
of doxorubicin infusions when combined with cyclophosphamide and fluoro-

uracil in patients with breast cancer (Table 1).

TABLE 1. Fluorouracil/Adriamycin/cyclophosphamide infusion protocol
(NYU-8103)

Eligibility	advanced breast cancer, evaluable or measurable; no prior chemotherapy
Treatment (3-week cycle)	fluorouracil, 500 mg/m^2, days 1 and 8; Adriamycin, 50 mg/m^2, day 1 by 6-hour infusion; cyclophosphamide, 500 mg/m^2, day 1
Monitoring	baseline ejection fraction (resting and exercise gated pool scan); repeat scan at 200, 300, 400, 500, . . . mg/m^2

3. _Special routes of administration._ Rationale and guidelines for
administration of doxorubicin into a peritoneal "compartment" have been
advanced by workers at the National Cancer Institute. Based on these
considerations and preliminary experience, we and others have designed
clinical studies in ovarian cancer. Such studies are based on 1) the
ability of non-doxorubicin combinations to produce in the majority of
patients with advanced ovarian cancer excellent clinical remissions; 2) the
supplementation of these remissions with doxorubicin administered intraperitoneally, with the goal of eliminating residual disease without additive
systemic toxicity; and 3) the otherwise prompt development of relative
doxorubicin resistance as documented by clonogenic assays requiring drug
concentrations greater than achievable intravenously. The intravesical
route is also receiving considerable attention. Pavone-Macaluso has
reviewed in detail the features that make doxorubicin particularly attractive for such use, and the preliminary data obtained.

4. _Combined modality therapy._ Advanced in the treatment of breast
cancer have potentially greater worldwide repercussions than do advances
made in less common malignancies. In spite of doxorubicin's well-documented
efficacy against this disease, its application has not been fully exploited.
Toxic manifestations such as cardiomyopathy, total alopecia, and the risk
of tissue necrosis from extravasation have greatly limited its use. More-

over, doxorubicin-containing combinations have not always been con-
vincingly superior to combinations lacking this agent. Nevertheless,
the evidence appears to be persuasive enough that the new direction of
adjuvant studies in breast cancer almost always includes the addition
of doxorubicin. If doxorubicin administered by infusion does modify its
cardiotoxic potential, we hope to reevaluate the regimen shown in Table 1
for adjuvant treatment.

In sarcomas, a treatment utilizing a combined modality and begun when
the disease is first diagnosed is likely to lead to improved results.
Doxorubicin constitutes the basic ingredient of current chemotherapeutic
regimens. Again, modifications of toxicity may enhance the applicability
of such strategy.

This section emphasizes the evolution of clinical investigation
with current anthracyclines. It represents a distillate of much clinical
and laboratory experience of the preceding section. It should also serve
as background for the clinical evaluation of new anthracyclines in the
subsequent section.

REFERENCES

1. Carter SK, Di Marco A, Ghione M, eds. 1972. International
    symposium on adriamycin. New York, Springer-Verlag, pp. 10270.
2. Crooke ST, Reich, SD. 1980. Anthracyclines: Current studies and
    new developments. New York, Academic Press, pp. 1-444.
3. Young RC, Ozols RF, Myers CF. 1981. The anthracycline anti-
    neoplastic drugs. New Engl. J. Med. 305: 139-152.
4. Legha SW, Benjamin RS, MacKay B, Ewer M, Wallace S, Valdivieso M,
    Rasmussen SL, Blumenschein AR, Freireich EJ. 1982. Reduction of
    doxorubicin cardiotoxicity by prolonged intravenous infusion. Ann.
    Intern. Med. 96: 133-139.

DOXORUBICIN IN THE 1980s: IS THERE STILL ROOM FOR CLINICAL INVESTIGATION?

C. PRAGA, G. BERETTA,* O. BAWA, D. TABANELLI, AND P. ZANON

1. INTRODUCTION

Doxorubicin (DXR) was a successful drug in its first decade, and, to
the present, it has seen an increasingly frequent use on a clinical level.
Certainly the major contribution to such increasing use has been the
continuing clinical investigation (1-7). The main strategic approaches
that were followed in the 1970s for the clinical development of DXR are
shown in Table 1.

Table 1: Clinical development of doxorubicin in the 1970s: Main
strategic approaches

Disease-oriented therapeutic evaluation

Empirical approach to best chemotherapy combinations

Incorporation into combined modality treatment

Cardiotoxicity studies

Looking at the 1980s, we should ask ourselves 1) whether the role of
DXR has been totally defined along these strategic lines; 2) whether any
complementary clinical approach exists today in which DXR may play an
important part; and, finally, 3) omitting cardiotoxicity, whether the
clinical pharmacology and toxicology profile of DXR is now so well defined
that further improvement in its therapeutic index is not possible.
Probably we should give a negative answer to the first question, a positive
one to the second, and, again, a negative answer to the third, this feeling
being substantiated by present clinical research with DXR.

---

*Consulting physician.

2. WHAT IS THE PRESENT SITUATION AS REGARDS CLINICAL RESEARCH AND DOXORUBICIN?

In order to have an idea of both the size and the targets of the on-going clinical research on DXR, we have reviewed the clinical protocols reported in a volume recently published by the National Institutes of Health (8). These protocols refer mainly to clinical studies that have been carried out independently in the United States by single institutions or by study groups. Three hundred fifty-two out of 1106 clinical protocols listed and illustrated in the volume indicated the use of DXR (Figure 1).

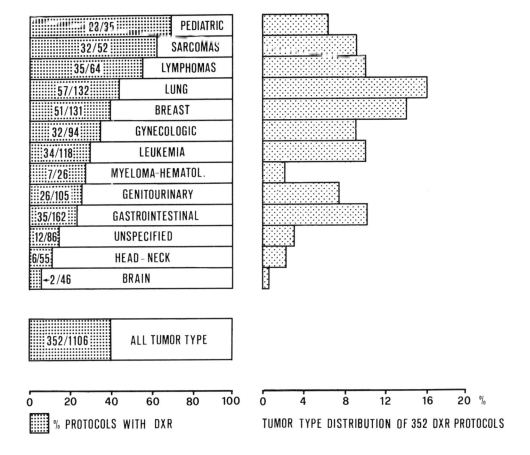

FIGURE 1.   Presence of doxorubicin in independent clinical protocols (Compilation of Experimental Cancer Therapy Protocol Summaries, National Institutes of Health, May 1981).

Doxorubicin was found especially often in treatment of the most classical and established indications (pediatric tumors, 23/35; sarcomas, 32/52; and lymphomas, 35/64), but it was also used in lung and breast cancer, which tumors had the highest number of DXR-containing protocols. It appears that present studies in the United States with DXR are particularly oriented toward a perfection of the established use of the drug. This is also true for lung cancer, if we consider that more than 50% of the studies were carried out in small-cell lung cancer. Ten percent of the studies dealt with leukemia; this seems quite impressive considering the effectiveness of daunorubicin (DNR) in this field even though several studies seem to show an activity similar to DXR at equitoxic doses (9).

Adjuvant studies are found more frequently in the most established indications (pediatric and sarcomas) and, in more than 90% of total studies, DXR was administered in combination with other anticancer agents. In lung cancer, for instance, all 57 protocols indicated the use of a DXR-containing combination even if the superiority of such protocols over DXR alone has never been demonstrated in randomized trials.

The number of drugs combined with DXR varied from one to five, with a prevalence of the protocols containing DXR plus two other drugs. Some of them also indicated the use of radiotherapy. The 10 anticancer drugs that were combined most frequently with DXR in ongoing trials are listed in descending order in Table 2.

Looking at the distribution by tumor type, we see that the empirical concept of combining agents that are active when used alone against the tumor in question is still the most frequently followed therapy. It is worthy of note that combinations with immunotherapy or with hormonotherapy are relatively few in these protocols.

An analysis of these data indicates that the body of ongoing clinical investigation with DXR is quite large, emphasizing that interest is still very high for this drug. Definitions of the best combinations for well-established indications seem to be the major targets of the ongoing trials in the United States, although a certain caution is being observed in the use of DXR in adjuvant treatment.

It is practically impossible to give a clear picture of the size and characteristics of the clinical research with DXR that is presently in progress in countries other than the United States. Nevertheless, a general impression may be derived by looking at the plan of the studies

Table 2. Anticancer drugs most frequently combined with doxorubicin in ongoing trials (compilation of Experimental Cancer Therapy Protocol Summaries, National Institutes of Health, May 1981)

	CLINICAL PROTOCOLS											
	BREAST	G.I.	G.U.	GYN.	MY.-H.	LUNG	LYNP.	SARC.	PED.	H.-N.	UNSPEC.	TOTAL
C T X	41		13	23	3	51	27	21	27	2	7	215
V C R	11		1	2	5	30	29	10	24		4	116
5 - F U	32	30	5	2		3			2	1		79
C D D P	1	3	15	18	1	24		4	3	4	5	78
P R E D	4		1		7		31				1	44
M T X	2	1				14	4	9	3		1	34
B L E O		3	3	1	5		21	1		1	1	34
V P - 16	1		2	2		24	4					33
M I T O - C	2	15	1	1		3						22
D T I C							3	11	5		1	20
IMMUNOTHERAPY	9			1		4	2	2	3		1	22
HORMONOTHERAPY	8											8

that Farmitalia Carlo Erba (FICE) was at least partly supporting internationally in 1981 (Table 3). The majority of these studies which, for reasons of internal organization, does not take into consideration those carried out in Italy and the United States, were concentrated in four tumor categories: genitourinary, gastrointestinal, breast, and lung cancer. Some different approaches were followed as far as the route of administration and combined modality treatment were concerned. Most studies in the genitourinary group comprised the use of topical intravesical administration of DXR for superficial bladder tumors, either as therapeutic treatment, especially in the tumors in situ, or as a prophylactic treatment after transurethral resection. A certain number of studies were carried out in liver cancer and two were carried out in bladder cancer where DXR was given by intraarterial infusion. About 50% of the studies in breast cancer utilized the combined use of DXR-containing combination with hormones, particularly with medroxyprogesterone acetate (MPA). Finally, as far as the gastrointestinal cancer group is concerned, some adjuvant studies in gastric cancer are still in progress.

The use of DXR by intravesical instillation is discussed in detail elsewhere in this volume (10); however, these clinical experiences bring forth in more general terms the problem of the topical use of DXR. Besides

Table 3. Farmitalia Carlo Erba-supported DXR clinical studies (1981)

P R O T O C O L S	G.U.	G.I.	BREAST	LUNG	GYN.	H.-N.	MY.-H.	LEUK.	TOTAL
	27 (25%)	25 (23%)	24 (23%)	15 (14%)	8 (7%)	3 (3%)	2 (2%)	2 (2%)	106
RANDOMIZED	8	13	16	7	6	2	1	1	54
NON RANDOMIZED	19	12	8	8	2	1	1.	1	52
EARLY OR ADVANCED									
- DXR Alone	5	6	1	-	-	-	-	-	12
- DXR in Combination	4	16	21	15	8	3	2	2	71
ADJUVANT									
- DXR Alone	18	-	-	-	-	-	-	-	18
- DXR in Combination	-	3	2	-	-	-	-	-	5
TOPICAL	21	-	-	-	-	-	-	-	21
INTRA-ARTERIAL	2	6	-	-	-	-	-	-	5
SYSTEMIC	4	19	24	15	8	3	2	2	77
MONOCHEMOTHERAPY	23	6	1	-	-	-	-	-	30
POLYCHEMOTHERAPY	2	18	12	10	6	3	2	2	55
POLYCHEMO-HORMONOTHERAPY	1	-	11	-	2	-	-	-	14
POLYCHEMO-RADIOTHERAPY	1	1	-	5	-	-	-	-	7

the intraperitoneal administration (11), DXR has been given intrapleurally (12) and, more recently, as an ointment (13) for the topical treatment of ulcerous skin metastases of breast cancer.

For many years it has been known that DXR is necrotizing and that it can sometimes induce a contact dermatitis (14) or a recall phenomenon (15). However, the present clinical experience with its topical use should indicate an extention of the research in this field at an experimental, pharmaceutical and clinical level. The new analogs, too, probably ought to be evaluated in this direction in the hope of detecting a lower tendency to damage normal tissues.

The use of chemohormonotherapy combination does not constitute a new approach for the treatment of advanced breast cancer. The different hypothes supporting this therapeutic approach are not specifically drug-related but refer generally to chemotherapy and hormonotherapy; on the contrary, very seldom has there been discussion about the combination of a particular antineoplastic drug with a given hormone.

The availablilty on the market in many countries of both DXR and MPA has allowed FICE to be interested in promoting both experimental and clinica research on combinations of these two drugs.

Some interesting experimental data which have recently been reported provide some new evidence on a possible synergistic effect of the two drugs (16). Actually MPA and DXR given simultaneously (but not sequentially) have shown an additive effect in 13726 mammary carcinoma and in its sublines responsive to MPA; however, some sublines not affected by MPA alone have shown sensitivity to the combined treatment with the two drugs.

Some multicenter cooperative studies that combine MPA to DXR-containing regimens are now in progress. One of these, comparing vincristine, Adriamycin, cyclophosphamide (VAC) with and without MPA in advanced metastatic breast cancer involves 10 oncological centers in Europe and Latin America (17). Two hundred fifty-six patients entered the study, and the preliminary results on 179 evaluable patients show that the median time to progression is significantly longer ($P < 0.05$) in the arm containing MPA (16+ versus 9 months). Moreover, the incidence of leucopenia is lower in the arm where MPA was associated with VAC. A total of 955 cycles have been evaluated so far: leucopenia, defined as a white cell number lower than $4000/mm^3$, was observed in 36% of the cycles without MPA and in 26% of cycles with MPA ($P < 0.01$).

Even if the role of DXR in adjuvant treatment of breast cancer has been, and still is, a matter of debate among different investigators, the present trend of the major institutes and study groups both in the United States and Europe is moving toward the introduction of DXR in the adjuvant combinations (18).

As far as gastric cancer is concerned, a very large multicenter trial in which surgery alone is compared versus surgery plus 5-fluorouracil, Adriamycin, and mitomycin C (FAM) has been recently activated in Europe and will involve more than 20 oncological centers (19). Similar studies are presently going on in Australia with active 5-fluorouracil, Adriamycin and BCNU (FAB) combination versus no treatment (20).

The basic problem common to all adjuvant treatments involving DXR is the possible risk of late toxicity in long-term survivors. Monitoring all of the late toxicities and, in particular, the cardiac risk both in already established or new indications of DXR is one of the most important objectives of a postmarketing surveillance program for DXR. In actual fact, a large survey parallel to the one performed in the United States by Von Hoff (21) was carried out in Europe 3 years ago (22), and the results of both studies were able to identify more clearly some important prognostic factors and to offer useful indications for the safer use of the drug or for further clinical evaluation.

We have now planned a new survey in some selected centers in Europe as well as in the United States in collaboration with Adria Laboratories with the objective of evaluating the clinical course and checking the present cardiac status of patients who have survived more than 5 years from the beginning of treatment with DXR. The late-toxicity study also intends to collect data concerning any other impairment of organ function and to survey the occurrence of a second tumor.

3. IS THERE STILL ROOM FOR FURTHER CLINICAL INVESTIGATION WITH DOXORUBICIN?

Over the past 10 years, DXR has been studied following the classical steps of clinical pharmacology, and now we can consider it to be established at the level occasionally referred to as phase IV. However, the phase I methodology of antitumoral drugs differs significantly from that of the other drugs. It is sufficient to remember that, while phase I is often done in healthy volunteers, the initial studies on antitumoral drugs are carried out, for obvious ethical reasons, in cancer patients with advanced disease and poor general conditions. Doxorubicin 10 years ago did not escape this rule, and this is true today for its analogs.

Looking at the 80s, one might wonder whether the present studies with DXR in early treatment could not give us an opportunity to define more clearl the clinical profile of the drug. In other words, the possibility of carryin out a correct drug-oriented research today is greater than it was 10 years ago, even though the possibility of administering the drug alone today is much less than 10 years ago. The advances in experimental chemotherapy and the increasing confidence in the predictability of animal models represent an additional advantage. In fact, DXR enters as the standard reference drug in almost all experimental pharmacological investigations with the anthracycline analogs which are presently in progress (23). This is not only a way to better evaluate the possible superiority of the analogs, but it also provides an additional opportunity to reevaluate and enlarge the preclinical knowledge on DXR. On the other hand, the technical achievements for the assays of DXR in biological fluids (24) and for the monitoring of cardiotoxicity in animals (25) and in man (7) have improved greatly in the last 10 years.

Besides the main problem of cardiotoxicity which is discussed elsewhere in this volume, some need for additional clinical pharmacology investigation exists today in several areas including toxicology, drug interaction, pharmac kinetics, and drug availability when DXR is bound to special carriers.

The problem of nephrotoxicity may represent a good example. At the experimental level, kidney damage after acute and chronic administration of DXR has been reported over the years by different authors (26,27). On the other hand, only one case of nephrotoxicity has been reported in humans (28), and renal function repeatedly has been normal after prolonged treatment with DXR. However, it is interesting to note that the biochemical changes observed in rats after exposure to high single doses of DXR are those of a nephrotic syndrome with progressively increased proteinuria, hypercholesterolemia, and hypercoagulability, with BUN and serum creatinine remaining almost unchanged (29). Again, a nephrotic syndrome has never been reported in humans treated with DXR; however, very seldom have proteinuria or the lipid pattern been systematically monitored in patients treated with DXR. Probably a careful clinical metabolic evaluation, which is not always possible in patients with advanced disease, would be advisable today in patients being subjected to adjuvant treatment; such an evaluation would eliminate any possible doubt about DXR nephrotoxicity in humans.

Another aspect which deserves some consideration and probably further investigation is related to the fact that potentially important interactions with commly employed drugs may occur (30). Heparin is a good example since there are several conditions where administration is clinically advisable and the drug is commonly given: when DXR is given by intraarterial infusion, heparin is necessary to keep the catheter open. The advantage of combining heparin with DXR or DNR in disseminated intravascular coagulation from acute promyelocytic leukemia has been claimed by many authors (31,32). Finally, there is a renewed interest in associating anticoagulants with chemotherapy in the treatment of some tumors (33).

It is well known that in vitro DXR forms a complex with heparin (34) with the disappearance of the anticoagulant activity of heparin (35). This has been confirmed also in vivo (36). Following its administration to heparinized patients, DXR is able to modify radically the anticoagulant activity of heparin for a short time (10-15 min), corresponding to highest concentration of DXR in plasma.

Whether DXR disposition and its eventual antitumoral activity could be changed by administration of the drug in combination with heparin is something that should be investigated in animals and possibly in humans. In actual fact, it cannot be excluded a priori that such an interaction might

even have a positive effect on DXR antitumoral activity. The possibility
that the therapeutic index of DXR may be improved in the clinics by a better
evaluation of new dosage schedules seems to be one of the most attractive
objectives of clinical investigation.

Even though a bolus every 3-4 weeks still is the standard method of DXR
administration, recent progress in analytical methods has allowed us to
obtain a number of pharmacokinetic data for DXR given by different schedules
(weekly injections or continuous infusions) or given by different routes
(intraarterial perfusion, i.p. dialysis, and intravesical instillation). A
number of clinical studies have already been carried out with the weekly
schedule and with the i.v. perfusion that show a decrease both in acute and
chronic toxicity (37-40). However, it remains uncertain whether the therapeutic activity associated with the weekly administration or with the i.v.
perfusion is at least equal to the bolus method. Obviously, prospective
randomized studies integrated by careful pharmacokinetic analyses are necessar

Treatment may possibly be made even safer in poor-risk patients (elderly
patients more than 70 years old; performance status $\sqrt{K.I.}\sqrt{}$ less than 50;
heavy pretreatment with other chemotherapeutic agents) by weekly administrations of low doses.

Optimal timing of surgery is an additional aspect which should be further
investigated. For some tumor types (osteosarcoma, inflammatory breast cancer)
DXR administration prior to surgery has been suggested mainly to facilitate
the subsequent operation (41). Some authors, however, have suggested the
possibility that metastatic spread might better be prevented by early chemotherapy given prior or during surgery (42).

The chronological aspects may be critical for some drugs or some specific
combinations. Quite interestingly, the combination DXR + ICRF 159 showed a
synergistic effect against lung metastases of MS-2 sarcoma when the drug
treatment was performed before surgery or both before and after surgery (43).
No synergistic effect was found when the MS-2 lung metastases were treated
only after surgery.

Some attempts have already been made to improve significantly the therapeutic index of DXR by development of a carrier system that would decrease
the DXR uptake by heart muscle without diminishing its antitumor activity.
Actually, DXR-DNA (44) or DXR-iron complexes (45) have been investigated in
the last few years, but the clinical investigation has not yet been conclusiv
More recently, the potential role of liposomes as drug carriers has been

extensively discussed (46,47) and data on the feasibility of this approach
for DXR have already been published (48). Liposomes offer the opportunity
of targeting substantial amounts of drug to liver and lung, which are two
common sites of metastatic growth. On the other hand, liposomes hardly reach
the extravascular compartment of tissues containing continuous capillaries
such as skeletal, cardiac muscle, and nervous tissue. The possibility of
gaining a selective drug distrubition with liposome-entrapped DXR may be of
great clinical importance; however, some other carrier systems such as those
utilizing monoclonal antibodies (49) or nanoparticles (50) are now being
studied at an experimental level and could become of clinical interest in
the coming years.

As far as the phase II disease-oriented approach is concerned, we should
also ask ourselves whether there is still room in the 1980s. One aspect
is related to the development of new predictive systems in vitro such as that
represented by the "human tumor stem-cell assay" (51), or in vivo such as that
represented by the "nude mouse-human tumor xenograft system" (52). Both
systems may be useful to allow us to investigate more thoroughly the spectrum
of antitumor activity of DXR itself and of DXR-containing combinations and
to provide useful information for a more extended disease-oriented clinical
investigation. For instance, the recent finding of a significant DXR activity
against various melanomas studied in xenografts (52) would deserve a further
clinical investigation in this type of tumor which has been considered till
now nonresponsive to DXR.

The geographical distribution of clinical investigations with DXR is
probably another important point to be taken into consideration. DXR has been
largely evaluated in almost all important tumor types in western countries;
however, with the worldwide use of this drug today, some new interesting
aspects related to the different cancer epidemiology found in African and
eastern areas have been encountered. Hepatoma, for instance, occurs frequently
in Africa, and Olweny, some years ago, reported promising results with DXR
treatment in Uganda (53). Falkson and the Eastern Cooperative Oncology Group
were able to confirm the good results in the African population, but noticed
that the hepatoma was much less responsive to DXR in American patients (54).
Results coming from Southeast Asia are, again, in agreement with a good
responsiveness to DXR treatment (55). Probably in the case of hepatoma
we are dealing with different types of tumor from the etiological point of
view; however, it may also be possible that racial differences and some

environmental factors play some role as far as drug responsiveness is concerned. Therefore, a disease-oriented clinical investigation in new geographical areas may represent an additional interesting approach for DXR in the 80s. Certainly one of the most interesting countries from the epidemiological point of view is China. Following a series of meetings with local investigators in Peking, Shanghai, and Canton (6), we were able to activate in the People's Republic of China some clinical trials with DXR in types of tumors with a very high incidence in that area, i.e., cancer of the esophagus, liver, and nasopharynx.

4. CONCLUSIONS

It is clear that the development of doxorubicin has provided the basis for significant improvements in cancer treatment in general. Because of the broad spectrum of activity that has been documented in a large number of clinical trials, DXR has become a "front-line" agent despite its typical side effects which include myelosuppression, nausea, vomiting, alopecia, and delayed cardiac toxicity. Instructions for a correct clinical use of the drug however, have rendered many of these toxicities either manageable or preventable. As a result, the use of DXR has progressively left the strictly investigational clinical institutes to reach to an ever-increasing extent the community hospitals. However, we are not at the end point of the clinical research with DXR; on the contrary, a number of investigational new approaches still remain open that will optimize its routine use.

It is important to avoid the risk of confusing what is still investigational with what is definitely accepted, not only to exploit in the best way the known properties of DXR for the medical benefit of patients, but also to establish strategic priorities in the clinical development of the new anthracycline analogs.

It would seem logical that the possible superiority of an analog both in terms of efficacy and toxicity can be documented more selectively and specifically in those areas where the pharmacotoxicological characteristics of the parent drug are well defined. Further drug-oriented clinical research with DXR, by clarifying those aspects still open to investigation, may also favor a rational identification of the best analogs.

REFERENCES

1. Tagnon H, Kenis Y, Bonadonna G, Carter SK, Sokal G, Trouet A, Ghione M, Praga C, Lenaz L, Karim OS, eds. 1975. Adriamycin review. E.O.R.T.C. International Symposium. Ghent, Belgium, European Press Medikon.
2. Füllenbach D, Nagel GA, Seeber S, eds. 1981. Adriamycin Symposium Ergebnisse und Aspekte. New York, S. Karger.
3. Carter SK, Di Marco A, Ghione M, Krakoff IH, Mathé, G, eds. 1972. International Symposium on Adriamycin. New York: Springer-Verlag.
4. Proceedings of the 5th New Drug Seminar on Adriamycin, Washington, D.C., 16-17 December 1974, and of the Adriamycin New Drug Seminar, San Francisco, California, 15-16 January 1975. 1975. Cancer Chemother. Rep. 6 (3). .
5. Proceedings of the International Symposium on Adriamycin and Related Drugs. Moscow, 30-31 March 1981. In press.
6. Huanxing W, Jiaxiang S, Nicolis FB, Changxiao L, Liang H, Gang F, Shaozhang S, Dechang W, Praga C, Beretta G, eds. 1981. Topics on cancer chemotherapy. Proceedings of the International Symposium on Adriamycin and Other Drugs in Antitumor Chemotherapy. China Academic Publishers.
7. Young RC, Ozols RF, Myers CE. 1981. N. Engl. J. Med. 305: 139.
8. U.S. Department of Health. 1981. Compilation of experimental cancer therapy protocol summaries. 5th ed. NIH publication 81-1116. Washington, D.C., National Institutes of Health.
9. Woodruff R. 1978. Cancer Treat. Rev. 5: 95.
10. Pavone-Macaluso M. 1981. Paper presented at the Symposium on Anthracycline Antibiotics in Cancer Therapy, New York, 16-18 September 1981.
11. Ozols R. 1981. Paper presented at the Symposium on Anthracycline Antibiotics in Cancer Therapy, New York, 16-18 September 1981.
12. Tattersall MH. 1980. Med. J. Aust. 2: 447.
13. Fukuda M, Yanagawa T, Ikari J, Komoriyama H, Hamaguchi M, Kanasugi K, Yamaguchi S, Tanaka Y, Arai S, Watanabe H. 1981. Gann 8: 134.
14. Etcubanas E, Wilbur JR. 1974. Cancer Chemother. Rep. 58: 757.
15. Phillips TL, Fu KK. 1977. Cancer 40: 489.
16. Formelli F, Zaccheo T, Casazza AM, Bellini O, Di Marco A. 1981. Eur. J. Cancer Clin. Oncol. 17: 1211.
17. Pellegrini A, Robustelli della Cuna G, Estevez R, Luchina A, Da Silva Neto JB, Lira Puerto V, Cortes-Funes H, Arraztoa J. 1982. U.I.C.C. International Symposium on Medroxyprogesterone Acetate, Geneva, 24-26 February 1982. Accepted abstract.
18. International Conference on the Adjuvant Therapy of Cancer (3rd). 1981. Tucson, Arizona. Abstract volume.
19. Schein P, Coombes C. 1981. Personal communication.
20. Levi JA. 1981. Proceedings of the International Congress on Diagnosis and Treatment of Upper Gastrointestinal Tumors (Friedman M, Ogawa M, Kisner D, eds.). Oxford, Excerpta Medica, pp. 370-380.
21. Von Hoff DD, Layard MW, Basa P, Davis HL Jr, Von Hoff AL, Rozencweig M, Muggia FM. 1979. Ann. Intern. Med. 91: 710.
22. Praga C, Beretta G, Vigo PL, Lenaz GR, Pollini C, Bonadonna G, Canetta R, Castellani R, Villa E, Gallagher CG, von Melchner H, Hayat M, Ribaud P, De Wasch G, Mattsson W, Heinz R, Waldner R, Kolaric K, Buehner R, Ten Bokkel-Huyninck W, Perevodchikova NI, Manziuk LA, Senn HJ, Mayr AC. 1979. Cancer Treat. Rep. 63: 827.
23. Casazza AM. 1979. Cancer Treat. Rep. 63: 835.
24. Eksborg S, Ehrsson H, Andersson I. 1979. Chromatogr. Biomed. Appl. 164: 479.
25. Bertazzoli C. 1981. Paper presented at the Symposium on Anthracycline

396

Antibiotics in Cancer Therapy, New York, 16-18 September 1981.
26. Fajardo LF, Eltringham JR, Stewart JR, Klauber MR. 1980. Lab. Invest. 43: 242.
27. Philips FS, Gilladoga A, Marquardt H, Sternberg SS, Vidal PM. 1975. Cancer Chemother. Rep. 6: 177.
28. Burke JF. 1977. Arch. Int. Med. 137: 385.
29. Bertani T, Poggi A, Pozzoni R, Delaini F, Sacchi G, Thoua Y, Mecca G, Remuzzi G, Donati MB. 1982. Lab. Invest. 46: 16.
30. Dorr RT, Fritz WL. 1980. Cancer chemotherapy handbook. New York, Elsevier Press, p. 388.
31. Drapkin RL, Gee TS, Dowling MD, Arlin Z, McKenzie S, Kempin S, Clarkson B. 1978. Cancer 41: 2484.
32. Dreyfus B, Varet B, Heilmann-Gouault M, Sultan C. Reyes F, Gluckman E, Basch A, Beaujean F. 1973. Nouv. Rev. Fr. Hematol. 13: 755.
33. Zacharski LR. 1981. Malignancy and the hemostatic system (Donati MB, Davidson JF, Garattini S, eds.). New York, Raven Press, pp. 113-127.
34. Menozzi M, Arcamone F. 1978. Biochem. Biophys. Res. Commun. 80: 313.
35. Cofrancesco E, Vigo A, Pogliani E, Polli EE. 1978. 17th Congress Int. Soc. Haemat. Abstract volume. Paris, p. 456.
36. Cofrancesco E. Vigo A, Pogliana E. 1980. Thrombos. Res. 18: 743.
37. Benjamin R, Legha S, Mackay B, .Ewer M, Wallace S, Valdivieso M, Rasmussen S, Blumenschein G, Freireich E. 1981. AACR-ASCO Proceedings, Abstr. 711.
38. Chlebowski RT, Paroly WS, Pugh RP, Hueser J, Jacobs EM, Pajak TF, Bateman JR. 1980. Cancer Treat. Rep. 64: 47.
39. Gercovich FG, Praga C, Beretta G, Morgenfeld M, Muchink J, Pesce R, Ho DHW, Benjamin RS. 1979. AACR-ASCO Proceedings, Abstr. C-337.
40. Weiss AJ, Manthel RW. 1977. Cancer 40: 2046.
41. Rosen G, Marcove RC, Caparros B, Nirenberg A, Kosloff C, Huvos AG. 1979. Cancer 43: 2163.
42. Papaioannu AN. 1981. Eur. J. Cancer 17: 263.
43. Giuliana F, Casazza AM, Di Marco A, Savi G. 1981. Cancer Treat. Rep. 65: 267.
44. Paul A, Lonnqvist B, Gharton G, Lockner D. Peterson C. 1981. Cancer 48: 1531.
45. Brugarolas A, Pachon N, Gosalvez M, Perez Llanderal A, Lacave AJ, Buesa JM, Gracia Marco M. 1978. Cancer Treat. Rep. 62: 1527.
46. Frühling J, Penasse W, Laurent G, Brassinne C, Hildebrand J, Vanhaelen M, Vanhaelen-Fastre R, Deleers M, Ruysschaert JM. 1980. Eur. J. Cancer 16: 1409.
47. Kaye SB, Richardson VJ. 1979. Cancer Chemother. Pharmacol. 3: 81.
48. Rahman A, Kessler A, More N, Sikic B, Rowden G, Woolley P, Schein PS. 1980. Cancer Res. 40: 1532.
49. Diamond BA, Yelton DE, Scharff MD. 1981. New Engl. J. Med. 304: 1344.
50. Couvreur P, Tulkens P, Roland M, Trouet A, Speiser P. 1977. FEBS Lett. 84: 323.
51. Salmon SE, ed. Cloning of human tumor stem cells. Progress in Clinical and Biological Research, vol. 48. New York, A. R. Liss.
52. Giuliani FC, Zirvi KA, Kaplan NO. 1981. Cancer Res. 41: 325.
53. Olweny CLM, Toya T, Katongole-Mbidde E, Mugerwa J, Kyalwazi SK, Cohen H. 1975. Cancer 36: 1250.
54. Falkson G, Moertel CC, McIntyre JM, Lavin P, Engstrom PF, Carbone PP. 1981. Proceedings of the International Congress on Diagnosis and Treatment of Upper Gastrointestinal Tumors (Friedman M, Ogawa M, Kisner D, eds.). Oxford, Excerpta Medica, pp. 455-459.

55. Oon CJ. 1981. Proceedings of the International Congress on Diagnosis and Treatment of Upper Gastrointestinal Tumors (Friedman M, Ogawa M, Kisner D, eds.). Oxford, Excerpta Medica, pp. 466-482.

A PHASE I/II STUDY OF 6-HOUR AND 24-HOUR INTRAVENOUS INFUSIONS OF DOXORUBICIN

J. L. SPEYER, M. D. GREEN, J. BOTTINO, J. WERNZ, R. H. BLUM, AND F. M. MUGGIA

1. INTRODUCTION

Cardiomyopathy related to the total cumulative dose is a major factor limiting the use of doxorubicin. This complication occurs in only a small percentage (7-15% of patients treated at a total cumulative dose of 550 mg/m^2) (1-3). However, its occasionally fatal outcome or otherwise disabling implications have restricted the use of doxorubicin. General practice has been to terminate therapy at a predetermined cumulative drug dose of 450-550 mg/m^2 and to exclude certain groups of patients from treatment with doxorubicin.

Retrospective reviews have identified groups of patients that are at relatively higher risk for the development of doxorubicin-induced cardiomyopathy (2,3). The risk factors include increased age, prior radiation to the heart, preexisting myocardial disease, and a high cumulative dose of doxorubicin. Endomyocardial biopsy (4) and measurement of left ventricular ejection fraction by radionuclide cardiac scans (5,6), particularly when determined during exercise-induced stress, more reliably identify patients with early cardiac muscle damage than do other available techniques.

Cardiac biopsy and radionuclide ventriculography may identify patients in whom doxorubicin should not be used or should be discontinued and also can be used to evaluate methods for preventing cardiomyopathy. We have sought to evaluate the effects of alterations in dose schedules with radionuclide monitoring on the development of cardiomyopathy. Preclinical and clinical studies have suggested that the administration of doxorubicin by continuous infusion may decrease the incidence of cardiac complications. Animal studies by Myers et al. (7) indicated that antitumor activity and cardiotoxicity may proceed by separable mechanisms.

Retrospective clinical studies of the Central Oncology Group (8) indicated that the weekly administration of doxorubicin resulted in fewer

Supported in part by a grant from The Chemotherapy Foundation, The Lila Motley Fund, and by NIH grant CA 16087-05.

cases of congestive heart failure than occurred when the drug was given on
a schedule of every 3 weeks, even though there was no apparent difference
in antitumor activity. Reviews of large numbers of patients have tended to
confirm this observation (2,3). These data suggest that cardiotoxicity may
be promoted by high peak blood levels that are not required to maintain
antitumor activity. The logical schedule that delivers adequate therapeutic doses but minimizes peak blood levels is a continuous infusion.
However, wide application of this schedule awaited development of techniques
and safe infusion to eliminate the danger of drug extravasation. Early
trials of infusion of doxorubicin have been reported from the M. D. Anderson
Hospital (9), Italy (10), and the Sidney Farber Cancer Center (11); and
its rationale has been reviewed in a previous report (12).

2. METHODS

Eighty-three patients with pathologically documented malignancies
were treated with doxorubicin by continuous infusion. A first group of
41 patients was treated for 24 hours and a second group of 42 patients
was treated for 6 hours in an effort to explore a schedule with greater
safety and convenience. The patients and types of malignancies are shown
in Tables 1 and 2.

Twenty-six of the 24-hour group (63%) and 28 of the 6-hour group (66%)
had received prior therapy with drugs or irradiation or both. Therapy was
begun at an initial dose of 60 mg/m^2 and escalated to 75 mg/m^2 and
90 mg/m^2 in subsequent cycles according to tolerance. Doses were escalated
if the nadir WBC exceeded 2500 and the nadir platelet count exceeded 100,000.
The drug was mixed in 500 cc of 5% dextrose and infused with the aid of an
infusion pump through indwelling catheters placed in high-flow blood vessels
(Table 3). The predominant catheter used (199 of 262 infusions) was the
femoral type (CTS 500 Cook, Inc., Bloomington, Indiana). This technique will
be described in detail in a subsequent publication. The catheter was
threaded over a guide wire placed through a no. 19 gauge needle that had
been inserted into a femoral vein. The guide wire and needle were removed,
leaving the catheter in place. The catheter was removed after each course
and was repeatedly reinserted for subsequent administration. Forty-one
infusions were given through peripherally inserted (Intrasil R) central
venous silicone elastomer catheters (13). Eighteen infusions were given
through Hickman R, Broviac R, or standard subclavian lines because of

prior existence of these lines or extensive local femoral/pelvic disease.

Table 1. Doxorubicin infusion--characteristics of patients

Characteristics of patients	Treatment with doxorubicin	
	24 hours	6 hours
Number of patients	41	42
Male:female	23:18	19:23
Number of infusions	145	117
Median number of infusions	2	2
Mean dose of doxorubicin (range)	70 mg/m^2(50- 90)	60 mg/m^2(40- 90)
Mean cumulative dose of doxorubicin (range)	243 mg/m^2(60-820)	161 mg/m^2(60-540)
Patients with dose greater than 450 mg/m^2	9	2
Patients currently on study	0	15*
Number with prior treatment	26	28
Chemotherapy	4	14
RT	12	7
Chem. RX and RT	10	7
No RX	15	14

* 9,9,7,4,4,4,3,2,2,1,1,1,1,1,1 cycles.

When possible, patients had baseline gated pool radionuclide cardiac scans (6). Exercise scans were performed before and after exercise to tolerance; a bicycle ergometer was used. Follow-up scans were obtained in patients at a cumulative dose of 240 mg/m^2, 450 mg/m^2, and every two cycles thereafter. Follow-up scans were also determined, if possible, 3-6 months after the patient was off study.

Therapeutic assessment was carried out by standard Eastern Cooperative Oncology Group criteria of response. A complete response was defined as a decrease of greater than 50% in all measureable disease as measured by the product of the largest two perpendicular diameters of all measureable lesions for at least 4 weeks.

Although the 24-hour infusions have been completed, patients are still being entered and treated on the 6-hour schedule. There are currently 15 patients who have received between one and nine courses of

Table 2. Objective responses to doxorubicin infusions

Tumor type	2 4 h o u r s			6 h o u r s		
	Patients entered	Patients evaluable	Responses	Patients entered	Patients evaluable	Responses
Breast	4	4	0	10	6	3
Long (non-oat-cell)	17	16	1	9	6	0
Endometrial	6	6	3	2	1	1
Sarcoma	4	4	0	6	2	0
Bladder	2	2	0	0	0	0
Head and neck	2	2	0	1	0	0
Prostate	2	1	0	1	0	0
Gastric	0	0	0	1	1	0
Adenocarcinoma, unknown primary	3	1	0	2	1	0
Cervix	0	0	0	1	1	0
Nephroblastoma	0	0	0	1	1	1*
Biliary	1	1	0	2	1	0
Testicular	0	0	0	1	1	0
Colon	0	0	0	1	1	0
Carcinoid	0	0	0	2	0	0
Thyroid	0	0	0	2	1	0
TOTAL	41	37	4	42	23	5

*Complete regression.

Table 3. Routes of administration of doxorubicin infusions

Route	24 hours	6 hours
Femoral	85	114
Brachial	41	0
Subclavian	19	3

therapy with cumulative doses between 60 to 540 mg/m^2. Preliminary findings were published in abstract form (14,15).

3. RESULTS

Eighty-three patients received a total of 262 infusions (Table 1). The median number of infusions for both schedules was 2, with a range of 1 to 11. For the 24-hour schedule, the mean dose was 70 mg/m^2 (range 50-90 mg/m^2) and the mean cumulative dose was 243 mg/m^2 (range 60-820 mg/m^2). The mean dose for the 6-hour schedule is 60 mg/m^2 (range 40-90 mg/m^2), with a mean cumulative dose of 161 mg/m^2 (range 60-540 mg/m^2). The number of infusions administered at each dose level is detailed in Table 4.

Table 4. Number of infusions of patients receiving doxorubicin at each dose level

	Duration of infusion				
	24 hours			6 hours	
Dose mg/m^2	60	75	90	60	75
Number of patients	32	26	8	36	9
Number of courses	63	56	21	92	13
Total number of courses	140			105	

Note that a small number of infusions were administered at lower doses because of early toxicity. The total number listed here (245) is only for infusions at the planned doses.

3.1. Local toxicity

The femoral vein catheter was most frequently used, followed by the Intrasil (Table 3). More recently, because of its convenience and our interest in this method, the femoral route has been used almost exclusively. There was no local, dermal, or subcutaneous irritation from the drug or catheter, even though the catheter leaked at the IV connection on three occasions. Three of the 199 femoral infusions (two 24-hour and one 6-hour) (1.5%) were followed by iliofemoral thrombophlebitis in the infused limb. In all three, the clinical findings were confirmed by venography and resolved with heparin therapy. In two of the three patients, repeated femoral vein catheterization was successfully accomplished in the contralateral leg without complication.

3.2 Systemic toxicity

The systemic side effects of the drug were similar by both schedules (Table 5). Doses were escalated within individual patients to tolerance of disease progression. The limiting toxicity was myelosuppression. White blood cell count nadirs of less than 2000 were observed in 50 of 187 (27%)

evaluable courses of therapy. Nadirs occurred between 10 and 20 days after therapy. In 11 of these courses (22%), there was fever-associated neutropenia, which was treated with antibiotics. Serious infections (two pneumonia and two sepsis) were observed in an additional four courses. Thirteen patients died during therapy, six with infection or fever. Progressive disease was, however, also observed in 10 of these patients. A breakdown of median WBC nadir by dose and schedule is given in Table 6.

Thrombycytopenia (platelet count less than 100,000) was noted in 20 of 187 evaluable courses (11%) and was associated with bleeding in one case. There were two episodes of gastrointestinal bleeding (one associated with decreased platelet count). Alopecia was common, occurring in over 50% (35 patients). Nausea and vomiting were recorded during 39 of 262 courses of therapy and were generally mild and limited to the end of the infusion or the 3 hours following it. No severe nausea and vomiting were noted. Six patients developed mild to moderate mucositis 1-2 weeks posttherapy. One patient developed angina pectoris during therapy, and three had a radiation recall reaction.

3.3. Cardiac toxicity

Acute arrhythmias were not observed, although monitoring was not carried out. Only two patients developed clinical signs of congestive

Table 5. Incidents of acute toxicity occurring with doxorubicin in cohort of 83 patients

Symptoms of toxicity	Duration of infusion	
	24 hours	6 hours
WBC less than 2000	31	19
Platelets less than 100,000	5	15
Infection	4	1
Fever with neutropenia	5	6
Alopecia	14	21
Nausea and vomiting	10	29
Angina pectoris	1	0
Gastrointestinal bleeding	1	1
RT recall	1	2
Mucositis	2	5
Total evaluable courses	118	69

Table 6. Hematologic side effects of doxorubicin infusion

Duration of infusion	(mg/m^2)	Number of evaluable courses	WBC x 10^3 median	range	Platelets x 10^3 median	range
24 hours	60	55	3.3	0.9-10.2	250	100-486
	75	46	3.0	0.8-13.5	220	45-810
	90	17	2.5	0.3-8.2	174	75-810
6 hours	60	59	2.5	0.4-7.0	219	31-554
	75	10	1.0	0.2-2.9	97	48-185

heart failure during or after therapy (Table 7). One patient, a 79-year-old woman with abdominal fibrosarcoma received a cumulative dose of 600 mg/m^2 of doxorubicin by 24-hour infusion. She developed cardiomegaly, an S_4 gallop, pedal edema, and pulmonary congestion. Within 1 month of her last treatment, she had a normal resting LVEF on two radionuclide ventriculography determinations performed while she was clinically compensated with digoxin and diuretics. An echocardiogram did, however, indicate a decrease in left ventricular performance as measured by systolic time interval. One patient developed congestive failure after two cycles of 6-hour therapy (cumulative dose 135 mg/m^2). One additional patient, on a dose of 585 mg/m^2 on the 24-hour schedule, developed increased heart size on X-ray and a fall in LVEF from 0.70 to 0.40 without clinical signs of congestive failure.

Baseline scans were performed in 30 patients (Table 8). The mean left ventricular ejection fraction was 0.64 (range 0.41 to 0.83). Follow-up scans were obtained only in patients at risk. These numbers are still small.

3.4. Antitumor activity

There was one complete response in a patient with Wilms' tumor on the 6-hour schedule which lasted for 2 months. Partial responses were observed in endometrial cancer, breast cancer, and lung cancer (Table 2).

4. DISCUSSION

All too often a patient who is responding to treatment or who might benefit from therapy with doxorubicin has therapy discontinued or withheld because of potential risk of cardiac damage. The importance of cardiotoxicity is especially evident when one considers this active agent for the adjuvant treatment of breast cancer, endometrial cancer, or sarcomas.

Table 7. Numbers of patients with altered cardiac function after
doxorubicin infusion

Patients' data	Duration of infusion	
	24 hours	6 hours
Number of patients with congestive heart failure (820 mg/m^2; 135 mg/m^2)	2	0
Number of patients with cumulative dose greater than 450 mg/m^2	8	3
Number of patients with decrease in LVEF by greater than .10	1	2
Number of patients with less than 0.05 increase in LVEF with exercise	0	0

Table 8. Changes in left ventricular ejection fraction in patients
receiving doxorubicin infusions

	24 hours		6 hours	
	Baseline	Follow-up	Baseline	Follow-up
Number of patients	10	5	20	6
Mean	0.57	0.52	0.68	0.56
Median	0.55	0.53	0.69	0.63
Range	0.4-0.83	0.35-0.67	0.50-0.83	0.25-0.73

Inasmuch as many of these patients will live for many years, the potential
risk of cardiac damage versus its antitumor effect is of major concern.

Approaches to this problem include 1) the development of analogs that
may have less cardiotoxic effects; 2) the use of agents such as alpha
tocopherol and N-acetyl cysteine as radical scavengers to block doxorubicin-
induced oxidative damage to the myocardium; 3) development of careful monitoring programs to select those patients who demonstrate a decrease in left
ventricular function and to discontinue treatment of them while permitting
the other patients to continue beyond 550 mg/m^2; and 4) new schedules.
Modification of schedule from bolus to continuous infusion is attractive
because it involves no new agents. Data to support the study of schedules
using prolonged infusion was provided by Legha et al. (9), who demonstrated
that peak blood levels of doxorubicin fall progressively as a function of
the duration of infusion. The largest relative drop in peak levels occurs

when the infusion time is extended from bolus to 1 or 2 hours. The long terminal half-life of the drug 17-22 hours, appears to keep drug detectable in serum for days following either bolus or infusion (16-18).

We first chose to test patients on a 24-hour schedule, and the treatment appeared acceptable in terms of toxicity and acceptance by patients. As a compromise between decreased peak levels and convenience, we then changed to a 6-hour schedule. The 6-hour schedule could be performed in an out-patient hospital setting and would not require overnight hospitalization and surveillance.

Early trials of doxorubicin did not pursue infusion schedules because of the long drug terminal half-life and because of the intense local sclerotic and inflammatory reactions associated with drug extravasation which rendered prolonged peripheral infusions unfeasible. The development and application of semipermanent peripherally inserted central venous catheters by Bottino et al. (13) and of femoral catheters for chemotherapy by our group (19) have now made prolonged infusions of doxorubicin both safe and convenient. Moreover, there is a high degree of acceptance by patients. No patient refused further therapy because of femoral vein catheterization. Only three (less than 2%) infusions were complicated by thrombophlebitis and these were resolved with treatment. There were no other catheter-related problems. Our preliminary experience with the use of these catheters with vesicant agents (vindesine, 4'epiadriamycin, and bisantrene) in patients with limited venous access has also been encouraging (20). Although the number of complications is small, we feel that special caution should be taken when considering for femoral catheterization those patients with bulk inguinal or femoral disease or other factors predisposing to thrombosis. Also, our findings may not necessarily apply to other drugs and longer durations of infusion.

The acute systemic side effects of the drug appear to be the same for both schedules and are similar to those seen with bolus administration. The limiting side effect was myelosuppression. The dose range of 60-90 mg/m^2 at which this occurred is also similar to that obtained with bolus adminis-tration, though escalation within patients makes a clear dose response relationship unlikely. There were some differences in characteristics of patients between the 24-hour and the 6-hour schedules. The former had a lower percentage of patients who had received prior chemotherapy (Table 9). Moreover, the treatment for many of the patients with lung cancer was local

Table 9. Numbers of patients who had received prior therapy

| Type of prior therapy | Schedule of doxorubicin infusions | |
	24-hour	6-hour
Chemotherapy	4	14
Radiation therapy	12	7
Both	10	7
No prior therapy	15	14

radiation therapy. The 6-hour group had more pretreated patients, and more of these had had extensive prior chemotherapy; e.g., CMF for the patients with breast cancer. These differences may explain in part the lower frequency of patients treated at higher doses in the 6-hour group. Inasmuch as patients treated by bolus administration can receive doses in excess of 75 mg/m^2, it seems unlikely that there is unique toxicity within 6-hour infusions when the data from the 24-hour infusions resemble those of patients treated by bolus injections (21). The nature of other side effects (mucositis in seven (49%) available infusions is less than that reported in the early bolus studies (21). Our impression is that the degree and frequency (21%) of nausea and vomiting were less than those usually observed in patients given doxorubicin by bolus administration.

The first premise of the study, i.e., that antitumor activity is maintained, appears to be established. The tumoricidal activity of doxorubicin given by continuous infusion in a spectrum of diseases appears similar to that observed by bolus administration. Other reports have also documented analogous efficacy (9-11). Without a randomized trial, it is impossible to state whether tumoricidal activity is equivalent to bolus administration. This group of patients was heavily pretreated. Our response rate of 25% for prior treated breast tumors is compatible with the reported range. Similarly, objective responses in only 2 of 22 evaluable and mostly pretreated non-small-cell lung tumors are not surprising. Considerable activity was documented in a small number of patients with endometrial cancer. Further testing of doxorubicin infusion therapy in untreated patients with doxorubicin-sensitive tumors will be required to verify further the activity of this schedule.

Although the infusion schedules appear relatively safe, they do have the disadvantage of being less practical in that they usually require treatment of patients in a hospital setting. Garnick et al. (11) have circumvented this problem by giving even longer (21-day) infusions through intravenous catheters with subcutaneously implanted pumps. Infusion schedules for doxorubicin will be worth their inconvenience and potential local side effects (though quite low) only if the incidence of drug-induced cardiomyopathy is reduced. Researchers at M. D. Anderson Hospital (9) have reported that patients treated with equivalent doses by infusion had less cardiac damage, as judged by endomyocardial biopsy, than did patients who received equivalent doses of drug by conventional bolus. The group at the Sidney Farber Cancer Center also reported a low incidence of cardiac changes as judged by biopsy score in patients treated with their prolonged infusion schedule (11). In these trials, we were unable to make a definitive statement about the degree of cardiotoxicity. Only two patients developed CHF, one probably with tumor progression at low dose and one at the time of tumor progression but at high dose; in this latter patient, the CHF was believed to be drug related. However, only 12 patients were treated to cumulative doses in excess of 450 mg/m^2 (range 480-820 mg/m^2). Follow-up studies in eight of these patients reveal a trend toward decreased left ventricular function. Mean follow-up LVEFs are 0.50. The degree of cardiac toxicity that results from the infusion schedule will be the subject of a subsequent publication as more patients become at risk. Studies of patients with breast cancer, by the 6-hour schedule alone and in combination with 5FU and cytoxan, are being continued to address this important issue.

In summary, using catheters placed into high-flow venous systems, we found that the administration of doxorubicin by 24-hour and 6-hour infusions was tolerable and well accepted. The incidence of local thrombosis with femoral vein infusions was less than 2%. The limiting systemic toxicity was myelosuppression. There was activity of the drug on these schedules but the exact amount and the degree to which infusions may protect against the development of dosorubicin-induced cardiotoxicity will require further investigation.

ACKNOWLEDGMENTS

The authors gratefully acknowledge support in data collection from Carolina Pinto and Ted Metzger, assistance with catheter placement from Dr. Bernard Nidus, and secretarial assistance from Peggy Nixdorf.

REFERENCES

1. Gottdiener JS, Mathisen DJ, Borer JS, Bonow RO, Myers CE, Barr LH, Schwartz DE, Bacharach SL, Green MV, Rosenberg SA. 1981 Doxorubicin cardiotoxicity: assessment of late left ventricular dysfunction by radionuclide cineangiography. Ann Int Med 94: 430-435.
2. Praga C, Beretta G, Vigo G, Lenaz GR, Pollini C, Bonadonna G, et al. 1979. Adriamycin cardiotoxicity: a survey of 1273 patients. Cancer Treat Rep 63: 827-834.
3. Von Hoff DD, Layard MW, Basa P, Davis HL Jr, Von Hoff AL, Rozencweig M, Muggia FM. 1979. Risk factors for doxorubicin-induced congestive heart failure. Ann Int Med 91: 710-717.
4. Bristow M, Mason J, Billingham M, Daniels J. 1978. Doxorubicin cardiomyopathy: evaluation by phonocardiography, endomyocardial biopsy, and cardiac catheterization. Ann Int Med 88: 168-175.
5. Alexander J, Dainiak N, Berger HJ, Goldman L, Johnstone D, Reduto L, Duffy, Schwartz P, Gottschalk A, Zoret B. 1979. Serial assessment of doxorubicin cardiotoxicity with quantitative radionuclide angiocardiography. New Engl J Med 300: 278-283.
6. Borer J, Bachrack S, Green M, Kent K, Epstein S, Johnston G. 1977. Real-time radionuclide cineangiography in the noninvasive evaluation of global and regional left ventricular function at rest and during exercise in patients with coronary-artery disease. New Engl J Med 039 844.
7. Myers C, McGuire W, Liss R, Grotzinger K, Young R. 1977. "Adriamycin": the role of lipid peroxidation in cardiotoxicity and tumor response. Science 197: 165-167.
8. Weiss A, Metter G, Fletcher W, Wilson W, Grage T, Ramirez G. 1976. Studies on adriamycin using a weekly regimen demonstrating its clinical effectiveness and lack of cardiac toxicity. Cancer Treat Rep. 60: 813-822.
9. Legha S, Benjamin R, Yap H, Freireich E. 1979. Augmentation of adriamycin's therapeutic index by prolonged continuous iv infusion for advanced breast cancer. Proc Am Assoc Cancer Res 20: A1059.
10. Gercovich F, Praga C, Beretta G, Morganfeld M, Muchnik J, Pesce R, Ho D, Benjamin R. 1979. Ten hour continuous infusion of adriamycin. Proc Am Soc Clin Oncol 20: 337.
11. Garnick M, Weiss G, Steele G, Israel M, Barry W, Billingham M, Sack M, Shade G, Canellos G, Frei E. 1981. Phase I trial of long term continuous infusion adriamycin administration. Proc Am Soc Clin Oncol 22: 106.
12. Muggia F, Speyer J, Bottino J. In press. Rationale for new clinical studies with doxorubicin. In: New approaches in cancer therapy. NY: Raven.
13. Bottino J, McCredie K, Groschel D, Lawson K. 1979. Long-term intravenous therapy with peripherally inserted silicone elastomer central venous catheters in patient with malignant disease. Cancer 43: 1937-1943.
14. Muggia FM, Levin M, Wernz J, Bottino J, Blum R, Speyer J. 1980. Continuous infusion adriamycin: rationale and preliminary results. Cancer Chemother and Pharm 5: A141.
15. Speyer J, Bottino J, Nidus B, Blum R, Wernz J, Levin M, Hymes K, Muggia F. 1981. Adriamycin 24-hour infusion: a phase I trial. Proc Am Soc Clin Oncol 22: 122.
16. Chan K, Cohen J, Gross J, Himmelstein K, Bateman J, Yen T, Marlis A. 1978. Prediction of adriamycin disposition in cancer patients using a physiologic pharmacokinetic model. Cancer Treat Rep 62: 1161-1171.
17. Chlebowski R, Paroly W, Pugh RP, Hueser J, Jacobs E, Pajak J, Bateman J. 1980. Adriamycin given as a weekly schedule without a loading dose: clinically effective with reduced incidence of cardiotoxicity. Cancer

410

Treat Rep 64: 47-51.

18. Creasey W, McIntosh S, Brescia T, Odjujinsin O, Aspnes G, Murray E, Marsh J.   1976.   Clinical effects and pharmocokinetics of different dosage schedules of adriamycin.   Cancer Res 36: 216-221.

19. Bottino J, Levin M, Hymes K, Pouillart P, Muggia F, Nidus B.   1980. Femoral venous cannulation for continuous Adriamycin and vindesine infusions.   Cancer Immunol and Immunther Supp 10: A22.

20. Nidus B, et al. Unpublished data.

21. Blum, RH, Carter SK.   1974.   Adriamycin: a new anti-cancer drug with significant clinical activity.   Ann Int Med 80: 249-259.

INTRAVESICAL CHEMOTHERAPY IN THE TREATMENT AND PROPHYLAXIS OF
BLADDER TUMORS, WITH SPECIAL REFERENCE TO DOXORUBICIN

M. PAVONE-MACALUSO

1. INTRODUCTION

Recurrence rate following complete removal of superficial
(TNM Ta and Tl categories; stages O and A) urotheliomas by
transurethral resection (TUR) is rather high. Patients, whose
tumors are recurrent or multiple are particularly at risk.
Various treatments have been employed to reduce recurrence rate
and to prolong disease-free interval. Such treatments include
hyperthermia, mucosal stripping, bladder distension, immunotherapy, local or distant irradiation, and systemic and intravesical chemotherapy. The latter method has been employed
most extensively.

2. INTRAVESICAL CHEMOTHERAPY

Diverse drugs have been employed for topical chemotherapy.
Among them, thiotepa, ethoglucide, doxorubicin, mitomycin C,
and bleomycin have enjoyed some popularity. Furthermore,
teniposide (VM-26) and cisplatin have also been employed in
recent clinical trials.

The various drugs may differ with regard to their efficacy
and their local and systemic toxicity as well as their cost.
Systemic absorption from the bladder leading to severe myelotoxi-
city has been observed only with thiotepa. Not only the choice
of the drug but also the modalities of treatment--such as the
optimal dose, concentration, contact time, intervals between
instillation, and total duration of the treatment--are still
controversial and deserve more detailed investigation. A
review of the literature and a discussion of the various
problems involved were given in a recent publication from

our Institute (1).

The data reported in the literature about the value of topical adjuvant ("prophylactic") chemotherapy are often contra-dictory. Extensive studies have been performed by two coopera-tive groups in Europe. A series of randomized trials has been implemented and led by the European Organization for Research on the Treatment of Cancer (EORTC), comparing different drugs and no adjuvant treatment following TUR of superficial urotheliomas, whereas an open study of doxorubicin, known as Blinst 1, has been carried out in several European centers. The first study of the EORTC urological group (protocol 30751), compared 30 mg thiotepa, 50 mg teniposide, and no treatment. This study has now been completed. Preliminary results have already been published (2). Data from a more recent analysis (December 1980 are shown in Tables 1 and 2.

The recent results can be summarized as follows: neither thiotepa nor teniposide, as employed according to the EORTC protocol, was successful in prolonging a recurrence-free in-terval or in reducing the number of patients affected by recur-rent tumors. However, both treatments showed some efficacy in

TABLE 1: EORTC trial 30751--Recurrence rate by treatment group (primary patients only)

Item	Thiotepa	VM-26	Control	Total
No. of patients randomized	77	76	78	231
No. of patients with follow-up	67	62	61	190
No. of patients with recurrences	35	38	36	109
Percentage with recurrences	52.2	61.3	59.0	57.4
Total no. of recurrences	51	62	66	179
Total months of follow-up	1295	1131	997	3423
Recurrence rate/100 patient months	3.94	5.48	6.61	5.22

Note: Comparisons--thiotepa versus VM-26, P = .136; thiotepa versus control, P = .004; VM-26 versus control, P = .40

TABLE 2:   EROTC trial 30751--Recurrence rate by treatment group
           (recurrent patients only)

Item	Thiotepa	VM-26	Control	Total
No. of patients randomized	45	48	46	139
No. of patients with follow-up	38	37	43	118
No. of patients with recurrences	27	30	36	93
Percentage with recurrences	71.1	81.1	83.7	78.8
Total no. of recurrences	54	49	76	179
Total months of follow-up	646	534	593	1773
Recurrence rate/100 patient months	8.36	9.18	12.82	10.10

Note: Comparisons thiotepa versus VM-26, P = .696; thiotepa versus control,, P = .048; VM-26 versus control, P = .124.

TABLE 3:   EROTC trial 30751--Recurrence rate by treatment
           (patients with more than one recurrence per year before
           entry into study)

Item	Thiotepa	VM-26	Control	Total
No. of patients randomized	27	23	26	76
No. of patients with follow-up	25	20	25	70
No. of patients with recurrences	18	17	24	59
Percentage with recurrences	72.0	85.0	96.0	84.3
Total no. of recurrences	37	29	57	123
Total months of follow-up	377	264	321	962
Recurrence rate/100 patient months	9.81	10.98	17.76	12.79

Note: Comparisons--thiotepa versus VM-26, P = .648; thiotepa versus control, P = .001; VM-26 versus control, P = .072.

decreasing the number of recurrences (or new occurrences) as expressed by the number of tumors per patients per time unit (100 patient months). This difference was significant only when thiotepa was compared over the other two arms, and it appeared particularly meaningful in patients who had recurrent tumors with multiple lesions in the year preceding the start of the treatment (Table 3).

The EORTC urological group is currently leading two further trials of intravesical adjuvant chemotherapy, as shown in Tables 4 and 5. Other trials in which thiotepa, doxorubicin, VM-26, and mitomycin C were compared are presently being conducted in Europe. In Germany, Engelman et al. (3) were unable to detect any significant difference in the percentage of recurrent tumors in patients treated postoperatively with 10 mg mitomycin C (28%), 50 mg Adriamycin (31%), or 50 mg VM-26 (33%).

3. INTRAVESICAL TREATMENT WITH DOXORUBICIN

The intravesical use of doxorubicin has continued to increase, following our preliminary report (4) and the subsequent work of Japanese workers (5, 6).

Doxorubicin (Adriamycin, Adriblastina, ADM) was reported to be active not only for prophylaxis of recurrent tumors (7) but also as a treatment for carcinoma in situ (Tis) and for multiple or diffuse urothelioma not amenable to TUR or other forms of conservative treatment (8). The efficacy of ADM against Tis is of particular interest, as a serious and mutilating procedure such as a total cyctectomy with urinary diversion can often be avoided under certain curcumstances, provided the patient can be kept under close supervision. This possibility emerges from the work of Edsmyr et al. (9) who obtained disappearance of atypical cells on cytology in 9 of 11 cases (91%) of primary Tis and 11 of 19 cases (74%) of secondary Tis. The cystoscopic findings were only slightly inferior to the cystoscopic results. Thses results have been confirmed by other investigators (10, 11). The Swedish workers (8, 9) have employed 80 mg per instillation, to be repeated at monthly intervals for 1 year and for every 3 months thereafter. The duration of the treatment should not be less than 3 years, since reappearance of atypical cells may occur after a premature interruption.

As neither radiation nor other drugs (thiotepa, ethoglucid) appear to be very efficacious for this indication, doxorubicin instillations can nowadays be considered the treatment of choic for carcinoma in situ of the bladder.

TABLE 4:   EROTC trial 30782--Study coordinators C. Schulman
           (Brussels) and M. Pavone-Macaluso (Palermo)

Recurrent papillary bladder tumors. Categories Ta and Tl

		thiotepa 50 mg
transurethral resection	randomization	Adriamycin 50 mg
		cisplatin 50 mg.

TABLE 5:   EROTC trial 30790--Study coordinator K. H. Kurth
           (Rotterdam)

Primary and recurrent papillary bladder tumors. Categories
Ta and Tl

		epodyl 1.13 g
transurethral resection	randomization	Adriamycin 50 mg
		no treatment

TABLE 6:   Cumulation results with topical doxorubicin

Dose (mg)	No. of patients	Results			
		Complete or partial regression >90%	Partial regression >50%	Partial regression <50%	No regression
10- 40	76	10 (14%)	12 (16%)	30 (77%)	24 (32%)
50-150	98	34 (34.3%)	43 (43.3%)	21 (21.3%)	0 (0%)

The use of ADM for the topical treatment of multiple or
diffuse superficial papillary bladder tumors has also proven
of value in the hands of Edsmyr et al. (9), though less useful
than for Tis. The response rate was 65%. Similar or even better
results were reported by Japanese workers (12).

It seems that the therapeutic efficacy of topical ADM is
dose-related, as shown in table 6, in which results from
several institutions were pooled together.

Other interesting features for the intravesical installa-
tions of ADM can be summarized as follows:

a. No systemic absorption and no meaningful systemic toxicity
    have been observed by various workers, who have employed
    different experimental techniques. Absorption is increased
    to some degree if instillations are given shortly after TUR
    or in the presence of cystitis or of infiltrating anaplastic
    cancer (13). No systemic side effects, however, have been
    reported, even under these circumstances.

b. Rapid fixation to the nuclei of neoplastic cells can be
    demonstrated under fluorescence microscopy after intravesi-
    cal ADM instillations (14). The penetration of ADM extends to
    a few cell layers but it does not reach therapeutic concen-
    trations in the muscular layer of the bladder wall (15).
    Only minimal traces, presumably devoid of any therapeutic
    action, can be found in the regional lymph nodes.

c. Lack of systemic absorption and toxicity of intravesical
    ADM may depend not only on rapid fixation to the cells but
    also and mainly on its high molecular weight.

d.   The efficacy of topical ADM can be increased by the ad-
    dition of Tween 80 to the diluting solution (16).

e. Topical side effects, under the form of chemical cystitis
    and/or hematuria, can occasionally occur. They can be
    very severe in previously irradiated bladders and in con-
    junction with bacterial cyctitis or other conditions respon-
    sible for local inflammation.

f.   In the few instances in which ADM instillations were per-
    formed in the presence of established **vesicoureteral reflux**,
    no side effects were found. Experimentally, vesicoureteral
    reflux is not associated with renal parenchymal damage in
    rabbits (17). This deserves further confirmation, in view
    of the fact that systemic toxicity was reported after
    instillations of thiotepa in patients with reflux.

g. The optimal dose and modalities of local administration of
    ADM will have to be found after more extensive investigation
    (1). The formula devised by Eksborg, who advises that the
    single doses should be selected for every individual patient
    according to the time-concentration area (16), must prove
    its superiority over the conventional schedule, since it

involves greater cost and complexity.

h.   Normal ABH antigens will reappear in the urothelium if the
     atypical ABH-negative cells of Tis respond to the treatment
     (18).

i.   Moderate morphological changes can be observed in the ex-
     foliated cells from the urothelium in ADM-treated patients,
     but such changes can be easily differentiated from neoplastic
     atypia if the smears are observed by an experienced
     cytologist (19).

4.   PROPHYLACTIC USE OF INTRAVESICAL DOXORUBICIN: THE BLINST
     STUDY

     The prophylactic value of intravesical ADM has been suggested
by various workers (7, 20, 21) but it was clearly demonstrated
by Jacobi and Thüroft (22), whose report is, to my knowledge,
the only controlled prospective trial that has been published
so far.   Jacobi's work compared ADM to no treatment.   The
present EORTC studies will also compare ADM with other established forms of local adjuvant treatment.

     The Blinst study, coordinated by Farmitalia Carlo Erba in
Milan, though suffering from the limitations inherent in an
open study without controls, has led to interesting preliminary
results (Table 7).   The standard treatment was 50 mg ADM dissolved in 50 ml sterile water or normal saline and retained
in the bladder for 1 hour.   The instillations were started at
variable intervals after TUR, from a few days to a month.   They
were performed at weekly intervals for a month, then at monthly
intervals.   Control cystoscopies were performed every 3 months.
Of 312 treated patients, chemical cystitis occurred in 16.6%,
and only 5% were obliged to stop the treatment as a consequence
of local toxicity.   The median follow-up was 7 months and the
total number of recurrences was 25%.   Recurrence rate was 35%
for those patients who were followed for 1 year.   Since the
general outline of the Blinst study was similar to the EORTC
protocols, it is tempting to compare results of this study
with those reported in the last analysis of the 30751 EORTC
trial.   In the latter trial, 60% of the patients had recur-

TABLE 7:   International Blinst study; local prophylactic
           treatment with doxorubicin after transurethral
           resection

Treated patients (Tl and Ta)	312
Lost to follow-up	5
Deaths during treatment	2
Cerebral vascular insufficiency	1
Acute renal failure	1
Local adverse reactions	52 (16.6%)
Dropouts for toxicity	16 (5.1%)
Local	15
Systemic (urea and creatinine increase)	1
Median follow-up	7 months
Total number of recurrences	85 (29%)

rences at 1 year from TUR, and no significant difference was
observed in the two treatment arms or in the control group.
However, we believe that conclusions based on historical
controls are arbitrary and must be confirmed by prospective
randomized trials.   Therefore, the real value of the prophylactic instillations of doxorubicin in comparison with other
treatment modalities will probably emerge from the current
EORTC intravesical studies.

5.   CONCLUSIONS

      Intravesical chemotherapy has been employed chiefly with
the aim of reducing recurrence rates of superficial urothelioma
after complete removal by conservative (usually transurethral)
treatment.   Doxorubicin appears to be effective in these cases
and is also capable of inducing the disappearance of atypical
cells in carcinoma in situ and of causing complete or partial
regression of multiple urotheliomas.   Doxorubicin presents
some interesting features which might be advantageous over othe
drugs that have been used for intravesical instillations.   In
particular, its high molecular weight appears to prevent
reabsorption and systemic toxicity, which is frequently

observed when agents with low molecular weight, such as thiotepa, are used (23).

Some studies are in progress and further research will be needed for a better evaluation of this promising therapeutic approach.

6. SUMMARY

After a brief discussion on the problem of recurrences of superficial urotheliomas, even when they are properly treated according to standard transurethral techniques, the use of intravesical chemotherapy is reviewed, with special reference to the trial performed in Europe by the EORTC urological group.

Intravesical instillation of doxorubicin appears to be a very promising form of treatment, not only in prophylaxis of recurrent papillary tumors, but also in the treatment of diffuse superficial papillary tumors and of carcinoma in situ. In the latter indication, it represents the treatment of choice if immediate cystectomy is not indicated.

The preliminary results of a large open study (Blinst 1) point to the prophylactic efficacy of doxorubicin, with an acceptable rate of local toxicity and without any systemic side effect attributable to the treatment.

REFERENCES

1. Pavone-Macaluso M, Ingargiola GB. 1980. Local chemotherapy in bladder cancer treatment. Oncology 37:71-76·
2. Schulman CC, Sylvester R, Robinson M, Smith P, Lachand A, Denis L, Pavone-Macaluso M, de Pauw M, Staquet M. 1981. Preliminary results from EORTC (European Organization for Research and Treatment of Cancer) studies for superficial bladder tumours. In: R.T.D. Oliver, W.F. Hendry and H.J.G. Bloom: Bladder cancer. Principles of combination therapy. Butterworth, London, pp. 75-84.
3. Engelman U, Thüroff J, Frohneberg D, Bauer HW, Jakse G, Jacobi GH. 1981. Wirkung von Adriamycin, Mitomycin C und VM 26 bei der intravesikalen instillations. Rezidivprophylaxe des oberflächlichen Harnblasenkarzinoms. Randomisierte Studie. In:D. Füllenbach, G.A. Nagel and S. Seeber: Adriamycin-Symposium. Ergebnisse und Aspekte. Beitr. Onkol. vol. 9, Karger, Basel p. 312-313.

4. Pavone-Macaluso M, Caramia G. 1972. Adriamycin and daunomycin in the treatment of vesical and prostatic neoplasias. Preliminary results. In: S. K. Carter, A. Di Marco, M. Ghione, I. H. Krakoff, and G. Mathé: International Symposium on Adriamycin. Springer Verlag, Berlin, pp. 180-187.
5. Matsumura Y. 1976. Intravesical infusion therapy with adriamycin. Nishi Nihon J. 38: 236-237.
6. Niijima T. 1978. Intravesical therapy with adriamycin and new trends in the diagnostics and therapy of superficial urinary bladder tumors. In: Diagnostics and treatment of superficial urinary bladder tumors. WHO collaborating centre for research and treatment of urinary bladder cancer. Montedison Läkemedel, Stockholm, pp. 37-44.
7. Banks MD, Pontes JE, Izbicki RM, Pierce JM. 1977. Topical instillation of doxorubicin hydrochloride in the treatment of recurring superficial transitional cell carcinoma of the bladder. J. Urol. 118: 757-760.
8. Edsmyr F. 1980. Intravesical therapy with adriamycin in patients with superficial bladder tumors. Eur. Urol. 6: 132-136.
9. Edsmyr F, Berlin T, Boman J, Duchek M, Esposti PL, Gustafson H, Wikstrom H. 1980. Intravesical therapy with adriamycin in patients with superficial bladder tumours. In: M. Pavone-Macaluso, P. H. Smith, and F. Edsmyr: Bladder tumors and other topics in urological oncology. Plenum Press, New York, pp. 321-322.
10. Glashan R. 1981. Personal communication.
11. Jakse G, Höfstadter F. 1980. Adriamycin therapy in carcinoma in situ: a preliminary report. In: M. Pavone-Macaluso, P. H. Smith, and F. Edsmyr: Bladder tumors and other topics in urological oncology. Plenum Press, New York, pp. 327-331.
12. The first conference on treatment of urinary tract tumors with adriamycin. Proceedings. 1979. Kyowa Hakko Kogyo and montedison Pharm., Tokyo.
13. Pavone-Macaluso M, Gebbia N, Biondo F, Bertolini S, Caramia G, Rizzo FP. 1976. Permeability of the bladder mucosa to thiotepa, adriamycin and daunorubicin in men and rabbits. Urol. Res. 4: 9-13.
14. Pavone-Macaluso M, Gebbia N, Biondo F, Rizzo FP, Caramia G, Rausa L. 1973. Experimental techniques of testing the sensitivity of bladder tumours to anti-neoplastic drugs. Urol. Res. 1: 60-66.
15. Jacobi GH, Kurth KH. 1980. Studies on the intravesical action of topically administered G 3H-doxorubicin hydrochloride in men. Plasma uptake and tumor penetration J. Urol. 124: 34-37.
16. Eksborg S. 1980. Intravesical instillation of adriamycin. Eur. Urol. 6: 132-136.

17. Rübben H. 1981. Topische Therapie beim Blasenkarzinom.1981
    In: D. Füllenbach, G.A. Nagel and S. Seeber: Adriamycin-
    Symposium. Ergebnisse und Aspekte. Beitr. Onkol. vol. 9,
    Karger, Basel pp.296-304.
18. Jakse G, Hofstädter F. 1981. ABH antigenicity of the in
    situ carcinoma of the urinary bladder during intracavity
    treatment with doxorubicin hydrochloride. Urol. Res. 9:
    153-156.
19. Esposti PL, Tribukait B and Gustafson H. 1978. Effect of
    local treatment with adriamycin in carcinoma in situ of
    the urinary bladder: cell morphology and DNA analysis for
    quantification of malignant cells. In: Diagnostics and
    treatment of superficial bladder tumors. WHO collaborating
    centre for research and treatment of urinary bladder cancer.
    Montedison Läkemedel, Stockholm pp. 71-77.
20. Pavone-Macaluso M. 1978. Intravesical treatment of superficial
    (T1) urinary bladder tumours. A review of a 15 year
    experience. In: Diagnostics and treatment of superficial
    urinary bladder tumors. WHO collaborating centre for
    research and treatment of urinary bladder cancer. Montedison
    Läkemedel, Stockholm pp. 21-36.
21. Burk K, Ulshröfer B, Hautum J, Herold W, Lymberopoulos E.
    1981. Intravesikale Adriamycininstillationen zur Rezidiv-
    prophylaxe bei nichtinvasiven Harnblasenkarzinomen. In:
    D. Fullenbach, G.A. Nagel and S. Seeber: Adriamycin-
    Symposium. Ergebnisse und Aspekte. Beitr. Onkol.vol.9,
    Karger, Basel pp.305-311.
22. Jacobi GH Thüroft JW, 1981. Prophylactic intravesical
    doxorubicin instillation after TUR of superficial transitional
    cell tumours: 3 years experience. In: R.T.D. Oliver,
    W.F. Hendry and H.J.G. Bloom: Bladder cancer. Principles
    of combination therapy. Butterworth, London, pp. 85-87
23. Hollister D, Coleman M. 1980. Hematologic effects of
    intravesicular thiotepa therapy for bladder carcinoma.
    J. Amer. Med. Assoc. 244: 2065-2067.

INTRAPERITONEAL ADRIAMYCIN IN OVARIAN CANCER

R. F. OZOLS, R. C. YOUNG, AND C. E. MYERS

INTRODUCTION

Ovarian cancer is the leading cause of death from a gynecologic malignancy in the United States, accounting for an estimated 11,000 deaths in 1980. Its natural history is characterized by a propensity to remain confined to the abdomen virtually throughout its entire clinical course. Malignant cells spread from their origin in an involved ovary via lymphatic drainage, contiguous spread,and by peritoneal seeding to serosal surfaces throughout the peritoneum. As a consequence of this pattern of metastases, therapeutic approaches have focused on the eradication of intraabdominal disease. Patients with advanced stage ovarian cancer (FIGO stage III-IV with disease outside the pelvis) have been treated with surgery to remove as much of the disease as technically feasible followed by postoperative chemotherapy or radiotherapy. Both of these modalities of treatment have been effective in controlling intraabdominal disease in patients with minimal residual disease (tumor masses less than 2.0 cm in diameter), i.e., a 100% complete response rate to HexaCAF combination chemotherapy (1) and a 65% 5-year survival with whole abdominal radiotherapy (2). However, patients with bulky residual disease have a markedly worse prognosis. Although the overall response rate to a variety of combination chemotherapy regimens is 60%-80% (3), the majority of these patients will not achieve a pathologically determined complete response to therapy and will eventually succumb to the regrowth of their intraabdominal disease. The Medicine and Pharmacology Branches at the National Cancer Institute have been examining the role of intraperitoneal chemotherapy in this group of patients with refractory intraabdominal disease. The intraperitoneal administration of adriamycin to patients with ovarian cancer has been based upon a pharmacokinetic rationale as well as upon experimental observations in both murine ovarian cancer and in human ovarian cancer cells.

PHARMACOKINETIC RATIONALE FOR INTRAPERITONEAL CHEMOTHERAPY

A pharmacokinetic model for the intraperitoneal administration of
antineoplastic agents in patients with ovarian cancer has been presented
by Dedrick et al.(4). The general features of their kinetic analysis can
be summarized by a two-compartment model of drug distribution between the
peritoneal cavity and the rest of the body. Drugs administered intraperitoneally will cross the peritoneal membrane and the product of the
permeability and the area of the membrane has the form of a clearance
expressed as ml/min. The peritoneal permeability of antineoplastic agents
decreases with increasing molecular weight. The pharmacologic advantage
of an antineoplastic drug i.e., the ratio of intraperitoneal levels to
corresponding peripheral drug levels, is based upon the slower clearance
of drug from the peritoneal cavity compared to clearance of the drug from
the systemic circulation.

Table 1. Intraperitoneal Administration of Antineoplastic Agents in
Ovarian Cancer

I. Theoretical Considerations for I.P. Therapy
  A. Pharmacologic advantage based on slower peritoneal clearance than
     systemic clearance.
  B. Drug should be administered in a large volume for uniform
     distribution.
II. Practical Considerations
  A. The antineoplastic agent should be cytotoxic to ovarian cancer
     cells.
  B. The drug does not cause excessive peritoneal irritation.

In addition, for an antineoplastic agent to be effective by intraperitoneal administration (Table 1), it should be:(1) administered in a
large volume to allow for uniform distribution throughout the abdomen and
(2) it should be cytotoxic to the tumor cells in the abdomen. The development of the human tumor stem cell assay (5,6) has allowed us to investigate
dose response relationships of antineoplastic agents in human tumor cells
(7,8). If intraperitoneal therapy is to be effective in ovarian cancer,
the levels of antineoplastic agents produced in the peritoneal cavity must
be cytotoxic to ovarian cancer cells and this can be directly assessed in
the stem cell assay.

ADMINISTRATION OF INTRAPERITONEAL CHEMOTHERAPY

We have utilized a Tenckhoff catheter to administer intraperitoneal chemotherapy. This catheter was initially developed for use in ambulatory peritoneal dialysis in patients with renal failure. It consists of a silastic rubber catheter with a Dacron cuff which can be implanted through a subcutaneous skin tunnel under local anesthesia. Patients are taught to change the catheter dressing on a daily basis and most patients are able to tolerate the catheter with minimal discomfort. The Tenckhoff catheter allows repeated administration of dialysate as well as a route to collect malignant tumor cells for in vitro chemotherapy sensitivity studies (7).

Three antineoplastic agents (methotrexate, 5-fluorouracil, adriamycin) have been evaluated in feasibility and toxicity studies of intraperitoneal chemotherapy at the NCI in refractory ovarian cancer patients. The initial 5 patients were treated with intraperitoneal methotrexate at a dose range of 7.5-50 μM (9). Local peritoneal irritation was dose limiting. In the phase I trial of intraperitoneal 5-fluorouracil hematologic suppression was dose limiting although peritoneal irritation was also observed (10). A phase II trial of 5-fluorouracil (4 mM) administered on a schedule of 8 consecutive 4-hr exchanges every 2 weeks is currently in progress.

RATIONALE FOR THE INTRAPERITONEAL ADMINISTRATION OF ADRIAMYCIN

The experimental rationale for the use of intraperitoneal adriamycin in ovarian cancer patients was provided by results of studies in a murine ovarian carcinoma and in human ovarian cancer cells and are summarized in Table 2.

Murine Ovarian Cancer

We compared the effects of i.p. and i.v. adriamycin in a transplantable murine ovarian cancer model which has a pattern of metastases similar to that observed in humans (11,12). Ascites develops within 6 days of administration of 10^6 tumor cells i.p. in C_3HeB/FeJ mice and this is followed by the appearance of subdiaphragmatic tumor deposits and intra abdominal carcinomatosis leading to death within 25 days of transplantation. The administration of i.p. adriamycin, 5 mg/kg, 2 days after transplantation of 10^6 tumor cells produced long term survival (>60 days) in 70% of the mice whereas an equitoxic i.v. dose, 10 mg/kg, was without therapeutic benefit. The survival advantage of i.p. adriamycin compared to the i.v.

route was due to: (1) increased levels of adriamycin in the peritoneal fluid (2) increased penetration of adriamycin into free-floating tumor cells in the ascites and (3) increased suppression of DNA synthesis in the tumor cells. In addition, the peak level of adriamycin in the hearts of tumor bearing mice was ten fold less after i.p. administration compared to i.v. adriamycin.

The pattern of metastases in murine ovarian cancer and the intrinsic fluorescence of adriamycin allowed us to compare the penetration of adriamycin into solid tumor masses after i.p. and i.v. administration(12). After i.p. administration (Figure 1),the outermost 4-8 cell layers of intra abdominal tumor masses had intense fluorescence while the cells in the bulk of the tumor mass did not fluoresce.

FIGURE 1.

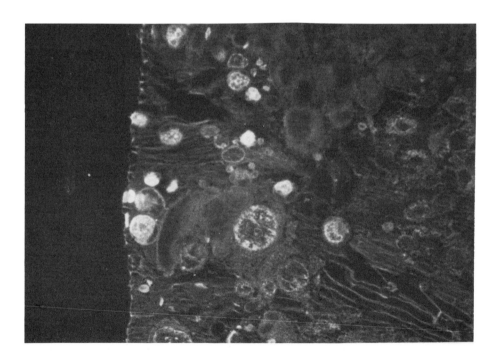

Legend For Figure 1.
    Intra abdominal tumor mass in a murine ovarian cancer demonstrating penetration of adriamycin into 4-8 outermost cell layers following IP therapy.

In contrast, after i.v. administration, the intra abdominal tumor masses had patchy, faint fluorescence through the center of the tumor mass indicating vascular distribution of adriamycin with less penetration into the outer cell layers. These results indicated that i.p. adriamycin does not penetrate deeply into large intra abdominal tumor masses and that therapeutic benefit from i.p. therapy would most likely result only in patients who had small serosal implants of tumor cells.

Dose Response Relationships in Human Ovarian Cancer

We examined the in vitro dose response relationships of adriamycin in human ovarian cancer cells which were obtained from three groups of patients: (1) untreated patients, (2) patients who had progressive disease on a non-adriamycin-containing regimen, and (3) patients who had progressive disease after primary treatment with an adriamycin-containing regimen (8). The ovarian cancer cells were obtained either from malignant effusion or peritoneal washings (7) and exposed to various concentrations of adriamycin for one hour after which they were washed and plated in soft agar as described by Hamburger and Salmon (5,6). The colony formation in the drug exposed cells was then compared to untreated controls. Three distinct patterns of in vitro sensitivity were observed (Figure 2).

The cells obtained from previously untreated patients demonstrated the greatest overall degree of in vitro sensitivity with cells from 40% of the patients having less than 30% colony survival after exposure for one hour to adriamycin at a concentration corresponding to 10% of the peak plasma level observed after i.v. administration of 60 mg/m^2. A 30% or less survival of colony-forming units after exposure to an antineoplastic agent of a concentration corresponding to 10% of the peak plasma level has been associated with a high likelihood of a clinical response (13). The greatest degree of resistance in vitro was observed in cells obtained from patients who had relapsed after primary induction with an adriamycin-based combination. Even at a concentration of 10 μg/ml, a dose level 10 times greater than achievable by i.v. administration, the mean percentage of survival of tumor colony-forming cells was 65%. In contrast, cells obtained from patients who had failed a non-adriamycin-containing combination demonstrated an intermediate pattern of sensitivity to adriamycin.

FIGURE 2

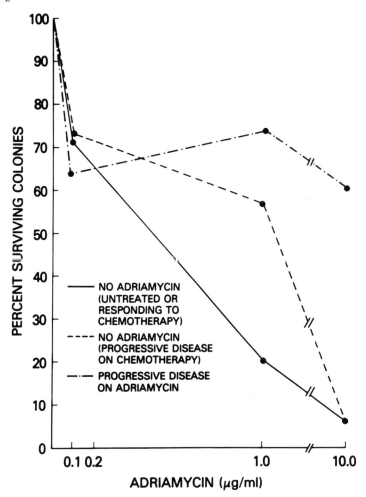

FIGURE 2. In vitro dose response curves to adriamycin in cells obtained from ovarian cancer patients. The cells were exposed to adriamycin and the tumor colony formation compared with untreated controls.

The degree of colony reduction observed with dose levels of 0.1 µg/ml and 1.0 µg/ml indicates that i.v. adriamycin would not likely be of benefit in ovarian cancer patients who had relapsed after treatment with a non-adriamycin-containing combination. These in vitro results demonstrated a cross-resistance between alkylating agents and/or antimetabolites and adriamycin and are in agreement with our clinical observations regarding the lack of benefit of i.v. adriamycin in patients who had relapsed after

therapy with melphalan or HexaCAF (14). However, at 10 µg/ml, a dose potentially achievable by i.p. administration of adriamycin via a Tenckhoff
catheter, the mean percent colony survival in cells from this group of
patients was 10%. These results suggested that patients who had not been
treated with i.v. adriamycin may derive benefit from the intraperitoneal
administration of adriamycin since by this route of therapy cytotoxic
levels could be achieved.

Table 2. Rationale for intraperitoneal adriamycin in ovarian cancer

---

I. Murine ovarian cancer
   A. I.P. adriamycin curative in 70% of mice whereas i.v. adriamycin
      was without benefit.
   B. Compared to equitoxic i.v. adriamycin, i.p. adriamycin
      resulted in:
      1. Increased permeation of adriamycin into ascites tumor cells
      2. Increased levels of adriamycin in ascites
      3. Increased suppression of DNA synthesis in tumor cells
      4. Decreased levels of adriamycin in cardiac tissue
   C. I.P. adriamycin penetrates readily into the outermost 4-6 layers
      of intraabdominal tumor masses.
II. Dose-response relationships in human ovarian cancer cells
   A. Ovarian cancer cells from patients who had been treated with a
      non-adriamycin-containing regimen were resistant in vitro to
      adriamycin doses achievable by i.v. administration but were
      sensitive at doses achievable by i.p. therapy.

Phase I Trial of I.P. Adriamycin

A phase I trial of intraperitoneal adriamycin in nine patients with
refractory ovarian cancer has been completed recently at the NCI (15).
All of the patients had refractory disease to combination chemotherapy
regimens and six of the patients also had received intraperitoneal
5-fluorouracil.

The dialysis procedure with adriamycin was carried out as follows: The
abdomen was washed with 2 liters of Inpersol via the Tenckhoff catheter. This
was followed by a 4-hour dwell of 2 liters of Inperson to which adriamycin had
been added. Samples of blood and dialysate were collected during the dialysis
for determination of adriamycin levels. At the completion of the 4-hour
dwell, the dialysate was drained and the peritoneal cavity washed with another 2 liters of Inpersol. This schedule was repeated every 2 weeks for a
total of six cycles of therapy unless disease progression was observed.

The results of the trial are summarized in Table 3.

Table 3. Phase I trial of i.p. adriamycin in ovarian cancer

Toxicity
 \Peritonitis dose limiting
 Nausea, vomiting, leukopenia, thrombocytopenia
Acceptable schedule
 40 mg adriamycin per 2 liters Inpersol for a 4-hour dwell every 2 weeks
Pharmacology (40 mg/2 liters Inpersol)

Peak intraperitoneal level	$1.2-2.7 \times 10^{-5}$ $\underline{M}$
Peak plasma level	$5.1-6.0 \times 10^{-8}$ $\underline{M}$
Pharmacologic advantage	
(peak dialysate level/peak plasma)	343
Mean % recovery following a 4-hour dwell	26%

The initial concentrations of adriamycin in the dialysate were 9 $\mu\underline{M}$ (10 mg adriamycin per 2 liters of dialysate). The doses were escalated until toxicity was observed. The maximum dose administered in this trial was 60 mg adriamycin per 2 liters of dialysate, which resulted in unacceptable toxicity in all three patients. A dose of 40 mg adriamycin per 2 liters of dialysate administered every 2 weeks produced acceptable toxicity.

The dose-limiting toxicity of i.p. adriamycin was a chemical peritonitis. The pain was dose-related and usually occurred 4 to 12 hours after administration of the adriamycin and persisted for 1 to 7 days. In addition to the peritonitis, nausea, vomiting, and myelosuppression were also observed.

The pharmacology of intraperitoneal adriamycin at 40 mg per 2 liters is also presented in Table 3. The pharmacologic advantage, i.e., the ratio of peak dialysate level to the peak plasma level was 343. The peak plasma levels were in the range of $5-6 \times 10^{-8}$ $\underline{M}$ and were approximately 10 times lower than were the peak levels observed after intravenous administration of adriamycin.

In these heavily treated ovarian cancer patients, antitumor activity was also observed. Two patients had a transient marked reduction in their ascites production; one patient had a conversion of positive cytology to negative cytology, which lasted 4 months; one patient had a partial response to therapy noted at a second-look laparotomy; and one patient has had a complete response (clinically but not pathologically documented) lasting 18+ months.

6. DISCUSSION

The results of the phase I trial with intraperitoneal adriamycin in refractory ovarian cancer patients has demonstrated that (1) adriamycin can be administered to patients in a large volume dialysis with acceptable toxicity at 40 mg/2 liters every 2 weeks; (2) cytotoxic levels of adriamycin to human ovarian cancer cells, as determined in the stem cell assay, can be achieved by the intraperitoneal administration of adriamycin; and (3) intraperitoneal adriamycin appears to have clinical activity in refractory ovarian cancer patients who have not been treated with systemic adriamycin. On the basis of these results the NCI has instituted a phase II trial of intraperitoneal i.p. adriamycin to define the response rate in ovarian cancer patients who have small volumes of disease (less than 2.0 cm masses) and who are refractory to therapy with a non-adriamycin-containing combination.

The actual role of intraperitoneal chemotherapy in the management of patients with ovarian cancer remains to be defined. From the results of the phase I-II studies at the NCI and from experimental studies regarding the penetration of adriamycin into tumor masses it appears that intra-peritoneal chemotherapy should be evaluated in the following clinical settings in ovarian cancer: (1) as an adjuvant to surgery in patients with localized disease; (2) in patients who have small volumes of disease follow-ing systemic chemotherapy; and (3) combined together with intravenous chemotherapy in an effort to maximize delivery of the drug to all parts of a tumor mass. In addition, the initial results with intraperitoneal metho-trexate, 5-fluorouracil and adriamycin have demonstrated that local toxicity can be dose limiting. Accordingly, if a drug can be identified which pro-duces less toxicity but which has activity against ovarian cancer, then such a drug could be administered at even higher doses. Aclacinomycin A is an anthracycline analog which is of particular interest since it may be markedly less irritating to tissue than adriamycin (16). Both experimental studies with the stem cell assay and clinical trials are currently in progress at the NCI with aclacinomycin A to determine if it has sufficient activity in ovarian cancer to warrant clinical study with intraperitoneal administration.

REFERENCES

1. Young RC, Chabner BA, Hubbard SP, et al. 1978, N Engl J Med 299: 1261-1266.
2. Dembo AJ, Bush RA, Beale FA, et al. 1979, Am J Obstet Gynecol 134: 793-800.
3. Young RC, Von Hoff DD, Gromley P, et al. 1979, Cancer Treat Rep 63: 1539-1544.
4. Dedrick RL, Myers CE, Bungay PM, et al. 1978, Cancer Treat Rep 62: 1.
5. Hamburger AW and Salmon SE. 1977, Science 197: 461-463.
6. Hamburger AW and Salmon SE. 1977, J Clin Invest 60: 846-854.
7. Ozols RF, Willson JKV, Grotzinger KR, et al. 1980, Cancer Res 40: 2743-2747.
8. Ozols RF, Willson JKV, Weltz MD, et al. 1980, Cancer Res 40: 4109 - 4112.
9. Speyer JL, Collins JM, Dedrick RL, et al. 1980, Cancer Res 40: 567-572.
10. Jones RB, Collins JM, Myers CE, et al. 1981, Cancer Res 41: 55-59.
11. Ozols RF, Grotzinger KR, Fisher RI, et al. 1979, Cancer Res 39: 3202-3208.
12. Ozols RF, Locker GY, Doroshow JH, et al 1979, Cancer Res 39. 3209-3214.
13. Von Hoff DD, Casper J, Bradley E, et al. 1981, Amer J Med 70: 1027-1032.
14. Hubbard SM, Barkes, P and Young RC. 1978, Cancer Treat Rep 62: 1375-1377.
15. Ozols RF, Young RC, Speyer JL, et al. 1980, Proc. Am. Soc. Clinical Oncology 21, Abstr. 423.
16. Young RC, Ozols RF and Myers CE. 1981, N Eng J Med 305: 139-148.

ROLE OF ADRIAMYCIN IN BREAST CANCER AND SARCOMAS

S. S. LEGHA, R. S. BENJAMIN, B. MACKAY, M. EWER, AND G. BLUMENSCHEIN

INTRODUCTION

Adriamycin is the most important component of present-day therapy for
carcinoma of the breast and sarcomas. For the treatment of breast cancer,
adriamycin is the most active single agent and is commonly used in combination
with other chemotherapeutic agents. The development of various combination
chemotherapy regimens incorporating adriamycin has resulted in objective
response in approximately 70% of the patients with advanced disease. For
advanced sarcomas, there was little useful therapy before adriamycin was
discovered. The utilization of adriamycin in combination with chemotherapeutic
agents has provided useful palliation in approximately one-half of the patient
with sarcomas. The major limitation of adriamycin therapy has been a dose-
dependent cardiomyopathy, which frequently precludes its continued use in the
responding patients beyond 6-9 months of treatment. Approximately 50% of the
patients on the standard 3-weekly schedule of adriamycin administration, up
to cumulative doses of 450 to 550 mg/m^2, develop evidence of cardiac toxicity,
either in the form of pathologic changes in the myocardial cells or reduction
in left ventricular function (1,2). Recently, we have explored the administration of adriamycin by continuous infusion and have found that this results
in a significant reduction of nausea-vomiting as well as cardiac toxicity
without compromising the therapeutic effect. This method of administration
also allows continued adriamycin therapy for a longer duration compared to that
of the standard schedule and has the promise of improving the duration of
response and survival of patients with breast cancer and sarcomas. We have
used continuous infusion of adriamycin in patients with breast cancer and
sarcomas, and our preliminary results are presented in this report.

ROLE IN BREAST CANCER

Adriamycin is the most active single agent in the treatment of breast
cancer. When used as a single agent in patients who have not had prior

chemotherapy, response rates have varied between 40% to 50% in different series (3). These response rates are similar to those achieved with many combination chemotherapy regimens. The response rates tend to be lower and have varied between 20% to 30% when the patients have had previous chemotherapy. Response duration in patients receiving adriamycin as a single agent are short, averaging 4 to 5 months. The response figures have been similar over adriamycin dose range of 45 mg/m^2 to 75 mg/m^2.

Based on the single-agent activity of adriamycin, a number of adriamycin-containing combination chemotherapy regimens have been developed over the past several years. One of the familiar regimens is a triple-drug combination of 5-fluorouracil, adriamycin, and cyclophosphamide (CAF), which was developed at the M. D. Anderson Hospital (5). In this regimen, adriamycin is used in a dose of 50 mg/m^2 on day 1, cyclophosphamide in a dose of 500 mg/m^2 on day 1, and 5-FU 500 mg/m^2 on day 1 and 8. The courses of treatment can be repeated at 3-week intervals in the majority of the patients, some requiring 4-week intervals between courses. Adriamycin is continued to a cumulative dose level of 450 mg/m^2, after which methotrexate is substituted in its place. The treatment is continued for a total of 2 years and therapy is then discontinued if the patient is in complete remission. Our experience with this regimen in over 600 patients resulted in objective responses in approximately 70% of the patients, stability of disease in an additional 20% of the patients, and failure to respond in approximately 10% of the patients (6). The median duration of response from the onset of therapy was 15 months and the survival of the total group was 21 months. Complete remission was observed in 20% of the patients and the median duration of response in these patients was 18 months. Although 80% of our patients in complete remission have relapsed over a period of 2 to 5 years, 20% of the patients have been in complete remission without any maintenance therapy over a period of 3 to 5 years (7). We anticipate that some of these patients are potentially cured of their disease.

Other combination chemotherapy regimens containing adriamycin include the cyclophosphamide plus adriamycin (AC) regimen developed by Jones and associates (8); adriamycin plus vincristine reported by Bonadonna and associates (9); and a five-drug regimen containing 5-fluorouracil, adriamycin, cyclophosphamide, vincristine, and prednisone reported by Mattson et al. (10). There is considerable controversy on whether adriamycin should be used in the primary combination regimens or whether patients should be treated initially with combination chemotherapy regimens without adriamycin, such as the triple com-

bination regimen containing cyclophosphamide, methotrexate, and 5-FU (CMF)
(11). A number of investigators have done comparative trials of adriamycin-
containing regimens with CMF or its modifications and have shown superior
results with adriamycin-containing regimens (12-14). For example, Bull and
associates have reported a randomized comparative trial of CAF versus CMF
and reported 20% higher response rate and a significantly longer duration of
remission as well as survival in patients treated with the CAF regimen (12).
A summary of various adriamycin-containing regimens reported to date is shown
in Table 1 and the non-adriamycin-containing regimens are summarized in Table 2.

Table 1. Response rates and survival of advanced breast cancer patients
treated with adriamycin-containing regimens

Source	Regimen	Number of patients	Response (%)	CR (%)	MST (mos)
Arizona	AC	51	80	20	17
Milan	AV	40	48	8	--
Arizona	VAC	32	72	28	24+
NCI	CAF	38	82	18	27
SEG	CAF	59	64	20	--
Yale	CAFM	22	55	32	18
CALGB	CAFVP	100	72	16	20
Bowman Gray	CAFVP	76	58	13	--
TOTAL		418	66	20	21

Table 2. Response rates and survival of advanced breast cancer patients
treated with non-adriamycin combination chemotherapy regimens

Source	Regimen	Number of patients	Response (%)	CR (%)	MST (mos)
NCI	CMF	40	62	8	17
Milan	CMF	53	49	10	18
ECOG	CMF	199	48	15	12
Mayo	CFP	49	59	10	24
ECOG	CMFP	88	59	25	17
NCI	CMFP	40	68	20	18
SWOG	CMFVP	106	59	19	14
CALGB	CMFVP	86	50	11	15
TOTAL		661	56	15	17

Attempts at reduction in adriamycin cardiotoxicity

Adriamycin is the most active drug in the treatment of breast cancer, and
it has been speculated that an extension of adriamycin therapy beyond the conventional cumulative dose level of 450 mg/m^2 might improve the results currently achieved with the CAF-CMF therapy. In this regard, there are a number
of efforts under way to find an antidote against adriamycin cardiac toxicity
or to manipulate adriamycin schedules to reduce the severity of cardiac toxicity. For example, a recent report by Weiss and associates has reported a
substantial reduction in adriamycin cardiac toxicity when the drug is administered in a weekly schedule (17). Following this lead, we have investigated
the efficacy and toxicity of adriamycin when it is delivered by continuous infusion schedule and have shown that adriamycin given as a 96-hour continuous
infusion was carried out in breast cancer patients who had been treated
previously with cytotoxic agents other than adriamycin. The dose of adriamycin
was 60 mg/m^2 and the drug was administered through a central venous catheter
in order to avoid extravasation. Initially, the duration of adriamycin infusion was 24 hours and later this was escalated by 100% increments to 96 hours
by the third course of treatment. The treatment with adriamycin infusion was
then maintained over 96-hour infusions as long as the patient's tumor was under
control. Adriamycin infusions were delivered either by means of a portable
infusion pump on an out-patient basis, or the patient was hospitalized and the
infusion delivered by means of a McGraw pump. Toxicity was monitored with
weekly blood counts and standred criteria were used to measure tumor response.
Cardiac toxicity was monitored by careful clinical examination of the heart
prior to each course of treatment, and this monitoring was supplemented with
serial determinations of the cardiac function by means of gaited cardiac blood
pool scans. To detect subclinical cardiac toxicity, we obtained serial endomyocardial biopsies from the right ventricle, using a percutaneous transjugular
approach. Cardiac biopsy was considered in the responding patients, initially
at a cumulative adriamycin dose of 200 to 250 mg/m^2 and, later, at dose levels
of 420-480 mg/m^2. Adriamycin therapy was continued in the responding patients
unless they developed either significant cardiac toxicity or progression of
their disease. Cardiac biopsy was repeated in responding patients at adriamycin dose increments of 200 to 250 mg/m^2. The pathologic changes in the cardiac biopsy were graded from 0 to 3 on a half-point scale adapted from criteria
developed by Billingham et al. (18). The development of grade 2 changes was
considered an indication that further adriamycin therapy be discontinued.

Results

A total of 27 patients were entered in this trial and 26 patients are evaluable. One patient achieved complete response and 12 patients achieved partial response for an overall objective response rate of 50% (95% confidence limits, 30% to 70%). The median time to progression of disease from initiation of therapy for patients who had an objective response was 7 months.

The acute gastrointestinal effects of adriamycin were markedly reduced. Twelve patients had no nausea or vomiting, 11 patients had mild nausea or occasional emesis and only 4 patients (15%) had significant nausea and vomiting. Four patients had mild degree of stomatitis, which occurred approximately 10 days following treatment. The nausea and vomiting were mostly observed with 24 and 48-hour infusions and were rarely observed during 96-hour infusions. The myelosuppressive toxicity of adriamycin infusion appeared to be similar to that observed with the standard schedule of adriamycin administration. The median lowest WBC count was 2000/µl and the median lowest granulocyte count was 900/µl. The median lowest platelet count was 150,000/µl and none of the patients had platelet counts less than 25,000. Blood counts were completely recovered by days 21 to 24, except in 2 patients who took 28 days. Other side effects associated with adriamycin infusion included total alopecia in all patients.

Evaluation of cardiac toxicity. Among the 19 patients who achieved some degree of therapeutic benefit from adriamycin therapy, cumulative adriamycin dose levels ranged from 180 to 1500 mg/m^2 (median 480 mg/m^2). Seven patients received a cumulative adriamycin dose level of 600 mg/m^2 or higher. Endomyocardial biopsies were performed in 11 patients who received a median cumulative adriamycin dose of 630 mg/m^2 (range 360–1500 mg/m^2). The pathologic changes in the biopsies were less than grade 2 in 9 of 11 patients and these patients could have received additional adriamycin if the tumor had not progressed. Two patients had significant pathologic changes (grade 2 and 3), preventing further adriamycin treatment. Both patients had received precordial irradiation in the past which is a known

risk factor for the development of adriamycin cardiomyopathy.
One patient with a biopsy grade of 1.5 developed mild congestive
heart failure 4 months after receiving her last adriamycin dose.

Retreatment with adriamycin infusions in relapsed patients

Although the long-term consequences of cardiac injury
from adriamycin are unknown, two bits of data indicate that the
damage may not be permanent. Firstly, it is rare to see congestive heart failure occurring beyond 1 year of the last dose of
adriamycin. Secondly, there is a gradual improvement in left
ventricle ejection fraction after termination of adriamycin
therapy. Based on these observations, we felt that it may be
possible to reuse adriamycin for the treatment of tumor recurrences in patients who had previously received what was considered
the maximum safe dose at the time of their first treatment
(450 to 500 mg/m^2). Accordingly, we undertook a prospective
study with the objective of determining the degree of residual
pathologic changes in the myocardium from previous adriamycin
therapy, and to determine the efficacy and cardiac toxicity of
adriamycin treatment in patients with breast carcinoma and
sarcomas. We selected patients who had previously responded
to adriamycin-containing regimens, and the disease was under
control when adriamycin was discontinued because of the stipu-
lated dose limitations. Patients who relapsed while receiving
adriamycin were considered unlikely to respond to treatment
and were not included in this study. Patients who had received
a cumulative adriamycin dose of 450 mg/m^2 or higher underwent
endomyocardial biopsies which were also done at lower dose
levels if the patient was suspected of being a high risk for
cardiac toxicity. Adriamycin was administered as a continuous
infusion over 96 hours and patients also received other cytotoxic agents such as 5-FU and cyclophosphamide for breast
carcinoma and cyclophosphamide and DTIC for patients with
sarcomas. Patients were monitored by means of radionuclide
angiography and cardiac biopsies which were done after every
4 to 5 courses of treatment unless other parameters indicated
possible cardiac toxicity which required confirmation by
cardiac biopsy.

A total of 25 patients with breast cancer underwent
endomyocardial biopsies and 4 patients had grade-2 changes
which precluded retreatment with adriamycin. Two others were
not treated because they opted to receive an alternative treatment
Among the 19 evaluable patients, 8 patients (42%) had objective
response and 3 patients showed minor responses. The median
duration of complete and partial responses was 11 months which
is significantly longer than the duration of 5 months for patients
with minor responses. The median retreatment dose of adriamycin
was 450 mg/m^2 (range 120+ - 850 mg/m^2). No patient developed
clinical evidence of congestive heart failure although 1 patient
developed grade-2 changes after receiving 600 mg/m^2 of additional
adriamycin. The probability of response to retreatment was
directly related to the interval between the previous adriamycin
treatment and retreatment. The response rate was lowest (8%)
for the group of patients retreated in less than 1-year interval.

ROLE OF ADRIAMYCIN IN SARCOMAS

Among the therapeutic agents with significant activity
against sarcomas, adriamycin has been studied most extensively.
In the treatment of bone sarcomas adriamycin has a response rate
of 20 to 30%. Other agents with response rates in excess of 20%
include high-dose methotrexate and cis-platin. Similarly in the
treatment of soft tissue sarcomas, adriamycin is the most active
single agent in addition to DTIC and methotrexate. Among the
bone sarcomas, chondrosarcoma is the least responsive and
Ewing's sarcoma, the most responsive to chemotherapy. For
osteosarcoma there is insufficient data to claim superiority
of results with any combination of drugs compared to single
agents. However, the availability of cis-platin in the recent
past might lead to improved results with combinations of adriamycin and cis-platin (19). Among the soft tissue sarcomas of
the adults, a cumulative response rate of 27% was reported
among a total of 357 patients treated with adriamycin (20).
The overall response rate with DTIC was 16% from a total of
61 patients (20). The combination of adriamycin and DTIC
proved to be synergistic and resulted in an overall response
rate of 47% out of 192 patients (21). The addition of

cyclophosphamide and vincristine to this combination (CYVADIC) further improved these results to a total of 59% out of 118 patients (21). Although there is some controversy about the role of cyclophosphamide and vincristine in this drug combination, other investigators have also reported a similar response rate with the triple-drug combination of cyclophosphamide, adriamycin and DTIC (22). With the combination chemotherapy regimens in soft tissue sarcomas, approximately 15 to 17% patients have achieved complete remissions and some of these patients have stayed in unmaintained complete remission for extended periods of time (23).

Over the past several years adjuvant chemotherapy studies have been carried out in patients with osteosarcoma. Most investigators compared the results of these trials to the previously untreated historical controls, where 20% of the patients had not relapsed over 2 years following resection of the tumor. Adjuvant chemotherapy regimens, both with the single-agent adriamycin chemotherapy and single-agent therapy with high-dose methotrexate had initially claimed substantial improvements in the disease-free survival of such patients. The 5-year follow-up of these studies, however, revealed that the proportion of disease-free survival had lowered to 30 to 40% of the patients, which has raised some doubt about the long-term benefit of adjuvant chemotherapy against osteosarcoma (24,25). Similarly, in soft tissue sarcomas, although there has been some improvement in the results with adjuvant cyclophosphamide, adriamycin and high-dose methotrexate (26), the ultimate role of an adjuvant therapy in these tumor types is not yet established.

Experience with continuous-infusion adriamycin against advanced sarcomas

Based on our findings of reduction in cardiac toxicity when adriamycin was used as continuous infusion in patients with breast cancer, we decided to conduct a prospective study using cyclophosphamide, adriamycin and DTIC in patients with advanced sarcomas. The dose schedule of drugs used is shown in table 3.

Table 3. Dose schedule for continuous infusion CYADIC

Drug	Schedule	Total Dose/Course in mg/m^2 Dose Levels		
		1	2	3
Cyclophosphamide	Day 1	600	750	900
Adriamycin	4-day infusion	60	75	90
Dacarbazine (DIC)	4-day infusion	1000	1000	1000

Based on a strong dose response relationship for adriamycin
in sarcomas (4) dose escalation was mandatory, and majority
of the patients received the middle dose level. Both adriamycin
and DTIC were mixed together and infused over a period of 4 days
and the courses of treatment were repeated at 3 to 4-week
intervals depending on the recovery from myelosuppression. In
the responding patients debulking surgery was carried out whenever
feasible after a total of 3 courses of CYADIC chemotherapy.

The preliminary results of this study show that treatment-
related nausea and vomiting were less severe than that observed
with the standard CYVADIC schedule. At the present time, 60
patients are evaluable for response, 51 of them have soft tissue
sarcomas and 9 patients have bone sarcomas. The response to
chemotherapy is summarized in table 4.

Table 4. Chemotherapy response of soft tissue sarcomas treated
with continuous infusion CYADIC

Sarcoma	Number of Patients	Number of Responses				
		Complete	Partial	Minor	Stable	Progression
MFH*	13	1	6	0	1	5
Angio	5	2	1	1	0	1
Leiomyo	5	0	3	0	1	1
Neurogenic	5	1	1	0	1	2
Unclassified	5	0	2	1	2	0
Other	18	3	7	2	4	2
Total	51	7(14%)	20(39%)	4	9	11
			53%			

*malignant fibrohistiocytoma

These response figures were achieved with the first 3 courses
of chemotherapy and may be lower than what would have occurred
if there was no intervening surgery for debulking the tumor.
The complete and partial remission rate (53%) appears to be

slightly higher than our previous experience with standard
schedules of adriamycin administration. Among the 9 patients
with bone sarcomas, 3 achieved complete and 4 achieved partial
remission for an overall response rate of 78%. Twenty-nine
patients underwent debulking surgery which converted a total
of 17 patients into complete remission and 12 patients to
partial remission. Final response figures are 24 CRs (40%)
and 20 PRs (33%), for an overall response rate of 73%. The
median duration of response has not yet been reached, but it
is estimated to be 9+ months. A total of 11 patients received
adriamycin dose levels in excess of 550 mg/m^2 (range 570 to
1365 mg/m^2). No patient experienced clinical evidence of congestive heart failure and all except 1 patient have had cardiac
biopsy changes of less than grade 2. The patient who developed
grade 2 changes in cardiac biopsy had received a total adriamycin
dose of 1305 mg/m^2. At the present time 5 patients have tolerated
adriamycin for a total of 18 months and have had their chemotherapy discontinued after they received total adriamycin dose
in excess of 1 gram/m^2.

Adriamycin retreatment for sarcomas

    A total of 21 patients with recurrent sarcomas were re-
evaluated with endomyocardial biopsies with a view to retreatment with adriamycin-containing chemotherapy. Two patients
showed-grade 2 changes and were accordingly not treated and
another patient was given alternative treatment leaving behind
18 patients who received ADIC or CYVADIC type of therapy. One
patient achieved a complete remission and 3 achieved partial
remissions and 7 patients had minor regressions. The overall
response rate was 28% which is lower than that achieved with
retreatment in patients with breast cancer. The median retreatment
adriamycin dose was 300 mg/m^2 (range 230 to 560 mg/m^2). Five
patients developed congestive heart failure, 1 of them died
as a result of congestive heart failure. The incidence of heart
failure is significantly higher than that observed in breast
cancer patients. This may be explained by higher adriamycin
dose per course of treatment in sarcoma patients.

Future prospects

Our experience with continuous infusion of adriamycin has shown clear evidence of reduction in cardiac toxicity of adriamycin. By combining the data of continuous-infusion adriamycin from the 2 studies discussed here, a total of 31 patients have been studied with endomyocardial biopsies. Three patients (10%) have shown significant changes in the cardiac biopsies and 1 patient has had mild heart failure. The median cumulative dose of adriamycin in this group is in excess of 675 mg/m^2 which is a 50% higher dose compared to the standard dose limitation of 450 mg/m^2 which has been our practice in the past. Using 450 mg/m^2 as our cutoff for standard schedule of adriamycin we have observed grade 2 biopsy changes in approximately 50% of the patients (1). Reduction in the incidence and severity of cardiac toxicity with 96-hour infusions may have considerable impact in the treatment of patients with breast cancer and sarcomas. In the case of breast cancer, the tumor is generally under control in approximately 2/3 of patients when the dose limit of 450 mg/m^2 is reached. This group of patients is likely to be benefited by continued adriamycin administration for an additional period of 3 to 6 months which could potentially convert a higher proportion of patients into complete remission. This possibility is under evaluation in our current protocol in which we use continuous administration of adriamycin in combination with 5-FU and cyclophosphamide. Furthermore, observations of reduced cardiac toxicity will encourage utilization of adriamycin in adjuvant chemotherapy for the high-risk patients with stage II and stage III breast carcinoma. Since adriamycin-containing regimens (FAC) which we have been using as adjuvant chemotherapy over the past 5 years have shown significant reduction in relapses in premenopausal as well as postmenopausal patients, many investigators are now evaluating the usefulness of adriamycin in the adjuvant therapy of breast cancer.

For patients with sarcomas, the impact of our findings may not be that great because of the lower response rate and generally shorter durations of remission (approximately 8 to 9 months), however, a small proportion of patients (approximately 20% of the patients) will have the opportunity of continued administration of adriamycin as long as their disease is responding for the treatment duration of approximately 18 months. Furthermore, for patients with locally advanced sarcomas delivery of adriamycin by continuous infusion may have considerable impact especially in patients where surgery has effectively removed the gross tumor. Finally, reduction of adriamycin cardiac toxicity has opened up the possibility of retreatment for patients who in the past had received what was considered to be their maximum tolerated dose and later developed recurrence and adriamycin-containing regimen offered the best probability of response.

REFERENCES

1. Legha S, Benjamin R, Mackay B, et al. Reduction of adriamycin cardiac toxicity using a prolonged continuous intravenous infusion. Ann. Intern. Med. In press
2. Gottdiener JF, Mathisen DJ, Borer JS, et al. Doxorubicin cardiotoxicity: Assessment of late left ventricular dysfunction by radionuclide cineangiography. Ann. Intern. Med. 94:430-435, 1981.
3. Tormey DC. Adriamycin in breast cancer: An overview of studies. Cancer Treat. Rep.6(3)319-327, 1975.
4. O'Bryan RM, Baker LH, Gottlieb JE, et al. Dose responsive evaluation of adriamycin in human neoplasia. Cancer 39: 1940-1948, 1977.
5. Blumenschein GR, Cardenas JO, Freireich EJ and Gottlieb JA. FAC chemotherapy for breast cancer. Proc. Am. Assoc. Clin. Oncol. 15:193, 1974.
6. Swenerton KD, Legha S, Smith T, et al. Prognostic factors in metastatic breast cancer treated with combination chemo-therapy. Cancer Res. 39:1552-1562, 1979.
7. Legha S, Buzdar AU, Smith TL, et al. Complete remissions in metastatic breast cancer treated with combination drug therapy. Ann. Intern. Med. 91:847-852, 1979.
8. Jones SE, Durie BG and Salmon SE. Combination chemotherapy with adriamycin and cyclophosphamide for advanced breast cancer. Cancer 36:90-97, 1975.
9. Brambilla C, De Lena M and Bonadonna G. Combination chemotherapy with adriamycin in metastatic mammary carcinoma. Cancer Treat. Rep. 58:251-253, 1974.
10. Mattsson W, Arwidi A, Eyben FV and Lindholm CE. Phase II study of combined vincristine, adriamycin, cyclophosphamide and citrovorum factor rescue in metastatic breast cancer. Cancer Treat. Rep. 61:1527-1531, 1977.
11. Canellos GP, DeVita VT, Gold GL et al. Combination chemo-therapy for advanced breast cancer: Response and effect on survival. Ann. Intern. Med. 84:389-392, 1976.

12. Bull JM, Tormey DC, Li SH,et al. A randomized comparative trial of adriamycin versus methotrexate in combination drug therapy. Cancer 41:1649-1657, 1978.
13. Muss HB, White DR, Richards F, et al. Adriamycin versus methotrexate in five-drug combination chemotherapy for advanced breast cancer, a randomized trial. Cancer 42:2141-2148, 1978.
14. Smalley RV, Carpenter J, Bartolucci A, et al. A comparison of cyclophosphamide, adriamycin, 5-fluorouracil (CAF) and cyclophosphamide, methotrexate, 5-fluorouracil, vincristine, prednisone (CMFVP) in patients with metastatic breast cancer. Cancer 40:625-632, 1977.
15. Legha S, Hortobagyi GN, Buzdar AU and Blumenschein GR. Unmaintained remissions in metastatic breast cancer treated with combination drug therapy. Proc. Am. Assoc. Cancer Res. 21:167, 1980.
16. Decker DA, Ahmann DL, Bisel HF, et al. Complete responders to chemotherapy in metastatic breast cancer, characterization and analysis. JAMA 242:2075-2079, 1979.
17. Weiss AJ, Metter GE, Fletcher WS, et al. Studies on adriamycin using a weekly regimen demonstrating its clinical effectiveness and lack of cardiac toxicity. Cancer Treat. Rep. 60:813-822, 1976.
18. Billingham M, Bristow M, Mason J, and Friedman M. Endomyocardial findings in adriamycin-treated patients. Proc. Am. Soc. Clin. Oncol. 17:281, 1976.
19. Ettinger LJ, Douglass HO, Higby DJ, et al. Adjuvant adriamycin and cis-diamminedichloroplatinum (cis-platinum) in primary osteosarcoma. Cancer 47:248-254, 1981.
20. Pinedo HM and Kenis Y. Chemotherapy of advanced soft tissue sarcomas in adults. Cancer Treat. Rev. 4:67-86, 1977.
21. Gottlieb JA, Baker LH, O'Bryan RM, et al. Adriamycin used alone and in combination for soft tissue and bony sarcomas. Cancer Chemother. Rep. 6(3):271-282, 1975.
22. Blum RJ, Corson JM, Wilson RE, et al. Successful treatment of metastatic sarcomas with cyclophosphamide, adriamycin and DTIC (CAD). Cancer 46:1722-1726, 1980.
23. Yap BS, Sinkovics JG, Benjamin RS, et al. Survival and relapse patterns of complete responders in adults with advanced soft tissue sarcomas. Proc. Am. Assoc. Cancer Res. and ASCO 20:352, 1979.
24. Jaffe N, Frei E, Watts H and Traggis D. High dose methotrexate in osteogenic sarcoma: A five-year experience. Cancer Treat. Rep. 62:259-264, 1978.
25. Cortes EP, Holland JF and Glidewell O. Amputation and adriamycin in primary osteosarcoma: A five-year report. Cancer Treat. Rep. 62:271-277, 1978.
26. Rosenberg SA, Kent H, Costa J, et al. Prospective randomized evaluation of the role limb-sparing surgery, radiation therapy, and adjuvant chemoimmunotherapy in the treatment of adult soft tissue sarcomas. Surgery 84:62-68, 1978.

PROSPECTS FOR DOXORUBICIN IN ADJUVANT BREAST CANCER TRIALS

G. BONADONNA, C. BRAMBILLA, A. ROSSI, R. BUZZONI, A. MOLITERNI, AND
P. VALAGUSSA

HISTORICAL BACKGROUND

More than a decade ago, our medical oncology team initiated the first
clinical studies on doxorubicin (1, 2) and, within the group of solid
tumors, breast cancer appeared to be one of the most responsive neoplasms
(3, 4). During the same years, combination chemotherapy for breast cancer
developed considerably through the administration of CMFVP, CMFP, and CMF
regimens (5, 6). Once the superiority of combination chemotherapy over
single-agent chemotherapy was clearly established also in breast cancer,
the attempt to improve the incidence and the duration of response by the
addition of doxorubicin in several drug combinations became the subsequent logical step. In more recent years, the change in the strategic
approach for primary breast cancer was soon followed by encouraging results
through the use of a combined modality approach. This led some research
institutions to utilize doxorubicin also in an adjuvant situation (7, 8).

Today, the knowledge achieved in about 2 decades with the clinical
study of several important anticancer drugs requires that the role of a
given compound in the treatment of a specific neoplasm must be clearly
defined following established parameters of evaluation. Table 1 lists
the useful parameters to determine the role of doxorubicin in advanced
and early breast cancer, respectively. With the available drugs, cure of
clinically advanced breast cancer appears to be a distant goal. Therefore, the application of systemic therapy early in the course of the disease, i.e., in an adjuvant situation, offers the only real possibility of
improving the survival rate of this important human neoplasm. Thus, it appears useful to review critically the role of doxorubicin in the multimodal therapy of mammary carcinoma.

Supported in part by Contract no. NO1-CM-33714 with DCT, NCI, and NIH.

Table 1.   Useful parameters in the determination of the role of doxorubicin
           in breast cancer

In advanced disease	In an adjuvant situation
Total response rate	Improved relapse-free survival
·Complete response rate	Survival benefit
Duration of response	Morbidity comparison
Survival from initiation of chemotherapy	
Acute and chronic toxicity	

DOXORUBICIN ACTIVITY IN ADVANCED BREAST CANCER

The activity of doxorubicin as single-agent chemotherapy in metastatic
breast cancer was tested through a wide range of treatment regimens by
numerous research groups. Table 2 summarizes some of the most representative results. The response rate ranged from 30% to 37% with a median duration of 4 months in patients refractory to alkylating agents, antimetabolites and Vinca alkaloids, whereas in patients previously untreated
with chemotherapy the response rate was definitely higher, ranging from
38% to 54% with the median duration of 3 to 9 months. As for other
drug treatments, the incidence of objective response and its duration was
also related to the pattern of metastatic disease. The conclusion from
Phase II studies was that doxorubicin represented the single most effective
drug for the treatment of advanced breast cancer and, as in other solid
tumors, the recommended dose schedule was that of 60-75 mg/m^2 i.v. every
3 to 4 weeks without exceeding the cumulative dose of 550 mg/m^2.

As previously mentioned, in the search for the optimal combination
regimen, doxorubicin was included in various multiple drug treatments
(6), and the results of prospective randomized studies versus regimens
not containing this drug, such as CMF and CMFVP, are reported in Table 3.
It appears that only CAF and CAFVP yielded a higher incidence of complete
remission (CR) plus partial (PR) remission; and in the study of NCI, a higher
median duration of survival, than did CMF. A higher CR plus PR rate
was also observed with the regimens designed at the University of Arizona
and utilizing a standard dose of doxorubicin (40 mg/m^2) as well as at the
M. D. Anderson Hospital and Tumor Institute (Table 4). Thus, the available
data suggest, but do not firmly establish, that combinations containing
doxorubicin are superior to those not including this agent.

Table 2. Doxorubicin activity in advanced breast cancer

Research group	Response rate (%)	Median duration (months)
Milan Cancer Institute	37	4
Cancer Therapy Evaluation Program, NCI (CTEP)	35	–
Albany Medical Center Hospital	38*	7.6
Southwest Oncology Group (SWOG)	40*	5
	30	4
Fox Chase Cancer Center		
20 mg/m^2, D 1 and 8, q 4 weeks	37*	6+
60 mg/m^2, D 1, q 3 weeks	42*	9+
Memorial Sloan-Kettering Cancer Center (MSKCC)	43*	7
Mayo Clinic	50*	8
Eastern Cooperative Oncology Group (ECOG)	54*	3+

* In patients previously untreated with chemotherapy.

Table 3. Doxorubicin-containing regimens in advanced breast cancer; randomized studies

Research group	Study design	CR+PR (%)	Median duration (months)	Median survival (months)
Milan Cancer Institute	CMF versus	55	10.5	22
	AV	55	11	20
	CMF-AV alternating combinations	61	12	23
ECOG	CMF versus	49	5.3	14.8
	CMFP versus	59	8.5	18.0
	AV	53	8.0	13.0
Bowman Gray School of Medicine	CMFVP versus	57	13.0	20.2*
	CAFVP	58	15.0	33.2*
Mayo Clinic	CFP versus	54	--	--
	AVM	48	--	--
Cancer and Leukemia Group B (CALGB)	CMFVP (continuous) versus	50	--	--
	CMFVP (intermittent) vs.	53	--	--
	CAFVP	72	--	--
Southeastern Cancer Group (SEG)	CMFVP versus	37	5.5	--
	CAF	64	8.0	--
National Cancer Institute (NCI)	CMF versus	62	9.0	17*
	CAF	82	11	27.2*

* Statistically significant.
Note: C, cyclophosphamide; M, methotrexate; F, fluorouracil; V, vincristine; P, prednisone; A, adriamycin (doxorubicin).

Table 4. Doxorubicin plus cyclophosphamide (AC) and fluorouracil (CAF)
          in advanced breast cancer; nonrandomized studies

Research group	Combination	CR+PR (%)	Median duration (months)	Median survival (months)
University of Arizona				
Standard dose ADM	AC	73	10	70% (1 yr)
Low dose ADM	AC	53	11.5	16.5
Yale University	AC	50	10	15
SWOG	AC	42	9.5	17
M. D. Anderson Hospital	CAF	73	8.5	15

ADJUVANT COMBINATIONS CONTAINING DOXORUBICIN

The same reasons that led to the inclusion of doxorubicin in combination with other drugs for advanced breast cancer formed the rationale for its use in an adjuvant situation in women with positive axillary lymph nodes. The drug regimens being tested in women with resectable disease and having positive axillary lymph nodes are reported in Table 5 and the study designs in Table 6, respectively. Essentially, the CAF and AC regimens are those that the M. D. Anderson Hospital, the University of Arizona, and Indiana University have tested in clinically advanced breast cancer. The Milan Cancer Institute is evaluating in an adjuvant situation the efficacy of sequential non-cross-resistant regimens to circumvent the problem of selective drug resistance. After radical mastectomy, postmenopausal women 65 years old or less were treated with six cycles of CMFP followed by four cycles of AV (9). The mathematical model proposed by Norton and Simon (10) was tested by a random allocation of the patients who were to receive chemotherapy with and without progressive intensification. Thus, in one of the treatment arms, the dose of the initial two cycles for CMFP and AV was lower than was the standard dose utilized for cyclophosphamide, methotrexate, fluorouracil, and adriamycin. To avoid excessive toxicity, prednisor and vincristine were not intensified. Furthermore, in both treatment groups, no drug attenuation schedule was utilized in the presence of transient myelosuppression, and the subsequent dose was delayed until full marrow recovery occurred (9). Sequential combination chemotherapy is also being tested by the research group at Indiana University where CMF is administered following a fixed number of AC given orally.

The essential 5-year results after CAF and AC are reported in Tables

Table 5. Doxorubicin-containing regimens being tested in the adjuvant treatment of breast cancer.

Acronym	Drugs	mg/m^2 and route	Days of administration	Repeat cycle at day
FAC	Fluorouracil	400 iv	1 and 8	29
	Doxorubicin	40 iv	1	
	Cyclophosphamide	400 iv	1	
AC	Doxorubicin	30 iv	1	22
	Cyclophosphamide	150 po	3 to 6	
CMFP**	Cyclophosphamide	100 po	1 ⟶ 14	29
↓	Methotrexate	40 iv	1 and 8	
	Fluorouracil	600 iv	1 and 8	
	Prednisone	40 po	1 ⟶ 14	
AV**	Doxorubicin	60 iv	1	29
	Vincristine	1.4 iv	1 and 8	

* After a total dose of 300 mg/m^2 of ADM change to CMF (CTX 500 mg/m^2 day 2; MTX 30 mg/m^2 days 1 and 8; FU 500 mg/m^2 days 1 and 8; all drugs given orally.
** Standard regimen.

Table 6. Operable breast cancer with positive axillary nodes examples of doxorubicin-containing adjuvant regimens

Research group	Regimen	Treatment duration	Follow up (yrs)
MD Anderson	FAC + BCG ± RT	2 yr	5
Univ. of Arizona	AC ± RT	8 cycles	5
Indiana Univ.	R⟨ A + BCG	2 yr	4
	AC + BCG ⟶ CMF**	2 yr	4
	AC + FU ⟶ CMF**	2 yr	3
Milan Cancer Inst.	CMFP ⟶ AV* with vs without progressive dose escalation	10 cycles	2.6

* In postmenopausal patients ≤ 65 yr.
** All drugs by mouth.

7 and 8. In both studies the relapse-free survival (RFS) was significantly improved over historical controls. Furthermore, in the subgroup with 1 to 3 histologically positive axillary lymph nodes there was no difference in the reported RFS between FAC and AC (77%), whereas the RFS after FAC (68%) appeared superior to that of AC (49%) in women with more than 3 involved nodes (7, 8). In the series being studied in Milan the 3-year actuarial

Table 7. MD Anderson Hospital. Adjuvant program
in breast cancer with N+.Percent 5-yr results with
FAC + BCG $\pm$ RT.

	Stage II	Stage III
RFS, Total series	72	49
Nodes 1-3	77	
4-10	75	
> 10	50	
Survival, Total series	84	60

Table 8. University of Arizona. Adjuvant program in
breast cancer with N+.Percent 5-yr RFS with AC $\pm$ RT

	Nodes 1-3		Nodes > 3	
AC	70	P < 0.05	59	P = 0.95
AC + RT	88		45	
Total series	77		49	

Total series: 1-3 vs > 3 nodes P < 0.001
AC vs AC + RT P = 0.92

results suggested that women with 1 to 3 positive nodes and who started
treatment with a full dose regimen had a higher RFS (95.8%) compared to
patients started on a low-dose chemotherapy (84.6%) as well as to those
given 12 or 6 cycles of CMF (Table 9). At this point in the analysis,
such a difference was not observed within the group with > 3 positive
nodes. The observed findings re-emphasize the importance of initial full-
dose chemotherapy (11).

Since it is well known that doxorubicin can induce myocardial damage,
it is important to know the incidence of cardiac toxicity observed so far
during adjuvant therapy. No episodes of congestive heart failure were reported in 115 patients who have completed CMFP and AV chemotherapy (cumulative dose of doxorubicin: 240-250 mg/m^2) or in 159 patients who received AC chemotherapy (cumulative dose of doxorubicin: 240 mg/m^2). On the
contrary, 3 of 222 women (13%) treated with adjuvant FAC (cumulative dose
of doxorubicin: 300 mg/m^2) developed congestive heart failure which was
fatal in one patient. At the time of present report, it is not known
whether patients who developed symptomatic cardiomyopathy had also received
postoperative irradiation to the left side of the thoracic wall.

Table 9. Milan Cancer Institute. Adjuvant programs in breast cancer with N+.Percent 3-yr results in postmenopausal women $\leq$ 65 years.

Adjuvant therapy	RFS			Survival
	Total	Nodes 1-3	Nodes > 3	
CMFP → AV				
Total series	72.2	90.5	52.9	86.1
Full dose	72.3	95.8	51.4	90.0
Low dose*	72.1	84.6	53.3	81.7
CMF 12 cycles	65.9	72.9	52.5	86.8
CMF 6 cycles	70.2	75.8	61.1	82.9
Control	51.9	55.1	44.9	79.1

* During first two treatment cycles.

FUTURE PROSPECTS

At the present, adjuvant chemotherapy for primary breast cancer with high risk of early relapse is an accepted reality. The 5-year results of the new generation of prospective clinical trials utilizing various drug combinations and regimens have indicated that both RFS and total survival were improved over surgery alone (12, 13). Future trials will have to focus on treatment improvement for various subsets, namely those with extensive nodal involvement, as well as on treatment refinements, namely optimal treatment duration, delivery of full dose regimens, psychological and socio-economic impact after prolonged systemic therapy.

As far as the specific role of doxorubicin is concerned, today there are no prospective randomized studies which have tested or plan to test the relative role of this drug in the adjuvant therapy of breast cancer. From the available results, AC and FAC combinations have apparently not improved the RFS rate over the classical CMF (13) or CMFVP (14) in the subgroup with 1 to 3 positive axillary nodes. However, the early results from the Milan research group would suggest that the RFS could be superior to that obtained with CMF utilizing a sequential non-cross-resistant combination such as CMFP → AV. Present results require confirmation on subsequent analyses and an appropriate comparison among menopausal age groups who received similar dose levels. In patients having more than three involved axillary nodes, the best published results appear to be those reported by the MD Anderson group with FAC (8). Whether the possible superiority of FAC over other tested regimens is entirely attributable to doxorubicin remains to be clearly demonstrated, for there is apparently no difference in the RFS between CMF and another doxorubicin containing combination such as AC. Thus, as previously mentioned, the critical role of doxorubicin within a single polydrug adjuvant therapy remains to be proven through a specifically designed randomized study.

There is probably another way to look at the future use of doxorubicin within a combined modality setting, and this involves the concept(s) of cell heterogeneity. As stressed by the mathematical model of Goldie and Coldman (15) and by numerous studies carried out in experimental animal systems (16), neoplastic cells have a tendency to mutate toward drug(s)-resistant phenotypes and a large fluctuation probably exists in the proportion and absolute number of drug-resistant tumor cells in comparative staged individuals. Considering (a) that at present similar treatment results are being achieved with various types of single polydrug regimens, both in advanced and in early breast cancer, and (b) the recent confirmation that 6 cycles of adjuvant CMF can yield almost identical 4-year RFS and survival rates as 12 cycles (17), the chances for improving current results through the prolonged administration of a single combination are practically nill.   Therefore, future studies should focus more attention on the appropriate use of multiple combination regimens (e.g. sequential vs alternating delivery). Utilizing non-cross-resistant drugs, subsequent treatments on the continually changing burden and mix of neoplastic cells have the potential for effectively increasing the tumor cell kill and thus offer the chance for improving current results. Within this strategy, doxorubicin, the single most effective drug for breast cancer, should find a more appropriate role. Figure 1   schematically represents the new adjuvant studies currently ongoing at the Milan Cancer Institute for resectable breast cancer (T_{2a}-T_{3a}) with histologically positive axillary lymph nodes. Within two to four weeks from modified radical mastectomy pre and postmenopausal women are started on chemotherapy. Patients with 1 to 3 nodes are given intravenous CMF (cyclophosphamide 600 mg/m^2, methotrexate 40 mg/m^2, fluorouracil 600 mg/m^2) every three weeks, one cycle consisting of two intravenous courses. In one arm CMF is followed by four cycles of doxorubicin (75 mg/m^2 every three weeks) to test whether the results will be improved by the sequential addition of this drug. In women having more aggressive disease i.e. with $\geq$ 3 axillary lymph nodes, sequential vs. alternating chemotherapy is randomly administered with the

Figure 1. Milan Cancer Institute. New adjuvant trials for resectable breast cancer with histologically positive axillary lymph nodes.

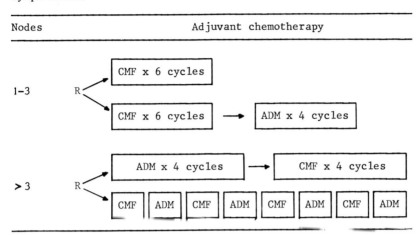

ADM: adriamycin (doxorubicin).

intent to explore the optimal treatment delivery. All patients are always given full dose chemotherapy and treatment is delayed of one to two weeks in the presence of myelosuppression on the planned day of drug administration.

In conclusion, although the present role of doxorubicin in the primary chemotherapy of breast cancer is still not clearly defined, the prospects for its use in an adjuvant situation should take into consideration the heterogeneity of breast cancer cells and selective drug resistance. Within this framework there is ample possibility to further test the role of this effective agent in high risk subgroups and to evaluate its relative therapeutic contribution through prospective randomized trials. For this reason, and considering the potential delayed toxicity, the adjuvant administration of doxorubicin should be confined to research institutions and its cumulative dose should not exceed 300 mg/m^2.

REFERENCES

1. Bonadonna G, Monfardini S, De Lena M, et al. 1969. Clinical evaluation of adriamycin, a new antitumor antibiotic. Br Med J 3:503-506.
2. Bonadonna G, Monfardini S, De Lena M, et al. 1970. Phase I and preliminary phase II evaluation of adriamycin (NSC-123127). Cancer Res 30:2572-2582.
3. Bonadonna G, Beretta G, Tancini G, et al. 1975. Adriamycin (NSC-123127) studies at the Istituto Nazionale Tumori, Milan. Cancer Chemother Rep, Part 3, Vol 6:231-245.
4. Proceedings of the Fifth New Drug Seminar on Adriamycin (Washington,

DC, Dec 16-17, 1974) and the Adriamycin New Drug Seminar (San Francisco, Jan 15-16, 1975). 1975. Cancer Chemother Rep, Part 3, Vol 6:83-397.

5. Canellos G, De Vita VT, Lennard Gold G, et al. 1974. Cyclical combination chemotherapy for advanced breast cancer. Br Med J 1:218-220.

6. Carter SK. 1976. Integration of chemotherapy into combined modality treatment of solid tumors. VII. Adenocarcinoma of the breast. Cancer Treat Rev 3:141-174.

7. Allen H, Brooks R, Jones SE, et al. 1981. Adjuvant treatment for stage II (node positive) breast cancer with adriamycin - cyclophosphamide (AC) ± radiotherapy (XRT). In: Adjuvant Therapy of Cancer III, SE Jones, SE Salmon (eds), Grune & Stratton, New York.

8. Buzdar AJ, et al. 1981. Adjuvant chemotherapy with Fluorouracil, Doxorubicin and Cyclophosphamide (FAC) in Stage II or III breast cancer. 5-year results. In: Adjuvant Therapy of Cancer III, SE Jones, SE Salmon (eds), Grune & Stratton, New York.

9. Bonadonna G, Valagussa P, Rossi A, et al. 1978. Are surgical adjuvant trials altering the course of breast cancer? Seminars Oncol 5:450-464.

10. Norton L, Simon R. 1977. Tumor size, sensitivity to therapy, and design of treatment schedules. Cancer Treat Rep 61:1307-1317.

11. Bonadonna G, Valagussa P. 1981. Dose-response effect of adjuvant chemotherapy in breast cancer. N Engl J Med 304:10-15.

12. Rossi A, Bonadonna G, Valagussa P, et al. 1981. Multimodal treatment in operable breast cancer: five-year results of the CMF programme. Br Med J 282:1427-1431.

13. Jones SE, Salmon SE (eds). 1981. Adjuvant Therapy of Cancer III. Grune & Stratton, New York.

14. Tormey DC, Holland JF, Weinberg V, et al. 1981. 5-drug vs 3-drug ± MER postoperative chemotherapy for mammary carcinoma. In: Adjuvant Therapy of Cancer III, SE Jones, SE Salmon (eds), Grune & Stratton, New York.

15. Goldie JH, Coldman AJ. 1979. A mathematical model for relating the drug sensitivity of tumors to their spontaneous mutation rate. Cancer Treat Rep 63:1727-1733.

16. Skipper HE. 1980. Reexamination of the problem of singly, doubly and multidrug-resistant neoplastic cells in cancer treatment. Birmingham, Ala.: Southern Research Institute (Booklet 15).

17. Bonadonna G, Valagussa P, Rossi A, et al. 1981. Multimodal therapy with CMF in resectable breast cancer with positive axillary nodes. The Milan Institute experience. In: Adjuvant Therapy of Cancer III, SE Jones, SE Salmon (eds), Grune & Stratton, New York.

CLINICAL EVALUATION OF 4'-EPI DOXORUBICIN AND 4-DEMETHOXY DAUNORUBICIN

G. BONADONNA AND V. BONFANTE

INTRODUCTION

The clinical activity of doxorubicin (DX), a daunorubicin (DNR) analog, was first demonstrated by the Medical Oncology Group in Milan at the end of the 1960s (1, 2, 3). Even from Phase I evaluation the main characteristics of this compound, namely broad spectrum of antitumor activity and cardiotoxicity, were clearly evident. In the subsequent decade, innumerable studies carried out all over the world, but particularly in the United States, have further defined the pharmacological properties, the specific antineoplastic activity as well as the risk of cardiomyopathy of DX. Thus, DX became an important, and for given tumors of adults and children an essential, component of many effective drug combinations. In spite of its proven wide spectrum of activity, DX is not active in some neoplasms (large bowel adenocarcinoma, malignant melanoma, renal cancer, malignant gliomas, and chondrosarcoma) where other compounds also have limited efficacy. Because the risk of myocardial toxicity poses known limitations to prolonged drug therapy with DX and since treatment of many solid tumors responsive to DX needs to be improved, the development of anthracycline analogs becomes one of the important directions of cancer chemotherapy. As indicated by Carter (4), there are four possible ways in which a new anthracycline analog could show superiority to its parent compound: a) increased efficacy in tumor responsive to DX; b) efficacy in tumors unresponsive to DX; c) diminished acute toxicity; and d) diminished chronic (cardiac) toxicity.

This paper will summarize the clinical results obtained so far in our Institute with two anthracycline analogs developed and kindly provided by the Farmitalia Carlo Erba Laboratories in Milan.

Table 1. Main preclinical characteristics of some anthracycline derivatives

		DX	4'-epi-DX	4'-deoxy-DX	4-dm-DNR
Acute toxicity LD_{50} in mice (mg/kg i.v.)	at 1 mo	20.3	20.8	6.5	4.8
	at 3 mo	13.8	19.0	6.2	4.9
Chronic toxicity (rabbits treated i.v. 3 times/wk x 6 wks)		+++	++	++++	++++
Cardiac toxicity (mice and rabbits)		+++	++	$\pm$	+++
Potency*		1	1	2	4
Therapeutic index		0,73	0,93	>1,57	3,11
Antitumor effect Leukemia		+++ .	+++	+++	+++
Solid tumors		+++	+++	++++	+

* Ratio between optimal antitumor doses.

MAIN PHARMACOLOGICAL CHARACTERISTICS

The 4'-epi doxorubicin (4'-epi DX) belongs to a group of analogs consisting of new glicosides modified in the position 4' of the amino sugar which were obtained by coupling the anthracyclinone with a modified aminosugar moiety, followed by chemical manipulation to achieve the desired final compound. The 4-demethoxy daunorubicin (4-dm DNR) is one of the derivatives of daunorubicin (DNR) obtained by removal of the methoxyl group at the C-4 position (5, 6).

The pharmacological studies of 4'-epi DX and 4-dm DNR, including their antitumor activity in vitro and in experimental animal systems were detailed in previous publications (6, 7). Table 1 summarizes the most important preclinical characteristics of DX and DNR derivatives which are currently being tested in our Institute in various types of human neoplasms. Suffice i to point out that, compared to DX, 4'-epi DX has a lower acute and chronic toxicity (including cardiac toxicity) and a higher therapeutic index. As far as 4-dm DNR is concerned, the most attractive preclinical characteristics are the higher potency and therapeutic index compared to DX. In mouse experimental systems, this drug was also found to be active when administered orally at doses which are about four times higher than those given intravenously (8). The 4'-deoxy daunorubicin (4'-deoxy DX), whose

Table 2. Summary of most important pharmacokinetic characteristics in mice of intravenous 4'-epi doxorubicin and deoxy-doxorubicin as related to equal doses of doxorubicin

Characteristics	4'-epi-DX	Deoxy-DX
Concentration 1-6 h	Equal in all organs	Equal in heart, liver, kidney, small intestine, and tumor Higher in spleen and lung
48-72 h	Lower in all organs except liver	Equal in spleen, and tumor Lower in other organs
Elimination	Slightly more rapid	More rapid
Plasma levels after 24 h	Slightly lower	Equal

Table 3. Summary of most important pharmacokinetic characteristics in mice of intravenous 4 demethoxy daunorubicin as related to equal doses of daunorubicin

Characteristics	4-dm DNR
Concentration 1-6 h	Higher in lung, spleen, small intestine and tumor Equal in other organs
48-72 h	Higher in all organs
Elimination	Slower
Plasma level 1 h	Lower
24 h	Higher

Phase I study, which will begin very soon in our Institute, has shown minimal cardiac toxicity in mice and rabbits as well as high effectiveness on human colon carcinoma in nude mice (5, 9, 10).

Tables 2 and 3 report the essential pharmacokinetic properties of the above-mentioned analogs as related to equal doses of their parent compounds (7, 11, 12). Compared to DX, the 4'-epi DX showed lesser tissue uptake and more rapid elimination. Recent studies in cancer patients reported in Italy by Natale et al. (12) have confirmed that the elimination of 4'-epi DX (half life 30h) was more rapid than that of DX (half-life 43h), probably due to a higher extrahepatic metabolism and/or renal excretion. The opposite findings were observed after intravenous administration of 4-dm DNR. As shown by Formelli et al. (11) in mice bearing solid tumors and

Table 4. Summary of clinical results obtained with 4'-epi doxorubicin at the Milan Cancer Institute in 116 patients with advanced neoplasms

Acute non hematological toxicity after 60 to 90 mg/m^2	Vomiting: about 50% Mucositis: < 10% Alopecia: about 70%
Hematological toxicity	Leukopenia*: about 50-60% Thrombocytopenia**: about 15%
Electrocardiographic abnormalities	Aspecific in 24% of patients and similar to those observed after doxorubicin
Responsive tumors	Lymphomas, chronic leukemias, Carcinomas of breast, urinary bladder, kidney, colorectal, and thyroid. Soft tissue sarcomas and malignant melanoma

*   Leukocytes < 4000/mm^3
**   Platelets < 110,000/mm^3

treated with equal doses of DNR and 4-dm DNR, the C x t values of 4-dm DNR equivalents were significantly higher than those found in DNR-treated mice in all organs tested except the heart. The prolonged higher plasma level of 4-dm DNR can be attributed to the fact that this analog is released more slowly than DNR from tissues.

INITIAL CLINICAL STUDIES

4'-epi Doxorubicin

Studies in man with 4-epi DX were started in July 1977, and the Phase I and preliminary Phase II results in a total of 108 patients with advanced neoplasms were previously reported (14, 15). Table 4 summarizes the essential findings observed in 116 patients (no prior chemotherapy 45, prior chemotherapy 71 including 8 patients who received DX). The drug was administered by rapid intravenous injection at three-week intervals. The highest single dose administered was 90 mg/m^2, and the highest total dose 630 mg/m^2, respectively. No significant toxic signs were observed with doses less than 50 mg/m^2. With doses ranging from 60 to 90 mg/m^2, vomiting occurred in about half of patients, oral mucositis and diarrhea in less than 10%, and pronounced alopecia in about 70% (80% in patients treated with 90 mg/m^2). Myelosuppression represented the dose-limiting toxicity, was apparently not dose dependent after 50 to 90 mg/m^2, and its incidence was more related to the extent of prior irradiation than to prior chemotherapy. Severe leukopenia (leukocytes < 1,500/mm^3) and severe thrombocytopenia (platelets < 75,000/mm^3) were extremely rare findings even after successive doses of 75 and 90 mg/m^2. The nadir of leukocyte and platelet fall occurred at about the second week from drug injection and complete return to normal blood values was observed by the third week in almost all instances. Aspecific electrocardiographic abnormalities, similar to those reported after conventional doses of DX (2, 3), were recorded in 24% of patients. Cumulative cardiac toxicity was evaluated only through variation of PEP/LVET ratio. The results indicated a lower toxic effect of 4'-epi DX on myocardial contractility compared to DX. However, the difference between 4'-epi DX and DX was not significant. No patient developed clinical or radiological signs of drug-induced cardiomyopathy.

Therapeutic activity was observed in a number of neoplasms (14), and the response rate (mostly partial remission or PR) was related to prior chemotherapy. In fact, in patients previously untreated with chemotherapy objective tumor regression, including all five patients achieving complete remission (CR), occurred in 44% (20 of 45) compared to 19% (14 of 71) for patients who were subjected to extensive prior drug therapy. In patients treated with 50-60-75-90 mg/m^2, both incidence and duration of response were apparently unrelated to the dose of 4'-epi DX. The overall tumor response, including objective improvement, was documented in 5 of 20 patients with malignant melanoma (CR 1, PR 1), in 7 of 20 with breast cancer (PR 3), in 3 of 10 with renal cancer (CR 1, PR 1), in 2 of 8 with colorectal cancer (CR 1), in 1 of 9 with soft tissue sarcoma (PR 1), in 1 of 2 with thyroid cancer (PR 1), and in 8 of 9 with non-Hodgkin's lymphomas (CR 2, PR 4). Tumor response was also observed in one patient with Kaposi's sarcoma (PR), polycythemia vera (CR), and chronic lymphocytic leukemia (PR) as well as in both patients with chronic myelogenous leukemia (PR). No tumor regression was observed in 8 patients who were previously treated with DX.

4'-demethoxy daunorubicin

Phase I study with 4-dm DNR was initiated in June 1980 and as of July 1981 a total of 46 patients with advanced cancer were considered evaluable. The main patient characteristics are shown in Table 5.

The drug for intravenous use was supplied as orange powder in 5-mg vials, reconstituted with distilled water, and administered by rapid injection every three weeks or upon recovery from myelosuppression. For

Table 5. Characteristics of patients
studied with 4-dmDNR

Total	29	27
Age (yr)		
Median	54	49
Range	18-71	14-68
Sex		
Male	11	12
Female	18	15
Prior therapy		
Chemotherapy	27	22
Radiotherapy	2	5
Prior doxorubicin	6	3
Mean tot. dose*	230	300
Range tot. dose*	150-470	300-400

* mg/m^2.

Table 6. Doses and courses of 4-demethoxy daunorubicin

Intravenous administration			Oral administration		
mg/m^2 q. 3 weeks*	Patients (29)	Courses (57)	mg/m^2 q. 3 weeks**	Patients (27)	Courses (51)
1.5	3	3	6	3	3
3	3	3	10	3	3
5	3	4	15	3	3
7.5	3	6	21	5	6
10.5	4	6	27	7	9
13.5	6	8	36	7	8
15	8	16	48	8	9
18	8	11	60	6	10

*   Cumulative dose: 84 mg/m^2
** Cumulative dose: 268 mg/m^2.

oral use, the drug was supplied as 5 and 10 mg capsules and the entire
dose was administered every three weeks. Table 6 indicates doses and number of courses given up to July 1981. The ratio between iv and oral doses
was about 1 to 4 because this was the therapeutic ratio observed in experimental animal systems utilizing equitoxic doses (11). For both routes
of administration, the Fibonacci scheme was utilized and for the first
three drug levels only one drug course was given.

The incidence of toxic manifestations after intravenous routes (Table

Table 7. Percent toxic manifestations after intravenous 4-demethoxy daunorubicin

mg/m^2	7.5	10.5	13.5	15	18
patients	3	4	6	8	8
Nausea		25	33	50	50
Vomiting			16		
Stomatitis				12	
Alopecia		25	16	50	37
Leukopenia*	66	75	66	100	100
Thrombocytopenia**				12	75

* Leukocytes < 4,000/mm^3
** Platelets < 110,000/mm^3.

Table 8. Percent toxic manifestations after oral 4-demethoxy daunorubicin

mg/m^2	21	27	36	48	60
patients	5	7	7	8	6
Nausea	20	14	57	87	100
Vomiting	20	14	57	62	66
Diarrhea				25	33
Alopecia				37	17
Leukopenia*	20	14	43	62	66
Thrombocytopenia**		14		12	17

* Leukocytes < 4,000/mm^3
** Platelets < 110,000/mm^3.

7) indicated that vomiting and stomatitis were infrequent. At this point in the evaluation, the incidence of alopecia cannot be fully documented because this side effect was already present in many patients as a result of prior combination chemotherapy. Myelosuppression, expressed in terms of mean nadir of leukocyte and platelet fall, was dose related and leuko- penia occurred more frequently than thrombocytopenia. There were three patients in whom leukocytes dropped below 500/mm^3 after 15 mg/m^2 (1 case) and 18 mg/m^2 (2 cases). In one patient receiving 18 mg/m^2 platelets drop- ped below 50,000/mm^3. In patients given the drug orally (Table 8) nausea, vomiting, and diarrhea were comparatively more frequent than observed after intravenous administration. Conversely, myelosuppression was more rarely

Table 9. Therapeutic activity of 4-demethoxy daunorubicin in patients heavily pretreated with chemotherapy

Tumor type	Partial response i.v.	p.o.
Malignant melanoma	0/10	1/14
Breast cancer	1*/5	0/3
Cancer of uterine cervix	0/1	0/3
Colorectal cancer	0/2	
Gastric cancer	0/1	
Testicular cancer	0/1	0/1
Bladder cancer	0/1	
Lung cancer	0/1	0/1
Soft tissue sarcoma	0/2	0/1
Osteosarcoma		0/2
Neuroblastoma	0/1	
Hodgkin's disease	2*/2	
Non Hodgkin's lymphoma	1*/1	0/1
Primary site unknown	0/1	0/1

* Prior chemotherapy included doxorubicin.

encountered after oral administration. Only the mean nadir of leukocyte fall appeared dose related with one patient showing 600 leukocytes/mm^3 after 60 mg/m^2.

Aspecific electrocardiographic changes were recorded in 13 of 47 patients (27%). They were observed in 4 of 29 patients given intravenous and in 9 of 27 given oral 4-dm DX, respectively. Comparative PEP/LVET studies are not available at the time of this writing. No patient showed clinical signs and symptoms of drug-induced cardiomyopathy, including patients who were previously treated with 400 mg/m^2 of DX.

Table 9 reports tumor response related to the route of drug administration. At the present moment, only PR was documented. Of five responsive patients, four were treated with intravenous drug administration. Tumor response was observed in patients receiving 15-18 and 60 mg/m^2. It is interesting to point out that PR was documented in four patients who were resistant to prior combination chemotherapy including DX.

COMMENTS

The findings reported in this paper are still in a preliminary stage, and very few aspects of the present trials allow us to draw conclusions. Both 4'-epi DX and 4-dm DNR are being studied in human cancers on the basis of results that emerged after their evaluation on experimental animal systems. The ultimate goals are qualitative and quantitative comparisons of toxic and therapeutic effects, with doxorubicin as the core drug upon which improvement must be made clinically. Thus, the superiority of a given analog versus doxurubicin, either because of its reduced toxicity or because of its improved antineoplastic efficacy as predicted by the existing systems, must be confirmed during Phase I and Phase II studies if chaos and anarchy are to be avoided during Phase III trials (16).

Compared with the results obtained with doxorubicin, available data from 4'-epi DX would suggest that a) acute toxicity is less at comparative doses in mg/m^2; and b) 4'-epi DX may be more active in unresponsive tumors. The clinical observation that 4-epi DX appears less toxic than does DX is in line with predictive toxicological and pharmacokinetic tests that showed less tissue uptake and more rapid elimination of the analog. It remains to be established whether treatment activity in susceptible tumors is really comparable in patients who have not been treated previously with chemo-therapy and whether there is absolute cross-resistance between DX and 4'epi DX. Last, but not least, the problem of cardiac toxicity remains to be fully evaluated through a prospective comparative analysis. Tests that utilize the same doses in mg/m^2 should allow us, using the techniques of endomyocardial biopsy, to evaluate the effects of the drugs on the heart.

As far as 4-dm DNR is concerned, the initial results indicate that the pattern of acute toxicity, namely myelosuppression, is rather similar to that of DNR and DX. However, nausea and vomiting were rare findings, even after high intravenous doses. The maximum tolerated dose appears to be 15 mg/m^2 after intravenous injection and 60 mg/m^2 following oral administration, respectively. The preliminary evidence that antitumor activity has been observed in patients who were resistant or had become resistant to DX would suggest at minimum that there is no absolute cross-resistance between DX and 4-dm DNR. This potentially useful observation deserves confirmation on large numbers of patients

464

REFERENCES

1. Bonadonna G, Monfardini S, De Lena M, et al. 1969. Clinical evaluation of adriamycin, a new antitumor antibiotic. Br Med J 3:503-506.
2. Bonadonna G, Monfardini S, De Lena M, et al. 1970. Phase I and preliminary phase II evaluation of adriamycin (NSC-123127). Cancer Res 30:2572-2582.
3. Bonadonna G, Beretta G, Tancini G, et al. 1975. Adriamycin (NSC-123127) studies at the Istituto Nazionale Tumori, Milan. Cancer Chemother Rep Part 3, Vol 6 (2):231-245.
4. Carter SK. 1980. The clinical evaluation of analogs. III. Anthracyclines. Cancer Chemother Pharmacol 4:5-10.
5. Arcamone F, Bernardi L, Giardino P, et al. 1976. Synthesis and antitumor activity of 4-demethoxy daunorubicin, 4-demethoxy-7,9-diepidaunorubicin, and their β anomers. Cancer Treat Rep 60:829-834.
6. Casazza AM, Di Marco A, Bonadonna G, et al. 1980. Effects of modifications in position 4 of the chromophore or in position 4' of the aminosugar, on the antitumor activity and toxicity of daunorubicin and doxorubicin. In: Crooke ST, Reich SD (eds) Anthracycline: current status and new developments. Academic Press, London, 403-430.
7. Casazza AM, Di Marco A, Bertazzoli C, et al. 1978. Antitumor activity, toxicity and pharmacological properties of 4'-epiadriamycin. Curr Chemother 2:1257-1260.
8. Di Marco A, Casazza AM and Pratesi G. 1977. Antitumor activity of 4-demethoxy-daunorubicin administered orally. Cancer Treat Rep 61:893-894.
9. Arcamone F, Penco S and Redaelli S. 1976. Synthesis and antitumor activity of 4'-deoxydaunorubicin and 4'-deoxy adriamycin. J Med Chem 19:1424.
10. Casazza AM, Bellini O and Savi G. 1981. Antitumor activity and cardiac toxicity of 4'-deoxy doxorubicin (4'-deoxy DX) in mice. AACR 22:267,1059.
11. Formelli F, Casazza AM, Di Marco A, et al. 1979. Fluorescence assay of tissue distribution of 4-demethoxy daunorubicin and 4-demethoxy doxorubicin in mice bearing solid tumors. Cancer Chemother Pharmacol 3:261-269.
12. Formelli F, Pollini C, Casazza AM, et al. 1981. Fluorescence assays and pharmacokinetic studies of 4'-deoxy doxorubicin and doxorubicin in organs of mice bearing solid tumors. Cancer Chemother Pharmacol 5:139-144.
13. Natale N, Brambilla M and Luchini S. 1981. 4'-Epidoxorubicin and doxorubicin: toxicity and pharmacokinetics in cancer patients. 12th International Congress of Chemotherapy 114,348.
14. Bonfante V, Bonadonna G, Villani F, et al. 1980. Preliminary clinical experience with 4'-epidoxorubicin in advanced human neoplasia. Recent Results in Cancer Research 74:192-199.
15. Bonfante V, Villani F and Bonadonna G. Toxic and therapeutic activity of 4'-epidoxorubicin. Cancer Chemother Pharmacol, in press.
16. Carter SK. 1981. The anthracyclines: historical perspectives. In: Symposium on Anthracycline Antibiotics in Cancer Therapy.

ACKNOWLEDGMENT

The authors are indebted to Dr. A.M. Casazza, A. Martini and F. Nicolis for helpful suggestions in the design of study protocols as well as to Dr. F. Villani, Cardiological Unit, Istituto Nazionale Tumori of Milan, for monitoring the cardiac tests during the entire period of study.

This work has been supported in part by a Research Grant from Farmitalia-Carlo Erba, Milano, Italy.

SECTION 6

CLINICAL STUDIES WITH NEW ANTHRACYCLINES
AND RELATED COMPOUNDS

INTRODUCTION

S. K. CARTER

The impressive broad-spectrum activity of Adriamycin has led
to a large-scale attempt to develop new analogs with a superior
therapeutic index. The goal of the new analogs is either to
improve efficacy or to diminish cardiac toxicity. Much emphasis
has been placed on the latter goal. A general rule in cancer
chemotherapy is that interest and excitement in a new drug exist
in inverse proportion to the amount of clinical data available.
All new drugs enter the clinic with a preclinical rationale that
is a mixture of experimental information and optimistic assump-
tions. The reality of clinical data usually mitigates the as-
sumptions and exposes the weaknesses in our experimental systems.
An analog is more difficult to evaluate clinically than is a
new structure. With an analog, all data must be compared to the
data on the parent structure. It is not enough to observe activity with an analog. A positive result demands activity that
is in some way superior to that observed with the parent. This
requirement for comparative analysis usually means that phase-one
and phase-two studies rarely provide much positive information
unless evidence of dramatic superiority is seen. The purpose
of these early-phase trials is to allow a decision to be made
as to whether the large-scale comparative phase-three studies
are worth attempting.
The phase-three trials of a new anthracycline can be designed
from the perspective of efficacy or cardiac toxicity. The design
of these studies will differ significantly, depending upon which
perspective is paramount. If superior efficacy is the goal, then
the end results of the trial will be response rates, time to
failure, and survival after treatment with the analog as com-

pared with Adriamycin. If dimished cardiac toxicity is the
goal, then equivalent efficacy is acceptable for the analog
in relation to Adriamycin. The trial will require an acceptable end point of cardiac toxicity or the lack thereof within
the framework of comparable efficacy. To make a study of
cardiac impact, one must have a large number of patients entered to achieve an adequate number of responders who can be
maintained for a sufficient period of time.

Given the requirement for well-designed phase-three studies
for new anthracyclines, it is important to understand how
little of practical importance, for oncologic practice, can be
learned from the preliminary reports included in this final
section. The fact that a new anthracycline results in objective
regressions in a few patients with breast cancer, bladder cancer,
lymphomas, or sarcomas is minimally exciting. The critical
question is, does the new drug demonstrate clear-cut superiority
to what can be accomplished with Adriamycin against the specific
tumor in question? When Adriamycin is used as a part of combination regimens, this demonstration is fraught with difficulty.

The fact that cardiomyopathy has not been reported in a phase-
one or phase-two study with a new anthracycline is also of minimal practical importance for long-term decision making. The
greatest importance of this observation is that further study is
not precluded. One should keep firmly in mind that no cardiomyopathy was reported in the early clinical trials with
Adriamycin.

In this section, data on a variety of new anthracyclines
will be presented. These include 4'-epiadriamycin and demethoxydaunorubicin from Italy, aclacinomycin from Japan, carminomycin
from the Soviet Union, and marcellomycin from the United States.
These drugs, taken together, offer the potentials of greater
potency, oral activity, superior efficacy, diminished marrow
suppression, and lessened cardiac toxicity. We can all hope
that their promises will be fulfilled, but we should temper
our enthusiasm with a patient demand for definitive data.

THE ANTHRACYCLINES—A HISTORICAL PERSPECTIVE

S. K. CARTER

The anthracyclines are now a 20-year-old story in drug development, a story of successes and disappointments which, in balance, has led to an improvement in cancer care for a great many patients. The anthracyclines currently represent one of the busiest areas of analog development in cancer chemotherapy, as fourth- and fifth-generation approaches struggle to improve the therapeutic index and grab a share of the lucrative commercial market.

So far, 10 anthracyclines have entered clinical trial in the United States, beginning with daunorubicin in the early 1960s (Table 1). An additional five analogs have entered clinical study in other parts of the world, predominantly in Europe, and more can be expected to enter trial in the United States (Table 2). Nearly all of these drugs have entered clinical study as part of an effort to improve the therapeutic index obtained with Adriamycin. Adriamycin is the core drug against which all other anthracyclines are compared, experimentally and clinically. It is worth noting that Adriamycin is one of the few examples in cancer chemotherapy where a second-generation compound was dramatically superior to the first-generation structure, in this case daunorubicin.

The massive developmental work that has gone into third-generation anthracycline analogs, and beyond, offers a gold mine of experimental and clinical data to be analyzed. If the gold can be extracted from the mine, the potential for a better jewel of an anthracycline drug will be significantly enhanced. Unfortunately, most of the anthracyclines placed into clinical trial strategy geared to a testing of the predictions of the experimental data used to select them for human use. This is particularly true in two broad areas: 1) the disease-oriented phase II studies, which are mainly a haphazard mix of patients and are with and without clearly defined prospective end-points, and 2) evaluation of cardiac toxicity, which requires unique designs and considerations related to the exigencies of the dose-related aspect of anthracycline cardiomyopathy.

Table 1. Anthracyclines that have had investigational new drug applications filed in the United States

Drug	Country of origin
1. Daunorubicin	Italy-France
2. Adriamycin	Italy
3. Rubidazone	France
4. Adriamycin-DNA	Belgium
5. AD-32	United States
6. Carminomycin	USSR
7. Dihydroxyanthracenedione (DHAD, mitoxantrone)[a]	United States
8. Anthracenedicarboxaldehyde (bisantrene)[a]	United States
9. Aclacinomycin A	Japan
10. 4'-epi-Adriamycin	Italy

a, Synthetic compounds sharing some common features with anthracyclines.

Table 2. Anthracyclines that have had some clinical study but not within the United States

Drug	Country of origin
1. Dubiromycin	France
2. Daunorubicin-DNA	Belgium
3. Quelamycin	Spain
4. Detorubicin	France
5. Marcellomycin	United States
6. Demethoxydaunorubicin	Italy

What currently exists is a large and ever-growing mass of data that are not collected and correlated in any single place and that are chaotic as to scope and definition of intent.

It is the purpose of this paper to review briefly the clinical data on the anthracyclines from a historical point of view.

Daunomycin was discovered in 1961 by Arcamone and colleagues and was isolated in 1963 from cultures of Streptomyces peucetius (1-5). In 1962, a French group of chemists isolated the same drug from cultures of Streptomyces caeruleorubidus and called it rubidomycin (6). The name daunorubicin has become a popular hybridization of the Italian and French names. It is interesting to note that in the Soviet Union the drug was called rubomycin (7).

The early clinical trials with daunomycin took place in Italy and France. These included studies by Bertazzoli (8) in 1965 and Bernard (9) in 1967, the latter study devoted exclusively to leukemia. The first report in the United States was by Tan et al. (10) from Memorial Sloan-Kettering Cancer Center (MSKCC). In 25 children with leukemia the maximal tolerated dose (MTD) was described as 1 mg/kg/day x 4-5 days, with a 3-day rest, then 1-1.5 mg/kg for 1 day, then 3 days rest, followed by 2 mg/kg once to twice a week. In 34 children with solid tumors the MTD was 1 mg/kg/day for 6-8 days, while the adult dose was 0.8 mg/kg/day x 4 days, rest for 5-10 days, followed by 0.5-0.8 mg/kg every 1-2 days.

Daunomycin was never extensively studied in solid tumors, although the clinical brochure of the National Cancer Institute does give a cumulative summary of solid tumor data (Table 3) (8). The reason why daunomycin was not studied extensively in solid tumors is difficult to elucidate from a perusal of the literature. It can be surmised that early attempts to use the drug in solid tumors ran into the problem of severe marrow toxicity. A partial reason for this may be that the doses utilized were derived from the studies in adult leukemia and may not have been moderated adequately at the beginning. This reason may have been enhanced by the fact that the dosages reported out of Europe for leukemia were higher than could be tolerated in this country. The initial trials of the then Acute Leukemia Group B (ALGB) used dosages as high as 60 mg/kg/day x 5 (11,12). They observed initially a complete response rate of 50%, with nearly all of the other patients expiring with marrow aplasia. In the studies of the ALGB, the dosage of daunomycin was progressively lowered. As this was done, both the complete response rate and drug-related mortality fell. Unlike daunomycin, Adriamycin was studied initially in solid tumors utilizing dose levels from European studies developed for solid tumors which were toxicologically reasonable.

Cardiac toxicity with daunomycin was first reported at MSKCC in 1966 (8). In an initial report, it was observed that cardiotoxicity had occurred in 3 of 18 patients receiving greater than 25 mg/kg total dose of the drug. A syndrome of tachycardia, dyspnea, tachypnea, cyanosis, gallop rhythm, and congestive heart failure (CHF) was described. In two of the three patients, EKG changes were found that consisted of T wave changes and sinus tachycardia.

Table 3. Daunomycin in solid tumors: Cumulative data from the 1975
clinical brochure of the National Cancer Institute

Tumor type	Number of studies	Number of patients	Number of responses
Colon and rectum	4	7	0
Breast	1	2	0
Lung	4	19	2
Melanoma	6	10	2
Stomach	1	1	0
Ovary	4	5	0
Renal	5	8	1
Testicular	5	8	0
Choriocarcinoma	1	1	1
Sarcomas	14	61	8
Hodgkin's disease	6	20	3
Lymphoma	9	25	3
Mesothelioma	1	2	0
Head and neck	2	5	3[a]
Liver	1	1	0

a, All intraarterial in early study by Bertazzoli.

All three of the patients expired.

At about the same time, Bernard (9) and his group, at the Hospital
Saint-Louis in Paris, were also observing cardiac toxic problems. They
reported congestive heart failure in 5 of 11 children with acute lymphocytic
leukemia (ALL) maintained on daunorubicin to total doses of 32-45 mg/kg.
All of the five patients died despite having had some response to digitalis
and diuretics.

In a large study by the Cancer and Acute Leukemia Group B (CALGB) in
children with ALL, Halazun et al. (13) compared induction with vincristine
and prednisone to induction with the same two drugs plus daunomycin. In 172
children treated with the anthracycline-containing combination, congestive
failure developed in 17, for an incidence of 9.9%. In comparison, no cases
developed in the 167 children treated with just vincristine + prednisone.
In the 17 children with cardiotoxicity, the mean total dose of daunomycin
was 780 mg/m^2.

Von Hoff (8) performed a retrospective analysis of the world literature and reported a total incidence of 1.96% (110) in 5613 cases. In 31 cases of CHF, where it could be analyzed, 84% were in remission at the time of onset and 79% died as a result of the toxicity. The daunorubicin cardiac toxicity demonstrates a dose-response effect with 22 to 25 mg/kg seeming to be the point at which a significant risk of clinically expressed damage occurs. Von Hoff constructed a dose-response curve for children, which indicates an incidence of cardiac toxicity of 2% at 600 mg/m^2 total dose, increasing to 15% at doses greater than 1000 mg/m^2. An analysis of EKG changes indicates a lack of dose-response effect with an incidence of 0.2% at total doses of only 50 mg/m^2. In adults the dose-response effect for cardio-myopathy is less clear.

Adriamycin was first clinically evaluated in Italy by Bonadonna (14) and associates at the Cancer Institute of Milan. Its first studies in the United States were at the MSKCC in New York City. Early in the course of its evaluation in the United States, the National Cancer Institute cross-filed with MSKCC's IND file and began sponsoring the widespread trials that rapidly occurred with this exciting drug.

In his initial study, Bonadonna reported on six different schedules for the drug (Table 4) (14). Nearly all of these schedules were tried in the United States by some cooperative group. The single dose every 3 weeks emerged as the generally accepted schedule of choice because it caused less stomatitis and appeared equivalently active to all the others. In the series by Bonadonna and in subsequent studies in the United States, no evidence of important schedule dependency for Adriamycin can be found with the schedules used (15-16).

Bonadonna reported a wide range of activities in solid tumors, which generated a massive interest in the drug. It is worth noting that all of the activity demonstrated by Bonadonna was confirmed by the large-scale American studies that followed.

The initial studies in which Adriamycin was utilized in adults at MSKCC were not encouraging. Krakoff (17), at the 1971 International Symposium, stated that the patients treated "were those with far advanced non-resectable malignant neoplasms for whom no conventional therapy was considered likely to be useful. In most instances patients had received extensive prior radiotherapy and chemotherapy." Utilizing a schedule of 0.3-0.4 mg/kg daily x 3, 3-day rest, and daily x 3, Krakoff observed

476

Table 4. Dose schedules of Adriamycin used in the initial phase I-II
          studies of Adriamycin at the National Cancer Institute, Milan (18)

A)	0.4-0.8 mg/kg	daily x 4, stop 3 days, then once or twice weekly
B)	0.4-0.8 mg/kg	every other day x 4-6 doses, stop 3 days, then once or twice weekly
C)	0.4-0.8 mg/kg	daily x 3, stop 4 days, daily x 3, stop 4 days, then once or twice weekly
D)	0.4-0.6 mg/kg	daily x 3, stop 7 days, daily x 3, stop 7 days, then once or twice weekly
E)	20-25 mg/m^2	daily x 3, repeated every 3 weeks

Objective responses in only 3 of 84 patients treated (of whom 50 were
labelled "adequate"). His paper states, "In adults at the present time, we
have seen little response of various solid tumors to treatment with Adriamycin." This is an instructive retrospective experience, which highlights
the importance of case selection in phase II studies. Had this type of
case selection been the sole phase II experience with Adriamycin in adult
solid tumors, a drug with its high level of activity would have been missed.
This is a sobering thought as we contemplate some of the case selections in
1981 (as compared to 1971) for the phase II studies of new drugs.

Fortunately, a different experience in adult tumors was occurring at the
M. D. Anderson Hospital and Tumor Institute. Frei, in his initial study at
M. D. Anderson, used three dose schedules: 1) 20-30 mg/m^2 1 d x 3 every 3
weeks; 2) 20-35 mg/m^2 1 week x 9; and 3) 60-105 mg/m^2 single dose every 3
weeks (17). Early in this study, it was observed that stomatitis occurred
in only 10% of patients treated with the single dose schedule and that this
figure was significantly less than that found on the other schedules. All
other toxicities did not appear to be schedule dependent. Thus, the logic
for the use of the single dose schedule in the United States was empirical
toxicologic observation, with a post hoc rationale provided by the
pharmacologic studies.

Early in the M. D. Anderson study, a wide range of activity was observed.
At the 1971 International Symposium held in Milan, Frei (18) reported responses in 6 of 11 patients with bladder cancer, 9 of 27 with sarcomas, 3 of
14 with thyroid, 3 of 3 with lymphomas, and 3 of 4 with breast cancer.

The toxic effects of Adriamycin are dose-related, predictable, and,
for the most part, reversible. The major toxicities are dose-limiting

myelosuppression in approximately 60%–80% of patients, stomatitis in as
many as 80%, nausea and/or vomiting in 20%–55%, and alopecia in virtually
all cases. Leukopenia is the predominant hematologic manifestation
of toxicity, and the severity depends on the dosage of Adriamycin and the
regenerative capacity of the bond marrow.

Drug-induced stomatitis typically begins as a burning sensation with
erythema of the oral mucosa, and in 2-3 days it may produce frank ulceration,
particularly in the sublingual and lateral tongue margins. Alopecia involving
the scalp, axillary, and pubic hair occurs in all patients. Growth of hair
usually resumes on cessation of the drug. Gastrointestinal toxicity evidenced
by nausea and occasional vomiting is associated with the drug but rarely
limits clinical use. Extravasation during IV administration can produce local
tissue necrosis, but normal precautions can prevent this toxic effect.

Despite the well-established cardiac toxicity with daunomycin, the
clinical evaluation of Adriamycin proceeded as if it were a completely new
drug rather than a second-generation compound. The acute large animal toxicology protocol in use at that time did not show any cardiac toxicity in dogs
and monkeys because of the lack of chronic dosing. In clinical trials of
Adriamycin, the drug was used continuously in patients who were showing
beneficial responses until evidence appeared of disease progression. This
followed accepted therapeutic guidelines then in vogue for patients treated
with palliative intent. With this approach, it was not too long before
evidence of cardiac toxicity was observed, which was in no way qualitatively
different than that which had been observed with daunomycin.

In this initial experience of 403 patients, Bonadonna (14) reported fatal
cardiac toxicity in seven for an incidence of 1.7%. The fatal cardiac toxicity
was described as abrupt, occurring only in adults (average age 48.5 years),
and apparently not related to the total dose in patients over the age of
60 years. In younger patients, however, cardiac toxicity was seen only with
total doses in excess of 600 mg/m^2. Reversible EKG changes were recorded
in about 30% of patients and almost always in adults. An analysis of the first
131 patients examined for EKG changes showed 68 individuals who had a normal
EKG prior to starting Adriamycin and 63 who had different types of abnormalities prior to starting the drug. Therefore, nearly one-half of the patients
had some EKG changes prior to starting the drug. In the 68 normal EKG
patients, Adriamycin led to abnormalities in 24, of which 10 were only
transitory. In the 63 abnormal EKG patients, Adriamycin therapy led to 20

being unchanged, 13 improved, and 30 with worsening, of which 9 were
transitory.

As evidence concerning cardiac toxicity began to be accumulated in ongoing clinical trials, the late Jeffrey Gottlieb (19), who was one of the
pioneers of Adriamycin study in the United States, developed an analysis
which indicated the critical importance of total dose. In his analysis, the
first evidence of cardiomyopathy was observed at total doses in excess of
500 to 550 mg/m^2. No cases were reported at total doses below these levels
and, for a period of time, it appeared that this would be an extremely valuabl
cutoff point for Adriamycin therapy. As a larger clinical experience evolved,
cases of cardiomyopathy began to be seen at total doses that were significantl
lower, particularly if they were associated with cardiac irradiation, as first
reported by Gilladoga and associates.

Von Hoff (16) has analyzed 4018 patients treated with Adriamycin in the
United States cooperative groups between March 1970 and March 1977. A range
of variables were recorded for all patients. These totalled 67 and included
age, sex, race, performance status, tumor type, and prior concomitant treatment with other drugs. Ten specific parameters were examined in relation to
the development of CHF caused by Adriamycin. These consisted of total
dose and schedule of drug adminiatration, concomitant chemotherapy, prior
radiotherapy to the mediastinum, prior cardiac disease, age, sex, race, type
of tumor, and performance status.

In this analysis, Adriamycin-induced CHF occurred in 88 cases (2.2%).
This was observed at intervals ranging from 0 to 231 days, with a median of
23 days, after the last administration of the drug. The mean and median
total dosages of the anthracycline received by the patient with CHF were 364
and 390 mg/m^2, respectively. Death occurred within 70 days after the
diagnosis of CHF in 63 of the 88 patients. In only 38 of the 63 was death
attributed to the CHF. In the others, it was attributed to progressive
disease. In these latter 25 cases, the CHF was stable but unresolved in 12,
partially resolved in 8, and totally resolved in 5. In this analysis, the
total dose of Adriamycin was strongly related to the development of CHF. The
cumulative probability of developing drug-induced CHF was 0.3 at 400 mg/m^2,
0.7 at 550 mg/m^2, and 0.18 at 700 mg/m^2. When the schedule was examined,
the weekly schedule had the lowest incidence of CHF at 0.8% (8/967), the
incidence with a single dose every 3 weeks was 2.9% (66/2262), and the three
consecutive daily doses repeated every 3 weeks involved an incidence of

2.5% (14/576)..

The endomyocardial biopsy technique developed at Stanford (20-25) has enabled a more specific approach to be made to total dose limitation than did the empiric limitation at 550 mg/m^2. This technique allows evaluation by electron microscope of tissue from the apical portion of the right ventricular septum. The material can be quantified as to the amount of pathologic damage; a system is utilized that has been described in the literature and that ranges from 0 to 3+. The studies at Stanford with the biopsy have demonstrated a morphologic basis for setting the empiric limit at 550 mg/m^2. At this total dose, the average biopsy score is 2+, which is a moderate amount of pathologic damage. As the dose goes up, a sngnificant amount of biopsies begin to show 3+ damage, which is the morphologic equivalent of heart failure. The data indicate, however, that some patients will develop severe damage at lower total doses, while others still will have only minimal (1+) damage when 550 mg/m^2 is reached. It appears that the empiric dose limit of 550 mg/m^2 is appropriate when no risk factors are present, but the limit should be modified in their presence. These risk factors are: 1) previous mediastinal radiation; 2) advanced age (greater than 70 years); and 3) underlying heart disease.

Currently at Stanford (26), the total dose limitators are 450 mg/m^2 for patients without any risk factors and 300 mg/m^2 for those who have received fewer than 3000 rads to the mediastinum and/or are over 70 years of age. In patients who have received over 3000 rads to the mediastinum or have a history of radiation carditis, the total dose limitation is only 150 mg/m^2. These dose levels may be modified upward, based on a cardiac monitoring protocol which may include endomyocardial biopsy.

Adriamycin rapidly became established as active against a wide range of tumors. Following its demonstration of activity in a given tumor, it moved along two broad lines of clinical research. The first was combination chemotherapy and the second, combined modality. The actual realization of the potential for Adriamycin in combination has varied disease by disease.

In breast cancer, Adriamycin alone is clearly the most active single agent (27). It has shown a nearly comparable response rate to combinations such as CMF,* CMFVP, and CFP in previously untreated patients. The potential for combinations has been somewhat disappointing. In combination with cyclophosphamide and 5-fluorouracil, it has shown overall response rates only slightly higher at best than have been observed in nonanthracycline-

*See end of chapter for definitions of abbreviations used for drugs.

containing combinations. What has been most disappointing is that the complete response rate has not improved with any of the recently tried combinations. There is evidence, however, from controlled trials that Adriamycin-containing combinations give a longer survival than do regimens such as CMFVP and CMF (28-29). In surgical adjuvant studies, many groups have not used Adriamycin because of concern over long-term cardiac toxicity (30). The relative efficacy of Adriamycin combinations in the adjuvant situation cannot be evaluated since there have been no studies reported which were designed with that question in mind. The earliest adjuvant studies with Adriamycin combinations such as the FAC-BCG (31) of M. D. Anderson Hospital and Tumor Institute and the Adriamycin plus cytoxan of the University of Arizona (32) suffer from a lack of randomized controls.

Adriamycin is the most active single agent against soft-tissue sarcomas in adults, with the response rate in most series in the range of 25% to 30% (33). There appears to be an important dose-response effect in sarcomas, and doses of 70 mg/m^2 or higher every 3 to 4 weeks are needed to achieve the highest response rates. Adriamycin combined with dacarbazine has been reported as having a higher response rate than does Adriamycin alone, but a controlled study in uterine sarcomas has not been able to confirm this. The addition of vincristine and cyclophosphamide to these two drugs to make CYVADIC combination has the highest response rate in sarcomas (34). Controlled studies have not yet definitively established this regimen as the combination of choice. Carminomycin has been reported as being active in sarcomas within the Soviet Union but trials in the United States or Europe confirming this have not yet been published.

In acute leukemia, Adriamycin and daunorubicin appear to have comparable activity and this is the only disease area where Adriamycin's superiority over daunorubicin is not clear-cut (35). Newer anthracyclines, particularly rubidazone and aclacinomycin A, have also shown evidence of comparable inducing power in adult acute leukemia. The ability (as well as the need) to treat the marrow to aplasia in adult acute leukemia seems to wipe out the superior therapeutic index, in relation to myelosuppression, which exists for Adriamycin in solid tumors. The standard induction therapy for adult acute leukemia is now a combination of anthracycline plus arabinosyl cytosine. This makes the phase II evaluation of new anthracyclines difficult. There has been a tendency with recent new anthracyclines to test them in patients who have been exposed previously to daunorubicin or Adriamycin.

Despite this, some evidence of activity has been observed. Whether this proves a lack of cross-resistance still remains highly debatable, since pretreatment with daunorubicin or Adriamycin might well show similar levels of activity.

In Hodgkin's disease, Adriamycin has become part of a four-drug regimen, ABVD, in which it is combined with bleomycin, vinblastine, and dacarbazine (36). The ABVD combination appears comparable to the standard MOPP regimen for induction and is valuable as a salvage approach in MOPP failures. Recently, impressive long-term results have been achieved by an approach that alternates ABVD with MOPP (37). Newer anthracyclines have not been extensively studied in Hodgkin's disease and their evaluation poses conceptual difficulties.

In the non Hodgkin's lymphomas, the role of anthracyclines is best established in the diffuse lymphomas. Adriamycin has been added to cyclophosphamide, vincristine, and prednisone to make the so called CHOP regimen which is perhaps the most commonly used combination in this group of diseases (38). Whether CHOP is clearly superior to C-MOPP or whether the addition of bleomycin to CHOP to make BACOP improves the efficacy is not clearly established by review of the currently available data.

In the nodular lymphomas, the value of aggressive chemotherapy has not been established (39), and the role of Adriamycin alone or in combination for these diseases also has not been established, although activity exists.

In non-oat-cell lung cancer, Adriamycin has been reported to achieve objective remission rates in the 20% range, but survival impact is minimal, as it is with all single-agent treatments (16). Adriamycin has been part of most recent combinations. These combinations all follow a pattern. In the pilot study of a single institution, it was found that this pattern began with a high initial response rate. Subsequent studies failed to reproduce the high response rate and meaningful survival advantages have not been observed. The current combinations of greatest interest are the CAP regimen (40) in which cyclophosphamide and cisplatin are combined with the anthracycline, and the FAM regimen (41) in which 5-FU and mitomycin C are added. In oat cell lung cancer, a significant complete response rate has been observed which is critically important in achieving survival gains. Unfortunately, complete responses are uncommon in non-oat-cell lung cancer.

In genitourinary malignancy, Adriamycin has demonstrated activity against all tumor types with the exception of kidney neoplasms (42). In bladder cancer, Adriamycin and cisplatin are the two most active drugs, and these drugs have been combined either with cyclophosphamide or 5-FU by various investigators. As yet, there is no combination that is clearly established as superior to single-agent treatment for metastatic disease. Intravesical therapy for early-stage disease is now receiving increasing emphasis and evidence exists that Adriamycin has activity in this situation which is comparable to that observed with thiotepa.

The activity of Adriamycin in cancer of the prostate appears to be among the highest recorded in studies in which clear-cut criteria of objective response have been used (43). Many groups include stable disease and use other criteria for response in this disease. Since there is no established criteria of response, comparability in the literature is difficult to achieve. Although some combinations have been attempted, none have been shown superior in controlled studies to single-agent usage.

In testicular cancer, Adriamycin has clear-cut activity. Attempts to add the anthracycline to the three-drug regimen of velban, bleomycin and cisplatin by Einhorn and colleagues (44) did not lead to an improved result. The major role for Adriamycin may turn out to be as part of a secondary salvage regimen along with a drug such as VP-16.

In ovarian cancer, Adriamycin has shown significant activity in patients who have not had previous exposure to cytotoxic drugs (45). In this situation Adriamycin activity is comparable to that observed with alkylating agents. In patients who have failed on alkylating agents, Adriamycin appears to have minimal activity. Adriamycin combined with cisplatin and cyclophosphamide, either as two-drug combinations or all three together, has become popular due to the high response rates that have been reported in single-arm studies. These regimens have been reported to have complete clinical remission rates of 30% to 40%, with overall response rates of 60% to 80%. The Northern California Oncology Group is currently comparing the three-drug regimen PAC to Adriamycin plus cyclophosphamide. At the National Cencer Institute, non-Adriamycin-containing combinations such as HexaCAF and CHexUP have given similar-type response rates (46-47). Newer anthracyclines have not been studied significantly in ovarian cancer. If they were to be tested in patients failing on a HexaCAF or CHexUP-type regimen, they would have to be significantly more active than than is Adriamycin to demonstrate any response rate.

A new investigative approach with Adriamycin in ovarian cancer involves the administration of this drug intraperitoneally where the peak level is

300 times greater than the peak plasma level. As reported by Ozols, Young, and coworkers, the drug is given through a semipermanent Tenckhoff dialysis catheter (48-49). The early results are encouraging but further study is needed.

If Adriamycin was a second generation of anthracyclines in clinical trial (daunorubicin being the first), then rubidazone began the third generation. Rubidazone is daunorubicin benzoyl-hydrazone and as such is an analog of daunorubicin, not of Adriamycin, which is one way of differentiating among the numerous anthracycline analogs (Table 5). The initial studies in France (50) indicated high activity in adult acute leukemia. This has been confirmed by the M. D. Anderson Group (51), although studies in the Southwest Oncology Group (52) have shown a somewhat lower ability to induce complete remissions.

Table 5. Anthracycline analogs divided as to whether they are identical to daunomycin or Adriamycin, as regards to the C-14 carbon

Related to daunomycin	Related to Adriamycin	Unrelated
1. Rubidazone	1. Adriamycin-DNA	1. AD-32
2. Carminomycin	2. Quelamycin	2. Aclacinomycin-D
3. Daunomycin-DNA	3. 4'-epi-Adriamycin	3. Marcellomycin
4. Dubiromycin	4. Detorubicin	4. Dihydroxyanthra-cenedione
5. 4-Demethoxy-daunorubicin		5. Anthracenediacarboxal-dehyde ("orange crush")
6. Demethydaunorubicin		6. 7-OMEN

Jacquillat et al. (50) achieved complete remission (CR) in 57% of 70 previously untreated adults with acute leukemia. Benjamin et al. (51) reported a 33% CR rate in 39 previously treated patients with rubidazone, which was raised to 53% in 19 patients receiving what was considered to be an optimal dose. The Southwest Oncology Group studied 126 patients, of whom 116 were evaluable (52). In 25 patients with blast crisis of CML, no complete responses were observed. In the remaining patients, the complete response rate was only 22%.

In solid tumors, rubidazone has not demonstrated any activity. At the

Mayo Clinic, a randomized comparison between Adriamycin and rubidazone demonstrated a response rate over 20% for Adriamycin, but no response for rubidazone.

Anthracyclines complexed with DNA have represented early third-generation approaches. Both daunomycin and Adriamycin have been complexed (53). These complexes are based on the hypothesis that tumor cells have a higher rate of endocytosis than does normal tissue, leading to a greater uptake of the complex and subsequent release of the free drug within the tumor cell. Clinical studies with the Adriamycin-DNA complex have been disappointing, since the complex is unstable and there is rapid release of Adriamycin (54). In studies in the United States, the acute toxicologic spectrum of the complex has been similar to that seen with free Adriamycin. The daunomycin-DNA complexes have been extensively studied in Europe with some positive data being reported, but definitive superiority has not been proven.

N-Trifluoroacetyladriamycin-14-valerate (AD-32) is a semisynthetic analog of Adriamycin synthesized by Israel et al. (55) in 1975. When tested against the L1210 and P388 leukemic models, AD-32 was found to be superior to Adriamycin (56). It is also active in the Ridgway osteogenic sarcoma and Lewis lung carcinoma. In contrast to Adriamycin, AD-32 rapidly enters cells and shows cytofluorescence localized within the cytoplasm. Adriamycin uptake is slower with cytofluorescence seen only in the nucleus (57).

Pharmacologically, AD-32 is extensively metabolized and its biotransformation products are rapidly eliminated. This again is in contrast to Adriamycin. Since AD-32 is relatively insoluble, it must be solubilized in a lipophilic solvent medium. The reconstitution for clinical administration involves the use of polyethoxylated vegetable oil (emulphor EL620) and absolute ethanol in equal volumes and then diluted to nine times its volume with 0.9% saline without preservatives. This solution is again diluted 1:10 with 5% dextrose or normal saline. AD-32, therefore, must be given by 24-hour continuous infusion. The emulphor solvent system has been associated with an acute systemic reaction involving chest pain, shaking chills, fevers, hypotension, and diffuse bronchospasm. Because of these reactions, IV hydrocortisone is administered to all patients receiving infusions of AD-32 (58).

Carminomycin is an anthracycline antibiotic isolated from the mycelium of Actinomadura carminata (59). It differs from Adriamycin by the substitution of a hydroxyl for a methoxy group on C-4 and the absence of the hydroxyl group on C-14 (60). However, unlike Adriamycin, carminomycin has been suggested to exert cytotoxicity by binding to DNA and inhibiting DNA and RNA synthesis (6

Carminomycin has a similar experimental antitumor spectrum in comparison
with Adriamycin and daunomycin (62). Merski et al. (63) have shown that the
dose of carminomycin required to produce nucleolar segregation in cardiac and
skeletal muscle is six times greater than is the dose of Adriamycin needed
to induce equivalent alterations.

Clinical evaluation in the Soviet Union (64) has shown that the acute
toxicity spectrum of carminomycin is similar to the other anthracyclines. It
has antitumor activity, again, with a similar spectrum to Adriamycin with
emphasis on sarcomas.

Carminomycin is being studied as a single IV injection every 3 to 4 weeks
by Abele et al. (65). The starting dose was 12 mg/m^2, which has been escalated up to 22 mg/m^2. A total of 21 courses has been administered to 15
patients. Leukopenia was dose limiting, with a median nadir greater than
4000 at 15 mg/m^2 and 700 at 22 mg/m^2, indicating a very steep dose-response
curve. The median day of nadir was day 12 with rapid recovery by day 17.
Thrombocytopenia below 100,000 was observed in three cases. The only other
toxicities were mild nausea, vomiting, and phlebitis. No antitumor effect was
observed and a dose of 20 mg/m^2 every 3 weeks is recommended for phase II
study. It appears that carminomycin is the most potent of all anthracyclines
clinically studied to date in terms of dose per course to achieved dose-
limiting leukopenia. What this means for therapeutic index and cardiac
toxicity remains to be determined.

Comis et al. (66) have also studied carminomycin on a dose schedule
of a single IV dose every 4 weeks. They started at a dose of 1 mg/m^2 and
escalated up to 15 mg/m^2. No toxicity was observed at doses lower than
15 mg/m^2. In six evaluable patients given 15 mg/m^2, a median WBC of 3800 was
observed on the first course with no thrombopenia. The lowest WBC nadir was
1000. Nausea and vomiting were seen in two patients, and there was no evidence of cardiac toxicity.

1,4-Dihydroxy-5,8-bis{{ {2-[(2-hydroxyethyl) amino] ethyl }amino}}-9,10-
anthracenedione dihydrochloride (DHAD) represents an attempt to develop a DNA
intercalating agent that will be devoid of the cardiac toxicity associated
with Adriamycin and daunomycin (67). The rationale behind this compound is
that the cardiac toxicity of the Adriamycin may require the amino sugar
moiety (65). DHAD is active against a wide range of experimental tumors and
is less cardiotoxic than is Adriamycin in the Zbinden rate cardiotoxicity
model (68).

Detorubicin (14-diethoxyacetooxydaunorubicin) is a new semisynthetic anthracycline derivative first described by Maral et al. (69). In vitro detorubicin remains stable under acidic conditions, whereas it is very quickly hydrolyzed into Adriamycin under neutral pH conditions. In vivo, the hydrolysis of detrorubicin into Adriamycin occurs in the bloodstream a few minutes after IV injection into mice (70). The tissue distribution of drug and metabolites differs significantly, however. In comparison with Adriamycin, significantly lower drug levels (parent drug plus metabolites) are found in various tissues, except for the heart and liver, 30 minutes after administration of detorubicin.

Jacquillat et al. (71) have reported on 111 patients treated with detorubicin. In leukemia the drug was given at a dose of 2 mg/kg/d x 56, whereas in solid tumors it was 1 mg/kg x 1 week, then 2 mg/kg every 3 weeks. As with other anthracyclines, myelosuppression is dose limiting. Nausea and vomiting were seen in one-half the patients. In this study, responses were seen in leukemias, lymphomas, and scattered solid tumors.

Quelamycin is a triferric derivative of Adriamycin developed by Gosalvez et al. (72) in Spain. The drug is prepared by neutralization of an aqueous solution of Adriamycin and ferric chloride with sodium hydroxide. The binding of ferric ion to Adriamycin modifies the properties of the drug in terms of cell uptake, distribution, and metabolism. The LD_{50} in mice is three times higher with Adriamycin than it is with quelamycin. Unlike Adriamycin, quelamycin does not inhibit cardiac Na-K ATPase, and so it is postulate that quelamycin is the less cardiotoxic drug (73). Despite this, histopathologic evidence of cardiomyopathy has been demonstrated in rats and rabbits following repeated administration of quelamycin (74). These changes occurred at doses that were twofold higher than were the Adriamycin doses that caused similar changes.

Cortes-Funes et al. (75) have reported the MTD of quelamycin in man to be 150 mg/m^2 as a 1-hour infusion every 3 weeks. The dose-limiting toxicity is leukopenia. Also observed have been gastrointestinal toxicity, alopecia, chills, and fever. Scattered objective responses were observed. Brugarolas et al. (76), in an early phase I study, saw a great deal of iron-related toxicity, including cardiac toxicity, with quelamycin. In a later study, 40 mg/m^2 d x 2-3 was seen to be better tolerated, with no iron-related toxicity. It remains yet to be seen whether quelamycin will be a viable approach to the improvement of the therapeutic index of Adriamycin.

4'-Epi-Adriamycin is a stereoisomer of Adriamycin. Despite its identical molecular weight, it shows less toxicity in mice in comparison with Adriamycin. Although qualitatively the two compounds show identical toxicity, 25% more drug is required to reach the toxicity with the 4'-epi-Adriamycin (77). This could be due to a lower concentration of the 4'-epi-Adriamycin in cardiac and splenic tissues at 1, 24, and 48 hours after drug administration in mice in comparison with Adriamycin. The two compounds have identical antitumor activity in the Ll210 and P388 leukemias.

Phase I studies with the drug show a toxicity spectrum similar to Adriamycin but with a somewhat lower incidence of vomiting and alopecia. At dose levels equivalent to the MTD of Adriamycin, the 4'-epi analog is only mildly myelosuppressive and its equivalently myelosuppressive dose appears to be 90 mg/m^2. Preliminary responses have been observed.

Aclacinomycin A is a trisaccharide anthracycline isolated from Streptomyces galilaeus by Japanese investigators (78). It is also of interest in being inactive in mutogenic assay systems in comparison with the positivity observed with Adriamycin. Clinical trials in Japan (79) have shown activity in leukemia and lymphoma but have been disappointing in solid tumors, particularly gastric cancer. Trials are now underway in the United States.

CONCLUSIONS

The future study of anthracyclines should build on the lessons of the past. Inasmuch as more than 10 anthracycline structures have entered clinical trial, the potential for integrating a vast data base into the design of future studies does exist. This data base exists to be used in approaching several critical areas. One of these is the predictive ability of the existing experimental systems. All of the drugs placed into clinical trial have an efficacy rationale based on murine transplantable systems. The activity of all these compounds can be compared qualitatively and quantitatively with the experimental data base on Adriamycin as the core drug that must be improved upon clinically. As a minimum we should be able to learn what kinds of experimental superiority have not translated into superior clinical efficacy so that these criteria are not utilized in future decision making. In a quantitative fashion, we should be able to learn about the potency prediction of existing systems. For all compounds clinically tested, we should be able to compare on a mg/m^2 basis the optimal dose in the active mouse tumor systems, the LD_{10} and LD_{50} doses in the mouse variety used, and the maximally tolerated dose in man. In the past, a great deal of emphasis has been placed on potency superiority for some analogs in experimental systems, particularly the acute cardiac toxicity models. The viability of this approach should be validated by a study of ratios derived from the experimental data base and the known clinical data. Again, as a minimum, a range or ratios which did not predict for any clinical benefit could be helpful in future decision making.

Based on the available clinical data, the predictability of the existing cardiac toxicity models should be evaluated closely. Data exist on nearly every compound placed into the clinic on an acute, EKG-related model; e.g., the Zbinden test and on a chronic toxicity model such as the rabbit. It would be important to study the appropriateness of the dose levels used in these tests in relation to the myelosuppression doses in the experimental systems compared with the myelosuppression doses found in man. In the acute systems the relative advantages for compounds over Adriamycin are potency advantages. These potency advantages in rats and hamsters may well be found to be meaningful when the varying ratios of experimental to clinical marrow suppressive doses are examined. In the rabbit model, the doses chosen for analogs of Adriamycin have been choses on the basis of what will be tolerated by the rabbit, with the emphasis on an initial choice based on myelosuppression. It is worth noting that over the last few years a wide range of compounds have gone into the clinic with the claim, based on experimental data, that they have less cardiac toxicity than does Adriamycin. To date none have been validated as being less toxic in the clinic, although most have been poorly evaluated from this point of view.

In terms of the clinical trial of new anthracyclines, we have chaos and anarchy. With the diversification inherent in multiple pharmaceutical companies' emphasizing the development of anthracyclines, multiple drugs have entered the clinic in overlapping fashion. These drugs compete for clinical trial resources and are, for the most part, totally uncoordinated in terms of the approaches used and the data that accumulate.

This situation is most acutely seen in the phase II arena. Within a given tumor, different groups test different drugs in a mix of patients who have been previously untreated or treated with drugs including or not including Adriamycin. It is obvious that the end results which would justify phase III study would differ based on the prior therapy of the patients used, but such criteria, if they exist at all, are difficult to find.

If the phase II area is marked by chaos and anarchy, the phase III area is a conceptual wasteland. The phase III trials can be geared to establishing either superior efficacy or diminished chronic toxicity or both. The design of efficacy trials, however, will be quite different from the design of toxicity trials. Both efficacy and toxicity trials are highly complicated by the common usage of anthracyclines in combination regimens in most of the diseases where activity for Adriamycin has been established.

The current clinical literature on anthracyclines is all too often characterized by an undigestable mass of data. New drugs enter clinical trial with no answers available or older analyses to help guide the studies. The "big hit" mentality that prays for the dramatic breakthrough and does not know what to do next when it does not materialize seems to predominate. This approach is a difficult one to defend, and one hopes that such failures will not turn off scientific groups from making continued contributions to this area.

ABBREVIATIONS USED FOR DRUG REGIMENS

ABVD = Adriamycin, bleomycin, vinblastine, dacarbazine

BACOP = bleomycin, Adriamycin, Cytoxan, Oncovin, prednisone

CAP = cyclophosphamide, Adriamycin, cisplatin

CFP = cyclophosphamide, 5-fluorouracil, prednisone

CHexUP = cyclophosphamide, hexamethylmelamine, 5-fluorouracil, cisplatin

CHOP = cyclophosphamide, hydroxyldaunorubicin (Adriamycin), vincristine (Oncovin), prednisone

CMF = cyclophosphamide, methotrexate, 5-fluorouracil

CMFVP = cyclophosphamide, methotrexate, 5-fluorouracil, vincristine, prednisone

C-MOPP = cyclophosphamide (Cytoxan), nitrogen mustard (Mustargen), vincristine (Oncovin), prednisone, procarbazine

CYVADIC = cyclophosphamide, vincristine, Adriamycin, dacarbazine

DHAD = 1,4-dihydroxy-5,8-bis{{ {2-[(2-hydroxyethyl)amino]ethyl}amino}}-9,10-anthracenedione dihydrochloride

FAC-BCG = 5-fluorouracil, Adriamycin, cyclophosphamide, bacillus Calmette-Guérin

FAM = 5-fluorouracil, Adriamycin, mitomycin C

HexaCAF = hexamethylmelamine, cyclophosphamide, methotrexate, 5-fluorouracil

MOPP = nitrogen mustard (Mustargen), vincristine (Oncovin), procarbazine, prednisone

PAC = cisplatin, Adriamycin, cyclophosphamide

490

REFERENCES

1. Arcamone F, Di Marco A, Gaetani M, Scotti T. 1961. Isolation of an antibiotic from Streptomyces species and its antitumorigenic activity. G. Microbiol. 9: 83-90.
2. Arcamone F, Franceschi G, Orezzi P, Cassinelli G, Barbieri W, Mandelli R. 1964. Daunomycin I. The structure of daunomycinone. J. Am. Chem. Soc. 86: 5334-5335.
3. Arcamone F, Cassinelli G, Mondelli R. 1964. Daunomycin II. The structure and steriochemistry of daunosamine. J. Am. Chem. Soc. 86: 5335-5336.
4. Di Marco A, Gaetni M, Orezzi P, Scarpinato BM, Silverstrini R, Soldati M, Dasdia T, Valentini L. 1964. Daunomycin, a new antibiotic of the rhodomycin group. Nature 201: 706-707.
5. Grein A, Spalla C, Di Marco A, Canevazzi G. 1963. Descrizione e Classificazione di un Attimomicete (Streptomyces peucetius sp. nova) Produttrice di una Sostaniza Attiva Antitumorale--la Daunomicina. G. Microbiol. 11: 109-118.
6. Dubost M, Ganter P, Maral R, Ninet L, Pinnert S, Prud'homme J, Werner GH. 1963. Rubidomycin: A new antibiotic with cytostatic properties. C. R. Acad. Sci. 257: 1813-1815.
7. Gause FG. 1966. Aspects of antibiotic research. Chem. Ind. 15061513, Sept. 3.
8. Von Hoff D, Slavik M. 1975. Daunomycin (NSC-82151), Clinical brochure, Investigational Drug Branch, Cancer Therapy Evaluation Progrom. Division of Cancer Treatment, National Cancer Institute, December.
· 9. Bernard J. 1967. Acute leukemia treatment. Cancer Res. 27: 2565.
10. Tan C, Hosaka H, Kov-Ping Y, Murphy ML, Karnofsky DA. 1967. Daunomycin an antitumoral antibiotic in the treatment of neoplastic disease. Clinical evaluation with special reference to childhood leukemia. Cancer 20: 333-353.
11. Weil M, Glidewell OJ, Jacquillat CL, Levy R, Serpick AA. 1973. Daunorubicin in the therapy of acute granulocytic leukemia. Cancer Res. 33: 921-928.
12. Cortes EP, Ellison RR, Yates JW. 1972. Adriamycin (NSC 123127) in the treatment of acute myelocytic leukemia. Cancer Chemother. Rep. 56: 237-243.
13. Halazun J, Wagner HR, Gaeta JF, Sinks LF. 1974. Daunorubicin cardiac toxicity in children with acute lymphocytic leukemia. Cancer 33: 545-554
14. Bonadonna G, Monfardini S, DeLena M, Fossati-Bellani F, Beretta G. 1972. Clinical trials of Adriamycin: Results of three years study. In: International Symposium on Adriamycin (Carter SK, Di Marco A, Krakoff IH, Mathé G, eds.). Springer-Verlag, New York, pp. 139-152.
15. Blum RH, Carter SK. 1974. Adriamycin: A new anthracycline drug with significant clinical activity. Ann. Intern. Med. 80: 249-259.
16. Von Hoff DD, Layard DD, Basa P, et al. 1979. Risk factors for adriamyci induced congestive heart failure. Ann. Intern. Med. 91: 710-717.
17. Krakoff IH. 1972. Adriamycin in adults with neoplastic disease. In: International Symposium on Adriamycin (Carter SK, Di Marco A, Krakoff IH, Mathé G, eds.). Springer-Verlag, New York, pp. 165-168.
18. Frei E, Luce JK, Middleman E. 1972. Clinical trials with adriamycin. In: International Symposium on Adriamycin (Carter SK, Di Marco A, Krakof IH, Mathé G, eds.). Springer-Verlag, New York, pp. 153-160.
19. Carter SK. 1975. Adriamycin--A review. J. Nat. Cancer Inst. 55(6): 1265-1274.
20. Billingham ME, Mason JW, Bristow MR, Daniels JR. 1978. Anthracycline cardiomyopathy monitored by morphologic changes. Cancer Treat. Rep. 62:

865-872.

21. Bristow MR, Mason JW, Billingham ME, Daniels JR. 1980. Doxorubicin cardiomyopathy: Evaluation by phonocardiography, endomyocardial biopsy, and cardiac catheterization. Ann. Intern. Med. 88: 168-175.

22. Bristow MR. 1980. Rational system for cardiac monitoring in patients receiving anthracyclines. Proc. Am. Assoc. Cancer Res./Am. Soc. Clinic. Oncol. 21: 356. /Abstr./

23. Bristow MR, Thompson PD, Martin RP, Mason JW, Billingham ME, Harrison DC. 1978. Early anthracycline cardiotoxicity. Am. J. Med. 65: 823-832.

24. Mason JW, Bristow MR, Billingham ME, Daniels JR. 1978. Invasive and non-invasive methods of assessing adriamycin cardiotoxic effects in man: Superiority of histopathiologic assessment using endomyocardial biopsy. Cancer Treat. Rep. 62: 857.

25. Billingham ME, Mason JW, Bristow MR, Daniels JR. 1978. Anthracycline cardiomyopathy monitored by morphologic changes. Cancer Treat. Rep. 62: 965-969.

26. Bristow MR. 1980. Pathophysiologic basis for cardiac monitoring in patients receiving anthracyclines. In: Anthracyclines: Current status and new developments (Crooke CT, Reich SD, eds.). Academic Press, New York, pp. 255-271.

27. Carter SK. 1977. The chemical therapy of breast cancer. Comin, Oncol. 1: 131-144.

28. Bull JM, Tormey DC, Li S-H, et al. 1978. A randomized comparative trial of adriamycin versus methotrexate in combination drug therapy. Cancer 41: 1649-1657.

29. Muss HB, White DR, Richards F II, et al. 1978. Adriamycin versus methotrexate in five-drug combination chemotherapy for advanced breast cancer: A randomized trial. Cancer 42: 2141-2148.

30. Carter SK. 1980. Surgery plus adjuvant chemotherapy: A review of therapeutic implications. I. Breast cancer. Cancer Chemother. Pharmacol. 4(3): 147-165.

31. Buzdar AU, Blumenschein G, Gutterman J, et al. 1979. Adjuvant therapy with 5-fluorouracil, adriamycin, cyclophosphamide and BCG (FAC-BCG) for stage II or III breast cancer. In: Adjuvant therapy of cancer II (Jones SE, Salmon SE, eds.). Grune & Stratton, New York, pp. 277-284.

32. Wendt AG, Jones SE, Salmon SE, et al. 1979. Adjuvant treatment of breast cancer with adriamycin-cyclophosphamide with or without radiation therapy. In: Adjuvant therapy of cancer II (Jones SE, Salmon SE, eds). Grune & Stratton, New York, pp. 285-293.

33. Pinedo HM, Kenis Y. 1977. Chemotherapy of advanced soft-tissue sarcoma in adults. Cancer Treat. Rev. 4: 67-86.

34. Gottlieb JA, Baker LH, O'Bryan RM, et al. 1975. Adriamycin used alone and in combination for soft tissue and bone sarcomas. Cancer Chemother. Rep. 6: 271-282.

35. Gale RP. 1979. Advances in the treatment of acute myelogenous leukemia. N. Engl. J. Med. 300: 1189-1199.

36. Bonadonna G, Zucali R, Monfardini S, DeLena M, Uslenghi C. 1975. Combination chemotherapy of Hodgkin's disease with adriamycin, bleomycin, vinblastine, and imidazole carboxamide versus MOPP. Cancer 252-259.

37. Santoro A, Bonadonna G, Bonfante V, Valagussa P. 1980. Non-cross resistant regimens (MOPP and ABVD) vs. MOPP alone in stage IV Hodgkin's disease (HD). Proc. Am. Assoc. Cancer Res./Am. Soc. Clin. Oncol. 21: 470. /Abstr./

38. McKelvey EM. 1978. Review of CHOP-HOP combination chemotherapy in malignant lymphoma. Proc. Am. Assoc. Cancer Res./Am. Soc. Clin. Oncol.

19: 310.

39. Portlock CS. 1980. Management of indolent non-Hodgkin's lymphomas. Semin. Oncol. 7: 292-301.

40. Eagan RT, Ingle JN, Frytak S, Rubin J, Kvols LK, Carr DT, Coles DT, O'Fallon JR. 1977. Platinum-based polychemotherapy versus dianhydrogalactitol in advanced non-small cell lung cancer. Cancer Treat. Rep. 61: 1339-1345.

41. Butler T, MacDonald JS, Smith FP, et al. 1979. 5-Fluorouracil, adriamycin, and mitomycin C (FAM) chemotherapy for adenocarcinoma of the lung. Cancer 43: 1183.

42. Carter SK. 1978. Chemotherapy and genitourinary oncology I. Bladder. Cancer Treat. Rep. 5: 85-95.

43. Torti FM, Carter SK. 1980. The chemotherapy of prostatic adenocarcinoma. Ann. Intern. Med. 92(5): 681-692.

44. Stoter G, Williams SD, Einhorn LH. 1980. Genitourinary tumors. In: Cancer chemotherapy (Pinedo HM, ed.). Excerpta Medica, Amsterdam-Oxford, pp. 306-320.

45. Young RC. Gynecologic malignancies. In: Cancer chemotherapy (Pinedo HM, ed.). Excerpta Medica, Amsterdam-Oxford, pp. 321-350.

46. Young RC, Chabner BA, Hubbard SP, et al. 1978. Advanced ovarian adenocarcinoma: A prospective clinical trial of melphalan (L-PAM) versus combination chemotherapy. N. Engl. J. Med. 299: 1261-1266.

47. Young RC, Howser DM, Myers CE, et al. 1981. Combination chemotherapy (CHEX-UP) with intraperitoneal maintenance in advanced ovarian adenocarcinoma. Proc. Am. Assoc. Cancer Res./Am. Soc. Clin. Oncol. 22: 465.

48. Ozols RF, Locker GY, Speyer JL, et al. 1980. Intraperitoneal (IP) Adriamycin (ADR) in ovarian carcinoma. Proc. Am. Assoc. Cancer Res./Am. Soc. Clin. Oncol. 21: 425. /Abstr./

49. Ozols RF, Locker GY, Doroshow JH, Grotzinger KR, Myers CE, Young RC. 1979. Pharmacokinetics of adriamycin and tissue penetration in murine ovarian cancer. Cancer Res. 39: 3209-3214.

50. Jacquillat CL, Weil M, Gemon-Auclerc MD, et al. 1976. Clinical study of rubidazone (22050 RP), a new daunorubicin derived compound in 170 patients with acute leukemias and other malignancies. Cancer 37: 653-659.

51. Benjamin RS, Keating MJ, McCredie KB, et al. 1977. A phase I and II trial of rubidazone in patients with acute leukemia. Cancer Res. 37: 4623-4628.

52. Bickers J, Benjamin RS, Wilson H, et al. 1981. Rubidazone in adults with previously treated acute leukemia and blast cell phase of chronic myelocytic leukemia: A southwest oncology group study. Cancer Treat. Rep. 65: 427-430.

53. Trouet A. 1978. Increased selectivity of drugs by linking to carriers. Eur. J. Cancer 14: 105-111.

54. Benjamin RS, Mason JW, Billingham ME. 1978. Cardiac toxicity of adriamycin-DNA complex and rubidazone: Evaluation by electrocardiogram and endomyocardial biopsy. Cancer Treat. Rep. 62: 935-939.

55. Israel M, Modest EJ, Frei E. 1975. N-trifluoroacetyladriamycin-14-valerate, an analog with greater experimental antitumor activity and less toxicity than Adriamycin. Cancer Res. 35: 1365-1368.

56. Parker LM, Hirst M, Israel M. 1978. N-trifluoroacetyl Adriamycin-14-valerate: Additional mouse antitumor and toxicity studies. Cancer Treat. Rep. 62: 119-127.

57. Krishan A, Israel M, Modest EJ, et al. 1981. Preclinical rationale and phase I clinical trial of an Adriamycin analog, AD32. In: Recent results in cancer research, vol. 76 (Carter SK, Sakurai Y, Umezawa H, eds.).

Springer-Verlag, New York.
58. Blum RH, Garnick MB, Israel M, Canellos GP, Henderson IC, Frei E. 1979. Initial clinical evaluation of n-trifluoroacetyl Adriamycin-14-valerate (AD-32), an Adriamycin analogue. Cancer Treat. Rep. 63: 916-923.
59. Braznikova MG, Zbarsky MK, Kudinova MK, Muravieava LI, Ponomakrenko VI, Potapova NP. 1973. Carminomycin, a new anthracycline antibiotic. Antibiotiki (Moscow) 18: 678-681.
60. Braznikova MG, Zbarsky VB, Ponomarenki VI, Potapova NP. 1974. Physical and chemical characteristics and structure of carminomycin: A new antitumor antibiotic. J. Antibiot. (Tokyo), ser. A, 27: 254-259.
61. Dudnik YV, Ostanina LN, Kozyman LI, Gause GG. 1974. Action mechanism of carminomycin. Antibiotiki (Moscow) 19: 514-517.
62. Perevodchikova NI, Gorbunova VA, Lichinitser MR, Borisov VI, Alekseyev NA, Vygovskaya YI. 1975. First phase of a clinical study of the antitumor antibiotic carminomycin. Antibiotiki (Moscow) 20: 853-856.
63. Merski JA, Daskal Y, Crooke ST, Busch H. 1979. Acute ultrastructural effects of the antitumor antibiotic carminomycin on nucleoli of rat tissues. Cancer Res. 39: 1239-1244.
64. Perevodchikova NI, Lichinitser MA, Gorbunova VA. 1977. Phase I clinical study of carminomycin: Its activity against soft tissue sarcomas. Cancer Treat. Rep. 61: 1705-1707.
65. Adamson RH. 1974. Daunomycin and adriamycin: Hypothesis concerning antitumor activity and cardiotoxicity. Cancer Chemother. Rep. 58: 293-294.
66. Comis RJ, Ginsberg S, Crooke ST. 1980. A phase I study of carminomycin administered by intravenous bolus every 4 weeks. Proc. Am. Assoc. Cancer Res./Am. Soc. Clin. Oncol. 21: 333.
67. Von Hoff D, Pollard E. Kihn J, Murray E, Coltman CA. 1980. Phase I clinical investigation of DHAD (NSC 301739), a new anthracenedione. Cancer Res. 40: 1516-1518.
68. Cheng CC, Zbinden G, Zee-Cheng Riley. 1979. Comparison of antineoplastic activity of aminoethylaminoquinones and anthracycline antibiotics. J. Pharm. Sci. 68: 393.
69. Maral R, Ducep JB, Farge D. 1978. Preparation et activite antitumorale experimentale d'un nouvel antibiotique semisynthetique: La kiethoxyaceto-xy-14-daunorubicine (33921 RP). C. R. Acad. Sci. Paris 286: 443-446.
70. Deprez-de Compeneere D, Baurain R, Trouet A. 1979. Pharmacokinetics, toxicologic and chemotherapeutic properties of detorubicin in mice: A comparative study with daunorubicin and adriamycin. Cancer Treat. Rep. 68: 861-867.
71. Jacquillat C, Auclerc MF, Weil M, Maral J, Degos L, Auclerc G, Tobelem G, Schaisan G, Bernard J. 1979. Clinical activity of detorubicin: A new anthracycline derivative. Cancer Treat. Rep. 68: 889-893.
72. Gosalvez M, Blanco MF, Vivero C. 1978. Quelamycin, a new derivative of adriamycin with several possible therapeutic advantages. Eur. J. Cancer 14: 1185-1190.
73. Gosalvez M, Von Rossum GDV, Blanco MF. 1979. Inhibition of sodium-potassium activated adenosine: 5'-Triphosphate and ion transport by adriamycin. Cancer Res. 39: 257-261.
74. Young DM, Ward JM, Pelham JF. 1978. Quelamycin induced cardiotoxicity in rabbits and rats. Proc. Am. Assoc. Cancer Res./Am. Soc. Clin. Oncol. 19: 56.
75. Cortes-Funes H, Gosalvez M, Moyano A, Manas A, Mendiola C. 1979. Early clinical trial with quelamycin. Cancer Treat. Rep. 63: 903-908.
76. Brugarolas A, Pachen N, Gosalvez M. 1978. Phase I clinical study of quelamycin. Cancer Treat. Rep. 62: 1527-1534.

494

77. Bonfante V, Bonadonna G, Villani F, DiFranzo G, Mareini A, Casazza AM. 1979. Preliminary phase I study of 4'-epi-adriamycin. Cancer Treat. Rep. 63: 915-918.

78. Oki T, Matsuzawa Y, Yoshimoto A, et al. 1975. New antitumor antibiotics, aclacinomycins A and B. J. Antiobiot. (Tokyo) 28(10): 830-834.

79. Wakabayashi T, Oki T, Tone H, Hirano S, Omori K. 1980. A comparative electron microscopical study of aclacinomycin and Adriamycin induced cardiotoxicities in rabbits and hamsters. J. Electron Micros. (Tokyo) 29: 106-118.

PHASE-I TRIAL WITH 4-DEMETHOXYDAUNORUBICIN

F. CAVALLI,* S. KAPLAN, M. VARINI, P. TOGNI, AND A. MARTINI

1. ABSTRACT

We report the results of a phase-I trial with the intravenous and oral formulation of a new analog of daunorubicin, 4-demethoxydaunorubicin. The study was conducted exclusively in patients suffering from solid tumors. Myelosuppression was the dose-limiting toxicity for both formulations. In the i.v. trial, the maximum tolerated dose was reached at 18 mg/m^2 with a single-dose administration being used; whereas, for the oral formulation, the maximum tolerated dose is between 50-60 mg/m^2. For this schedule, 15 mg/m^2 i.v. and 45 mg/m^2 oral are proposed as starting doses for phase-II trials in solid tumors. However, the drug seems to be more suitable for the treatment of hematologic malignancies.

2. INTRODUCTION

Much endeavor is continuously being devoted to the development of new analogs of chemotherapeutic agents in the search for new compounds with broader antitumor activity and a better therapeutic index. The anthracyclines, particularly doxorubicin and daunorubicin, are being extensively investigated for this purpose.

4-Demethoxydaunorubicin (IMI-30) is a new analog of daunorubicin, which lacks the methoxyl group at the C-4 position of the tetracyclic aglycone (1,2). IMI-30 was shown to be effective in a variety of experimental mouse tumors. In the L1210 model and in Gross leukemia tumor, IMI-30 showed an antitumor activity similar to that of daunorubicin at doses 5-8 times lower. IMI-30 is also active by the oral route. At doses that are about four times higher than the optimal i.v. doses, oral IMI-30 reaches the same antitumor activity as it does when administered i.v., and it is as effective as doxorubicin i.p. in ascitic P388 leukemia and as effective as doxorubicin i.v. in L1210 leukemia

---

* Author to whom requests for reprints should be sent.

(3,4). Initial toxicologic data hint to a better therapeutic index, mainly as regards cardiotoxicity, when IMI-30 is compared with the parent compound (5).

In this paper we report the results of a phase-I trial with 4-demethoxy-daunorubicin that aimed to define the maximum tolerated dose (MTD) and the acute toxicity in man when the drug is given in one single dose intravenously and orally. These studies were undertaken within the framework of the new drugs program of the Early Clinical Trials Group of the European Organization for Research on the Treatment of Cancer.

3. MATERIALS AND METHODS

All patients selected for this trial (see Table 1) had histologically confirmed solid malignancies no longer suitable for conventional therapy. They had completely recovered from major toxic effects induced by prior treatment. All patients had white blood cell (WBC) counts of at least $4000/mm^3$, platelet count of $100,000/mm^3$ or more, maximum serum creatinine and bilirubin levels of 1.5 mg%. Expected survival upon entry into the trial was longer than 6 weeks. Three complete blood cell counts and one SMA 12 chemistry panel were scheduled per week. Poly-EKG was performed before the drug administration, 1 hour, 24 hours, and 1 week thereafter.

Table 1. Characteristics of patients

Characteristics	Oral	Intravenous
Number	14	14
Male/female	8/6	8/6
Median age	59 (50-75)	57 (43-74)
Median Karnofsky	70 (40-90)	80 (40-90)
Number prior CT	0	1
Primary tumor		
NSCLC (lung)	4	6
Colorectal	2	5
ENT	2	2
Breast	2	-
Melanoma	2	-
Ovarian	1	-
Renal	1	-
Soft tissue sarcoma	-	1

In patients with measurable disease, tumor response was assessed according to conventional response criteria (6). The starting doses were 5 mg/m^2 for the i.v. formulation and 10 mg/m^2 for the oral trial. These doses corresponded roughly to 1/5-1/7 of the LD10 (mg/m^2) in dogs. For escalation, a modified Fibonacci scheme was used, which is presented in Table 2. Twenty-eight patients with far-advanced malignancies entered the study between November 1980 and April 1981. Fourteen patients entered the i.v. trial, and the same number of cases was considered for the study with the oral formulation. The patients' characteristics are listed in Table 1. The protocol called only for one course of therapy; if continuation of the treatment was medically indicated, the courses were repeated once every 3 weeks. In the trial with the i.v. formulation, all but one patient received one sole course of treatment; evaluation of the toxicity will be presented per patients. On the contrary, in the trial with the oral formulation, in six cases the patients received two courses of therapy; that evaluation will be presented per courses.

Table 2. Patients' entry

Level	Oral mg/m^2	N	Intravenous Mg/m^2	N
I	10	3	5	2
II	20	3	10	2
III	30	1	15	5
IV	40	3	18	5
V	50	4	–	–
Total		14[a]		14[b]

a, Three patients treated at two levels; one patient treated at three levels.
b, One patient treated at two levels.

4. RESULTS

The dose-limiting toxicity was clearly myelosuppression, both for the i.v. as well as for the oral formulation.

4.1. The intravenous trial

The dose-limiting factor was clearly myelosuppression. Twelve patients are completely evaluable for hematologic, gastrointestinal, and cardiac acute toxicity. One patient treated at the first dose-level died of disease progression on day 9 after treatment, another patient treated at 18 mg/m^2 expired on day 16 because of septicemia while in agranulocytosis.

No relevant acute hematologic toxicity was observed among the patients treated at 5 mg/m^2 and 10 mg/m^2. The data are summarized in Table 3. Hematologic toxicity was observed in all five patients treated at 15 mg/m^2. The median nadir of WBC was 1.5 x 10^3/mm^3 (range 0.6-2.0 x 10^3/mm^3) and its median occurrence was on day 9. At this level, thrombocytopenia less than 75.0 x 10^3/mm^3 occurred in three patients; the median nadir of PLT was 66.0 x 10^3/mm^3 (range 42.0-130.0 x 10^3/mm^3) with median occurrence at day 13. WBC and platelet values recovered within 3-6 days. A decrease in hemoglobin levels was constantly observed in all 5 patients, with a median decrease of 1.8 g (range 0.6-5 g) occurring at day 15. At least three of the five patients treated at this level had had a very extensive prior treatment and were known to have reduced bone-marrow resistance to cytotoxic drugs. Four of the five patients had colorectal tumors with liver metastases. All presented at the beginning of the study with an alkaline phosphatase slightly over the upper normal value, while biliburin, GOT, and GPT were in normal ranges.

At 18 mg/m^2, one patient was without prior treatment and the others were known to have a fair hematologic tolerance to chemotherapy. Only two of the five patients had known liver metastases with a minimal increase of alkaline phosphatase. At this level, the median nadir of WBC was 1.0 x 10^3/mm^3 (range 0.1-2.1 x 10^3/mm^3). The median nadir of PLT was 65.0 x 10^3/mm^3 (range: 28-116 x 10^3/mm^3). Both nadirs occurred at day 15 with a recovery within 2-7 days. All five patients showed an important decrease in Hb levels with a median value of 3 g% (range 1.8-3.9 g%). One toxic death occurred on day 16 in a 75-year-old male with an epidermoid carcinoma of the lung. On day 14, he developed septicemia while WBC was 0.1 x 10^3/mm^3.

The nonhematologic toxicity is summarized in Table 4.

At all levels gastrointestinal toxicity was not impressive. No stomatitis was registered. Mild nausea occurred erratically in two patients treated at 10 mg/m^2 and 15 mg/m^2, respectively. At 18 mg/m^2 one patient complained about moderate nausea and vomiting lasting for 3 days. Nausea was generally registered 3-4 hours after the drug administration.

None of the patients showed electrocardiographic changes at the poly-EKG investigations. No objective tumor responses were observed in this trial.

Table 3. Hematologic toxicity in the intravenous trial

Level	Number of patients	Nadir WBC (range) $\times 10^3/\mathrm{mm}^3$	Nadir TC $\times 10^3/\mathrm{mm}^3$
5 mg/m^2	2[a]	7.5	139
10 mg/m^2	2	3.75 (3.5-4.0)	220 (190-250)
15 mg/m^2	5	1.5 (0.6-2.0)	66 (42-130)
18 mg/m^2	5	1.0 (0.1-2.1)	65 (28-116)

a, One patient only partially evaluable (early death).

Table 4. Nonhematologic toxicity in the intravenous trial

mg/m^2	Number of patients	Nausea	Vomiting	Stomatitis	Poly-EKG changes
5	2[a]	0	0	0	−
10	2	2	0	0	−
15	5	0	0	0	0/2
18	5	0	1	0	0/3

a, One patient only partially evaluable (early death).

4.2. The oral trial

Thirteen patients are completely evaluable for hematologic and gastro-intestinal toxicity. One patient treated at the first dose-level died of disease progression on day 8 after treatment; on the second dose-level, one patient died of disease progression on day 16. Six patients received two courses of treatment; therefore, the evaluation is based on 20 courses of therapy. No relevant or consistent acute hematologic toxicity was observed among the patients treated up to 30 mg/m^2. The data are summarized in Table 5. Some hematologic toxicity was observed in three out of five courses carried out with 40 mg/m^2. The median nadir of WBC was 3.8 x 10^3/mm^3 (range 2.5-7.0 x 10^3/mm^3), while the median nadir of platelets was 140.0 x 10^3/mm^3 (range 99.0-205.0 x 10^3/mm^3). At 50 mg/m^2 myelosuppression became prominent. Hematologic toxicity was observed in all seven courses. The median nadir of WBC was 1.1 x 10^3/mm^3 (range 0.2-3.0 x 10^3/mm^3) and its median occurrence was at day 12 (range 9-15) with a median recovery at day 21 (range 19-37). The

Table 5. Hematologic toxicity in the oral trial

Level	Number of courses	Nadir WBC (range) x 10^3/mm^3	Nadir platelets (range) x 10^3/mm^3
10 mg/m^2	3	>4.0	>150.0
20 mg/m^2	3	>4.0	>150.0
30 mg/m^2	2	3.9	>150.0
40 mg/m^2	5	3.8 (2.5-7.0)	140 (99.9-205.0)
50 mg/m^2	7	1.1 (0.2-3.0)	83 (29.0-203.0)

median nadir of platelets was 83.0 x 10^3/mm^3 (range 29.0-203.0 x 10^3/mm^3).
The occurrence of the nadirs and their recovery was similar for the platelets
to the values observed in the case of the WBC. Also for the oral formulation
an important decrease in the Hb levels with a median value of 2.5 g% (range
1.5-3.5 g%) was observed in the seven courses of therapy carried out at
50 mg/m^2.

Only one of the four patients entered at 50 mg/m^2 had known liver metastases with a minimal increase of alkaline phosphatase. However, two of the
patients entered at this level were known to have a suboptimal bone marrow
resistance to cytotoxic drugs.

The nonhematologic toxicity for the oral formulation is summarized in
Table 6. Gastrointestinal toxicity occurred erratically up to 30 mg/m^2. At
40 mg/m^2, patients complained in four instances of mild nausea and vomiting.
Those disturbances, mainly vomiting, became moderate in four out of seven
courses, when the patients received 50 mg/m^2. None of the patients showed
electrocardiographic changes at the poly-EKG investigations. No objective
tumor responses were observed in the trial with the oral formulation; however,
in one case with an ill-defined abdominal mass from a colorectal cancer a
stabilization of the disease (or a minimal tumor regression) with a subjective
improvement of the patient was registered.

5. DISCUSSION

The anthracyclines presently have a major role in the treatment of a
large variety of malignant diseases (7,8). Nevertheless, the long-term use
of these drugs is limited because of their peculiar cardiac toxicity. The
acute toxicity also remains troublesome for many patients. These facts
prompted in the last years a continuous search for analogs having a broader

Table 6. Nonhematologic toxicity in the oral trial

Dose (mg/m^2)	Courses	Nausea/Vomiting	Stomatitis	Poly-EKG changes
10	3[a]	0	0	--
20	3[a]	1	0	--
30	2	1	0	--
40	5	4[b]	0	0/2
50	7	5[c]	1	0/3

a, At this level one drug-unrelated early death.
b, Mild.
c. One-fifth mild, four-fifths moderate.

spectrum of activity and a higher therapeutic index.

4-Demethoxydaunorubicin is a new analog of daunorubicin that showed a definite antitumor activity in experimental animal tumors. Early toxicologic data hint also to a reduced cardiotoxicity as compared to doxorubicin and daunorubicin (5). The possibility of a reduced cardiotoxicity was the main reason that prompted the clinical evaluation of this new analog. Another motivation was clearly the availability of an oral formulation. This route of administration could have a very important practical impact in the treatment of many tumors, provided that the oral formulation proves to have a consistent rate of gastrointestinal absorption.

The results of our phase-I trial with both formulations show that the hematologic toxicity is dose-limiting. The limited difference observed in the intravenous trial in the median nadirs of the blood value registered at 15 mg/m^2 and 18 mg/m^2 can easily be explained by the different characteristics of the patients entered at the two levels. The patients treated with the higher dosage were known to have a better tolerance to chemotherapy and also a somewhat better liver function than did the patients entered at 15 mg/m^2. This observation underscores once more the well-known correlation between hematologic toxicity and liver function in patients treated with anthracyclines. With the oral administration of IMI-30 the pattern of the hematologic toxicity is somewhat less consistent. Particularly at 50 mg/m^2, we observed a nadir similar to the one registered with 18 mg/m^2 given i.v. But the range of the toxicity was wider both for the WBC and for the platelets. Differences in the characteristics of the patients account only partially for this broad range of hematologic toxicity observed with the oral formulation.

This finding probably must be viewed as the result of a somewhat erratic gastrointestinal absorption of the compound. In our patients, we were not able to escalate further the dosage of the oral formulation. Because of the wide range in hematologic toxicity, we feel that we cannot define a maximal tolerated dose sensu stricto.

Compared with doxorubicin and daunorubicin, 4-demethoxydaunorubicin permits a somewhat slower recovery of WBC and platelets and a slightly more pronounced thrombocytopenia.

The finding of an important decrease in the median level of hemoglobin without clinical evidence of hemorrhagic or hemolytic events was surprising. Further investigations of these observations are warranted.

The gastrointestinal toxicity registered in the i.v. trial was less pronounced than is the one normally registered for the parent compound. As expected, the gastrointestinal side effects were more pronounced with the use of the oral formulation. In some patients treated with the oral drug, nausea and vomiting were moderate, if not severe. With the oral formulation, the gastrointestinal toxicity seemed to occur earlier than it did with the drug given i.v. The gastrointestinal toxicity may account, at least partially, for the somewhat more erratic hematologic toxicity that occurred with the oral formulation.

No acute cardiotoxicity was detected, but studies on the chronic cardiotoxicity of this compound still need to be performed.

In conclusion, the toxicity pattern observed in this trial suggests that this analog should be particularly suitable for further clinical evaluation in the treatment of hematologic malignancies. In the therapy of solid tumors, we suggest that 18 mg/m^2 is the maximum tolerated dose for this drug given intravenously. Using the same formulation, we can propose 15 mg/m^2 as a safe starting dose for phase-II trials, provided that the patient has normal liver function and a fair hematologic tolerance for chemotherapy. For the oral formulation, the maximum tolerated dose is in the range of 50-60 mg/m^2; for the single administration, a safe starting dose for phase-II trials in solid tumors with the oral formulation could be 45 mg/m^2. We feel, however, that more experience should be accumulated with the oral formulation before phase-II trials are begun. Particularly, the possibility of dividing the dosage over 2-3 days should be explored in order to avoid or at least to decrease the degree of gastrointestinal toxicity. We are presently completing our pharmacokinetic studies, performed in patients treated with i.v.

and oral formulations (9).

It is hoped, therefore, that these pharmacokinetic results will lead to a better definition of the treatment schedule, mainly for the oral formulations.

REFERENCES

1. Arcamone F, Bernardi L, Biardino P, Patelli B, Di Marco A, Casazza AM, Pratesi G, Reggiani P. 1976. Synthesis and antitumor activity of 4'demethoxydaunorubicin, 4-demethoxy-7,9-diepidaunorubicin, and their β-anomers. Cancer Treat. Rep. 60: 829-834.
2. Supino R, Necco A, Dasdia T, Casazza AM, Di Marco A. 1977. Relationship between effects on nucleic acid synthesis in cell cultures and cytotoxicity of 4-demethoxyderivatives of daunorubicin and adriamycin. Cancer Res. 37: 4523-4528.
3. Di Marco A, Casazza AM, Pratesi G, 1977. Antitumor activity of 4'-demethoxydaunorubicin administered orally. Cancer Treat. Rep. 61: 893-894.
4. Casazza AM. 1979. Experimental evaluation of anthracycline analogues. Cancer Treat. Rep. 63: 835-844.
5. Casazza AM, Bertazzoli C, Pratesi G, Bellini O, Di Marco A. 1979. Antileukemic activity and cardiac toxicity of 4-demethoxydaunorubicin (4-DMD). Proc. Am. Assoc. Cancer Res. 20: 16.
6. WHhandbook for reporting results of cancer treatment. 1979. WHO, Geneva.
7. Carter SK. 1980. The clinical evaluation of analogues. III. Anthracyclines. Cancer Chemother. Pharmac. 4: 5-10.
8. Young RC, Ozols RF, Myers CE. 1981. The anthracycline antineoplastic drugs. New Engl. J. Med. 305: 139-153.
9. Martini A, Cavalli F. In preparation. The pharmacokinetic of 4-demethoxydaunorubicin.

CLINICAL STUDIES OF NEW ANTHRACYCLINE ANALOGS

C. W. YOUNG, R. WITTES, P. DEESEN, B. JONES, E. CASPER, AND
R. WARRELL

1. INTRODUCTION

Daunorubicin and doxorubicin (or adriamycin) are among
the most important of our current cancer chemotherapeutic
drugs. They are key components in current therapy of acute
leukemia, malignant lymphoma, breast cancer, thyroid cancer,
and a variety of sarcomas. Although they are valuable therapeutic tools, they do have limitations and liabilities that
have stimulated intense efforts to obtain analogues having
a broader therapeutic spectrum and reduced toxicity; in
particular, there is a desire to acquire drugs with a lessened cardiac toxicity. A remarkable number of analogues with
diverse structural variations on the anthracycline theme have
been isolated or synthesized. A smaller number of these have
entered into clinical trial. This communication will examine
studies at the Memorial Sloan-Kettering Cancer Center and
summarize the current status of Phase II and clinical pharmacologic evaluation of 4'-epi-doxorubicin, Phase I and Phase II
evaluation of aclacinomycin in leukemia, and the early results
of our Phase I trial of 4-demethoxy-daunorubicin.

2. PHASE II STUDIES OF 4'-EPI-DOXORUBICIN

4'-Epi-doxorubicin was selected for advancement to clinical
trial because of its broad spectrum of antitumor activity, comparable to that of doxorubicin in animal tumor systems, and its
lessened overall toxicity (1,2). It was somewhat less cardiotoxic
in model systems (2). Phase I studies showed myelosuppression to
be the dose-limiting acute toxic effect (3,4,5); antitumor effects
were seen in patients with cancer arising in the kidney or colon
and in malignant melanoma (3,4).

At the Memorial Sloan-Kettering Cancer Center disease-oriented Phase II evaluation has been initiated in patients with non-small-cell lung carcinoma, colorectal carcinoma, renal carcinoma, head and neck carcinoma, breast carcinoma and malignant melanoma. The breast cancer study is constructed as a randomized comparison of 4'-epi-doxorubicin with doxorubicin in previously treated patients with advanced disease who have not received prior anthracycline therapy; the other trials are non-randomized evaluations. All patients had bidimensionally measurable disease; all had a Performance Status capable of out-patient therapy. Sixty-two of the 129 patients had received no prior chemotherapy. The drug was administered by brief intravenous infusion over 15 minutes every 21 days. The initial dosage was $85mg/m^2$; the dose was escalated at a rate of $15mg/m^2$/cycle in the absence of significant myelosuppression. The criteria employed for Complete Remission (CR), Partial Remission (PR), Minor Response (MR), No Change (NC) and Progression are those in general use at the present time. The therapeutic results in five cancer varieties are provided in Table 1.

Table 1. Therapeutic response in Phase II evaluation of 4'-epi-doxorubicin in 129 patients with advanced cancer.

Diagnosis	# of Pts Entered	No Prior Chemo Rx	Median PS	PR	MR	NC	PROG
Non-small cell lung ca	39	15	70	1	1	2	31
Colorectal ca	32	11	90	1	0	1	30
Renal ca	18	10	80	0	0	0	15
Melanoma	25	15	80	1	3	4	12
Head and neck ca	15	11	80	2	0	0	6
Totals:	129	62	--	5	4	7	94

Isolated Partial Remissions were observed in the previously untreated patients with non-small-cell lung cancer and 1 previously treated patient with colorectal cancer. Although the NSC lung cancer study is not yet concluded, it appears unlikely that 4'-epi-doxorubicin will have major therapeutic activity in these two disorders. Similarly, although patient accrual will continue in renal cancer because of the favorable reports from Phase I and II studies in Europe, our failure to observe objective antitumor effect in 15 evaluable patients is not encouraging.

The still preliminary results with melanoma and with head and neck cancer are somewhat more encouraging. Objective antitumor effect was seen in 4 of 20 evaluable patients with malignant melanoma and in 2 of 8 evaluable patients with head and neck carcinoma. These responses were observed in patients receiving 4'-epi-doxorubicin as initial therapy. Although not dramatic these results fully justify more extended study of the drug in these two disorders.

2.1 Studies in breast cancer. Randomized comparison of 4'-epi-doxorubicin with doxorubicin has been initiated enlisting previously treated patients with advanced breast cancer. None of the patients had received exposure to anthracyclines prior to entering this comparative trial. Both drugs were given by 15-minute intravenous infusion every 21 days; the starting dosages were: 4'epi-doxorubicin $85mg/m^2$, doxorubicin $60mg/m^2$. In the absence of myelosuppression each drug could be escalated by 20% of the prior dose. We are following the patients for therapeutic and toxic effects. We are monitoring for cardiotoxic effects by obtaining gated cardiac blood pool scans without and with exercise after drug dosages 3, 5,7,8,9, etc. The therapeutic results are shown in Table 2. Clear cardiac toxicity has not yet been reached with either drug.

Table 2. Comparison of 4'epi-doxorubicin and doxorubicin in previously treated patients with advanced breast cancer: preliminary results

	# of Patients		Best Response Observed				
	Entered	Eval	CR	PR	MR	NC	PROG
4'Epi-doxorubicin	13	9	--	2*	--	5	2
Doxorubicin	12	8	--	2*	2	2	2

*Duration: 4'Epi-doxorubicin 7+ and 7+ months, Doxorubicin 9 and 2+ months

2.2 Toxic effects of 4'Epi-doxorubicin. 4'Epi-doxorubicin produced mild to moderate nausea and vomiting, alopecia, mucositis, fatigue and occasional fevers. Although not fully quantifiable these side effects appeared somewhat less severe than what would be expected from comparably myelosuppressive doses of doxorubicin. As illustrated in Table 3 the acute dose-limiting side effect was myelosuppression: leukopenia usually exceeded thrombocytopenia.

Table 3. Hematopoietic effects of therapy with 4'epi-doxorubicin

Diagnosis	Hematologic Nadirs* Leukocytes Median	Thrombocytes Median	Gms ↓ in Hemoglobin Median
Lung cancer	3.6	250	2.1
Colorectal cancer	2.6	184	1.6
Renal cancer	3.2	255	2.2
Melanoma	2.7	203	1.6
Head and Neck cancer	3.5	223	1.9
All diagnoses *x 10^3	3.1	203	1.9

3. CLINICAL PHARMACOLOGIC STUDIES OF 4'EPI-DOXORUBICIN

We have developed a high pressure liquid chromatography (HPLC) method for the measurement of 4'epi-doxorubicin and its metabolites in plasma and urine of patients receiving the drug. The extraction procedure the HPLC conditions and the retention times for various standards are provided in Table 4.

Table 4. Extraction procedures, HPLC conditions and elution volumes of 4'epi-doxorubicin and known metabolites.

Extraction procedure

0.5ml or 1.0ml plasma with 150ng or 300ng daunorubicin as an internal standard

2ml 1:1 methylene chloride:isopropanol

1.0-1.5g ammonium sulfate

Centrifuge at 2000g for 15 min

The top (organic) layer is removed and taken to dryness under N_2 at 25°

The extract is dissolved in the initial buffer A

HPLC conditions

Column: μBondapak phenyl' (Waters Associates)

Mobile phase: A: .05M KH_2PO_4 pH 3.0

B: 65:35 CH_3CN: .05M KH_2PO_4 pH 3.0

Gradient: Linear from 0 to 60% B over 25 minutes

```
Flow rate: 2.5ml/minute
Injection volume: 100μl
Detection: Fluorescence. Ex 470nm Em 585nm
Detection limit: 1ng/injection, 5ng/ml out of plasma
```

Retention times

4'Epi-doxorubicinol E2	17.9 min
Doxorubicinol aglycone A2a	18.8 min
4'Epi-doxorubicin E1	19.4 min
7 Deoxydoxorubicinol aglycone dA2a	20.4 min
Doxorubicin aglycone Ala	20.4 min
Daunorubicin DN	21.2 min
7 Deoxydoxorubicin aglycone dAla	22.8 min

The pharmacokinetic studies are still in their initial phase; the three patients studied to date received 50,60 and 60mg/m^2 4'epi-doxorubicin respectively. The mean terminal half-life of the parent compound was 499 ± 182 (SD) minutes. The mean apparent volume of distribution was 3214 ± 1546ml/kg. The mean metabolic clearance rate was 4.3 ± 1.0 (ml/min)/kg. We have also observed 4'epi-doxorubicinol, 7 deoxy-doxorubicin aglycone and one, as yet uncharacterized metabolite in plasma of patients receiving 4'epi-doxorubicin; definition of the relative proportions of these metabolites will require further patient studies. Figure 1 demonstrates the pharmacokinetic pattern in a patient who received 60mg/m^2 of 4'epi-doxorubicin.

4. PRELIMINARY RESULTS OF THE PHASE I TRIAL OF 4-DEMETHOXY-
    DAUNORUBICIN

4-Demethoxydaunorubicin has been advanced to clinical trial because of its therapeutic superiority on intravenous administration, to either daunorubicin or doxorubicin against intravenously administered Ll210 leukemia and Gross leukemia. Moreover, 4-demethoxydaunorubicin was also therapeutically highly active against transplanted murine leukemia when administered by the oral route (6,7). In addition, 4-demethoxydaunorubicin is significantly less cardiotoxic than is daunorubicin; by the oral route it appears to be devoid of cardiac toxicity in rats and dogs (6).

To date in the Phase I study at the Memorial Sloan-Kettering Cancer Center 4-demethoxydaunorubicin has been

Figure 1.

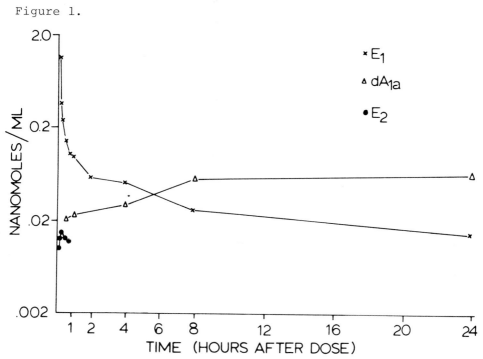

administered by 15 minute intravenous infusion at intervals
of 21 days. Following completion of the intravenous study,
we will initiate dose finding by the oral route. Twenty-
two patients have been enlisted in the study; these include:
carcinoma of the lung 12, of the breast 2, of the colon 3,
of head and neck 1, of ovary 1, of pancreas 1, unknown
primary 1, and melanoma 1. The median (Karnofsky) Performance Status was 70%. Seventeen patients had received prior
chemotherapy; only two were previously untreated.

Although we have not fully defined a maximally tolerated
dose it appears likely that the acute dose-limiting toxic
effect of this drug will be myelosuppression. The detailed
results for the first three dosage levels are provided in
Table 5. Our data are consistent with the reports from
Europe wherein a MTD of 15 to 18mg/m^2 was observed. To
this date we have not observed significant mucositis, nausea,
vomiting or fatigue or change in cardiac funtion. A
separate further escalation sequence will be required to

define a proper dosage schedule for treatment of acute
leukemia.

Table 5. Hematopoietic toxicity of 4 demethoxydaunorubicin
in patients with advanced cancer

Drug dosage*	# of Pts Ent	Eval	Median WBC	Day	Nadirs** Plt	Day
5mg/m^2	4	4	4.7	-	302	-
10mg/m^2	10	9	3.1	15	206	-
12.5mg/m^2	8	7	2.4	15	187	13

*Intravenous administration q 21 days   **x 10^{-3}

As yet we have not observed objective antitumor effects
in these patients.

5. EARLY CLINICAL STUDIES OF ACLACINOMYCIN A

5.1. Phase I studies in non-leukemic patients

Aclacinomycin A possesses 3 sugars, rhodosamine, 2-
deoxyfucose and cinerulose, linked by glycosidic bonds,
attached to the anthracycline ring at C-7 (8). Aclacinomycin
A was chosen for advancement to clinical evaluation because
of its antitumor activity against a spectrum of transplanted
murine tumors (9) and its apparently reduced cardiac toxicity
in the golden hamster model (10). Although transient
electrocardiographic changes were noted both in preclinical
toxicology and in earlier clinical studies cardiomyopathy
has not been reported as a significant clinical problem
to date.

Phase I evaluation at the Memorial Sloan-Kettering
Cancer Center included 25 adult patients with solid tumors.
Exploring a dosage range of aclacinomycin A of 60 to 120mg/m^2
intravenously every 3 to 4 weeks, we observed myelosuppression to be the dose-limiting toxic effect (11). Drug induced leukopenia and thrombocytopenia were comparably severe;
120mg/m^2 every 3 weeks appears to be a reasonable Phase II
dosage for good-risk patients. The drug also produced
moderate nausea and vomiting but negligible mucositis; alopecia was seen in approximately one-third of treated patients.
In this limited trial we observed only minor therapeutic

effects in one patient with breast cancer; in the majority
of the patients the disease was non-measurable.

5.2. Phase I-II evaluation in acute leukemia

Aclacinomycin-A has been reported to be an active antileukemic agent in clinical studies both in Europe (12) and
Japan (13). We are carrying out an evaluation of aclacinomycin A in heavily pretreated patients with acute leukemia
using a daily x 3 schedule that began with twice a dose that
produced marrow hypoplasia in patients with solid tumors (14).
The drug was given intravenously daily for 2 or 3 days; the
bone marrow was assessed for the degree of hypoplasia 7 to 10
days following the last dose of chemotherapy. The marrow was
repeated at 7 to 10 day intervals thereafter to assess therapeutic response. A complete remission was defined as $\leq$ 5%
blasts on two determinations at least 7 days apart with peripheral hemoglobin $\geq$ 10gm%, leukocyte count $\geq$ 4,000 with a
normal differential smear and platelets $\geq$ 100,000.

The population of 21 patients with acute non-lymphoblastic leukemia had a median Karnofsky Performance Status of
40%, median age of 31 and a median prior total anthracycline
dose of 360mg/m^2. All patients had relatively normal hepatic
and renal function (bilirubin and creatinine < 1.5 mg/dl), and
gated cardiac blood pool scan, a resting left ventricular
ejection fraction $\geq$ .5.

It required at least 100mg/m^2/day x 3 days of aclacinomycin therapy to clear the tumor cells from the bone marrow
(Table 6). Since not all patients obtained clearing of tumor
cells even at that dosage we have begun exploring a dose of
120mg/m^2/day x 3 days. We have observed complete remission
of leukemia in 3 patients; although our response percentage
is lower than that reported elsewhere (12,13) it may reflect
differences among the groups with regard to the intensity
of prior therapy.

512

Table 6. Response to aclacinomycin-A of 21 heavily pretreat-
          ed patients with acute non-lymphoblastic leukemia

Dose (mg/m^2/day)	# of Pts Entered	Hypoplastic	CR	Remission Duration (wks)
100 x 2	2	0	0	
100 x 3	16	10	3	4, 10+, 24+
120 x 3	3	1	0	

The major toxic effect of this therapy has been profound and prolonged bone marrow depression. The hemorrhagic
and infectious consequences of leukemia and of its treatment
present severe management problems. The degree and duration
of myelosuppression we observed in these patients treated
with aclacinomycin is comparable to that we have observed in
similar patients treated with other new drugs such as AMSA
or combination regimens. We did observe abnormalities in
liver function tests in many of these patients but hepatotoxicity was not a serious problem. Perhaps of greater concern was that serial electrocardiograms revealed a reversible
pattern of acute cardiac injury (T-wave inversion, ST-T
depression and, in some patients, transient elevation of cardiac enzymes in peripheral blood), in the majority of patients
receiving 100 to 120mg/m^2/day x 3 days. We have not as yet
observed progression to congestive failure or a typical
anthracycline cardiomyopathy.

6.   COMMENTARY
     We are in an exciting period with regard to drug
development in anthracyclines at the clinical level. There
appears to be a real possibility that the differing therapeutic and toxic effects that characterize the activity of
doxorubicin and daunorubicin can be separated by a series of
structural modifications of the drug molecules. 4'Epi-
doxorubicin appears to be less toxic in animal models with
comparable activity to doxorubicin. Similarly, 4-Demothoxy-
daunorubicin is active by mouth and clearly less cardiotoxic
than daunorubicin in mice, rats and dogs.
     The clinical studies are still early but there is clear
evidence that 4'epi-doxorubicin has activity against

breast cancer and promising activity also in head and neck
cancer and possibly melanoma. In time we should be able to
define in breast cancer patients the comparative utility
and cardiotoxicity of 4'epi-doxorubicin with the newer tools
of the gated cardiac blood pool scan and endomyocardial
biopsy. The more subjective toxicities of malaise, nausea
and vomiting and alopecia are also susceptible to quantitation by an objective observer and proper protocol design.
The time seems favorable for significant progress in this
important area of cancer therapeutics.

REFERENCES

1. Arcamone F, Penco S, Vigevani A, Redaelli S, Franchi S,
    DiMarco A, Casazza AM, Dasdia T, Formelli F, Necco A,
    Soranzo C: Synthesis and antitumor properties of new
    glycosides of daunomycinone and adriamycinone. J Med
    Chem 18: 703-707, 1975.
2. Casazza AM, DiMarco A, Bertazzoli C, Formelli F,
    Giuliani F, Pratesi G: Antitumor activity, toxicity and
    pharmacological properties of 4'Epiadriamycin. In:
    Proceedings of the 10th International Congress of
    Chemotherapy, Zurich, Switzerland, Sept 1977 Washington,
    DC, American Society of Microbiology 1978, vol 2, p
    1257-1260.
3. Bonfante V, Bonadonna G, Villani F, DiFronzo G, Martini
    A, Casazza AM: Preliminary phase I study of 4'-epi-adria-
    mycin. Cancer Treat Rep 63: 915-918, 1979.
4. Bonfante V, Bonadonna G, Villani F, Martini A: Pre-
    liminary clinical experience with 4'-epi-doxorubicin in
    advanced human neoplasia. In Recent Results in Cancer
    Research (eds): Springer Verlag, vol 74 1980, p 202-209.
5. Schauer P, Wittes R, Gralla R, Young C: A phase I trial
    of 4'-epi-adriamycin. Cancer Clinical Trials, in press.
6. Casazza AM: Experimental evaluation of anthracycline
    analogs. Cancer Treat Rep 63: 835-844, 1979.
7. Casazza AM, Pratesi G, Giuliani F, DiMarco A: Anti-
    leukemic activity of 4-demethoxydaunorubicin in mice.
    Tumori 66: 549-564, 1980.
8. Oki T, Matsuzawa Y, Yoshimoto A, Numata K, Kitamura I,
    Hori S, Takamutsu A, Umezawa J, Ishizuka M, Naganawa H,
    Suda J, Hamada M, Takenchi T: New antitumor antibiotics
    aclacinomycins A and B. J Antibiot (Tokyo) 28: 830-834,
    1975.
9. Oki T: New anthracycline antibiotics. Japan J Antibiot
    30(Suppl): 70-84, 1977.
10. Dantchev D, Sliousartchouk V, Paintrand M, Hayat M,
    Bourut C, Mathé G: Electron microscopic studies of the
    heart and light microscopic studies of the skin after
    treatment of golden hamsters with adriamycin, deto-

rubicin, AD-32 and aclacinomycin. Cancer Treat Rep 63: 875-888, 1979.

11. Casper ES, Gralla RJ, Young CW: Clinical phase I study of aclacinomycin A by evaluation of an intermittent intravenous administration schedule. Cancer Res 41: 2417-2420, 1981.

12. Mathé G, Bayssas M, Gouveia J, Dantchev D, Ribaud P, Machover D, Misset JL, Schwarzenberg L, Jasmin C, Hayat M: Preliminary results of a phase II trial of aclacinomycin in acute leukemia and lymphosarcoma. Cancer chemother Pharmacol 1: 259-262, 1978.

13. Suzuki H, Kwashima K, Yamada K: Aclacinomycin-A, a new antileukemic agent. Lancet 2: 870-871, 1979.

14. Warrell RP Jr, Arlin Z, Gee T, Lacher M, Young C: Phase I-II evaluations of aclacinomycin-A in acute leukemia. Proc Amer Assoc Cancer Res 22: 191, 1981.

A CLINICAL OVERVIEW OF ACLACINOMYCIN A IN JAPAN

M. OGAWA

1. INTRODUCTION

A new anthracycline, aclacinomycin A (ACM-A), was isolated from a
culture filtrate of Streptomyces galilaeus, MA144-M1, by Oki, Umezawa,
and coworkers (1-3). The compound is one of the class II anthracyclines,
which mainly inhibit RNA synthesis (4,5); class I anthracyclines, such as
Adriamycin and carminomycin, mainly inhibit DNA synthesis.

In various animal tumors tested (3,4,6,7), ACM-A demonstrated
antitumor activity superior to Adriamycin in human xenograft tumors,
CD mouse mammary carcinoma, and colon 38, although it was less active
in L1210 and P388 leukemias.

Comparative toxocological studies (3,4,6,8) of EKG abnormalities
and histopathological findings, and electron microscopic examination
of myocardial changes in hamsters demonstrated that ACM-A produced a
milder cardiac toxicity than did Adriamycin or daunomycin; in addition,
there are indications that these myocardial changes are reversible up to
certain cumulative doses (8).

Furue et al. (9,10) reported on an initial clinical study, and
large-scale phase I-II studies have been performed since then. Several
reviews were published previously (4,6,11,12); however, I will summarize
in this chapter the results collected from published literature in which
assessments of responses were clearly described. Patients treated with
local injections including intraperitoneal and intraarterial infusion
or bladder instillation were excluded from the analysis.

Criteria to assess responses in solid tumors and lymphomas were
basically identical to those documented in the WHO handbook (13). Karnofsky's
method (14) arranges responses as follows: 1-C, complete response (CR);
1-B, partial response (PR); and 1-A, minor response (MR). MR was listed
in tables but it was not included in calculations of response rate. For
acute leukemias, all investigators employed Kimura's criteria (15) to assess

remissions, but these criteria are nearly identical to ALGB criteria described by Ellison (16) for acute leukemias.

2. PHASE I STUDY

The results obtained in four phase I studies are summarized in Table 1.

Table 1. Phase I study of aclacinomycin A

Author	Year	Schedule	Maximum tolerated dose	Recommended dose for phase II study	Dose-limiting toxicity
Furue	1977	daily	30 mg/day	20 mg/day	gastrointestinal toxicity
Sakano	1978	a single dose	70 mg/m^2	70 mg/m^2	leukopenia, thrombocytopenia
Majima	1978	weekly	3.75 mg/kg (120 mg/m^2)*	2.5 mg/kg (80 mg/m^2)*	leukopenia, thrombocytopenia
Ogawa	1979	a single dose	133 mg/m^2	100-120 mg/m^2	leukopenia, thrombocytopenia, hepatotoxicity

*Approximate values calculated by author.

Furue et al. (9,10) conducted a preliminary phase I study in 22 patients with various malignant tumors. Using daily dosages ranging from 10 mg to 30 mg, they administered a total dose exceeding 300 mg. They found that nausea and vomiting were frequently seen in a daily dose of 30 mg; furthermore, hepatic dysfunction was observed in five patients administered a total dose of more than 200 mg; and mild hematologic toxicity occurred from administration of a total dose of 300-350 mg. They concluded, therefore, that gastrointestinal toxicity was the dose-limiting factor of ACM-A.

Sakano et al. (17) administered ACM-A to 22 patients, using a single dose that escalated from 15 mg/m^2 to 70 mg/m^2. They observed mild gastrointestinal toxicity in five patients and mild hepatotoxicity in three patients; dose-limiting toxicities in this study were leukopenia and thrombocytopenia, which were significant from 50 mg/m^2. Thus, they concluded that the hematologic toxicity was dose dependent.

Majima et al. (18), employing weekly dosages ranging from 20 mg to 180 mg, gave ACM-A to 11 patients. These researchers found that dose-limiting toxicities were leukopenia and thrombocytopenia, which were seen in patients who had received a cumulative dose of approximately 10 mg/kg. They recommended use of 2.5 mg/kg weekly for four times up to a total dose of 10 mg/kg for phase II study.

My colleagues and I (19) administered a single dose, gradually escalating it from 0.4 mg/kg to 4 mg/kg in 3- to 4-week intervals, to a total of 15 patients with various advanced tumors. We found gastrointestinal toxicity to be mild to moderate and not related to dose escalations. Since previous studies (9,10,17) had indicated hepatotoxicity, we carefully monitored changes of hepatic enzymes. In four patients who had been administered a single dose of 3.5-4 mg/kg, the SGOT, the SGPT became significantly higher in 3-7 days; however, these parameters returned to normal levels within 7-11 days thereafter. Leukopenia and thrombocytopenia occurred in all of the patients who had been given drug dosages of more than 3.0 mg/kg. Leukopenia reached a nadir in 13-18 days, whereas nadirs of thrombocytopenia had occurred approximately 1 week earlier. Thus, we concluded that both hematologic and hepatic toxicities were dose limiting, and 2.5-3.0 mg/kg (100-120 mg/m^2) administered in 3-week intervals was the recommended dose for phase II study.

In the phase I studies shown in Table 1, EKG changes, including abnormality of ST-T waves and sinus tachycardia, were observed in a few patients, but these abnormalities were transient and reversible. Epilation was also extremely mild.

3. ANTITUMOR EFFICACY

3.1. Hematologic tumors

Suzuki et al. (20) reported a complete regression (CR) in a patient with acute myeloblastic leukemia that had become refractory to a combination chemotherapy consisting of daunomycin, cytarabine, 6-mercaptopurine, and prednisolone (DCMP). They infused 20 mg daily for 20 days and obtained CR on day 30. Thereafter, two institutions (18,19) and a cooperative study group (30) performed phase II studies in acute leukemias. The results are summarized in Table 2.

In a previously untreated cohort of 24 patients with acute nonlympho-cytic leukemia (ANNL), there were nine CRs (37.5%) and four PRs; whereas in 46 patients who had been treated previously, there were nine CRs (19.6%) and six PRs.

Nearly all patients who had had prior chemotherapy were treated with

Table 2. Phase II study in hematologic tumors

Disease	Prior chemo- therapy		Number of patients	Responders		Response rate (%)		References
				CR	PR	CR	CR+PR	
Acute	ANNL	(−)	24	9	4	37.5	54.2	21,22
leukemias	ANNL	(+)	46	9	6	19.6	32.6	21-23
	ALL	(+)	16	2	0	12.5	12.5	21-23
Lymphomas	NHL	(±)	15	4	3	26.7	46.7	18,19,21,24,25
	HD	(±)	4	0	1	0	25.0	9,24,26

Note: ANNL, acute nonlymphocytic leukemia; ALL, acute lymphocytic leukemia; NHL, non-Hodgkin's lymphoma; HD, Hodgkin's disease

combinations similar to DCMP containing daunomycin, cytarabine, and others, so that the results indicate that ACM-A has no clinical cross-resistance to these agents.

In a total of 16 patients with acute lymphocytic leukemia (ALL) who had been treated previously with various regimens containing vincristine (VCR) there were two CRs (12.5%).

The median duration of remissions of these patients who had attained CR is not known, because they were subsequently treated with various combinations containing other antileukemic agents as early intensification treatment.

Takubo et al. (19) and Furue et al. (9,10) reported hematological improvements accompanying shrinkage of splenomegaly in three out of four patients with chronic myelogenous leukemia. In a total of 15 patients with non-Hodgkin's lymphomas, of whom the majority had had prior chemotherapy, there were four CRs (26.7%) and three PRs; the median duration of the remissions was approximately 4 weeks. It is interesting to note that among six patients who had had previous regimens containing Adriamycin, one CR and two PRs were attained. This suggests that ACM-A has no cross-resistance to Adriamycin. Only four patients with Hodgkin's disease were treated with ACM-A alone and, of these, one PR was reported.

3.2. Solid tumors

3.2. Solid tumors

In a total of 100 patients with advanced gastric cancer, there were eight PRs (8%) and 16 MRs (16%), and the duration of PRs ranged from 4 to 6 weeks (Table 3).

The largest phase II study in solid tumors was performed by Kikuchi and coworkers (24) in the Tohoku area study group. They used four different

Table 3. Clinical efficacy of aclacinomycin A in solid tumors

Disease	Number of patients	Responders CR	PR	MR	CR+PR (%)	Reference
Gastric cancer	100	0	8	16	8.0	24,26-31
Breast cancer	37	0	4	7	10.8	9,10,18,19,24-26,31,32
Ovarian cancer	15	0	0	3	0	18,24,26,31,33
Colorectal cancer	13	0	0	2	0	24,26-29,31
Esophageal cancer	3	0	1	0	33.3	26,28,31
Lung cancer, small-cell	6	0	0	2	0	28,34
Lung cancer, non-small cell	18	0	1	4	5.6	28,34
Leiomyosarcoma	4	0	1	1	25.0	18,24,28
Pancreatic cancer	3	0	0	0	0	28,29,31

weekly schedules: 40 mg, days 1 and 4; 40 mg, days 1 and 2; 50 mg, days 1 and 2; and 40 mg, day 1 and 60 mg, day 4. Although this study was not a randomized trial, it did indicate that the first schedule, 40 mg on days 1 and 4 until total dosages of 300-500 mg had been reached, was the most effective of the four regimens.

In a total of 37 patients with advanced breast cancer, there were four PRs (10.8%) and seven MRs (18.9%), but durations of PRs were not described.

Nomura et al. (32) administered daily dosages of 20 mg for 5 days or 20 to 60 mg two to three times per week to 13 patients with advanced breast cancer. Ten patients had been treated with regimens containing Adriamycin, and two patients had had prior chemotherapy containing mitomycin C. None of the previously treated patients responded, whereas one patient who had had no prior chemotherapy showed a PR that continued for 4 months. This indicated that ACM-A has clinical cross-resistance to Adriamycin at the dose schedules used in this study.

No PR was seen in a total of 15 patients with ovarian cancer, but three MRs were reported. No PR was seen in a total of 13 patients with colorectal cancer, but two MRs were observed.

Yokoyama et al. (26) reported that one patient with esophageal cancer had shrinkage of more than 50% in metastasis to the abdominal wall. In a total of 24 patients with various histological types of lung cancer, one PR

was seen in a patient with adenocarcinoma and another six patients had MRs.
In a total of four patients with leiomyosarcomas, there was one PR that
continued for more than 1 month.

4. TOXICITY

4.1. Hematologic toxicity

As previously described in phase I studies, hematologic toxicity is a
dose-limiting toxicity, one seen in the three major dose schedules investigated, as summarized in Table 4.

Table 4. Hematologic toxicity

Dosage and schedule	Nadir $(X10^3/mm^3)$	Days to nadir	Days to recovery	Reference
L e u k o p e n i a				
20 mg/body,* daily	1.2 (0.2-6.7)**	20	--	22
20-60 mg, 2-3/week	1.9 (0.8-6.8)	48 (27-123)	--	31
100-120 mg/m^2	0.3-2.1	13-18	7-16	19
T h r o m b o c y t o p e n i a				
20 mg/body,* daily	9 (2-46)	18	--	22
20 mg/body, 2-3/week	39 (8-68)	33 (17-90)	--	31
100-120 mg/m^2	4-35	7-15	4-16	19

* Patients with acute leukemias.
** Range in parentheses.

Yamada et al. (22) used a daily schedule of 20 mg/body in patients
with acute leukemias in order to induce remissions and, in this schedule,
the nadir of peripheral leukocytes occurred in a median day of 20 and
that of platelets, in a median day of 18; thus, the median total dose required
to reach this target point was more than 200 mg, and recovery was not clearly
documented. Remissions were attained in days ranging from 1 to 2 weeks after
cessation of treatment.

Nakai et al. (31) administered 20 or 40 mg two to three times weekly to
most patients and, if tolerated, 60 mg twice weekly was given. Hematologic
toxicity was related to a total dose, and most patients who received a dose
of more than 300 mg developed leukopenia and thrombocytopenia that reached
nadirs at median days 48 and 33, respectively. In this study, anemia was

noted in nine patients (16%).

4.2. Nonhematologic toxicity

Nonhematologic toxicities seen in two large studies are summarized in Table 5.

Table 5. Clinical toxicity of aclacinomycin A

Toxicities	D o s a g e s	
	0.4-1.0 mg/kg, 2-3X/week (%)	20 mg/body, daily (%)
Nausea and vomiting	55.4	38
Anorexia	45.4	32
Fever	7.6	--
Lassitude	5.0	--
Phlebitis	5.0	10
Stomatitis	4.2	32
EKG changes	3.4	10.6
Hepatotoxicity	3.4	6
Renal dysfunction	--	3
Diarrhea	1.7	12
Alopecia	0.8	1
TOTAL NUMBER OF PATIENTS	119	62

Kikuchi et al. (27) employed four different methods of administration, as previously described. The overall incidence of toxicities did not differ greatly in the various schedules. They noted gastrointestinal toxicities such as anorexia, nausea, and vomiting in about one-half of the patients but these symptoms were generally mild. Phlebitis and stomatitis were observed in a few patients.

Yamada et al. (22) found a slightly lower incidence of gastrointestinal toxicity but noted a higher incidence of phlebitis and stomatitis. It is possible that a daily chronic schedule may damage veins more frequently and also may cause more stomatitis.

Hepatotoxicity in both studies was mild and reversible, but, because these researchers used relatively lower doses of ACM-A, the incidence of hepatotoxicity in higher intermittent doses remains unknown. The incidence of EKG abnormality seen in both studies was 3.4 and 16.6%, respectively. In other studies (18,21,23,24,28,31), EKG changes ranged from 0% to 10%. Abnormalities related to ACM-A were sinus tachycardia, changes of ST-T waves, or arrhythmias. These abnormalities occurred in cumulative dosages ranging from 120 to 240 mg. The highest incidence was reported by Yamada et al. (22) in patients with acute leukemia, but this finding may relate partially either to the natural history of the disease or to previously administered daunomycin. These EKG abnormalities were reported to be transient and reversible, and none of the patients developed congestive heart failure.

5. DISCUSSION

5.1. The optimal dose for clinical use

When a daily continual schedule of 20 mg was administered, ACM-A had to be discontinued at cumulative doses between 300 and 400 mg because of hematologic toxicity. This method has proven successful in treatment of acute leukemias and lymphomas, and similar response rates have been attained in other countries.

In solid tumors, various schedules have been tested: mostly daily continual doses, as previously described, or 20-60 mg two to three times weekly. Overall, there has been no clear-cut relationship between antitumor efficacy and dosages employed.

There has been no published phase II study that employed either a 5-day schedule or a high-dose, intermittent schedule.

5.2. Antitumor efficacy

Table 2 summarizes the antitumor activity of ACM-A in hematologic tumors. In ANNL, ALL, and non-Hodgkin's lymphomas, the response rates reported here are similar to those reported from France (35). In the French studies, the complete response rate for ANNL was 23% (4/17) in previously treated patients (35), while the complete response rate in previously treated patients with ALL was initially 11% (1/9) (36), and at a later follow-up was 10% (2/19) (35). Taken together with the data reported here, it appears that the clinical efficacy of ACM-A in ALL may be inferior to that in ANNL. In non-Hodgkin's lymphoma, the 46% CR+PR from our group compares favorably with the 50% response (CR+PR) rate in the French studies (35).

In solid tumors, ACM-A has obtained a response rate of 8% in advanced gastric cancer and 10.8% in breast cancer. However, most patients with breast cancer in Japan had had prior chemotherapy with drugs containing Adriamycin; thus, this previous treatment may have adversely affected the outcome for ACM-A.

There have not been sufficient numbers of patients with other malignant tumors to allow us to evaluate the clinical effectiveness of ACM-A in their treatment. It may be mentioned, however, that this drug does not appear to be so active for ovarian cancer, colorectal cancer, and non-oat-cell cancer of the lung, although the latter two malignancies are known to be unresponsive to chemotherapy.

It is of interest that PR was seen in one patient with esophageal cancer and one with leiomyosarcoma.

5.3. Toxicity

Hematologic toxicity is a dose-limiting toxicity of ACM-A. When used continually in a schedule of 20 mg/day and when used intermittently at a dose of 100-120 mg/m^2 every 4 weeks, leukopenia reached a nadir in about 2 weeks, with recovery within 2 weeks. Thrombocytopenia reached a nadir about 1 week earlier but time required for recovery was similar to that needed with leukopenia.

Recently two phase I studies (37,38) were reported that used escalating schedules of a single dose of ACM-A; in these studies, the limiting toxic dose was 100 mg/m^2 in good-performance-status patients.

Nonhematological toxicities of ACM-A have been generally milder than those of Adriamycin, with only mild to moderate gastrointestinal toxicity and rare episodes of alopecia. Hepatotoxicity may be dose-limiting above 120 mg/m^2; however, as most investigators have used smaller doses, this is still uncertain.

Most patients with solid tumors, except breast cancer, had not previously been exposed to regimens containing Adriamycin, whereas nearly all patients with acute leukemia had been treated with regimens containing daunomycin. Therefore, the increased rate of change of EKG seen in leukemic patients may be related to additive adverse effects of both drugs. None of these patients have developed congestive heart failure, however. It is important to note that DeJager et al. (35) reported congestive heart failure in two patients who had been previously treated with Adriamycin. The results suggest, therefore, that careful monitoring of clinical signs and EKG signs should be done if ACM-A is to be used in the second-line treatment of the disease if the patient has already received prior chemotherapy with drugs containing anthracyclines. In this analysis, a few patients have received cumulative doses exceeding 550 mg/m^2, which is a threshold of total dose to induce cardio-myopathy with Adriamycin (39,40).

In animal systems, the drug has shown lower cardiac toxicity. Biopsies of myocardium or a randomized trial will be necessary to allow a comparison to be made of the chronic cardiac toxicity of Adriamycin and ACM-A.

REFERENCES

1. Oki T, Matsuyama A, Yoshimoto A, et al. 1975. New antitumor antibiotics, aclacinomycin A and B. J. Antibiot. 28(10): 830-834.
2. Oki T. 1977. New anthracycline antibiotics. J. Antibiot. 30(suppl.): 70-84.
3. Hori S, Shirai M, Hirano S, et al. 1977. Antitumor activity of new anthracycline antibiotics, aclacinomycin A and its analogs, and their toxicity. Gann 68: 685-690.
4. Oki T, Takeuchi T, Oka S, Umezawa H. 1980. Current status of Japanese studies with the new anthracycline antibiotics, aclacinomycin A. In: Recent results in cancer research, vol. 74 (G. Mathé and F. Muggia, eds.), pp. 207-216.
5. Crooke ST, Duvernay VH, Galvan L, et al. 1978. Structure-activity relations of anthracyclines relative to effects on macromolecular synthesis. Molec. Pharmacol. 14: 290-298.
6. Oki T, Takeuchi T, Oka S, and Umezawa H. 1981. New anthracycline antibiotic, aclacinomycin A: Experimental studies and correlation with clinical trials. In: Recent results in cancer research, vol. 76 (SK Carter, Y Sakurai, H Umezawa, eds.), pp. 21-40.
7. Fujimoto S, Inagaki J, Horikoshi N, Ogawa M. 1979. Combination chemotherapy with a new anthracycline glycoside, aclacinomycin-A and active drugs for malignant lymphomas in P388 mouse leukemia system. Gann 70: 411-420.
8. Dantchev D, Siloussartchouk V, Paintrand M, et al. 1979. Electron microscopic studies of the heart and light macroscopic studies of the skin after treatment of golden hamsters with adriamycin, detorubicin, Ad-32, and aclacinomycin. Cancer Treat. Rep. 63: 875-888.
9. Furue H, ukukawa K, Nakao I, et al. 1977. Clinical information of aclacinomycin A. Gan to Kagakuryoho 4(1): 75-79.
10. Furue H, Komita T, Nakao I, et al. 1978. Clinical experiences with aclacinomycin-A. In: Recent results in cancer research, vol. 63 (SK Carter, H. Umezawa, J. Douros, Y Sakurai, eds.). Springer-Verlag, Berlin, Heidelberg, New York.
11. Oka S. 1978. A review of clinical studies on aclacinomycin A--phase I and preliminary phase II evaluation of ACM--. Sci. Rep. Res. Inst. Tohoku Univ. - C 25(3-4): 37-49.
12. Furue H. 1981. Aclarubucin. Gan to Kagakuryoho 8(2): 329-331.
13. WHO. 1979. WHO handbook for reporting results of cancer treatment. WHO offset publication no. 48. World Health Organization, Geneva.
14. Karnofsky DA. 1961. Meaningful clinical classification of therapeutic responses to anticancer drugs. Clin. Pharmacol. Ther. 2: 709-712.
15. Kimura K. 1965. Chemotherapy of acute leukemia with special reference to criteria for evaluation of therapeutic effect. In: Advances in chemotherapy of acute leukemia under the JAPAN-U.S. Cooperative Science

Program. September 27-28, Bethesda, Maryland, U.S.A., pp. 21-23.

16. Ellison RR. 1973. Acute myelocytic leukemia in cancer medicine (JF Holland and E Frei III, eds.), Lea & Febiger, Philadelphia, pp. 1199-1234.

17. Sakano T, Okazaki N, Ise T, et al. 1978. Phase I study of aclacinomycin A. Jpn. J. Clin. Oncol. 8(1): 49-53.

18. Majima H, Ogawa M, Takagi T. 1978. Aclacinomycin A is new antitumor antibiotic of the anthracycline group. Gan to Kagakuryoho 5(6): 141-145.

19. Ogawa M, Inagaki J, Horikoshi N, et al. 1979. Clinical study of aclacinomycin A. Cancer Treat. Rep. 63: 931-934.

20. Suzuki H, Kawashima K, Yamada K. 1979. Aclacinomycin A, a new anti-leukemic agent. Lancet, April 21: 870-871.

21. Takubo T, Sonoda T, Namiuchi S, et al. 1980. Clinical results of aclacinomycin-A in haematatopoietic malignancies. Gan to Kagakuryoho 7(8): 1361-1365.

22. Yamada K, Nakamura T, Tsuruo T, et al. 1980. A phase II study of aclacinomycin A in acute leukemia in adults. Cancer Treat. Rev. 7: 177-182.

23. Kitajima K, Takahashi I, Yorimitsu S, et al. 1980. Treatment of refractory adult acute leukemia with aclacinomycin A: Phase II study. Gan to Kagakuryoho 7(7). 1220-1227.

24. Ishibiki H, Enomoto K, Kumai K, et al. 1980. A clinical study of an anthracycline, aclacinomycin A. Shinyaku to Rinsho 29(1): 2-18.

25. Nakano Y, Jikuya K, Ohoshima K, et al. 1980. A clinical study of new antitumor antibiotic, "aclacinomycin A." Gan to Kagakuryoho 7(6): 1007-1012.

26. Yokoyama M, Wakui A, Saito T. 1979. Clinical study of aclacinomycin A. Presentation to the Fifth Group Study Meeting of Aclacinomycin, Tokyo.

27. Kikuchi K. 1980. Evaluation of aclacinomycin A in patients with advanced gastric and colorectal cancer. Gan to Kagakuryoho 7(3): 425-434.

28. Maeda M, Izumi A, Yoshida H, et al. 1980. Clinical evaluation of new anticarcinogen, aclacinomycin A. Gan to Kagakuryoho 7(5): 875-880.

29. Hiramoto Y, Kumashiro R, Tamada R, et al. 1980. A new schedule of aclacinomycin-A administration and its effectiveness. Gan to Kagakuryoho 7(6): 1002-1006.

30. Mizuno I, Tanada , Okumura K, et al. 1980. Clinical evaluation of aclacinomycin A on advanced or recurrent gastric cancer. Gan to Kagakuryoho 7(8): 1366-1372.

31. Nakai Y, Ishikawa T, Koinumaru S, et al. 1980. Clinical effect of aclacinomycin A on lung cancer. Gan to Kagakuryoho 7(4): 645-656.

32. Nomura Y, Yamagata A, Takenaka K, et al. 1980. Effect of aclacinomycin A on advanced recurrent breast cancer. Shinyaku to Rinsho 29(1): 27-30.

33. Suzuki M, Shogime M, Masuda T, et al. 1980. Clinical effect of aclacino-mycin A on gynecological malignant diseases. Gan to Kagakuryoho 7(6): 1013-1020.

34. Konno K, Motomiya M, Nakai Y, et al. 1978. Clinical effect of aclacinomycin on lung cancer. Gan to Kagakuryoho 5(4): 119-126.

35. De Jager R, Delgado M, Bayssas M, et a. 1981. Phase II study of aclacinomycin A (ACM) in acute leukemia (AL) and leukemic lympho-sarcoma (LSL). Proc. 72nd Ann. Meeting Am. Assoc. Cancer Res. & 17th Ann. Meeting Am. Soc. Clinic. Oncol., vol. 22, abstr. 680.

36. Mathe G, Bayssas M, Gonveia J, et al. 1978. Preliminary results of phase II trial of aclacinomycin in acute leukemia and lymphosarcoma. Cancer Chemother. Pharmacol. 1: 259-262.

37. Casper ES, Gralla RJ, Young CW. 1981. Clinical phase I study of

aclacinomycin A by evaluation of an intermittent intravenous administration schedule. Cancer 41: 2417-2420.

38. Egorin MJ, Van Echo DA, Whitacre MY, et al. 1981. A phase I trial of aclacinomycin-A (ACM-A). Proc. 73th Ann. Meeting of Am. Assoc. Cancer Res. and 17th Ann. Meeting Am. Soc. Clinic. Oncol., vol. 22, abstr. C-80.

39. Praga CG, Beretta G, Vigo PL, et al. 1979. Adriamycin cardiotoxicity a survey of 1273 patients. Cancer Treat. Rep. 63(5): 827-834.

40. Von Hoff DD, Layard MW, Basa P, et al. 1979. Risk factors for doxorubicin-induced congestive heart failure. Ann. Int. Med. 91: 710-717.

THE CLINICAL PHARMACOLOGY OF ACLACINOMYCIN-A

M. J. EGORIN, D. VAN ECHO, P. A. ANDREWS, B. M. FOX, H. NAKAZAWA, M. WHITACRE, AND N. R. BACHUR

Aclacinomycin-A (Acm) (Figure 1), an anthracycline antibiotic produced by Streptomyces galilaeus (1), has proven active against a number of animal and human tumors (2,3).

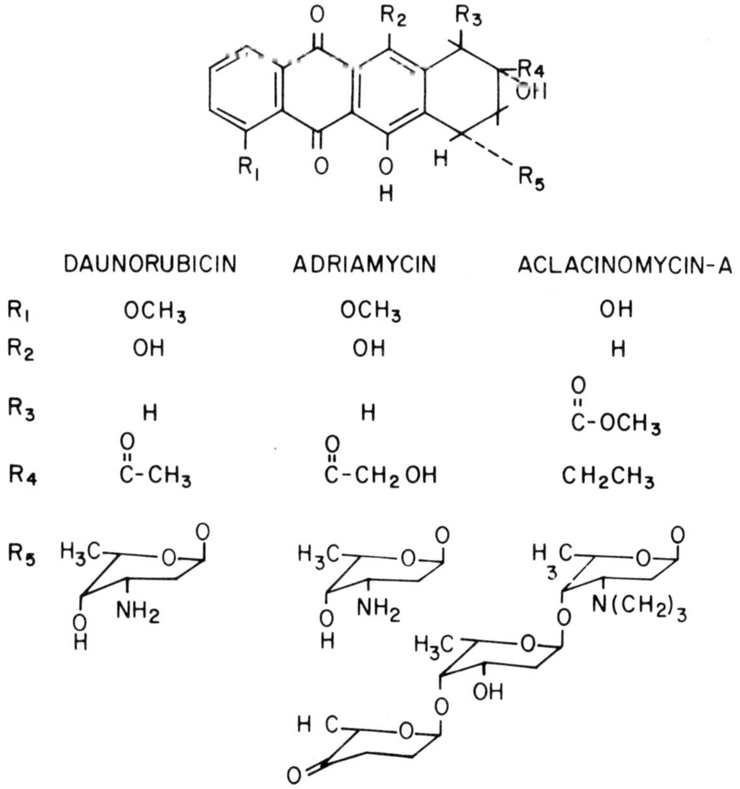

	DAUNORUBICIN	ADRIAMYCIN	ACLACINOMYCIN-A
R_1	OCH_3	OCH_3	OH
R_2	OH	OH	H
R_3	H	H	$\overset{O}{\overset{\|\|}{C}}-OCH_3$
R_4	$\overset{O}{\overset{\|\|}{C}}-CH_3$	$\overset{O}{\overset{\|\|}{C}}-CH_2OH$	CH_2CH_3

FIGURE 1. The structures of aclacinomycin-A, daunorubicin, and adriamycin.

Acm differs from the commonly employed anthracyclines daunorubicin (Dnr) and adriamycin (Adr), both structurally (Figure 1) and, to some extent,

528

mechanistically, inhibiting RNA synthesis more efficiently than DNA synthesis (4,5). On the basis of its inhibition of radionucleoside incorporation, Acm has been described as a Class II anthracycline (4,5), and as such, is the first of this group of drugs to be used clinically.

Oki and co-workers in Japan have carefully characterized the many Acm metabolites found in fermentation broths (6,7) and have investigated the enzymatic pathways that produce a number of these metabolites in animals (1,8,9). These studies have shown the metabolism of Acm to proceed in two main directions. There can be enzymatic reduction of the terminal keto sugar to form the stereoisomeric metabolites M_1 and N_1 or there can be reductive enzymatic cleavage of the trisaccharide to liberate the aglycone, 7-deoxyaklavinone (C_1) or its dimer, metabolite E_1 (Figure 2).

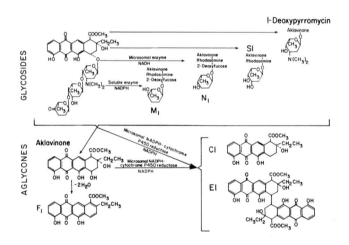

FIGURE 2. The proposed metabolic pathways of aclacinomycin (after Oki).

Also, there is a certain amount of sequential cleavage of Acm's sugars producing first the disaccharide metabolite, S_1, and then the monosaccharide, aklavin, which is also called deoxypyrromycin (Figure 2). Further, the aglycones, aklavinone and bisanhydroaklavinone (F_1) have been described (Figure 2).

Despite these extensive metabolic studies, there is little information on the disposition of Acm in animals and even less information (4,6,10) on the metabolism and disposition of Acm in humans (4,11). We have investigated the latter of these two problems in patients receiving

Acm in a Phase I clinical trial at our institution (12).

Acm, provided by the Developmental Therapeutics Branch, DCT, NCI, Bethesda, MD, was administered as an i.v. bolus to 12 patients, 4 female and 8 male, aged 43-70 years (median 52 years), at dosages of 60 to 120 mg/square meter. All patients had advanced-stage neoplasms that were not amenable to control by surgery, radiation therapy, hormonal therapy, or accepted chemotherapeutic agents. All patients had received prior chemotherapy and 8 had received Adr. No patient was of Oriental or Hispanic descent.

Plasma was assayed for total Acm-derived fluorescence and for individual Acm metabolites. In order to determine total Acm-derived fluorescence in plasma, samples were extracted with 0.45 $\underline{N}$ HCl in 50% ethanol as described previously (13). Fluorescence was then determined with an Aminco SPF 125 spectrofluorometer (American Instrument Co., Silver Spring, MD) at 450 nm excitation and 585 nm emission (14), and plasma Acm equivalents were determined by comparison with a series of freshly prepared Acm standards.

During the first 60 minutes after drug administration, plasma total drug fluorescence, which was accounted for by parent compound only (see below) declined very rapidly (Figure 3).

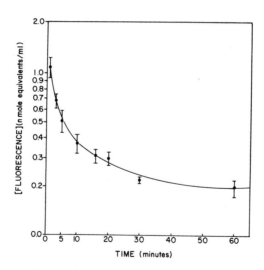

Figure 3. Concentrations of aclacinomycin-A derived fluorescence present in plasma during the first hour after aclacinomycin injection.

This rapid decline is well described by the equation, plasma concentration $C_p = 0.989e^{-0.0.519}$ $0.345e^{-0.0668t} + 0.190e^{-0.000t}$ and agrees well with

530

earlier reports of plasma studies done in rabbits, a dog and a human by Oki
and coworkers (4,6,10). In addition, Malspeis and coworkers have confirmed
the rapid disappearance of Acm from the plasma of five patients treated
with 60 mg/m^2 Acm as 4-16 min infusions (11). As can be inferred from the
composite curve presented in Figure 3, there was close agreement among the
individual patients' studies, and there was close agreement in the value of
concentration times time for the 0-60 minute portion of each patient's
studies (18.42 ± 2.0 μM min, mean ± S.D.).

After this initial decay, plasma total drug fluorescence rose progressively from 2-24 hours before finally declining slowly (Figure 4).

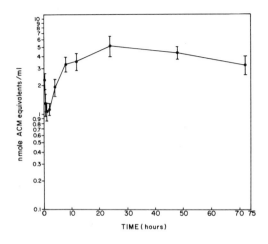

FIGURE 4.   Concentrations of aclacinomycin-A derived fluorescence present
in plasma.

In every patient studied, this secondary peak in plasma drug fluorescence
exceeded the amount of total fluorescence measured in the first sample
drawn after Acm administration (Figure 4). This rebound in plasma total
drug fluorescence has not been reported for animals treated with Acm. In
order to characterize further the individual fluorescent species responsible for the observed pattern of total drug fluorescence, Acm and its
metabolites were measured separately.

Plasma was extracted with two volumes of chloroform:isopropanol (1:1) as previously described (15), and this extract was analyzed by thin layer chromatography on 250 µm silica gel G plates (E. Merck, Darmstadt, Germany) that were developed first in diethyl ether, air-dried, and then developed in an ascending fashion to a solvent front of 15 cm with chloroform:methanol:water (80:20:3) as a solvent system (Solvent System I). In some cases, aliquots of plasma extracts were also developed in chloroform:methanol:glacial acetic acid (100:2:2.5) (Solvent system II). Chromatographic standards of Acm and metabolites M_1, N_1, C_1, F_1, S_1, E_1, deoxypyrromycin and aklavinone (15) (Figure 2), kindly provided by Dr. T. Oki of the Sanraku-Ocean Co., Ltd, Fujisawa, Japan, were run on each plate. Drug fluorescence on TLC plates was detected with 2537 Å light (UVS-54 Mineralight, Ultra-Violet Products, San Gabriel, Cal) and fluorescent regions of the plates were scraped. Drug was then eluted from the silica gel with 0.3 $\underline{N}$ HCl in 50% ethanol and quantified fluorometrically by comparison with a series of fresh Acm standards (16).

When the plasma samples were extracted and analyzed in this fashion, we found that the rebound in plasma drug fluorescence was not due to reappearance of parent Acm, but rather, represented the appearance of two metabolites.

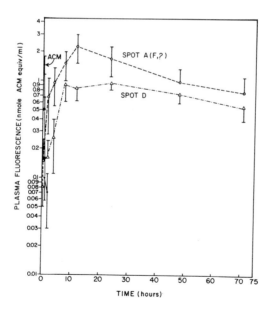

FIGURE 5. Plasma concentrations of aclacinomycin-A and its metabolites. One of these (spot A) was less polar than Acm and cochromatographed with

532

known metabolite F_1 (Figure 5, Table 1). The other metabolite (spot D) was much more polar than Acm in solvent system I but less polar than Acm in solvent system II, and did not cochromatograph with any previously described Acm metabolite (Table I). Both Acm metabolites persisted in plasma for long periods of time and their slow decline was not associated with the appearance of any new fluorescent species (Figure 5). Malspeis and co-workers have also noted the production of long-lived metabolites of Acm, which are likely to correspond to those observed in our patients (11). There is, however, one discrepancy between our observations and those of Malspeis et al. in that we do not observe any metabolite M_1 in plasma, while they do. The basis for this difference is unclear and we are currently attempting to resolve this disparity.

When activated by 450 nm light and measured at 585 nm, more fluorescence was measured in spot A than in spot D (Figure 5). However, when TLC plates were examined with 2537 Å u.v. light prior to scraping, spot D appeared brighter than did spot A. As might be expected, this discrepancy, to some degree, reflects different fluorescent spectra for the metabolites (Figure 6).

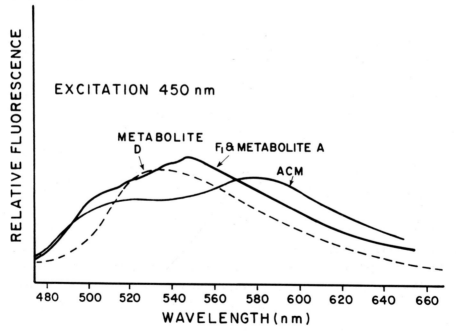

FIGURE 6. Fluorescence emission spectra of Acm, metabolite F_1, and plasma metabolites A and D.

The fluorescent spectrum of the metabolite in spot A was identical to that of metabolite F_1, with maximum excitation at 450 nm and maximum fluorescence at 552 nm (Figure 6). On the other hand, the metabolite in spot D, while exciting maximally at 450 nm, had a maximum emission at 538 nm, emitting much less at 585 nm, the wavelength measured in our studies (Figure 6). Small amounts of metabolites "A" and "D" were isolated and purified from pooled plasma by extraction with chloroform:isopropanol and subsequent TLC. The TLC behaviour of these materials was not altered by treatment at $100^{\circ}C$ with 0.2 $\underline{N}$ HCl, or by incubation at $37^{\circ}C$ for 24 hours with bacterial β-glucuronidase (Type VII, Sigma Chemical Co., St. Louis, MO) or limpet aryl sulfatase (Type V, Sigma Chemical Co.) (Table II). Unfortunately, the quantities of pure metabolites A and D that were isolated were insufficient for mass spectral analysis.

There may be several explanations for why plasma fluorescence due to Acm metabolites reaches levels greater than the amount of Acm fluorescence measured one minute after I.V. injection of Acm. It is not likely that one mole of Acm is converted to more than one mole of fluorescent metabolites. Rather the 2 Acm metabolites observed may have smaller volumes of distribution than does Acm and appear to be produced more rapidly than they are excreted and metabolized. Alternatively, the two metabolites may have greater quantum fluorescence efficiencies than does Acm. At this time we are unable to define whether either, or both, of these mechanisms actually explain our observations. Although these plasma studies of Acm and its metabolites demonstrated new patterns of pharmacokinetic behavior and new metabolites, they were relatively restricted by the paucity of available biological material. In addition, the number of Acm metabolites observed in plasma were far fewer than those proposed by Oki and co-workers. Therefore, we turned our attention to urine, a biological fluid which was not only more abundant but from which drug could be extracted and concentrated.

During the first 72 hours after Acm administration, urine was collected in opaque plastic bottles. At the conclusion of the 72-hour collection period, urinary drug was extracted into butanol with a horizontal flow-through coil planet centrifuge that was kindly provided by its inventor, Dr. Yoichiro Ito of the National Heart and Lung Institute, Bethesda, MD (17). The butanol extract was concentrated by flash evaporation (Buchler Instruments, Ft. Lee, N.J.). The dried butanol extracts were redissolved in small amounts of methanol and were purified by repeated thin layer chromatography on 250 μm silica gel 60 plates (E. Merck, Darmstadt, Germany). In additon to solvent systems I and II, chloroform:methanol:glacial acetic acid:water (80:20:14:6) (Solvent system III) was used to separate very polar metabolites. Purified samples of Acm and metabolites were run as standards on appropriate TLC plates.

Drug standards and urinary fluorescent species were also characterized by HPLC. The HPLC system consisted of a Model 3500B HPLC (Spectrahysics, Santa Clara, Cal.) Fitted with a μ-Bondapak phenyl column (3.9 mm x 30 cm) (Waters Associates, Milford, Mass.). A 10-min gradient of 30-70% tetrahydrofuran in 0.1% (w/v) ammonium formate buffer, pH 4.0 was used at a flow rate of 2 ml/min (18).

The chromatographic behavior of urinary species, I, II, III, and IV was not altered by treatment at 100°C for 60 min with 0.25 $\underline{N}$ HCl, or at 37°C for 24 hours with β glucuronidase or aryl sulfatase (Table II). This was expected in view of their appearing to be aglycones F_1, E_1, C_1, and aklavinone, respectively. The chromatographic behavior of urinary species, VI, VI, VII, VII, IX, and X was not affected by treatment with either β glucuronidase or aryl sulfatase (Table II). For species V, VI, VII, IX and X, this was expected since they appeared to be glycosides without conjugated glucuronic acid or sulfate groups. As expected, in view of their hypothesized structures, i.e. aklavinone with various glycosically linked sugar moieties, species, VI, VI, VII, VIII, IX, and X were all converted by acid hydrolysis to a material that cochromatographed with aklavinone standard in TLC systems I and II (Table II). The chromatographic behavior of species XI was not altered by acid hydrolysis or by incubation with β glucuronidase or aryl sulfatase. This is consistent with its tentative correspondence to human plasma metabolite "D." Finally, the chromatographic behavior of urinary species XII was not altered by incubation with aryl sulfatase; however, on treatment with 0.25 $\underline{N}$ HCl or β glucuronidase, species XII was completely converted to a material that cochromatographed with species XI, implying it was a β glucuronide conjugate of species XI.

Mass spectral analysis of purified urinary metabolites was undertaken to confirm their proposed identities. These studies have confirmed the identities of urinary species I, III, IV, VI, VIII, and IX as F_1, C_1 aklavinone, M_1, N_1 and S_1, respectively. Mass spectral studies of urinary

TABLE I
THIN LAYER CHROMATOGRAPHIC RF'S AND HIGH PERFORMANCE
k' 's OF ACLACINOMYCIN AND ITS METABOLITES

	RF		k'
COMPOUND	SYSTEM I[a]	SYSTEM II[b]	HPLC[c]
F_1	0.89	0.77	8.9
E_1	0.86	0.38	9.8
C_1	0.83	0.49	8.2
Aklavinone	0.80	0.40	7.1
ACM	0.77	0.00	6.7
M_1	0.64	0.00	5.5
N_1	0.57	0.00	5.3
S_1	0.36	0.00	4.4
Aklavin	0.22	0.00	4.9
Plasma Metabolite A	0.87	0.77	—
Plasma Metabolite D	0.24	0.34	6.7
Urinary Species			
I	0.89	0.70	8.8
II	0.85	0.39	9.8
III	0.84	0.50	8.0
IV	0.80	0.41	7.0
V	0.76	0.00	6.7
VI	0.63	0.00	5.5
VII	0.63	0.00	5.5
VIII	0.47	0.00	5.3
IX	0.36	0.00	5.1
X	0.22	0.00	4.9
XI	0.24	0.00	6.7
XII	0.11	0.00	0.52

[a] Chloroform: methanol:distilled water (80:20:3).

[b] Chloroform:methanol: glacial acetic acid (100:2:2.5)

[c] 3.9 mm x 30 cm μ-Bondapak phenyl column with mobile phase of 15-50% tetrahydrofuran in 0.1% (w/v) ammonium formate buffer pH 4.0 pumped at 2 ml/min.

TABLE II
ACID AND ENZYMATIC HYDROLYSIS OF ACM, ITS METABOLITES AND URINARY SPECIES

COMPOUND	0.25N HCl	β GLUCURONIDASE	ARYL SULFATASE
F_1	No change	No change	No change
E_1	No change	No change	No change
C_1	No change	No change	No change
Aklavinone	No change	No change	No change
ACM	Converted to akalvinone	No change	No change
M_1	Converted to alkavinone	No change	No change
N_1	Converted to alkavinone	No change	No change
S_1	Converted to alkavinone	No change	No change
Aklavin	Converted to aklavinone	No change	No change
Plasma Metabolite A	No change	No change	No change
Plasma Metabolite D	No change	No change	No change

Urinary Species

I	No change	No change	No change
II	No change	No change	No change
III	No change	No change	No change
IV	No change	No change	No change
V	Converted to aklavinone	No change	No change
VI	Converted to aklavinone	No change	No change
VII	Converted to aklavinone	No change	No change
VIII	Converted to aklavinone	No change	No change
IX	Converted to aklavinone	No change	No change
X	Converted to aklavinone	No change	No change
XI	No change	No change	No change
XII	Converted to XI	Converted to XI	No change

species II, V, VIII, X and XII are still incomplete.

We have directed particular effort at defining the structure of urinary metabolite XI in view of its apparent correspondence to plasma metabolite D. The mass spectral analysis of urinary metabolite XI was not definitive for bisanhydroaklavinic acid but was compatible with bisan-hydroaklavinic acid, less the carboxyl moiety at carbon 10. We, therefore, attempted to esterify the postulated carboxyl group and convert urinary species XI to the-known metabolite F_1. Reaction of urinary species XI with diazomethane (19) produced a material that cochromatographed with F_1 in TLC systems I and II and in the HPLC system described above. Reaction of F_1, aclacinomycin, C_1, aklavinone, and E_1 with diazomethane produced no alteration of the chromatographic characteristics of these Acm metabolite standards.

These studies of the urinary metabolites of Acm complement and extend our observations of Acm's plasma behavior. Unlike plasma, in which we observed only three fluorescent species, urine appears to contain all of the previously described metabolites of Acm. Although many of these have been isolated from Streptomyces galilaeus broths and in vitro reactions, many have never been documented previously as human metabolites. It is likely that the failure to observe these metabolites in plasma reflects their very low concentrations. Their isolation from urine was greatly facilitated by the application of the new extraction methodology made available by the horizontal flow-through coil planet centrifuge (17). This technique allowed the rapid, convenient and simultaneous extraction and concentration of drug from many liters of urine into a small volume of organic solvent. The observation of these multiple Acm metabolites in urine lends further support to the studies of Oki et al. which elucidated the various pathways of Acm biotransformation.

In addition to documenting the generation in humans of all of the previously described Acm metabolites, our urinary studies establish F_1 as the identity of plasma metabolite A. They also indicate bisanhydroakla-vinic acid as the likely identity of the previously unidentified plasma metabolite D. Moreover, the demonstration in the urine of a glucuronide conjugate of bisanhydroaklavinic acid, provides additional evidence of the production of bisanhydroaklavinic acid by humans. Establishing the identity of plasma "metabolite D" as the acid portion of F_1 is of practical importance since it represents one of the two major fluorescent species present in plasma after the initial rapid disappearance of Acm. The other major plasma Acm metabolite, F_1 itself, is an aglycone. Demonstration of the other major plasma species as another aglycone, bisanhydroaklavinic acid, means that beyond two hours after Acm injection, all of the drug fluorescence measured in plasma is due to aglycones which are claimed to be relatively inactive compounds. This is in contrast to other clinically used anthracyclines such as daunorubicin, adriamycin, rubidazone, AD 32, 4' epi-adriamycin and carminomycin in which parent or active glycosidic metabolites are the major plasma species (15,20-23).

REFERENCES

1. Oki T, Matsuzawa Y, Yoshimoto A, Numata K, Kitamura I, Hori S, Takamatsu A, Umezawa H, Ishizuka M, Naganawa H, Suda H, Hamada M, Takeuchi T. 1975. New antitumor antibiotics aclacinomycins A & B. J. Antibiot XXVIII:830.

2. Hori S, Shirai M, Hirano S, Oki T, Inui T, Tsukagoshi S, Ishizuka M, Takeuchi T, Umezawa H. 1977. Antitumor activity of new anthracycline antibiotics, aclacinomycin A and its analogs, and their toxicity. GANN 68:685.

3. Ogawa M, Inagaki J, Horikoshi N, Inoue K, Chinen T, Ueoka H, Nagura E. 1979. Clinical study of aclacinomyin A. Cancer Treat. Rep 63:931.

4. Oki T, Takeuchi T, Oka S, Umezawa H. 1979. Current status of Japanese studies with the new anthracycine antibiotic, aclacinomycin A. In Mathé G, Muggia FM, Editors: Recent Results In Cancer Research, New York, Springer-Verlag.

5. Oki T. 1977. New anthracycline antibiotics. Japanese J. Antibiot. XXX Supplement:570.

6. Oki T, Kitamura I, Yoshimoto A, Matsuzawa Y, Shibamoto N, Ogasawara T, Inui T, Takamatsu A, Takeuchi T, Masuda T, Hamada M, Suda H, Ishizuka M. Sawa T, Umezawa H. 1979. Antitumor anthracycline antibiotics, aclacinomycin-A and analogues, I. J. Antibiotics XXXII:791.

7. Oki T, Kitamura I, Matsuzawa Y, Shibamoto N, Ogasawara T, Yoshimoto A, Inui T, Naganawa H, Takeuchi T, Umezawa H. 1979. Antitumor anthracycline antibiotics, aclacinomycin A and analogues, II. J. Antibiotics XXXII:801.

8. Oki T, Komiyama H, Tone H, Inui T, Takeuchi T, Umezawa H. 1977. J. Antibiotics 30:613.

9. Komiyama T, Oki T, Inui T. 1979. A proposed reaction mechanism for

the enzymatic reductive cleavage of glycosidic bond in anthracycline antibiotics. J. Antibiotics XXXII:1219-1222.

10. Ogasawara T, Masuda Y, Goto S, Mori S, Oki T. 1981. High performance liquid chromatographic determination of aclacinomycin A and its related compounds. II reverse phase HPLC determination of aclacinomycin A and its metabolites in biological fluids using fluorescence detection. J. Antibiotics. 34:52.

11. Malspeis L, Neidhart J, Staubus A, Kear T, Booth J. 1981. HPLC determination of aclacinomycin A (NSC 208734, Acm) in plasma and application to preliminary clinical pharmacokinetic studies. Proc. Am. Assoc. Cancer Res 22:242.

12. Egorin MJ, Van Echo DA, Whitacre MY, Fox BM, Aisner J, Wiernik PH, Bachur NR. (in press). A phase I trial of aclacinomycin A. Proc. Am. Assoc. Cancer Res. & Amer. Soc. Clin. Oncol.

13. Benjamin RS, Riggs CE, Bachur NR. 1973. The pharmacokinetics and metabolism of adriamycin in man. Clin. Pharmacol. Ther. 14:692.

14. Egorin, MJ, Clawson RE, Ross LA, Schlossberger NM, Bachur NR. 1979. Cellular accumulation and disposition of aclacinomycin A. Cancer Res. 39:4396.

15. Benjamin RS, Riggs CE, Bachur NR. 1977. Plasma pharmacokinetics of adriamycin and its metabolites in humans with normal hepatic and renal function. Cancer Res. 37:1416.

16. Bachur NR, Gee M. 1971. Daunorubicin metabolism by rat tissue preparations. J. Pharmacol. Exper. Therap. 177:567.

17. Ito Y. 1981. New continuous extraction method with a coil planet centrifuge. J. Chromatog. 207:161.

18. Andrews PA, Brenner DE, Chou FE, Kubo H, Bachur NR. 1980. Facile and definitive determination of human adriamycin and daunorubicin metabolites by high pressure liquid chromatography. Drug metab. Dispos. 8:152.

19. Huffman DH, Benjamin MD, Bachur NR. 1972. Daunorubicin metabolism and acute non-lymphocytic leukemia. Clin. Pharmacol & Ther. 13:895-905.

20. Kovach JS, Ames MM, Sternad ML, O'Connell MJ. 1979. Phase I trial and assay of rubidazone (NSC 164011) in patients with advanced solid tumors. Cancer Research 39:823-828.

21. Blum RH, Garnick MB, Israel M, CAnellos GP, Henderson IC, Frei III, E.
     1979. Initial clinical evaluation of N-trifluoroacetyl adriamycin-
     14-valerate (AD-32), an adriamycin analog. Cancer Treat. Rep.
     63:919–923.

22. Pittman KA, Fandrich S. Rozencweig M, Baker LH, Lenaz L, Crooke ST.
     1980. Clinical pharmacologic studies of carminomycin C carubicin.
     Proc. Am. Assoc. Cancer Res. 21:180.

23. Broggini M, Colombo T, Martini A, Donelli MG. 1980. Studies on the
     comparative distribution and biliary excretion of doxorubicin and 4'
     epi-doxorubicin in mice and rats. Cancer Treat. Rep. 64:897–904.

PHASE II EVALUATION OF N-TRIFLUOROACETYLADRIAMYCIN-14-VALERATE (AD 32)

M. B. GARNICK, J. D. GRIFFIN, M. J. SACK, R. H. BLUM, M. ISRAEL, AND E. FREI III

INTRODUCTION

The synthesis, development and evaluation of doxorubicin (Adriamycin) analogs with greater clinical efficacy and less acute and chronic toxicity than the parent drug continue to be a major challenge in cancer chemotherapy. As part of ongoing studies in anthracycline analog development at the Sidney Farber Cancer Institute, N-trifluoroacetyladriamycin-14-valerate (AD 32) (Figure 1) was found to be superior to Adriamycin in murine L1210, and P388 leukemias, Ridgeway osteogenic sarcoma, and Lewis lung carcinoma in preclinical studies (1-5). The initial clinical evaluation of AD 32 (6,7) indicated that dose-limiting toxicities were leukopenia and thrombocytopenia. The administration of AD 32 was associated with less gastrointestinal toxicity and alopecia in comparison to Adriamycin. Inadvertent paravenous extravasation of AD 32 did not produce local tissue damage. Also, preliminary evaluation suggested that

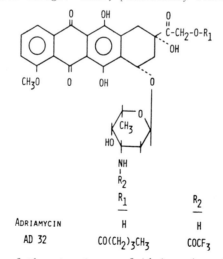

	R_1	R_2
ADRIAMYCIN	H	H
AD 32	$CO(CH_2)_3CH_3$	$COCF_3$

Figure 1. Comparison of the structures of Adriamycin and AD 32.

AD 32 may be less cardiotoxic than is Adriamycin. This theory is based on the observation that patients receiving cumulative doses of AD 32 equivalent to cardiotoxic doses of Adriamycin do not demonstrate cardiac damage on endomyo-cardial biopsy.

In contrast to Adriamycin, AD 32 is lipid soluble and only minimally solu-ble in aqueous media. The drug is thus formulated in a polyethoxylated vegetable oil (Emulphor EL620) and absolute ethanol for parenteral adminis-tration. A separate spectrum of toxicities resulted from this drug vehicle, including hypotension, arterial hypoxemia, oliguria, fever, chest pain, and bronchospasm. All of these latter manifestations which may, in part, be related to fat emboli were preventable and reversible with concomitant hydrocortisone administration (8,9,10,11,12).

We subsequently undertook a phase II study of AD 32 that was based upon our phase I investigation and that used a starting dose of 600 mg/m^2 of AD 32 given as a 24-hour continuous infusion, repeated every 21 days. The following report describes the results of this study.

MATERIALS AND METHODS

Drug Administration

The AD 32 used in the clinical trial was manufactured in bulk by Farmatalia S.p.A., Milan, Italy, through a joint agreement between the Sidney Farber Cancer Institute, Adria Laboratories, and the National Cancer Institute.* AD 32 was formulated as a lyophilized powder in 200-mg vials. As AD 32 is insoluble in aqueous phase, a lipophilic solvent medium (equal volumes of absolute ethanol and polyethoxylated vegetable oil (Emulphor EL620) is used to solubilize the drug. This solution is then diluted in aqueous medium, yielding a final clinical formulation of 0.35 mg AD 32/ml, in 0.5% absolute alcohol, 0.5% Emulphor, and 99.0% aqueous medium. AD 32 was administered by IMED pumps (San Diego, California), protected from light, as a 24-hour continuous infusion. Treatments were repeated at 21-day intervals. The initial starting dose was 600 mg/m^2 of AD 32 as previous work had shown that this dose results in myelosuppression equivalent to 90 mg/m^2 of Adriamycin. Dose deescalations were carried out according to the following schema:

---

*We also wish to acknowledge the assistance of J. Paul Davignon and the Pharma-ceutical Resources Branch, Developmental Therapeutics Program, Division of Cancer Treatment, National Cancer Institute, in the formulating process of AD 32.

Resultant WBC	AD 32 Reduction
>2000 ≤ 3000	No change
≥1000 ≤ 2000	25%
≥ 500 < 1000	50%

Because of the acute toxicity encountered in our phase I study which was apparently related to the Emulphor, all patients in this study received hydrocortisone, 100 mg IV over one hour at time 0 hours (initiation of treatment), and then at hour 6, 12, 18, and 24 during treatment, and a final hydrocortisone dose at 6 hours following completion of therapy.

Selection of Patients

All patients had histologic confirmation of cancer which had become refractory to other therapies or for which there was no therapy of proven clinical benefit. All patients were ambulatory, had an estimated survival of greater than 2 months, and had normal hematologic, renal, cardiac, pulmonary, and hepatic functions. Objective bidimensionally measurable disease was required. Patients previously treated with other anthracyclines or with a history of left ventricular dysfunction were not excluded from the study, although response to therapy was analyzed accordingly. Written informed consent was obtained from all patients prior to treatment.

A total of 56 patients was evaluable both for response to therapy and toxicity. Patients' characteristics and histologic diagnoses are seen in Tables 1 and 2.

Table 1. AD 32 Phase II Study

Number patients entered	56
Male/Female	22/34
Median age (range)	56 (19-69)
Total courses of AD 32 given	173
median courses/patient	3
Previous Therapy	
chemotherapy with Adriamycin	27
chemotherapy without Adriamycin	21
radiation therapy	25
no previous treatment	6
Performance status (ECOG)	
0-1	48
2-3	8

Table 2. AD 32 Phase II: Histologic Diagnoses

Primary Site	N	Efficacy Partial Response
Lung		
non-small cell	10	1
small cell	2	
Breast	11	
Soft tissue sarcoma	10	1
Colorectal	7	
other GI	3	
Genitourinary	4	1
Gynecologic	4	
Miscellaneous	5	

A single course of therapy was defined as one completed 24-hour infusion of AD 32. While evaluation of response usually required completion of two full courses, there were instances in which an assessment of both response and toxicity were made following just a single course. Definitions of response for patients in this study were as follows:

Complete response - The disappearance of all clinical, biochemical or radiographic evidence of disease for greater than or equal to 4 weeks.

Partial response - A greater than 50% decrease in the product of the longest perpendicular diameters of the most measurable areas of tumor for greater than or equal to 4 weeks.

Stable disease - No significant change in measurable disease (minor disease regression failing to meet the requirements of partial response are included in this category).

Progressive disease - A greater than 25% increase in the product of two perpendicular diameters, or the development of new lesions. Treatment of individual patients generally was continued until there was clear evidence of disease progression or until the patient requested that therapy be discontinue

RESULTS

Pretreatment Characteristics

Fifty of 56 patients (89%) had received extensive chemotherapy and/or radiation prior to entry in this study, while 6/56 (11%) were previously untreated. Thirty of the 48 previously chemotherapy-treated patients (63%) had received at least 4 antineoplastic agents in combination programs as part of their original treatment program. Likewise, 18 of 25 patients (72%) received radiation therapy to more than one bodily site prior to entrance on the AD 32 protocol. Of the 27 patients who had had prior Adriamycin exposure, Adriamycin had been discontinued in 23/27 (85%) because of progressive disease. Four out of 27 patients (15%) had demonstrated a response either to single-agent Adriamycin or Adriamycin in combination programs and had received a cumulative dose of between 450-500 mg/m^2 when treatment was withdrawn.

Therapeutic Efficacy of AD 32

Responding Group

Complete response - No patient achieved a complete response. Partial response - Three patients achieved a well-documented partial response. The diagnoses were lung adenocarcinoma, liposarcoma, and transitional cell carcinoma of the renal pelvis.

A 61-year-old male presenting with lung adenocarcinoma had marked (greater than 70%) resolution of a large hilar lesion and shrinkage of an ipsilateral supraclavicular lymph node. He received a total of 16.5 gm/m^2 of AD 32 over a period of 15 months, during which time the response was maintained. He had not received any prior antineoplastic agents.

A 60-year-old male with a retroperitoneal liposarcoma had greater than 50% reduction in the mass as measured by physical examination and ultrasound following his second course of AD 32. The duration of response is 5+ months. The patient had received prior Adriamycin-containing chemotherapy with cyclophosphamide, Actinomycin-D, DTIC, as well as irradiation, and was refractory to such treatment.

A 61-year-old female with grade II-III transitional cell carcinoma of the renal pelvis with biopsy-proven metastasis to a supraclavicular lymph node had a greater than 90% reduction in the lymphadenopathy during AD 32 chemotherapy. She is currently receiving her tenth course of drug and has maintained a remission for greater than 8+ months. Her previous treatment included cis-platinum and methylglyoxal-bis-guanylhydrazone.

Nonresponding Group

Stabilization - There were four patients who demonstrated a biological effect of chemotherapy, although they did not fulfill the criteria of objective disease regression. Disease stabilization or minor disease regression was documented in two patients with breast cancer (duration of stabilization of 9 and 30 weeks), hepatoma (duration 27 weeks), and renal cancer (12 weeks). All 4 of these patients had rapidly progressive disease prior to AD 32 administration. Following treatment, there was either cessation of disease progression, or less than 50% regression of measurable lesions.

Progressive Disease - Förty-nine of the 56 patients (88%) had clear-cut disease progression occurring after 2-3 courses of AD 32. Four of the 27 patients had had a partial response to Adriamycin prior to AD 32, including patients with sarcoma, breast (2), and small-cell lung carcinoma. None of these patients responded to AD 32 following their initial response to Adriamycin. Although the numbers are small, it is of note that we have not seen a response with AD 32 in Adriamycin-refractory cancers such as colorectal carcinoma, melanoma, or renal cell cancer.

Toxicity

Myelosuppression - The toxicity resulting from AD 32-Emulphor administration has been well described in previous communications where leukopenia was the dose-limiting toxicity (6,7). In the current study, twenty of 173 courses (12%) were associated with severe myelosuppression (i.e. white blood cell count of less than 1,000) which occurred a median of 11 days following drug administration. Forty-three of 173 courses (25%) resulted in white blood cell counts between 1000 and 2000, median nadir day 12; and 46/173 courses (27%) produced a WBC nadir of greater than 2,000, but less than 3,000, also occurring on Day 12. Thus, 109 of 173 courses (64%) were associated with myelosuppressio Overall, 46/56 patients (82%) experienced myelosuppression during their treatment. Thrombocytopenia with platelet counts less than 100,000 occurred in 10% of courses, and in no instances were platelet transfusions required.

Acute Systemic Toxicity - The acute systemic reaction characterized by dizziness, wheezing, fever, and oliguria occurred in 8 out of 56 patients (14%) despite hydrocortisone prophylaxis. This syndrome was self-limited in all patients. One episode of paroxysmal atrial tachycardia was observed during treatment.

Cardiac Toxicity - None of the patients had clinical or electrocardiographic evidence of cardiac dysfunction, including patients who had received prior Adriamycin chemotherapy. There was no evidence of cardiac dysfunction during the period of AD 32 administration, including 3 responding patients who received cumulative doses of 2.9, 6.0, and 16.5 gm/m^2. One episode of cardiac arrhythmia occurred during drug administration as noted above.

<u>Other</u> - Other reversible toxicities included partial to total alopecia and mild gastrointestinal side effects. Inadvertent paravenous extravasation of AD 32 has not been associated with skin ulceration.

DISCUSSION

The data of this phase II study in selected solid neoplasms indicate that AD 32 does possess anti-neoplastic properties in lung cancer, soft tissue sarcoma, and transitional cell carcinoma of the renal pelvis. As with any phase II study, the majority of patients entered in this trial had received a significant amount of prior chemotherapy, radiation therapy, or both. It is still too preliminary to make generalizations regarding the drug efficacy in any tumor types as the number of patients was small. Duration of response in those patients demonstrating partial regression of disease is now 5+, 5+, and 16 months.

The toxicity from AD 32 in this study parallels that demonstrated in earlier studies. Myelosuppression was dose limiting and was moderate or severe in 63 out of 173 courses (36%). The time course of myelosuppression and recovery is similar to that of Adriamycin. The acute systemic vehicle reaction, observed in 8 patients, was reduced, but not eliminated by hydrocortisone prophylaxis. AD 32 administration was not continued in those patients.

A variety of anthracycline antibiotic agents has been developed. While AD 32 was synthesized as an analog of Adriamycin, the pharmacologic and mechanism-of-action studies performed to date suggest that it is not a pro-drug of Adriamycin (5,13,14). Additional studies are necessary and are currently ongoing to fully describe the clinical efficacy and spectrum of activity of AD 32. Our ongoing studies will evaluate AD 32 in additional patients with lung cancer, urothelial cancer, sarcoma, and breast cancer. Also, in an effort to reduce vehicle-related toxicity, studies are underway with another solvent, Cremaphor.

REFERENCES

1. Israel M, Modest EJ, and Frei E, III: N-Trifluoroacetyladriamycin-14-valerate, an analog with greater experimental antitumor activity and less toxicity than Adriamycin. Cancer Res. 35:1365-1368, 1975.
2. Parker LM, Hirst M, and Israel M: N-Trifluoroacetyladriamycin-14-valerate: additional mouse antitumor and toxicity studies. Cancer Treat. Rep. 62: 119-127, 1978.

3. Vecchi A, Cairo M, Mantovani A, et al: Comparative antineoplastic
    activity of Adriamycin and N-trifluoroacetyladriamycin-14-valerate.
    Cancer Treat. Rep. 61:111-117, 1978.

4. Sengupta SK, Seshadri R, Modest EJ, et al: Comparative DNA-binding studies
    with Adriamycin (ADR), N-trifluoroacetyladriamycin-14-valerate (AD 32) and
    related compounds. Proc. Am. Assoc. Cancer Res. and ASCO 17:109, 1976.

5. Krishan A, Israel M, Modest EJ, et al: Differences in cellular uptake and
    cytofluorescence of Adriamycin and N-trifluoroacetyladriamycin-14-valerate.

6. Blum RH, Garnick MB, Israel M, et al: Initial clinical evaluation of N-
    Trifluoroacetyladriamycin-14-valerate (AD-32), an Adriamycin analog.
    Cancer Treat. Rep. 63:919-923, 1979.

7. Blum RH, Garnick MB, Israel M, et al: Preclinical rationale and phase I
    clinical trial of an Adriamycin analog, AD 32. In: Recent Results in
    Cancer Research, S.K. Carter, Y Sakurai, H Umezawa, editors. Springer-
    Verlag, New York, 1981, Vol. 76, pp 7-15.

8. Ashbaugh DG, and Petty TL: The use of corticosteroids in the treatment
    of respiratory failure associated with massive fat embolism. Surg.
    Gynecol. Obstet. 123:493-500, 1966.

9. Wertzberger JJ and Peltier LF: Fat embolism: the effect of corticosteroids
    on experimental fat embolism in the rat. Surgery 64:143-147, 1968.

10. Peltier LF, Collins JA, Evarts CM, et al: Fat embolism. Arch. Surg. 109:
    12-16, 1974.

11. McKeen CR, Brigham KL, Bowers RE, et al: Pulmonary vascular effects of
    fat embolism infusion in unanesthetized sheep. J. Clin. Invest. 61:1291-
    1297, 1978.

12. Haas CD, Stephens RL, Leite CT, et al.. Letter: Unexpected pain syndrome
    during a phase I study of iv methyl-CCNU. Cancer Treat. Rep. 61:1413-
    1415, 1977.

13. Israel M, Garnick MB, Pegg WJ, et al: Preliminary pharmacology of AD 32
    in man. Proc. Am. Assoc. Cancer Res. and ASCO 19:160, 1978.

14. Garnick MB, Israel M, Pegg WJ, et al: Hepatobiliary pharmacokinetics of
    AD 32 in man. Proc. Am. Assoc. Cancer Res. 20:206, 1979.

PRELIMINARY EXPERIENCE WITH MARCELLOMYCIN: PRECLINICAL AND CLINICAL ASPECTS

M. ROZENCWEIG, C. NICAISE, P. DODION, M. PICCART, D. BRON, M. MATTELAER, P. DUMONT, G. ATASSI, P. STRIJKMANS, and Y. KENIS.

1.   INTRODUCTION

Marcellomycin is a pyrromycinone glycoside isolated by fractionation of the bohemic acid complex, an anthracycline mixture obtained from fermentations of *Actinosporangium* sp. (1). Its chemical structure is closely related to that of aclacinomycin A (Fig. 1). The antitumor effect of the drug has been ascribed, at least in part, to its ability to inhibit nucleolar RNA synthesis (2). In Novikoff hepatoma ascites cells, this inhibition requires concentrations more than 1000-fold lower than those necessary to inhibit DNA synthesis whereas doxorubicin as well as pyrromycin inhibit DNA and nucleolar RNA synthesis at similar concentrations (3).

Marcellomycin was found to be active against various i.p. implanted tumors in mice i.e. the P388 leukemia, the L1210 leukemia, the B16 melanoma, the Lewis lung carcinoma, and the colon 26 carcinoma (4). This antitumor efficacy was comparable to that achieved with aclacinomycin A but somewhat lower than that of doxorubicin. No schedule dependency could be detected in the L1210 system with marcellomycin (5). In this system, there was no increase in life span after oral administration (6).

The authors are grateful to Dr. Marc Buyse (EORTC Data Center) for statistical analyses and to Mrs Geneviève Decoster for secretarial assistance.

This work was supported in part by contract NIH NO1-CM 53840 from the National Cancer Institute (NCI, Bethesda, Maryland) and by grant n° 3.4535.79 of the "Fonds de la Recherche Scientifique Médicale" (FRSM, Brussels, Belgium).

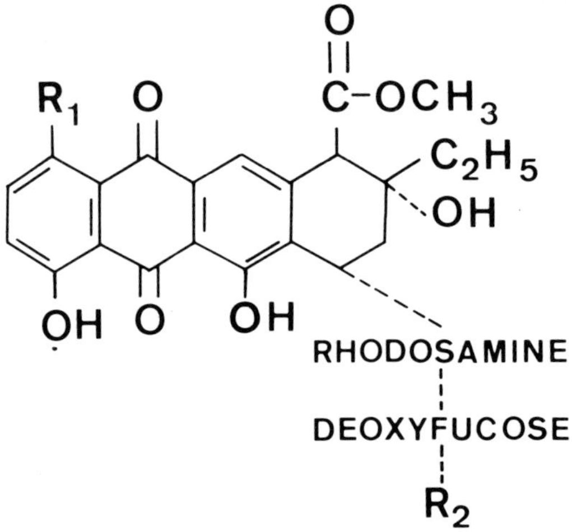

	R_1	R_2
MARCELLOMYCIN	OH	DEOXYFUCOSE
ACLACINOMYCIN A	H	L-CINERULOSE

FIGURE 1. Chemical structure of marcellomycin and aclacinomycin A.

Acute toxicity studies in animals indicated a steep dose-response relationship. In Swiss Webster mice, the LD_{50} and the LD_{10} after i.v. administration were 19.9 and 17.4 mg/kg respectively. In Beagle dogs, a single i.v. dose resulted in no deaths at 2.87 mg/kg whereas all animals died at 3.69 mg/kg. Administration of lethal doses to dogs produced severe intestinal toxicity which appeared to be the cause of acute death (7). Minimal leukocyte depression was noted with marcellomycin in BDF1 mice even at the LD_{50} and in Beagle dogs at nonlethal doses (6). In the agar diffusion chamber precursor cell assay, the sensitivity to marcellomycin of leukocyte-committed colony-forming cells from dogs was found to be similar to those from man (8). The relative cardiotoxicity of doxorubicin and marcellomycin was investigated with inconclusive results by measuring the CPK-MB isoenzyme in mice and by serially recording EKGs in rats (9, 10).

This paper summarizes additional screening data comparing marcellomycin and aclacinomycin A in murine tumors and a study on the inhibitory effect of these compounds against normal human myeloid stem cells. Preliminary findings of a phase I clinical trial with marcellomycin given at a single dose schedule are also reported.

2. MATERIALS AND METHODS

2.1 <u>Drugs</u>: Marcellomycin, aclacinomycin A and doxorubicin were kindly supplied by the Bristol-Myers Co, Syracuse, NY, USA, the Sanraku Ocean Co, Tokyo, Japan, and Farmitalia-Carlo-Erba, Brussels, Belgium respectively.

2.2 Animals and murine tumors

CDF1 and BDF1 mice of both sexes, weighing 20-22 g at the start of the experiments were supplied by Charles River Breeding Laboratories (Wilmington, Mass, USA). Tumor cell lines were obtained from Dr. A. Bogden (Mason Research Institute, Worcester, Mass, USA). The P388 and the L1210 leukemias were maintained in ascitic form by weekly transfer in DBA/2 mice. The Lewis lung carcinoma was maintained by the s.c. implantation of tumor fragments in C57B1/6 hosts.

2.3 Cloning assay

Bone marrows were sampled from 7 normal volunteers or cancer patients with marrows free of tumor cells. All donors had normal hematologic values. Samples were anticoagulated with 10 U heparin/ml (The Upjohn Company, Kalamazoo, Michigan, USA). Mononuclear cells were isolated by centrifugation on Ficoll-Hypaque for 20 min at 1,800 g. The cells in the interface were collected, washed twice in Dulbecco's tissue culture medium and resuspended in the same medium containing 20% fetal calf serum (GIBCO, Grand Island, NY, USA) (Solution A). All drugs were dissolved in dimethylsulfoxide (DMSO) and further diluted in solution A; the volume of DMSO was calculated so that its final concentration did not exceed 0.025%.

Mononuclear marrow cells (5.10^5) were incubated in a 7% CO_2 atmosphere at 37°C for 30 min in a 2-ml final volume of solution A containing various concentrations of drug. This incubation was terminated by the addition of an excess of Dulbecco's tissue culture media followed by centrifugation for 10 min at 1,800 g. The cloning assay developed by Pike and Robinson was used to determine the survival of myeloid colony-forming cells (CFU-C)(11). Human placental conditioned medium (HPCM) was used as a source of colony-stimulating activity at the concentration of 10%. The cells were mixed with a solution A-HPCM mixture containing 0.28% liquid agar and then plated in triplicate in 1-ml aliquots into 35-mm Petri dishes. Cells were incubated for 7 days at 37°C in a 7% CO_2 humidified atmosphere. Colonies (> 40 cells) were counted with an Olympus inverted microscope at 40-fold magnification. Statistical determinations were done with the t-test and an analysis of variance.

2.4 Phase I clinical trial

Seventeen patients with histologically confirmed solid tumors, mainly squamous cell carcinomas of the head and neck, were entered in the trial. All had diseases not or no longer suitable for conventional therapy. There were 11 men and 6 women with a median age of 53 years (range: 35-70) and a median performance status on the Karnofsky scale of 60 (range: 40-100). All but one had received prior radiotherapy (3 patients), prior chemotherapy (5 patients), or both (8 patients). None had received cytotoxic therapy during the 4 weeks prior to entering the trial. Eligibility criteria included a life expectancy of at least 4 weeks, WBC $\geq$ 4,000/mm^3, platelet counts $\geq$ 100,000/mm^3, normal serum bilirubin (< 1.5 mg/dl), and normal serum creatinine (< 1.5 mg/dl). Patients with a history of cardiac disease or prior therapy with a total dose of doxorubicin exceeding 300 mg/m^2 were excluded from the study.

Initial work-up included complete history and physical examination, complete blood cell counts, SMA-12 chemistries, urinalysis, chest radiograph, and 12-lead electrocardiogram. The electrocardiogram was repeated within 2 and 24 hours of drug administration. Blood cell counts were scheduled 3 times per week and biochemical profiles once weekly. Other investigations were performed and repeated as indicated.

For this trial, marcellomycin was supplied by the Bristol-Myers Company, International Division, as a tartrate salt, each vial containing 10 mg of marcellomycin base plus L (+) tartaric acid for injection. The drug was reconstituted with 10.3 ml of sterile water for injection; each vial yielded 10 mg deliverable dose containing 1 mg/ml of marcellomycin. The solution after reconstitution is stable for at least 24 hours at room temperature. The drug was given i.v. over 15-30 min. Drug administration was followed by an infusion of fluids for at least 2 hours.

The starting dose was 5 mg/m^2 corresponding to 1/10 of the LD$_{10}$ in mice, as currently recommended (12). Doses were escalated by increments of 100% up to 40 mg/m^2 and by one increment of 50% thereafter. At the level of 60 mg/m^2, severe toxicity was encountered and dosage in subsequent entries was reduced to 40 or 50 mg/m^2. Patients were retreated at higher dose levels when no significant toxic effects were encountered in previous courses. Four patients received 1 course, eight patients received 2 courses, and the remaining patients received 3 or 4 courses for a total of 37 courses. The study was designed to define a maximum tolerated dose for single dose intermittent treatments.

Patients were carefully monitored to identify drug efficacy. Response to therapy was assessed according to WHO criteria (13).

3. RESULTS

3.1 Animal data

Results of the experiments in P388 leukemia, L1210 leukemia, and Lewis lung carcinoma are summarized in Tables 1-3. No increase in life span was achieved with i.p. marcellomycin against advanced i.p. P388 leukemia in CDF1 mice; i.p. treatment with this compound was also ineffective against L1210 ascitic leukemia at a 5-day schedule and against i.v. inoculated Lewis lung carcinoma at a 9-day schedule. Aclacinomycin A achieved borderline activity against the advanced P388 leukemia whereas definite antitumor effect was seen with doxorubicin in this system. Aclacinomycin A was effective after i.p. administration against i.p. L1210 leukemia but failed to achieve significant activity against i.v. Lewis lung carcinoma.

Table 1. Effect of marcellomycin, aclacinomycin A, and doxorubicin on the survival of CDF1 mice bearing advanced P388 ascites.

Marcellomycin		Aclacinomycin A		Doxorubicin	
Dose (mg/kg/d)	ILS (%)	Dose (mg/kg/d)	ILS (%)	Dose (mg/kg/d)	ILS (%)
7	5	32	24	16	37
3.5	7	24	5	8	32
1.75	3	16	3	4	12
0.87	2	12	13	2	5

CDF1 mice were inoculated i.p. with 10^6 leukemic cells on day 0. Drugs were injected i.p. in saline on days 5, 9, 13 to groups of 10 mice. ILS: Percent increase in life span relative to untreated controls.

Table 2. Effect of marcellomycin and aclacinomycin A on the survival of
CDF1 mice bearing L1210 ascites.

Marcellomycin		Aclacinomycin A	
Dose (mg/kg/d)	ILS (%)	Dose (mg/kg/d)	ILS (%)
3.5	18	8	41
1.75	8	6	21
0.87	11	4	7
0.43	7	2	1

CDF1 mice were inoculated i.p. with 10^5 leukemic cells on day 0. Drugs
were injected i.p. in saline once daily from day 1 to day 5 to groups
of 6 mice.
ILS: Percent increase in life span relative to untreated controls.

Table 3. Effect of marcellomycin and aclacinomycin A on the survival of
BDF1 mice bearing Lewis lung carcinoma i.v.

Marcellomycin		Aclacinomycin A	
Dose (mg/kg/d)	ILS (%)	Dose (mg/kg/d)	ILS (%)
3	tox	6	9
2	- 48	4	- 1
1	5	2	- 4
0.5	- 4	1	1

BDF1 mice were inoculated i.v. with 2.10^5 tumor cells on day 0.
Drugs were injected i.p. in saline once daily from day 1 to day 9 to
groups of 10 mice.
ILS: Percent increase in life span relative to untreated controls.

3.2 Cloning assay

The inhibiting effect on colony growth at a given concentration was
measured by the percentage of formed colonies at this concentration relative to untreated controls. The graphic data were plotted as means plus
or minus the standard error of all experiments performed with a particular concentration of medication. Marcellomycin and aclacinomycin A yielded dose-dependent CFU-C inhibition with similar slopes (Fig. 2). Up to
0.10 µg/ml, the dose-response curve of marcellomycin did not display any
evidence of a plateau suggestive of relative drug resistance. Aclacinomycin A showed significantly greater potency against CFU-C as compared
to marcellomycin ($p < 0.005$). A 2- to 3-fold higher concentration (µg/ml)
of marcellomycin was required to reduce colony survival to 50%.

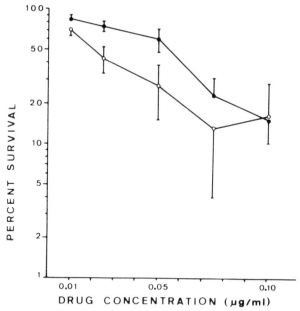

FIGURE 2. Comparison of dose-response curves of CFU-C after 30-min incubation with increasing concentrations of marcellomycin (●—●) and
aclacinomycin A (O—O). Bone marrows were obtained in 7 patients.
Data are plotted as means ± S.E. These curves are different at
the level of 0.005.

3.3 Phase I clinical trial

Patients selected for this trial represented a relatively unfavorable
population (Table 4). Myelosuppression was clearly dose-related and dose-
limiting (Tables 5 and 6). It was characterized by early thrombocytopenia
with a nadir on days 10-13 and a somewhat delayed leukopenia with a maximum WBC depression between days 14 and 22. In the vast majority of patients, recovery of myelosuppression occurred within 3 weeks of drug
administration. Life-threatening toxicity was encountered at the three
highest dose levels; leukopenia probably contributed to death in two patients with far-advanced disease treated at 40 and 60 mg/m² respectively.

At doses $\geq$ 40 mg/m², considerable variations in myelosuppression were
seen at the same dose levels. This observation could be related, at least
to some extent, to wide variations in pretreatment risk factors. Few patients were retreated at the same toxic dose levels and, among these, there
was a strong suggestion of cumulative myelosuppression as exemplified in

Table 4. Characteristics of patients

Total number of patients		17
Male / Female		11 / 6
Age	Median	53
	Range	35 - 70
Performance status	Median	60
	Range	40 - 100
Prior radiotherapy		3
Prior chemotherapy		5
Prior radiotherapy and chemotherapy		8
Tumor types	Head and neck	5
	Lung	3 (3)
	Gastrointestinal	2
	Kidney	2
	Cervix	1
	Ovary	1
	Adrenal gland	1
	Melanoma	1
	Bladder	1

( ) = second primary: head and neck (2), cervix (1)

Table 5. Drug-induced leukopenia

Dosage (mg/m^2)	N° of Patients/ N° of courses	Median nadir x10^3/mm^3		Median day to	
		W B C	P M N	Nadir	Recovery
5	2 / 2	8.0 (6.9-9.1)	5.9 (4.2-7.6)		
10	3 / 3	11.1 (10.8-13.4)	9.5 (7.2-11.0)		
20	3 / 3	9.2 (5.5-11.8)	7.3 (4.2-10.7)		
40	1 0 / 1 2	3.0 (0.1-14.7)	1.6 (0.1-12.9)	16 (14-22)	19 (17-25)
50	7 / 1 1	1.6 (0.9-4.2)	0.8 (0.1-1.3)	17 (14-19)	20 (16-22)
60	3 / 3	2.4 (0.4-5.8)	0.8 (0.2-3.4)		

Table 6. Drug-induced thrombocytopenia

Dosage (mg/m^2)	N° of patients/ N° of courses	Median platelet nadir x10^3/mm^3	(Range)	Median day to Nadir	Median day to Recovery
5	2 / 3	225	(200-250)		
10	3 / 3	360	(190-490)		
20	3 / 3	250	(250-330)		
40	1 1 / 1 3	158	(5-418)	12 (10-13)	14 (13-16)
50	7 / 1 1	62	(25-176)	11 (10-12)	14 (14-15)
60	3 / 3	35	(0.4-271)	12 (11-12)	

Fig. 3. These characteristics make difficult a correct interpretation of the dose-effect relationship on WBC and platelets, as tabulated here. Of seven patients treated at 50 mg/m^2 with no prior exposure to marcellomycin,

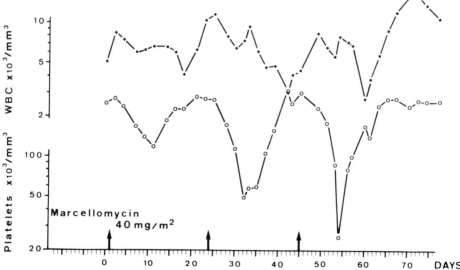

FIGURE 3. Possible cumulative myelosuppression in a patient with extensively pretreated ovarian cancer who received 3 courses of marcellomycin at a dose of 40 mg/m^2 each.

three good-risk patients had WBC and platelet nadirs x 10^3/mm^3 of 3.8
(2.0-4.7) and 95 (63-179) respectively whereas four poor-risk patients
had corresponding figures of 1.1 (0.9-1.6) and 75 (35-109) respectively.

Nausea and vomiting occurred frequently and were occasionally severe
(Table 7). Stomatitis was also common and sometimes dose-limiting. Phlebitis at the injection site was noted in nine patients. One of these presented severe dermatitis following extravasation of dextrose 5% in water
2 hours after drug administration. Infections and hemorrhages (hematochezia)
in relation to myelosuppression were observed in a total of four patients.
Transient EKG abnormalities consisting of alterations in the ST-T wave,
supraventricular extrasystoles and sinus tachycardia were detected at doses
$\geq$ 40 mg/m^2. Clearly drug-induced fatigue was noticeable in three patients
at least. Negligible alopecia was also encountered. No other toxic effects
were found in this trial.

Table 7. Non-hematologic toxic effects.

	Dosage in mg/m^2					
	5	10	20	40	50	60
Number of courses	3	3	3	13	11	4
Number of patients	2	3	3	11	7	3
Number of toxic patients	0	1	3	8	7	3
Nausea and vomiting	0	1	3	7(2)	6(2)	2
Stomatitis	0	0	0	2(1)	4(1)	1(1)
Phlebitis	0	0	0	3	7(1)	0
Infection	0	0	0	2(1)	1(1)	1(1)
Hemorrhage	0	0	0	1	1	1
EKG	0	0	0	3	2	1
Fatigue	0	0	0	2	1	0
Alopecia	0	0	0	0	2	1

Note: Figures in parentheses represent numbers of severe reactions.

Few patients had evaluable or measurable disease and experienced
nificant toxicity. None of these showed evidence of antitumor activity.

4. DISCUSSION

Marcellomycin was primarily introduced into clinical trials because of its potential for reduced myelosuppression. Our limited screening data in animals are consistent with its previously reported lower antitumor activity in experimental models relative to doxorubicin. Our experiments further suggest decreased activity in murine leukemias as compared to aclacinomycin A, a structurally related analog which might also act through interference with the metabolism of nucleolar RNA (3). Minimal or no activity in the L1210 system has been proposed to be predictive for lack of myelosuppression in man (14). Accordingly, our negative results with marcellomycin in this system were in agreement with the rationale for developing this new anthracycline.

The cloning assay indicated that marcellomycin was toxic for human myeloid stem cells and that CFU-C inhibition with this drug occurred at significantly higher doses than with aclacinomycin A. The maximum tolerated dose (MTD) of aclacinomycin A at a single dose intermittent schedule was 100-120 mg/m^2 in several phase I clinical trials (15-17). Based on our in vitro results, the clinical MTD of marcellomycin could have been expected to be higher in the event of dose-limiting leukopenia. This erroneous prediction must be analyzed in the light of comparative clinical pharmacology investigations, but the pharmacokinetic behavior of marcellomycin remains to be determined. Conclusions regarding the relevance of this cloning assay to assess hematologic tolerance to marcellomycin must also await results of ongoing studies correlating in vitro and in vivo drug effects in the same patients.

Clinically, marcellomycin may produce substantial bone marrow toxicity at least with the schedule selected for this trial. It would appear that the maximum tolerated dose is approximately one-half of that reported for aclacinomycin A (15-17). Both drugs produce early thrombocytopenia and delayed leukopenia, but cumulation has been documented with marcellomycin only. All nonhematologic toxic effects encountered with this new derivative seem qualitatively similar to what may be observed with conventional anthracyclines. Alopecia is rare and minimal. Drug-induced congestive heart failure has not been noted in this trial. However, more prolonged treatments and larger patient populations are required to evaluate chronic heart damage clinically.

As yet, there was no evidence of anticancer effect in this clinical trial. This fact could result from an unfavorable selection of patients with far-advanced malignancies often treated at suboptimal dosages.

Additional experience is still necessary to recommend a dosage for phase II trials. Such recommendation should take into account the steep dose-response relationship of marcellomycin and the possibility of cumulative myelosuppression. In any event, 50 mg/m^2 appears to be the maximum tolerated single dose for poor-risk patients. This phase I study is still ongoing.

REFERENCES

1. Nettleton DE Jr, Bradner WT, Bush JA, Coon AB, Moseley JE, Myllymaki RW, O'Herron FA, Schreiber RH, Vulcano AL. 1977, New antitumor antibiotics: Musettamycin and marcellomycin from bohemic acid complex. J. Antibiotics, 30, 525-529.
2. DuVernay VH, Essery JM, Doyle TW, Bradner WT, Crooke ST. 1979. The antitumor effects of anthracyclines. The importance of the carbometoxy-group at position-10 of marcellomycin and rudolfomycin. Molecular Pharmacol., 15, 341-356.
3. Crooke ST, Duvernay VH, Galvan L, Prestayko AW. 1978. Structure-activity relationships of anthracyclines relative to effects on macromolecular syntheses. Molecular Pharmacol., 14, 290-298.
4. Bradner WT, Rose WC. 1980. Antitumor testing in animals. In: Anthracyclines: Current Status and New Developments. Crooke ST and Reich SD (Eds). Academic Press, New York, pp. 125-140.
5. Bradner WT, Misiek M. 1977. Bohemic acid complex. Biological characterization of the antibiotics, musettamycin and marcellomycin. J. Antibiotics, 30, 519-522.
6. Reich SD, Bradner WT, Rose WC, Schurig JE, Madissoo H, Johnson DF, DuVernay VH, Crooke ST. 1980. Marcellomycin. In: Anthracyclines: Current Status and New Developments. Crooke ST and Reich SD (Eds) Academic Press, New York, pp. 343-364.
7. Hirth RS. 1980. Other toxicities associated with anthracyclines in animal systems. In: Anthracyclines: Current Status and New Developments. Crooke ST and Reich SD (Eds). Academic Press, New York, pp. 221-240.
8. Marsh JC. 1981. Bone marrow colony forming cell sensitivity to carminomycin, marcellomycin and spirogermanium. Proc. Am. Assoc Cancer Res. and ASCO, 22, 241.
9. Schurig JE, Bradner WT, Huftalen JB, Doyle GJ. 1980. Screening anthracyclines for side effects in mice. In: Anthracyclines: Current Status and New Developments. Crooke ST and Reich SD (Eds). Academic Press, New York, pp. 141-149.
10. Buyniski JP, Hirth RS. 1980. Anthracycline cardiotoxicity in the rat. In: Anthracyclines: Current Status and New Developments. Crooke ST and Reich SD (Eds) Academic Press, New York, pp. 157-170.

11. Pike BL, Robinson WA. 1970. Human bone marrow colony growth in agar-gel. J. Cell Physiology, 76, 77-84.
12. Rozencweig M, Von Hoff DD, Staquet MJ, Schein PS, Penta JS, Goldin A, Muggia FM, Freireich EJ, DeVita VTJr. 1981. Animal toxicology for early clinical trials with anticancer agents. Cancer Clin Trials, 4, 21-28.
13. WHO Handbook for Reporting Results of Cancer Treatment. WHO Geneva, 1979.
14. Rozencweig M, Von Hoff DD, Cysyk RL, Muggia FM. 1979. m-AMSA and PALA: Two new agents in cancer chemotherapy. Cancer Chemother. Pharmacol., 3, 135-141.
15. Ogawa M, Inagaki J, Horikoshi N, Inoue K, Chinen T, Ueoka H, Nagura E. 1979. Clinical study of aclacinomycin A. Cancer Treat. Rep., 63, 931-934.
16. Casper E, Gralla RJ, Young CW. 1981. Clinical phase I study of acla-cinomycin A by evaluation of an intermittent intravenous administra-tion schedule. Cancer Res., 41, 2417-2420.
17. Egorin MJ, Van Echo DA, Whitacre MY, Fox BM, Aisner J, Wiernik PH, Bachur N. 1981. A phase I trial of aclacinomycin-A (ACM-A). Proc. Am. Assoc. Cancer Res. and ASCO, 22, 353.

PRELIMINARY PHASE II EXPERIENCE WITH 4'EPIDOXORUBICIN

E. FERRAZZI, O. NICOLETTO, O. VINANTE, G. MARAGLINO, A. FORNASIERO,
P. PAGNIN, G. DAGNINI, AND M. V. FIORENTINO

1. INTRODUCTION

4'Epidoxorubicin (4'-epi-DXR) is a new stereoisomer of Adriamycin that
is currently undergoing clinical phase II testing at several cancer centers.
Although the antitumor activity has been reported equal to that of DXR in
animal models, the drug has a possible reduced cardiac toxicity (1). Early
studies in humans (Istituto Tumori Milan) have shown that 4'-epi-DXR
has an interesting activity on melanoma as well as on renal and colorectal
carcinoma (2,3).

In June 1980, we undertook a clinical phase II study to assess: 1) the
activity of 4'-epi-DXR in tumors sensitive to Adriamycin, that is, breast
cancer, gastric cancer, and sarcomas; and 2) the effectiveness of 4'-epi-DXR
in tumors resistant to Adriamycin (and to other conventional agents as well),
that is, melanoma, colorectal cancer, and renal cell carcinoma. We also
sought to define parameters of acute toxicity (nausea, vomiting) and
acute and chronic cardiotoxicity.

In addition, in a selected group of patients suffering from neoplastic
pleural effusion, we injected the drug directly into the pleural space in
an effort to achieve and/or improve local control of the malignant disease.

2. PATIENTS AND METHODS

4'-Epi-DXR was supplied by Farmitalia Carlo Erba, Milan, Italy, as a
sterile powder in 10 mg and 50 mg vials for i.v. administration. The drug
was reconstituted with twice-distilled water and given as a bolus injection,
usually at the dose of 75 mg/m^2 every 21 days for a minimum of two courses.

The patients comprised 26 males and 31 females; median age was 55 years
(range 27-70 years); 31.6% of the patients had been pretreated, and 68.4%
had received no previous treatment. Five patients had also received doxorubicin previously, for a mean total dose of 138 mg/m^2 (range 40-230).

Partial remission was defined as a regression of tumor mass of more than 50%; minor response, a regression of more than 25% but less than 50%. Stabilization or no change was defined as an increase or decrease of measureable lesions of less than 25% for 1 month.

For intrapleural administration, the drug was dissolved in twice-distilled water at a concentration of 5 mg/ml and was generally injected at a dose of 50 mg at intervals of 1 to 5 days.

3. RESULTS

3.1. Therapeutic activity of 4'-epi-DXR administered intravenously

The general therapeutic activity of 4'-epi-DXR is presented in Table 1.

Table 1. Therapeutic activity of 4'epidoxorubicin at 75 mg/m^2 given every 3 weeks

Type of tumor	Number of evaluable patients	Partial remission	Improvement	No change or subjective improvement
Breast	14	6	5	2
Sarcoma (mixed)	5	1	1	–
Gastric	4	–	2	1
Esophagus	1	–	–	–
Hepatoma	1	–	–	–
Lung	1	–	–	–
Cholangiocarcinoma	1	–	–	–
Head and neck	1	–	–	–
Renal cell	3	–	–	–
Colon-rectum	15	2	3	2
Melanoma	9	1	2	–
Pancreas	2	1	1	–

3.1.1. Breast cancer (14 patients). The median age of the 14 evaluable patients, 10 of whom had received no previous treatment, was 52 years, and nine were in advanced postmenopausal status. Dominant site of disease was the liver in five cases, lung in three, skin and nodes in four, and bone in one. There were two cases of inoperable primary cancer.

We achieved major responses in six of the 14 patients. Median duration of response, however, was only 10 weeks (range 5-20 weeks).

In one patient with pulmonary and peritoneal involvement, there was a

a complete disappearance of pulmonary nodules and a complete scarring
of peritoneal implants. Only bronchoscopy revealed a persistence of
bronchial infiltration. A "clinical improvement" (more than 25% decrease)
was noted in five patients and a stabilization in two. In this group, the
duration of response could not be measured exactly because we chose to
switch to a multidrug and/or hormonal program whenever a partial remission
after two courses had not been achieved. Our clinical series, however,
even though the number was small, has confirmed clearly that 4'-epi-DXR has
a good effectiveness in mammary cancer. We conclude that 4'-epi-DXR is
active in this neoplasm and is able to induce useful clinical remissions,
with at least the same probability as its parent compound, DXR.

3.1.2. Melanoma (nine patients). In a female patient with local
recurrence and inguinal node involvement, we observed a major response that
lasted 16 weeks. A clinical improvement (greater than 25%) was observed
in a female patient with regional dissemination of subcutaneous nodes in
one leg and in a male patient with inguinal and gross pulmonary involvement.
In addition, an objective reduction of measureable tumor was observed in
three other patients. This objective improvement was very short, however,
lasting only a few weeks.

We conclude that 4'-epi-DXR is a useful agent in advanced melanoma.
Further study is necessary to assess its role, possibly in synergistic
combination (with DDP and/or VDS, for example).

3.1.3. Colorectal cancer (15 patients). A major response was obtained in a female patient with liver involvement and in a male patient with
a liver metastasis and a palpable abdominal mass. A "clinical improvement"
was observed in three other patients: metastasis reduction was apparent
at liver CT scan in one case; small reduction of lung metastases in another
female patient, and shrinkage of a perineal subcutaneous mass in a male
patient, associated with pain relief. In addition, a dramatic pain relief
associated with weight gain was observed in another patient.

These very encouraging results, although preliminary, favor further
study and deeper investigation.

3.1.4. Sarcomas (five patients). In a female patient with gross
pulmonary involvement from uterine leiomyosarcoma, we observed an almost
complete disappearance of lung metastases (more than 90% decrease). A
minimal reduction of an abdominal mass was seen in another male patient
with leiomyosarcoma that had originated in the prostate. Two other soft

parts and one bone sarcoma showed no improvement.

3.1.5. Gastrointestinal--miscellaneous (eight patients). A "minor response" was seen in two gastric patients.

3.1.6. Pancreatic cancer. A very important reduction of an abdominal mass (more than 40 decrease as measured by CT scan) was seen in a female patient and a very impressive reduction (greater than 50% of palpable abdominal mass) in another.

In view of the poor sensitivity of pancreatic cancer to conventional agents, these results, although preliminary, seem very promising.

3.2 Clinical toxicity of 4'-epi-DXR administered intravenously

3.2.1. Acute toxicity (Table 2). The most common complaints were of nausea (65%) and vomiting (39%). Hair loss was observed in 49% and total alopecia in 35%. Stomatitis occurred in 26%. Other side effects were anorexia and diarrhea. Chemical phlebitis was observed in 6% of the patients and transient fever in 9%. Two patients developed transverse pigmentation striae of the fingernails. This effect has been described previously in breast cancer patients treated with Adriamycin (4).

3.2.2. Hematologic toxicity. The degree of myelosuppression was mild, with a median leucocyte nadir of 3800 cells/mm^3 (range 700-9500) and a median platelet nadir of 198,000 (range 50,000-350,000).

3.2.3. Cardiotoxicity. In the EKG, the most common abnormality seen was a flattening of the T waves, observed in 24.6% of the patients. Tachycardia was seen in 7%, atrial premature beats in 8.8%, and ST segment depression in 3.5%. A combination of these various EKG changes was seen in 8.8% of the cases.

A pilot study of the changes in systolic time intervals during 4'-epi-DXR treatment was also carried out in 14 patients. The PEP-LVET ratio increased within 1 hour after drug injection and returned to near-normal values 24 hours later. These findings suggest that 4'-epi-DXR induces acute but reversible damage of myocardial function.

Data for chronic toxicity are not available at present time. Only a few patients reached the threshold cardiotoxic dose that could be inferred by DXR data.

In the present study, no patient developed clinical signs or symptoms of congestive heart failure. One female patient, however, who had received a total dose of 600 mg/m^2 had a normal PEP-LVET ratio but showed enargement of cardiac diameters on a chest X-ray that was suggestive of initial damage.

3.3. Intrapleural 4'-epi-DXR (seven patients)

Therapeutic results of 4'-epi-DXR are presented in Table 3. Out of seven evaluable patients, a minimal response was observed in one malignant breast cancer effusion (duration 4 weeks). Stabilization was obtained in one patient with breast cancer and one with melanoma.

Table 2. Acute toxicity resulting from the use of 4'epidoxorubicin

Toxicity	Number of patients	Percentage
Nausea	37	65
Vomiting	22	39
Loss of hair	28	49
Total alopecia	20	35
Stomatitis	15	26
Asthenia	23	40
Anorexia	15	26
Diarrhea	7	12
Phlebitis	6	10
Fever	9	16
Pigmented nails	2	4
Recall dermatitis	1	--

Table 3. Results of direct pleural injection of 4'epidoxorubicin

Case number	Age	Diagnosis	Dose	Response
1	47	melanoma	50 mg x 4	no change 4 weeks
2	64	breast	50 mg x 2	minimal change; duration 4 weeks
3	60	adenocarcinoma (gastric)	50 mg x 1	progression
4	68	breast (or lung adenocarcinoma	50 mg x 1	progression
5	49	small cell	50 mg x 1	progression
6	52	large bowel	50 mg x 1	not evaluable
7	46	breast	20 mg day 1; 35 mg day 30	no change duration 7 weeks

4. CONCLUSIONS

The pattern of general toxicity of 4'epidoxorubicin is similar to that of its parent compound, doxorubicin. It is too early for us to make definite conclusions about cardiotoxicity. Therapeutic evaluation of our limited series suggests a spectrum of activity with 4'-epi-DXR that is broader than that of DXR, with encouraging results obtained in the treatment of melanoma, colorectal carcinoma, and pancreatic carcinoma. Further study of its usefulness in treating these neoplasms is desirable.

In breast cancer, 4'-epi-DXR is able to induce useful clinical remission at the same rate as DXR.

Our experience with intrapleural injection of 4'-epi-DXR was not encouraging.

REFERENCES

1. Bonfante V, Bonadonna G, Villani F, Di Fronzo G, Martini A, Casazza AM. 1979. Preliminary phase I study of 4'-epi-doxorubicin. Cancer Treat. Rep. 63: 915-918.
2. Bonfante V, Bonadonna G, Villani F, Martini A. 1980. Clinical experience with 4'-epi-doxorubicin in advanced human neoplasia. Rec. Results Cancer Res. 74: 202-209.
3. Casazza AM, Di Marco A, Bertazzoli e Coll C. 1977. Antitumor activity toxicity and pharmacological properties of 4'-epi-adriamycin. 10th International Congress of Chemotherapy, Zurich.
4. Priestman TJ, James KW. 1975. Adriamycin and longitudinal pigmented banding of fingernails. Lancet 1 (June 14): 1337-1338.